John W. Davis
Editor

Robot-Assisted Radical Prostatectomy

Beyond the Learning Curve

Springer

Editor
John W. Davis
Department of Urology
Uro-surgical Prostate Cancer Program
The University of Texas M.D. Anderson Cancer Center
Houston, TX, USA

ISBN 978-3-319-32639-9 ISBN 978-3-319-32641-2 (eBook)
DOI 10.1007/978-3-319-32641-2

Library of Congress Control Number: 2016936375

Printed on acid-free paper

This Springer imprint is published by Springer Nature
The registered company is Springer International Publishing AG Switzerland

Preface

Perspectives of the Robot-Assisted Radical Prostatectomy Learning Curve 10 Years Later

Welcome to the Springer Publishing series on robot-assisted urologic surgery. In this textbook, we are generously given an entire agenda for the radical prostatectomy operation. The genesis of the project started with our post-graduate course at the American Urological Association meeting of the same name. We are grateful to Springer Publishing for noticing the content and inviting us to develop this book. Of course the real thanks then goes to the multiple and talented authors who have signed on to the project and donated their uncompensated time and endless creativity. We all share a common goal of performing this operation at a high volume and excellent quality. Most of us have worked together at various international conferences and continuing medical education events. We hope you find this a valuable resource for study and one to augment your case observations, videoconferences, and video self-review.

In the forthcoming Chap. 2, you can review the objectives of the original course and this textbook. As stated, this will be an advanced textbook for surgeons who know basic docking, port placement, and the basic steps of a well-selected case. Before we dive into this advanced content, we would like to do a little story telling for your interest and background. As many have said, the present and future make more sense when we understand the past.

Before there was a surgical robot and a learning curve, there was a desire to develop a better way to perform a radical prostatectomy. As surgeons in our late 40s who trained in the 1990s, we had the joy of learning mostly open surgery—especially in oncologic procedures. However, the field of urinary stones had made a complete transition to minimally invasive surgery, and the field of laparoscopy was emerging in general surgery and basic extirpative procedures. The initial laparoscopic nephrectomy was performed in 1990 by Clayman and Kavoussi [1]; however the operative time of >6 h certainly led to a slow roll out of the procedure. In the late 1990s, Gill et al. reported laparoscopic renal cryoablation [2], and Clayman's group had progressed with oncologic applications for renal neoplasms—radical, nephroureterectomy, and partial [3-5].

Therefore it made perfect sense that radical prostatectomy would go the same route. But could a surgeon really do all of that reconstruction in the

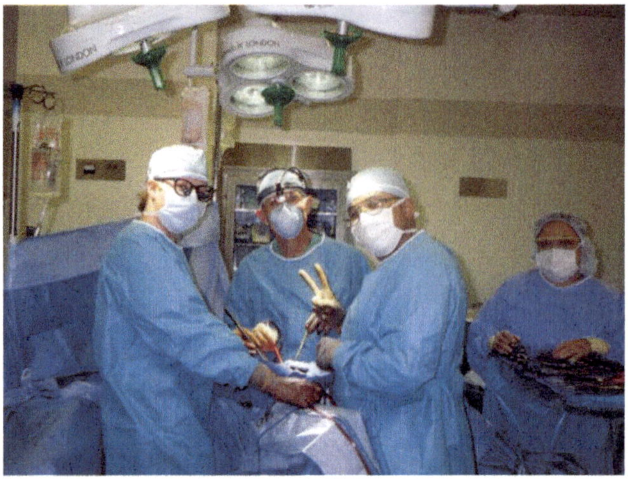

Fig. 1 Open radical prostatectomy at Sentara Norfolk General Hospital, 1999

male pelvis with a pure laparoscopic approach? The open operation itself was fraught with a long learning curve, blood loss, difficult exposure, and a very fine line between success and failure in the now termed "trifecta" of oncologic control, potency, and continence. Training was also a difficult area. Although we were not formally trained in laparoscopy at a high level as residents, at least we were trained in radical prostatectomy. Our mentors, however, were likely not formally trained. Our colleague Paul Schellhammer was one of the first fellows at Memorial Sloan Kettering Cancer Center in the early 1970s and performed only node dissections and open brachytherapy for prostate cancer. His training in radical prostatectomy was postgraduate and often involved case observations with Patrick Walsh at Johns Hopkins.

The problem with training in the 1990s was that the open operation was difficult for trainees to visualize. In Fig. 1, you can see Paul Schellhammer (Center) operating with John Davis (left) and an assistant in 1999. Can you see any anatomy? Definitely not, and most trainees only saw drapes and retractors until their chief resident year. Unless you were at an unusually high volume center, most residents scrubbed on anywhere from 25 to 75 cases. Expertise often required a fellowship, and in Fig. 2, you see the same setup at MD Anderson Cancer Center: lights, retractors, instruments, but no anatomy except for the two surgeons. From my personal standpoint (JWD) I am not sure I ever saw the apical dissection as a trainee. Richard Babaian (Fig. 2, left) would put his hands in the wound and manipulate the apex with his thumb and index figure, and voila! The dorsal vein stitch was ready.

It was no surprise and somewhat refreshingly honest to see the now famous 1997 paper from Schuessler et al. [6] on the first experience of laparoscopic radical prostatectomy. The group performed nine cases with an average time of 9.4 h and typical outcomes otherwise. The published conclusion was that it was "feasible but offers no advantage over open surgery…" Off the record, the authors were quoted as saying the operation was possible but "don't do it."

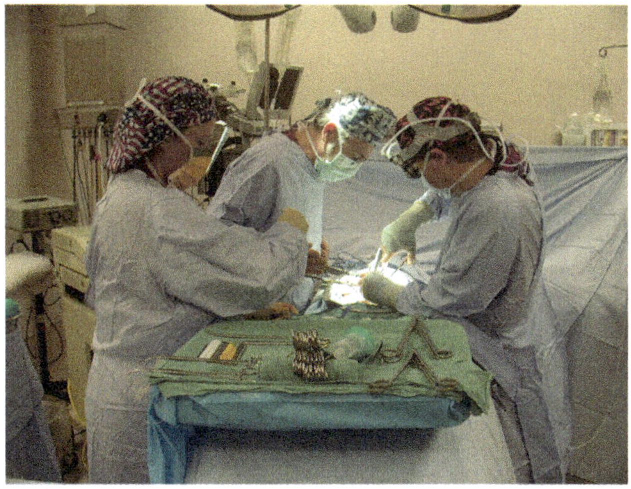

Fig. 2 Open radical prostatectomy at MD Anderson Cancer Center in 2002. Richard Babaian, *left*, and John Davis, *right*

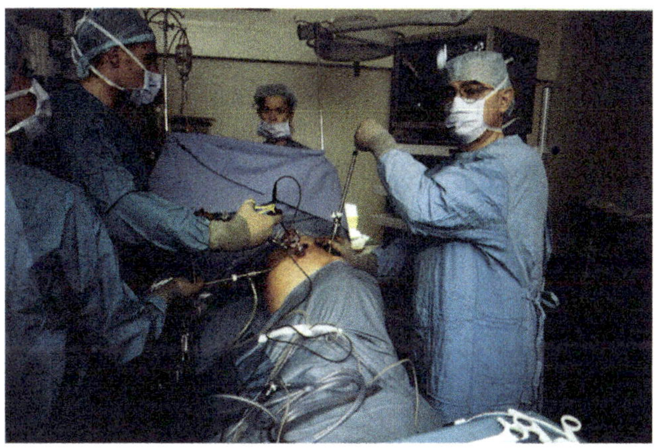

Fig. 3 Early experience with laparoscopy at Charité Hospital, Berlin, Germany. Professor-Chief Stephan Loening, *right*, and Oberartz Ingolf "Harry" Tuerk *left*

But as with many things in surgery and medicine, persistence can pay off. Only 2 years later, Guillonneau and Vallancien [7] published a series of 65 procedures with an average operative time of 4.4 h. How long did my residency and fellowship cases take? 4 hours. So now we are on to something—minimally invasive radical prostatectomy with the possibility of less bleeding, faster recovery, and better surgical vision.

From my perspective (MDF), laparoscopic radical prostatectomy was not part of the fellowship at Johns Hopkins, but rather a challenge from Paul Schellhammer as a junior associate in his group. Early attempts were long, as with the Schuessler group, and led to open conversion for the anastomosis. Clearly, additional training was needed. Fortunately, another colleague in the Norfolk group, Gerald Jordan, met with a colleague at a meeting in Hamburg Germany—Stephan Loening, Fig. 3. Professor Loening is a German native

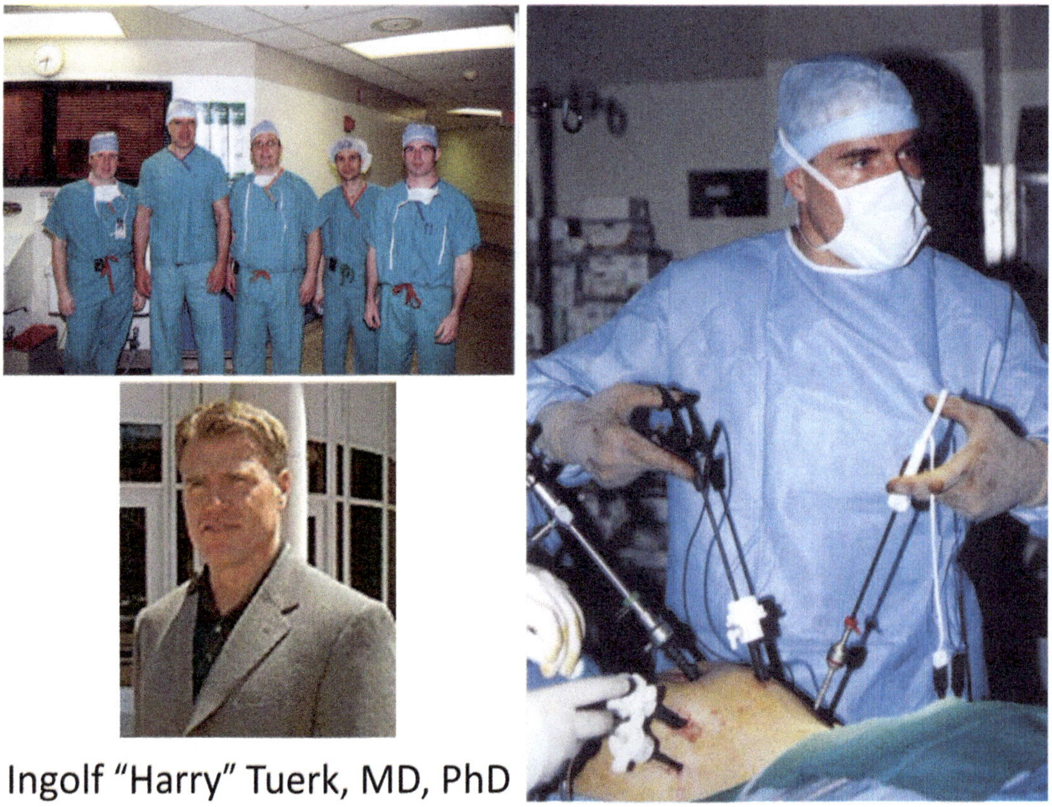

Fig. 4 Surgical team for the first laparoscopic radical prostatectomy at Sentara Norfolk General Hospital in 2001 led by Ingolf "Harry" Tuerk. Group photo *left* to *right*: John Davis, Harry Tuerk, Michael Fabrizio, Filippos Kondlyis, and Mike Pryor

but trained in the USA and practiced at the University of Iowa for many years before deciding to return to Germany as chair of urology at the famous Charité Hospital in Berlin. He had trained a young faculty member, Ingolf "Harry" Tuerk, Fig. 3, in laparoscopy and eventually he was able to master the prostatectomy operation. By 2000, he had performed over 150 operations, and could complete them in an eye opening 2 h. Plans were quickly made for a joint international training exchange: Tuerk would train Fabrizio in Norfolk for 6 months, and then would train Davis back in Berlin for 6 months following his MD Anderson fellowship. Additionally, Fabrizio traveled to Paris and spent a week with Drs. Vallancien and Guillonneau when the largest series in the world was 160 cases.

The first laparoscopic radical prostatectomies at Sentara Norfolk General were performed by Tuerk and Fabrizio in March 2001, and a short series of just under 50 were performed in the next 6 months. Figure 4 shows the team for the inaugural case. Eventually, this extensive training method was successful, and both of us were able to perform the operation independently. A typical operation with time splits (ideal):

- 30 min: position, ports.
- 30 min: mobilize vas/SVs.

- 30 min: drop bladder, endopelvic fascia, sew DVC.
- 30 min: divide bladder.
- 60 min: prostatectomy—to apex.
- 30 min: place and tie posterior two interrupted stitches.
- 30 min: place anterior four stitches.

That adds up to 4 h, but could be 5–6 h in the early cases. Obviously one case/day was very tiring and that was the end of the surgical schedule, or followed with minor procedures. If we both helped each other, we could pull off two cases. Fellow/resident training was possible but took a few years before they could play a meaningful role.

During this same 2-year period, a similar tale of complex training and planning was developing at Henry Ford Hospital in Detroit. In January 2001, Mani Menon was our visiting professor in Norfolk, and he outlined his plans for working with the French group [7] who would essentially spend 1 week a month doing cases with him with the idea of independence growing over time. Figure 5 shows the social time we had together at the recently relocated Battleship Wisconsin in downtown Norfolk.

As we will summarize at the end of this piece, all of this training was feasible, but very elaborate, and highly impractical for the rest of the practicing world. We knew minimally invasive surgery was going to succeed, but there had to be some additions to our technology.

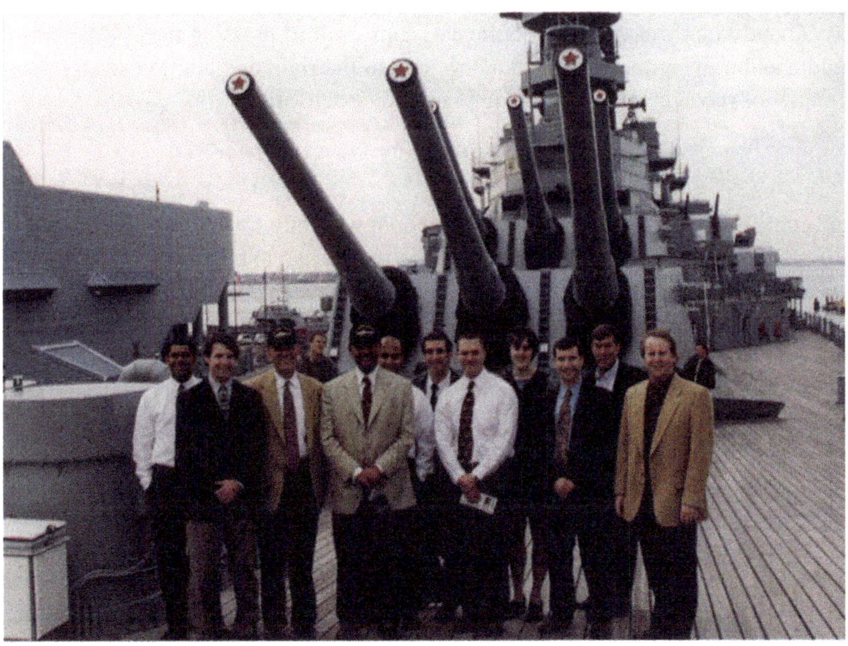

Fig. 5 Visiting Professor Mani Menon visits the Battleship Wisconsin, January 19, 2001: *Left* to *Right*: Roy Brown, Mike Pryor, Paul Schellhammer, Mani Menon, Naeem Rahman, Dan Rosenstein, Paul McAdams, *rotating intern*, Filippos Kondylis, Sture Sigfried, and John Davis

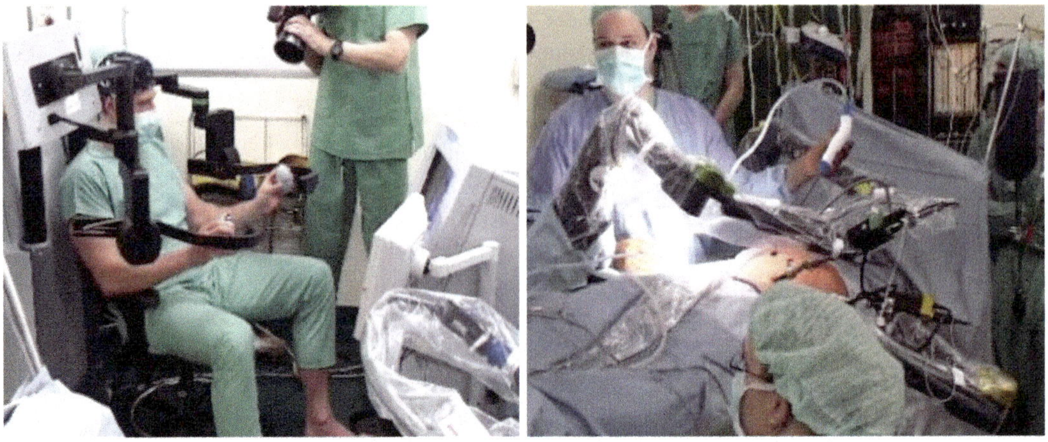

Fig. 6 The Computer Motion robotic platform Zeus, coupled with the Aesop camera robotic arm, and the Socrates telementoring system. *Upper right*—Harry Tuerk operates the console in Berlin, Germany. *Lower*—the surgical team assists with the robotic arms attached to the table. Not-pictured—Mike Fabrizio is using the telementoring system Socrates from his office in Norfolk, Virginia. From his console, he can drive the camera and draw on the screen

What did we do in Norfolk? We partnered with the now defunct company Computer Motion to be part of their FDA trials to be an approved surgical robot called Zeus. The platform looked really neat—you sat in a chair with 3D glasses and manipulated two robotic arms that latched to the rails of a standard operating room table. The camera was driven voice activated by the company's Aesop camera robot that we had used independently for laparoscopic prostate and kidney cases. For robotic surgeons used to pressing the daVinci peddle and moving the camera to a new spot to the right and a little down in a matter of seconds, imagine having to use voice activation:

> *"Aesop." [Aesop Beeps that he is awake]. "Move Right." [Aesop pans right slowly]. "Stop." [He stops]. "Move down." [He moves down.] "Stop."*

The hand controls worked but the degree of freedom was only 6° and certain areas like the bladder drop step were out of range so you had to mix laparoscopy and robotics back and forth. Eventually your hands became very sore using the grips. Figure 6 shows the platforms from Computer Motion in action—including the telementoring Socrates system. As you can probably Google online—Computer Motion and Intuitive Surgical sued each other over patent infringement—almost to the point of bankruptcy. However, in the one of the greatest business decisions on record, Intuitive bought Computer Motion (its sole competition) and shut the company down. The meteoric rise of "ISRG" is well known. Oh well. At least Mike got his picture in the local newspaper—Fig. 7. Aesop had one memorable feature: You could say "Zeus—Compliment." And it would say "You are the greatest surgeon in the world."

What did Mani Menon do in Detroit? Eventually, he determined that he just could not do laparoscopic RP to his satisfaction—despite all of the fine French training. A generous donor gave him the opportunity to invest in the daVinci platform from the outset, and he soon published that the learning

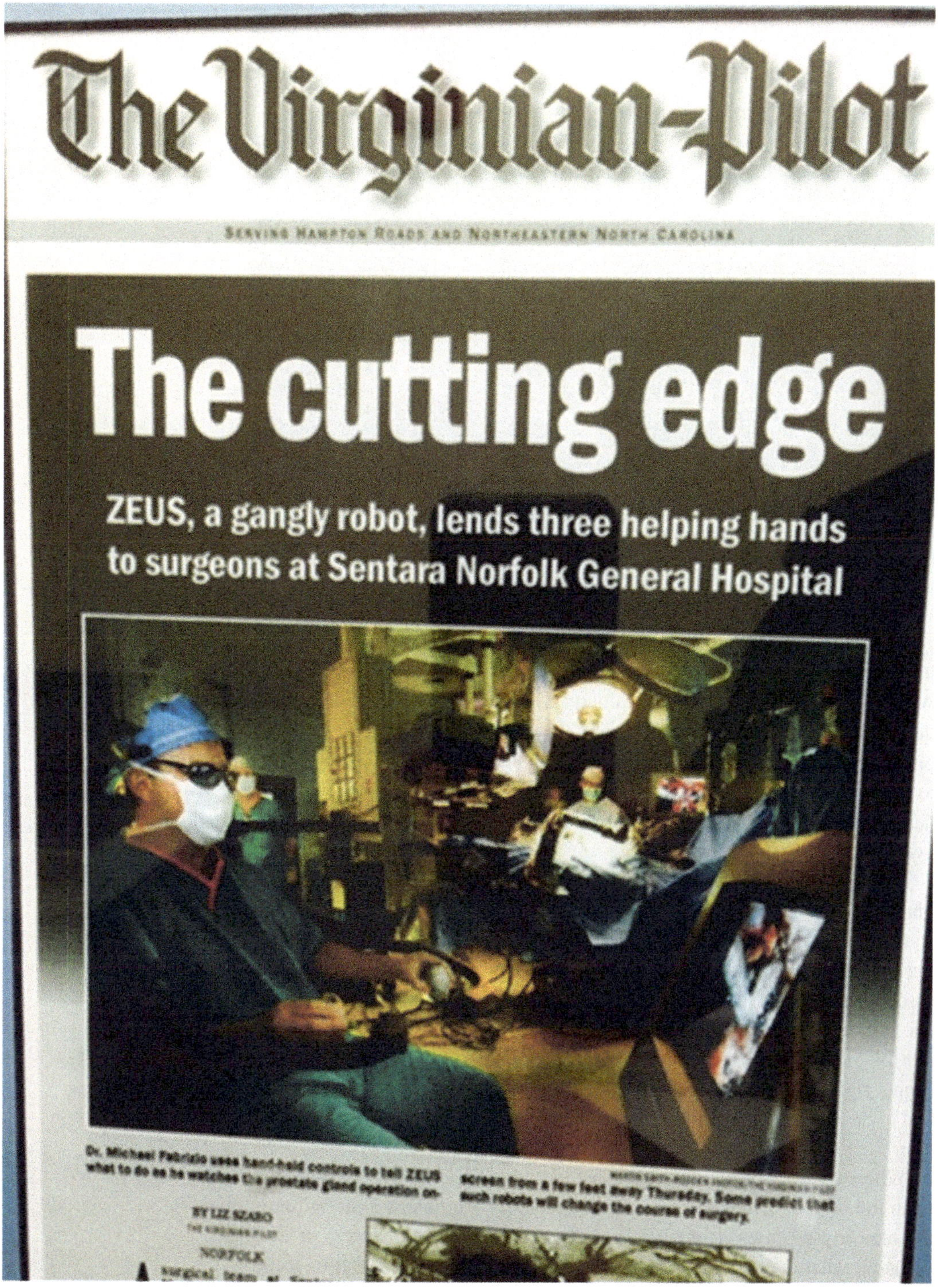

The Virginian-Pilot

SERVING HAMPTON ROADS AND NORTHEASTERN NORTH CAROLINA

The cutting edge

ZEUS, a gangly robot, lends three helping hands to surgeons at Sentara Norfolk General Hospital

Dr. Michael Fabrizio uses hand-held controls to tell ZEUS what to do as he watches the prostate gland operation on-screen from a few feet away Thursday. Some predict that such robots will change the course of surgery.

BY LIZ SZABO

NORFOLK

A surgical team at ...

Fig. 7 Novel technologies like Zeus and its futuristic vision made it through our local papers years before da Vinci was found to be superior

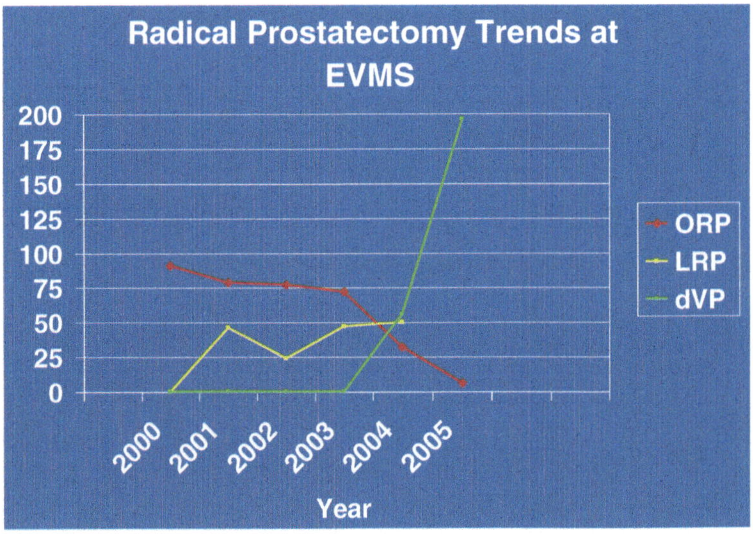

Fig. 8 The da Vinci platform changed our volumes like never seen previously. *ORP* = open radical prostatectomy, *LRP* = laparoscopic radical prostatectomy, *dVP* = da Vinci Radical Prostatectomy

curve was now feasible—even for an open surgeon. Two years later, we also had to make the switch to daVinci for the impending robotic arms race. Although as urologists we were trained and ready with a high volume procedure, many surgeons who lived through this era will recall that most hospitals bought these robots in the off chance that their cardiac surgeons would want to touch them. Most did not, and a few programs had unused robots in their departments ready to use now that the technique was described and proctors available.

Now we had not only a technique but also a company with a marketing plan. Websites came to light and billboards could be seen with surgeons standing in front of new console units. Our volumes exploded like never seen before. Figure 8 shows typical patient treatment selections overlapping laparoscopy, while Fig. 9 shows the surgical choices into the first 2 years of robotics. Figure 10 parallels Fig. 4 in showing the initial robotic case at Sentara Norfolk General Hospital in August, 2004—also made the local papers (upper right image of Adam Ball at bedside). Once again, attending surgeons had to be learners again, and fellow/residents had to revert to supporting cast (sorry guys, but thank you for your sacrifices).

Where does all of that history leave us today? The debate on how to perform the perfect technical radical prostatectomy continues, although now in the majority of cases it involves a daVinci robot. The debates now mostly focus on what techniques to apply, how to measure outcomes, how to train, how to troubleshoot, and how to introduce new concepts.

In this textbook, you will see chapters organized by theme—technique, perioperative care and safety, outcomes, and patient education. To conclude this highly personal introduction and move on to the formal presentations, we

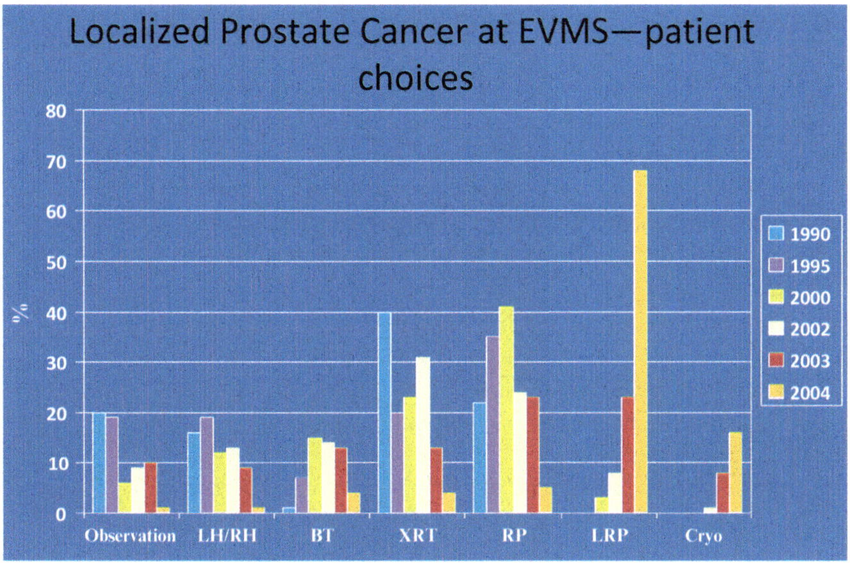

Fig. 9 Localized Prostate Cancer Choices at Eastern Virginia Medical School 1990–2004

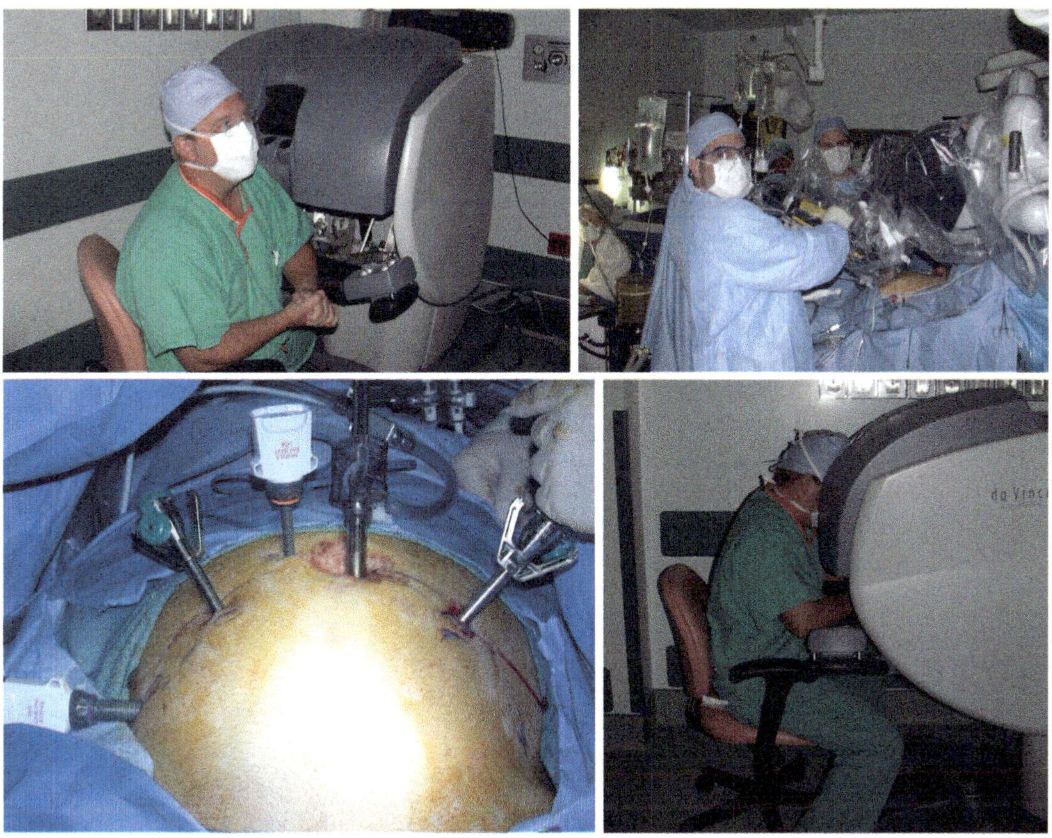

Fig. 10 The initial robot-assisted radical prostatectomy at Sentara Norfolk General Hospital, August 2004. *Upper left*—surgeon Mike Fabizio, *upper right*—fellow Adam Ball (*left*) and chief resident Kevin Bordeau (*right*). *Lower left*—typical port placement. Note we did not use the fourth arm for this standard system. We had one but did not know how to dock it or use it. *Lower right*—the era of surgeon ergonomics begins

can give you a series of bullet points on the impact of robotic surgery after >10 years of experience:

- The training is improved—everyone can see, learn to dissect, and learn to sew. Training can be stepwise starting early residency.
- The timing of training is improved—feasible for residents, fellows, and not requiring extraordinary training efforts as we experienced
- The ergonomics is improved—3–4 cases per day feasible compared to 1 long, tiring case of LRP.
- The anatomy is clear—techniques can be described from the central camera frame of reference and transferred surgeon to surgeon.
- The platform can improve—standard to S, to Si, to Xi, with improved instrumentation and assistant surgeon high definition video.
- Simulation is here—Mimic, etc.
- The cost is higher—but improves with efficiency and reduced complications. Of course proton therapy makes everything else appear reasonable.

Enjoy the textbook and thank you for reading. Thank you again to all of our coauthors.

Houston, TX John W. Davis, M.D.
Norfolk, VA Michael D. Fabrizio, M.D.

References

1. Clayman RV, Kavoussi LR, Soper NJ, et al. Laparoscopic nephrectomy: initial case report. J Urol. 1991;146: 278.
2. Gill IS, Novick AC, Soble JJ, et al. Laparoscopic renal cryoablation: initial clinical series. Urology. 1998; 52:545–51.
3. Kavoussi LR, Kerbi K, Capelouto CC, et al. Laparoscopic nephrectomy for renal neoplasms. Urology. 1993;42: 603–9.
4. Kerbi K, Clayman RV, McDougall EM, et al. Laparoscopic nephroureterectomy: evaluation of first clinical series. Eur Urol. 1993;23: 431–6.
5. McDougall EM, Clayman RV, Anderson K. Laparoscopic wedge resection of a renal tumor: initial experience. J Laparoendosc Surg. 1993;3:577–81.
6. Schuessler WW, Schulam PG, Clayman RV, et al. Laparoscopic radical prostatectomy: initial short-term experience. Urology. 1997;50: 854–7.
7. Guillonneau B, Vallancien G. Laparoscopic radical prostatectomy: initial experience and preliminary assessment after 65 operations. Prostate. 1999;39:71–5.

Acknowledgements

To my wife Deborah Kinney Davis, M.D., who has supported me through my years of fellowships, relocations, and long work days. She keeps our lives going while I am traveling the world to teach robotic surgery and work with outstanding collaborators. In addition, I am proud that our daughters Hannah and Rachel have matured into lovely young women. I hope they write their own books some day.

To my mentors Paul Schellhammer, Gerald Jordan, Stefan Loening, Ingolf Tuerk, and Mike Fabrizio who helped me put together an early vision for combining urologic oncology and minimally invasive surgery.

To my colleagues Colin Dinney, Richard Babaian, and Surena Matin who offered me the opportunity to bring robotics to MD Anderson Cancer Center.

Contents

Contributors

Newaj Abdullah, M.D. Vattikuti Urology Institute, Henry Ford Health System, Detroit, MI, USA

Piyush K. Agarwal, M.D. Urologic Oncology Branch, Center for Cancer Research, National Institutes of Health, National Cancer Institute, Hatfield Clinical Research Center, Bethesda, MD, USA

Vineet Agrawal, M.D., FRCSEd (Uro)., FEBU Department of Urology, The Guthrie Clinic, Sayre, PA, USA

Kamran Ahmed, M.B.B.S., M.R.C.S., Ph.D. MRC Centre for Transplantation, NIHR Biomedical Research Centre, Guy's Hospital, King's College London, London, UK

David M. Albala, M.D. Department of Urology, Crouse Hospital, Syracuse, NY, USA

Giancarlo Albo Department of Urology, University of Milan, Milan, Italy

Abdullah M. Alenizi, M.D. Department of Surgery, Section of Urology, Centre Hospitalier de l'Université de Montréal, Montréal, QC, Canada

Fatih Atug Professor of Urology Istanbul Bilim University School of Medicine, Istanbul, Turkey

Janet E. Baack Kukreja, M.D. Department of Urology, University of Rochester Medical Center, Rochester, NY, USA

Christopher E. Bayne, M.D. Department of Urology, The George Washington University, Washington, DC, USA

Cooper R. Benson, M.D. Department of Urology, MD Anderson Cancer Center, University of Texas-Houston Division of Urology, Houston, TX, USA

Claudia Berrondo, M.D. Department of Urology, University of Rochester Medical Center, Rochester, NY, USA

Burkhard Beyer Martini-Clinic, Prostate Cancer Center, University Medical Center Hamburg-Eppendorf, Hamburg, Germany

Ashley J.F. Brandon Department of Urology, Eastern Virginia Medical School, Norfolk, VA, USA

Erik P. Castle Department of Urology, Mayo Clinic Arizona, Phoenix, AZ, USA

Brian F. Chapin, M.D. Department of Urology, The University of Texas MD Anderson Cancer Center, Houston, TX, USA

Christopher Cheng, M.D. Professor and Senior Consultant, Singapore General Hospital, Singapore

Jonathan Clavell-Hernandez, Division of Urology, Department of Surgery, University of Texas Medical School at Houston MD Anderson Cancer Center, Houston, TX, USA

Maria Chiara Clementi Department of Urology, University Vita-Salute, Milan, Italy

Gabriele Cozzi Clinica Urologica I, Ospedale Maggiore Policlinico, Fondazione IRCCS Ca' Granda, Università degli Studi di Milano, Milan, Italy

Prokar Dasgupta, M.D., F.E.B.U., F.R.C.S. (Urol) MRC Centre for Transplantation, NIHR Biomedical Research Centre, Guy's Hospital, King's College London, London, UK

John W. Davis, M.D. Department of Urology, Uro-surgical Prostate Cancer Program, The University of Texas M.D. Anderson Cancer Center, Houston, TX, USA

John Michael DiBianco, M.D. Urologic Oncology Branch, Center for Cancer Research, National Institutes of Health, National Cancer Institute, Hatfield Clinical Research Center, Bethesda, MD, USA

Michael D. Fabrizio, M.D. Eastern Virginia Medical School, Urology of Virginia, PLLC, Virginia Beach, VA, USA

Arvin K. George, M.D. Urologic Oncology Branch, Center for Cancer Research, National Institutes of Health, NationalCancer Institute, Hatfield Clinical Research Center, Bethesda, MD, USA

Markus Graefen Martini-Clinic, Prostate Cancer Center, University Medical Center Hamburg-Eppendorf, Hamburg, Germany

Alexander Haese Martini-Clinic, Prostate Cancer Center, University Medical Center Hamburg-Eppendorf, Hamburg, Germany

Philipp M. Huber Department of Urology, University Hospital of Bern, University of Bern, Bern, Switzerland

Matthew D. Ingham, M.D. Department of Urology, Eastern Virginia Medical School, Norfolk, Virginia, USA

Jean Joseph, M.D., M.B.A. Departments of Urology and Oncology, Center for Robotic Surgery and Innovation, University of Rochester Medical Center, Rochester, NY, USA

Jeri Kim, M.D. The University of Texas MD Anderson Cancer Center, Houston, TX, USA

Tae-Kyung Kim, M.D. Department of Urology, University of Michigan Health System, Ann Arbor, MI, USA

Anup Kumar Global Robotics Institute, Florida Hospital-Celebration Health, University of Central Florida School of Medicine, Orlando, FL, USA

David M. Latini, Ph. D., M.S.W. Baylor College of Medicine, Houstony, TX, USA

Catherine Elizabeth Lovegrove, B.Sc. (Hons.) MRC Centre for Transplantation, NIHR Biomedical Research Centre, Guy's Hospital, King's College London, London, UK

Surena F. Matin MD Anderson Cancer Center, The University of Texas, Houston, TX, USA

Maxim J. McKibben, M.D. Department of Urology, University of North Carolina at Chapel Hill, Chapel Hill, NC, USA

Tobias A. Metzger Department of Urology, University Hospital of Bern, University of Bern, Bern, Switzerland

Francesco Alessandro Mistretta Department of Urology, Fondazione IRCCS Ca, GrandaOspedale Maggiore Policlinico, University of Milan, Italy

Daniel A. Moon Division of Cancer Surgery, Peter MacCallum Cancer Centre, University of Melbourne, Melbourne, Australia

Epworth Healthcare, Epworth Prostate Centre, Richmond, Melbourne,VIC, Australia

Eric Moskowitz Mount Sinai Health System, New York, NY, USA

Vladimir Mourviev Global Robotics Institute, Celebration Health, Orlando, FL, USA

Declan G. Murphy, M.D. Division of Cancer Surgery, Peter MacCallum Cancer Centre, University of Melbourne, Melbourne, Australia

Epworth Healthcare, Epworth Prostate Centre, Richmond, Melbourne, Australia

Daniel P. Nguyen Department of Urology, University Hospital of Bern, University of Bern, Bern, Switzerland

Marcelo A. Orvieto Department of Urology, Clinica Alemana, Santiago, Chile

Patricia A. Parker, Ph. D. Department of Psychiatry & Behavioral Sciences, Memorial Sloan-Kettering Cancer Center, New York, NY

Vipul R. Patel Global Robotics Institute, Florida Hospital-Celebration Health, University of Central Florida College of Medicine, Orlando, FL, USA

James O. Peabody, M.D. Vattikuti Urology Institute, Henry Ford Health System, Detroit, MI, USA

Raj S. Pruthi, M.D. Department of Urology, University of North Carolina at Chapel Hill, Chapel Hill, NC, USA

Avinash Reddy Mount Sinai Health System, New York, NY, USA

Koon Ho Rha Department of Urology, Urological Science Institute, Yonsei University College of Medicine, Seoul, South Korea

Bernardo Rocco Clinica Urologica I, Ospedale Maggiore Policlinico, Fondazione IRCCS Ca' Granda, Università degli Studi di Milano, Milan, Italy

Mathew Goland-Van Ryn Mount Sinai Health System, New York, NY, USA

Sunil Kumar Sahai, M.D., F.A.A.P., F.A.C.P Department of General Internal Medicine, The Internal Medicine Perioperative Assessment Center, The University of Texas MD Anderson Cancer Center, Houston, TX, USA

Srinivas Samavedi Global Robotics Institute, Florida Hospital-Celebration Health, University of Central Florida college of Medicine, Orlando, FL, USA

Kristen R. Scarpato, M.D., M.P.H. Urologic Surgery, Vanderbilt University Medical Center, Nashville, TN, USA

Jay B. Shah Department of Urology, MD Anderson Cancer Center, Houston, TX, USA

Joseph A. Smith Jr., M.D. Urologic Surgery, Vanderbilt University Medical Center, Nashville, TN, USA

Dylan Stoy Associated Medical Professionals, Syracuse, NY, USA

D. Telonis Associated Medical Professionals, Syracuse, NY, USA

Ash Tewari Mount Sinai Medical Center, New York, NY, USA

George N. Thalmann Department of Urology, University Hospital of Bern, University of Bern, Bern, Switzerland

Côme Tholomier Department of Surgery, Section of Urology, Centre Hospitalier de l'Université de Montréal, Montréal, QC, Canada

Patrick H. Tuliao Department of Urology, Urological Science Institute, Yonsei University College of Medicine, Seoul, South Korea

Mark D. Tyson, M.D. Department of Urology, Mayo Clinic Arizona, Phoenix, AZ, USA

Roger Valdivieso, M.D. Department of Surgery, Section of Urology, Centre Hospitalier de l'Université de Montréal, Montréal, QC, Canada

Run Wang Division of Urology, Department of Surgery, University of Texas Medical School at Houston and MD Anderson Cancer Center, Houston, TX, USA

Michael B. Williams, M.D. Department of Urology, Eastern Virginia Medical School, Norfolk, Virginia, USA

Stephen B. Williams, M.D. Department of Urology, The University of Texas MD Anderson Cancer Center, Houston, TX, USA

Eric S. Wisenbaugh, M.D. Department of Urology, Mayo Clinic Arizona, Phoenix, AZ, USA

Michael E. Woods, M.D., F.A.C.S Department of Urology, University of North Carolina at Chapel Hill, Chapel Hill, NC, USA

Pascal Zehnder Department of Urology, University Hospital of Bern, University of Bern, Bern, Switzerland

Kevin Zorn, M.D. Department of Urology–Director of Robotic Surgery, University of Montreal, Montreal, Canada

Part I

Robot-Assisted Radical Prostatectomy: Step by Step

Minimally Invasive Access to the Prostate: The Concept of Surgical Space Creation

1

John W. Davis

Introduction

Surgical space creation can involve several concepts including pneumoperitoneum access, transperitoneal versus extraperitoneal space creation, port placements, creating anatomic planes around key steps of the operation, and troubleshooting hostile anatomy. For this chapter, we will step outside of the traditional format of an original research article or structured review, and discuss straightforward "how I do it" descriptions with illustrations. A key take home message is that minimally invasive radical prostatectomy (MIRP—laparoscopic or robot-assisted) skills are like a toolbox of tips and tricks, and surgeons should learn all of them, and employ them when the anatomy calls for them. This mentality is distinct from other situations where one would believe or interpret from evidence that specific techniques are superior in all circumstances and should be executed the same way every time with more efficiency. As an analogy, if one drives from home to work the exact same route every day, you don't know your city and neighborhoods as well as if you try different routes. You may still prefer one route to another, but the diversity improves your orientation and over time your efficiency.

J.W. Davis, M.D. (✉)
Department of Urology, Uro-surgical Prostate Cancer Program, The University of Texas M.D. Anderson Cancer Center, Houston, TX, USA
e-mail: jdhdavis@aol.com

Establishing Pneumoperitoneum, Ports, and Docking in <8 min

By now, most surgeons attempting MIRP will have formal training in establishing pneumoperitoneum, but a few options are worth a brief description. The most common method would be Veress needle access. The device includes a sharp needle with a hollow bore and inner blunt portion that retracts upon perforating tissue. Therefore the sharp edge is exposed when perforating fascia and subcutaneous tissue and then the blunt edge slides forward after entering the abdominal cavity. In the supraumbilical position, the surgeon should feel two distinct "pops" going in: upon passing fascia, and again through pneumoperitoneum. It is important to gauge depth expected based upon patient size, and not to overly penetrate and damage bowels. I lift up on the fascia with a blunt towel clip—one blade inside the umbilical circle, and the other blade subcutaneous. This elevates the fascia off the bowels [1]. You can do the water drop test if you prefer, but with a clean entry and initial pneumoperitoneum measurement of <5, you are likely in every time. See Figs. 1.1 and 1.2.

J.W. Davis (ed.), *Robot-Assisted Radical Prostatectomy*, DOI 10.1007/978-3-319-32641-2_1

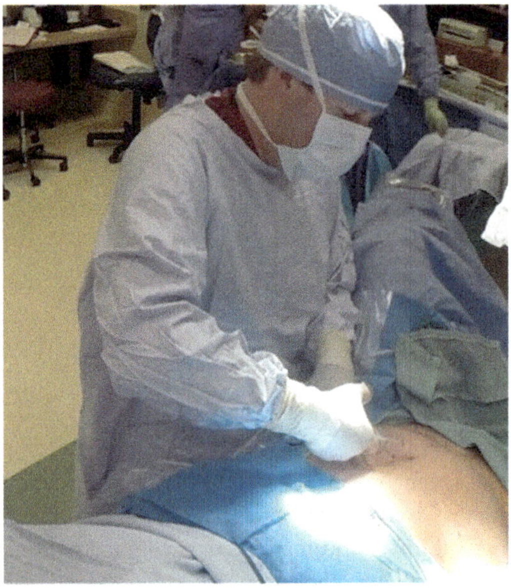

Fig. 1.1 Through a supra-umbilical vertical incision, a blunt towel clip is placed with 1 blade in the umbilicus and one subcutaneous with vigorous lift

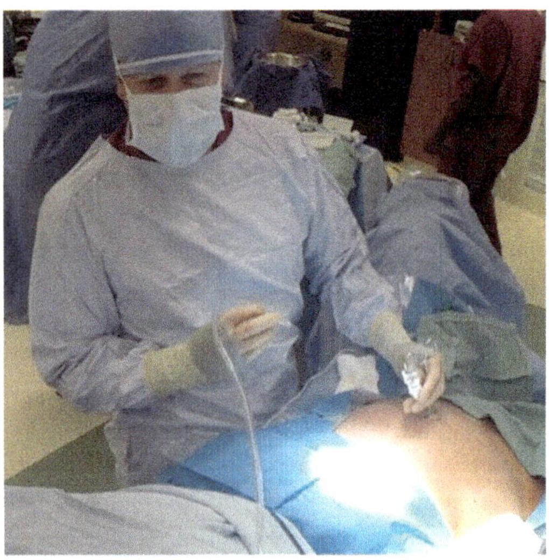

Fig. 1.2 The Veress in inserted, feeling the 2 "pops" on entry, and the entry pressure will be measured. The clamp is pulled up with force to separate fascia from bowels

Next, keep momentum going rather than watching the pneumoperitoneum measurements. We roll the robot into place while the gas is flowing. If you roll the robot to your arms reach with the patient flat, you can reach and pull the arms out wide, then go steep Trendelenberg, and then fining rolling to the final position—Fig. 1.3.

For port placement, the basic rules for transperitoneal are:

- Camera is supra-umbilical, slightly to the patient left in the right side assistant configuration—Fig. 1.4.
- Robot arm/left—15 cm up from the pubic bone, and 9 cm (4 fingers) wide from the camera—Fig. 1.4.
- Robot arm/Far Left (Often referred to as the "3rd arm for daVinci Si or "4th" arm for daVinci standard and S models)—place 2–3 fingers angled up from the left anterior superior iliac spine—Fig. 1.5.
- Robot arm right—mirror image for robot arm left—Fig. 1.6.
- Assistant port—suction—triangulate up from the camera and robot arm right—Fig. 1.6.
- Assistant port—12 mm—mirror image to the robot arm/far left. Figure 1.7—final configuration.

It is noteworthy that for very thin patients with less width, the robot arm/far left can go very vertical from the anterior superior iliac spine—keep three finger breadths from robot arm/left. For the assistant port 12 mm—keep somewhat close to the right anterior superior iliac spine as a high placement might keep clips out of range unless using special designs for obese patients.

Intuitive makes obesity trocars for such patients, and most vendors have disposable extra long trocars for such patients.

In general, if you can insufflate while positioning, place ports with basic hand measurements, and keep multi-tasking, you can be on consult in <8 min.

If the patient has significant scar, or the Veress needle technique does not give you low entry pressures, then convert to an open access technique. We use the balloon port from Applied Medical (Rancho Santa Margarita, CA). To explore for adhesions right under the camera port, place holding stitches in the outer fascia and gently dissect/probe into the ensuing layers. Use finger dissection to feel for adhesions and stuck

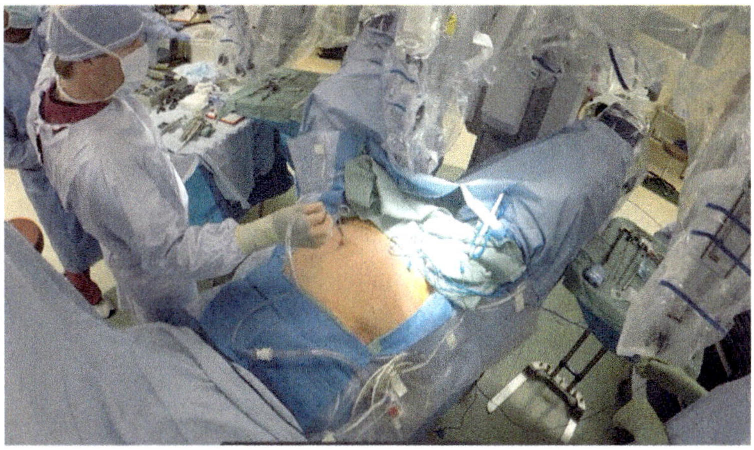

Fig. 1.3 While the pneumoperitoneum is coming up to 15 mmMg, the robot is simultaneously rolled into position and the patient placed into steep 25° Trendelenberg position

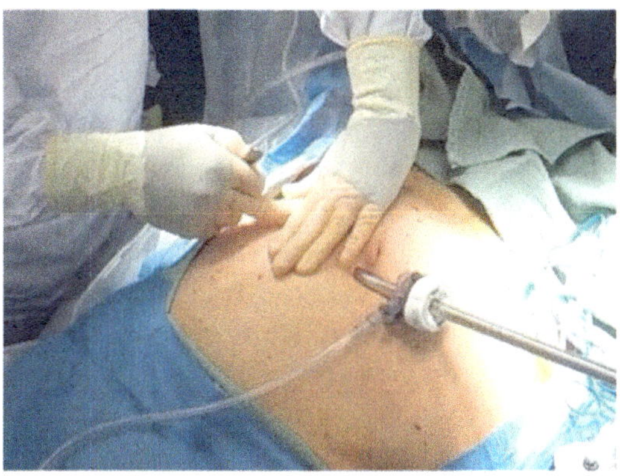

Fig. 1.4 Camera position and initial left side port measurements

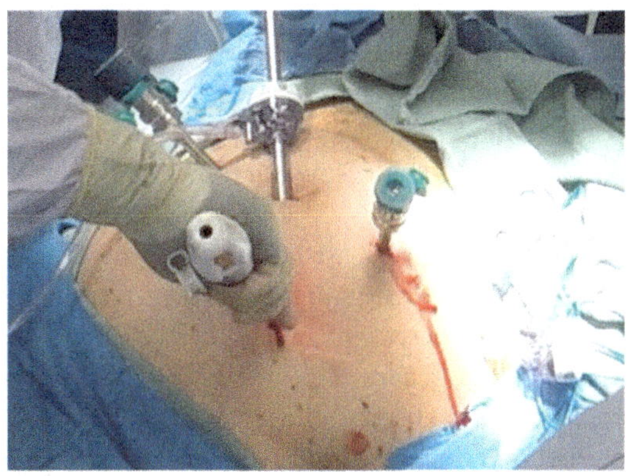

Fig. 1.6 Patient right ports are placed: robot, 5 mm assistant suction, and 12 mm assistant port

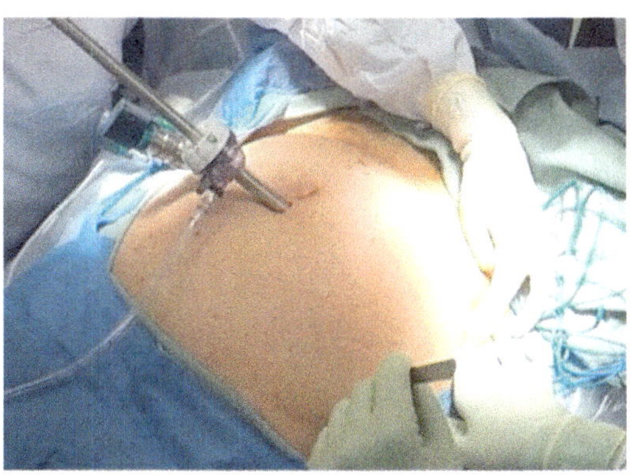

Fig. 1.5 Left-sided ports are in and starting to measure the right

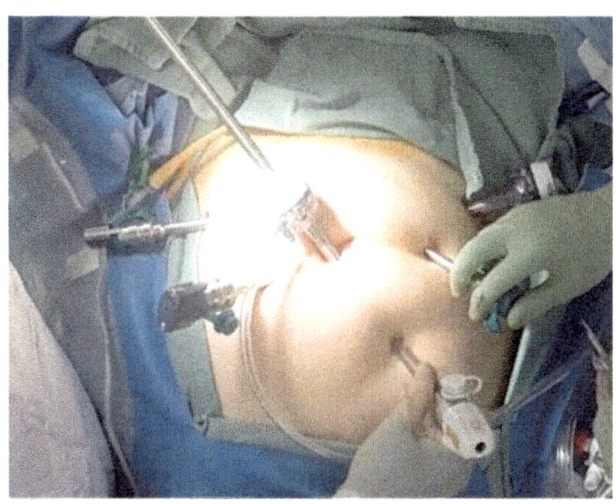

Fig. 1.7 Final configuration for transperitoneal ports-pubic bone is top of image, head down

bowel. An alternate entry pathway may be in the lateral port regions similar to renal surgery. Overall, the surgeon should be cautious, and some authors report overall safety superiority with routine open access techniques [2].

If you must take down adhesions from prior surgery, it may be best to setup a standard laparoscopic camera kit with 5 and 10 mm lenses Fig. 1.8. The 5 mm lenses can fit through a daVinci port using its adapter ring. This allows camera access to all ports and viewing for sharp dissection. If the adhesions are thin, then sharp dissection is reasonable, but if thick tissue with vascularized omental pedicles, then consider a bipolar or Ligasure device. These bleeders are hard to find later if they drop down and migrate into the upper quadrants. Therefore it is better to seal them up front.

Often the 5 mm assistant port has a good overall view of the lower quadrants for finding and lysing adhesions.

We previously published a guide to extraperitoneal access training, including resources needed, equipment changes, and pitfalls to avoid [3]. In general, a kidney balloon dilator creates the extraperitoneal spaces, and the ports move down from 15 to 8 cm up from the pubic ramus—Fig. 1.9. This technique needs some hands on training or case observations, but is feasible and a good tool-box technique to have in case of adhesions or need to reduce Trendelenberg requirements (15° rather than 25°).

Basic Space of Retzius Space Creation

If the sigmoid colon is in the way, then mobilize it. This will free space for a posterior Pouch of Douglas dissection of the seminal vesicles and/or free space to access left pelvic lymph nodes. Otherwise, if ready to proceed into the pelvis, here are some tips and tricks:

- The urachus and medial umbilical ligaments have a few bleeders—get them sealed well or the bleeding drips onto the camera—Fig. 1.10.
- Once these are divided, use sharp/cautery dissection to divide laterally to the vas—Fig. 1.11.
- Stay medial to the vas and you will avoid the iliac vessels.
- If no lymph node dissection or minimal planned, you can leave the vas intact. For extended nodes, you will eventually divide them laterally.
- Medial to the vas, separate the planes down low and can go straight to the endopelvic fascia.
- De-fat over the prostate and bladder neck.
- Be careful and seal the superficial dorsal vein—this bleeds and is hard to control if avulsed and retracts back—Figs. 1.12 and 1.13.

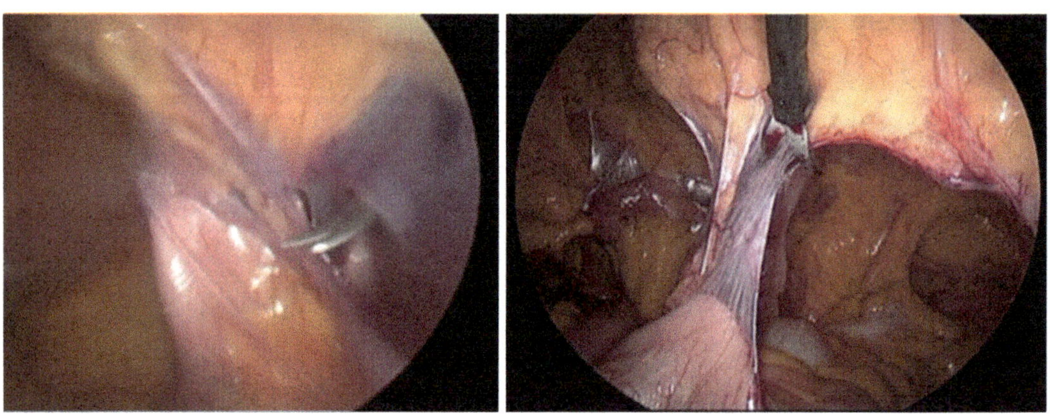

Fig. 1.8 Lysis of adhesions holding a standard laparoscope and hand held instruments

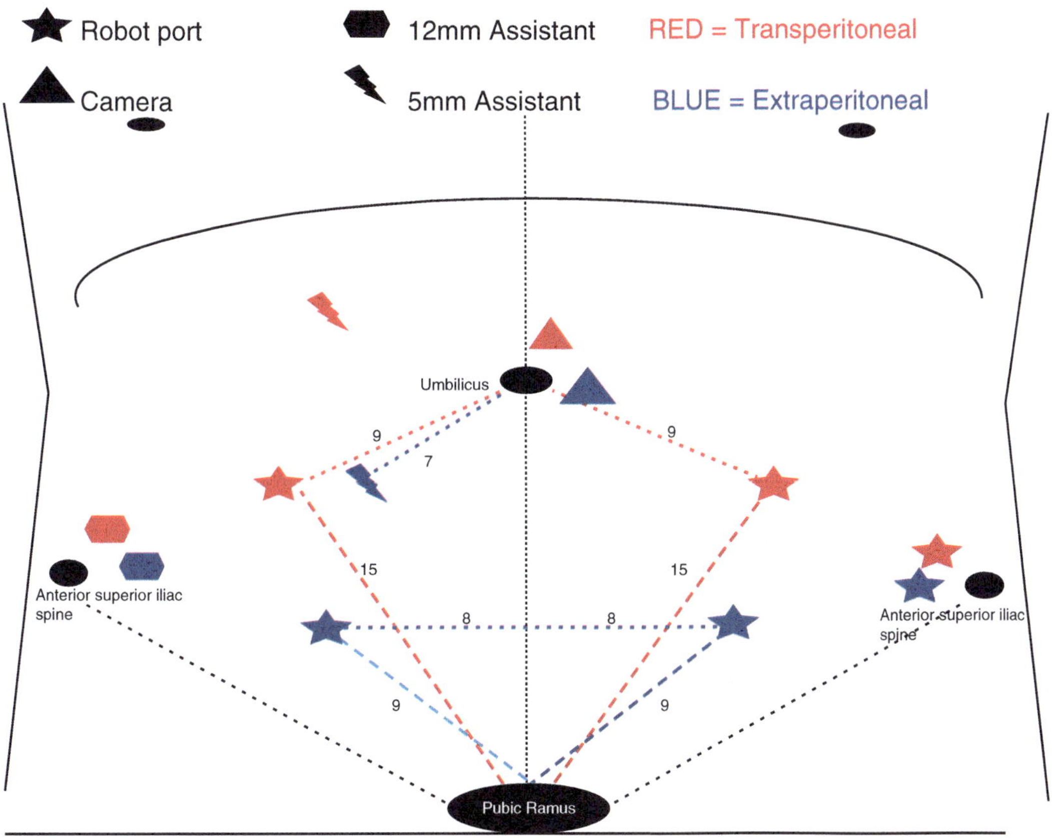

Fig. 1.9 Diagram

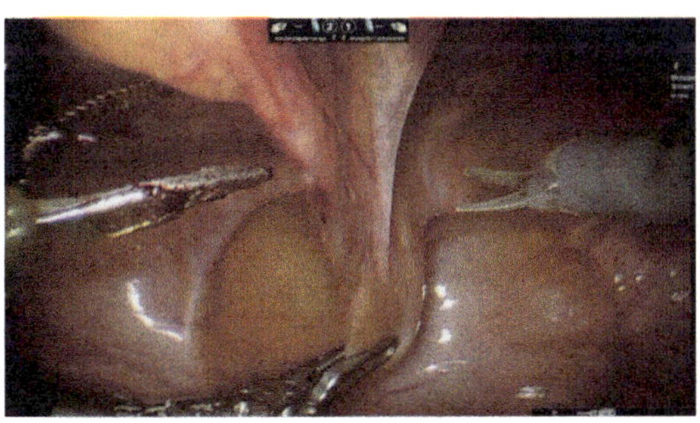

Fig. 1.10 Basic initial space of Retzius creation. Pull down on the midline with the Prograsp™ and the divide the urachus/median ligaments. Use good bipolar current to seal the vessels while in view

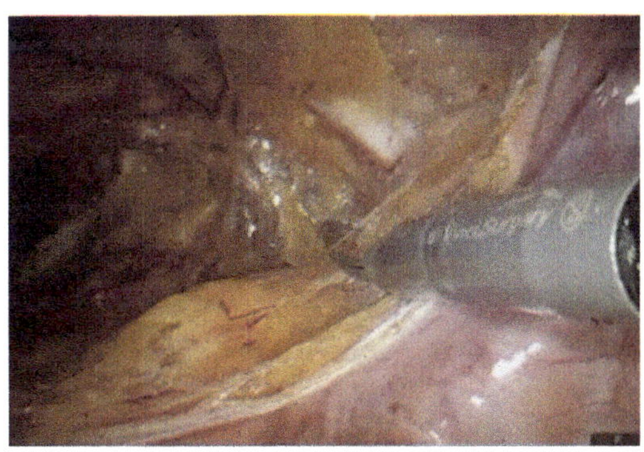

Fig. 1.11 The peritoneum is cut on the right side to the vas. The pubic bone is seen in the distance, and once exposed symmetrically on both sides, you can proceed to de-fat over the prostate

Urachal Stitch Trick

In some cases, the bowel is just in the way, and rides up in your field. This may be a variant anatomy or related to obesity. In other cases, you may wish to reduce Trendelenberg position due to cardiac risk. One method of interest plays upon the concept of externalized sutures to add to exposure. Guru et al. [4] published this concept as a Marionette nomenclature in its use for setting up robotic ileal conduit. The basic concept is

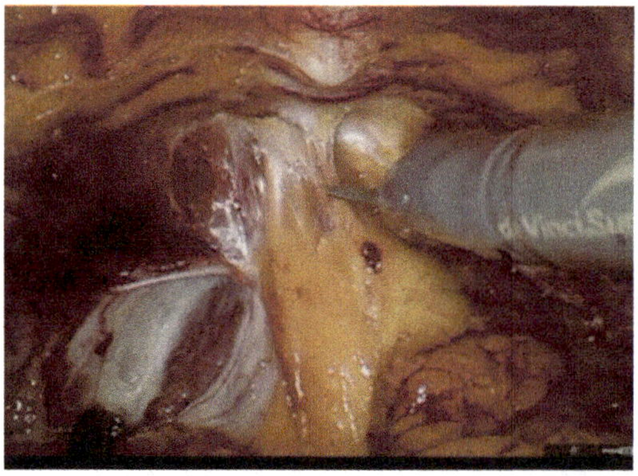

Fig. 1.12 The fat of the bladder needs removing, taking care to avid the superficial dorsal vein and the tip of the scissor

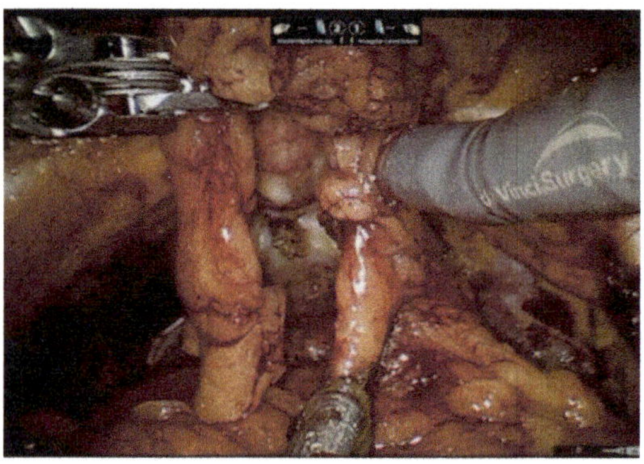

Fig. 1.13 The perivesical fat is exposed, sealed, and sent for a specimen

to sew a long 2-0 Vicryl to several spots on the cut urachus. Then use a Carter Thomason® device to perforate over the camera port and exteriorize the string. Clamp the string under tension for additional cephalad retraction without using an instrument for the purpose—Fig. 1.14.

Seminal Vesicle Exposure: Anterior or Posterior

The posterior approach goes through the Pouch of Douglas and was popularized in the pre-robotic era by the Montsouris group in Paris [5]. As mentioned, the sigmoid colon might need mobilizing first—Fig. 1.15. This approach is easier on beginners in terms of getting to the tip

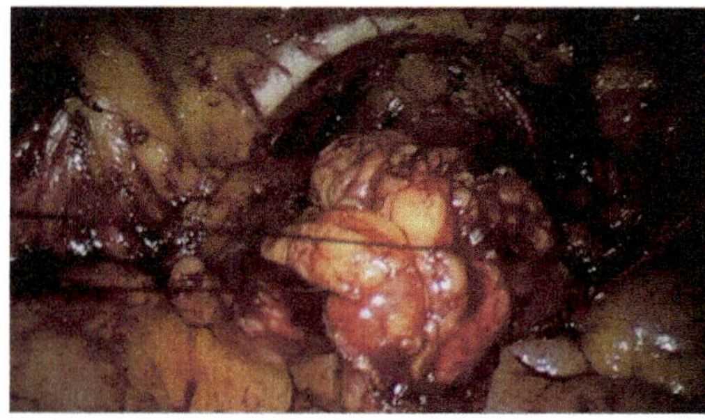

Fig. 1.14 Urachal stitch trick. The full-length 2-0 Vicryl is sewn around the urachus, exteriorized with a Cater-Thomason®, and retracted cephalad to keep the bowels out of the field or for reduced Trendelenberg position

of the seminal vesicle and effective clipping or bipolar sealing the small arteries here. The pouch is incised about 2 cm up from its lowest point, and for about 6–8 cm in width (Fig. 1.16). The 3rd arm lifts the upper peritoneal surface and the space is bluntly opened. In thin patients you will see the vas and SVs quickly such as with Fig. 1.16 but in some patients you have to look around. Always track the vas down from the sides to stay oriented. A ureteral injury could result from disoriented dissection in this space.

Essentially, a normal SV that is not affected by infection, biopsies, neoadjuvant treatments, or cancer should just tease out of its bed. The vessels hold it in place, and as you seal them, the SV rotates out. It is fragile and therefore too much traction before releasing the vessels results in significant tearing injury. The cut vasa can be good retraction points. Most of the vessels run posterior, and just lateral to the SV tip. An available retraction instrument (3rd arm or assistant) can grasp the bare surface of the SV and start the dissection while the robotic arms seek out and seal/cut the small vessel. Once the tip is free, a few lateral attachments remain and then the step is completed—Figs. 1.17 and 1.18. In some cases, the very large SV tip is easier to dissect from this angle than anterior.

In summary, the posterior dissection:

- Easier to learn.
- Very low tension on the SV/nerves.
- Facilitates bipolar or clip-free dissection.

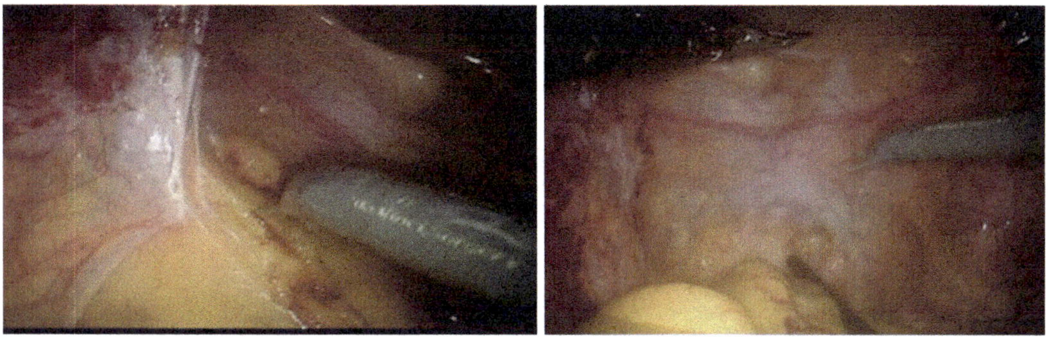

Fig. 1.15 The sigmoid colon may be in the way for a posterior approach. Once free, the sigmoid should straighten out and show you the full pouch

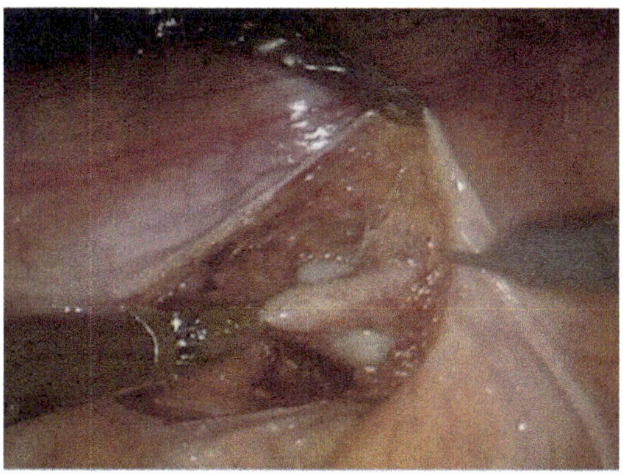

Fig. 1.16 Incise the pouch 2 cm or so above the lowest point. Lift up with the 3rd arm and open the space. In thin patients, the vas/SV should be seen soon

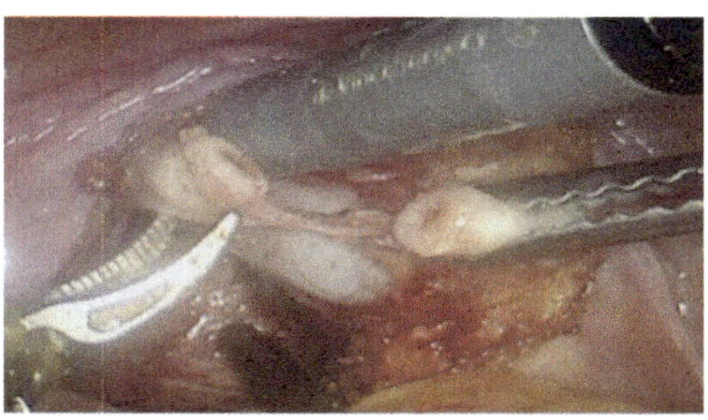

Fig. 1.17 Divide the vas. There is always an artery right behind it that needs sealing with clip or bipolar

- Step times equal to anterior if initial exposure learned.
- Possibly faster for larger SVs.

The anterior approach is required for extraperitoneal access, and can also be efficient. In theory, it is slightly less invasive, as the pouch barrier remains intact and might keep operative site bleeding or urine like out of the abdominal spaces. I have also wondered if bleeding from the SV's would be harder to tamponade if the Pouch is opened up. On the other hand, the exposure to the SV tips is trickier with the bladder now in the way, and additional challenges can add to the complexity such as long SV tips, peri-SV scarring, and a large prostate volume.

The principles of dissection are the same for either approach, and the adjacent neurovascular bundle lateral to the SV tip mandates no monopolar cautery in these areas. A few tips/tricks and figures are useful:

- Gauge the viewing angle. In some patients there is a naturally downward angle and you can remain in zero lens. However if you cannot see down well at the bladder neck division step, then change to a 30° down angle—Fig. 1.19.
- The bladder neck step needs to be completed to the point that the vasa are seen in the midline.
- Additional space is created by taking down some of the bladder pedicle and clipping the lateral branches of the Santorini plexus that runs in the lateral thirds of the bladder neck region—Fig. 1.20.
- The key to setting up the clips on the SV's is to find the medial tip of the SV and get the Dennonvilliers fascia off of it. A single hemo-lock™ or two can then fire around the lateral sides and complete the step—Figs. 1.21 and 1.22.

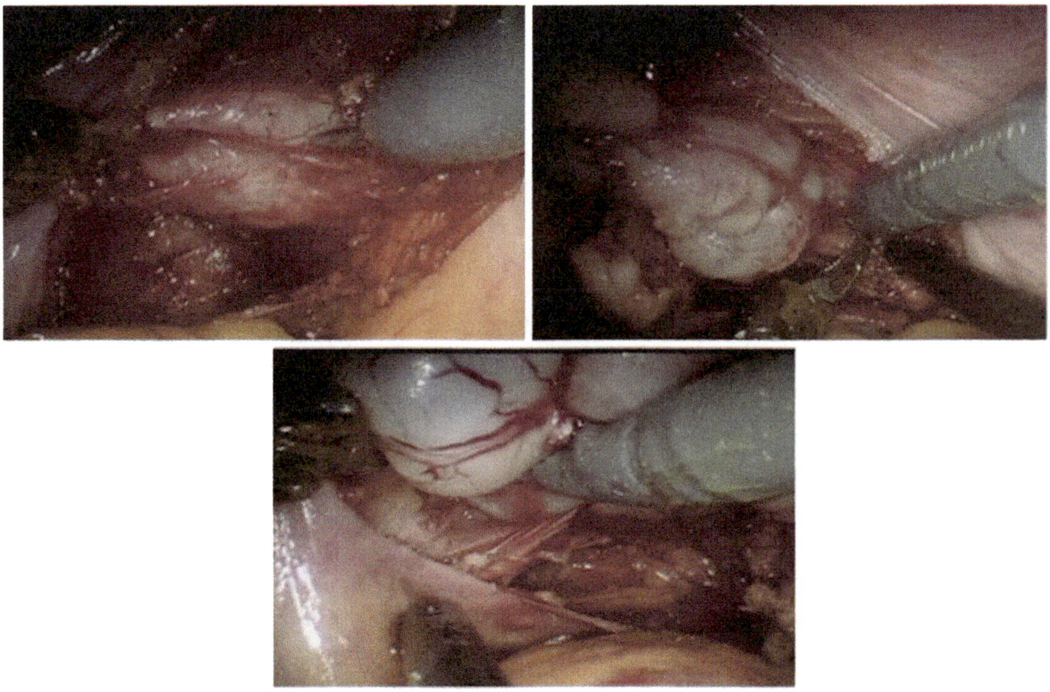

Fig. 1.18 Grasp the bare surface of the seminal vesicles and rotate medial. Push the Dennonvilliers fascia down and isolate the small arterial pedicles for clipping or brief bipolar sealing

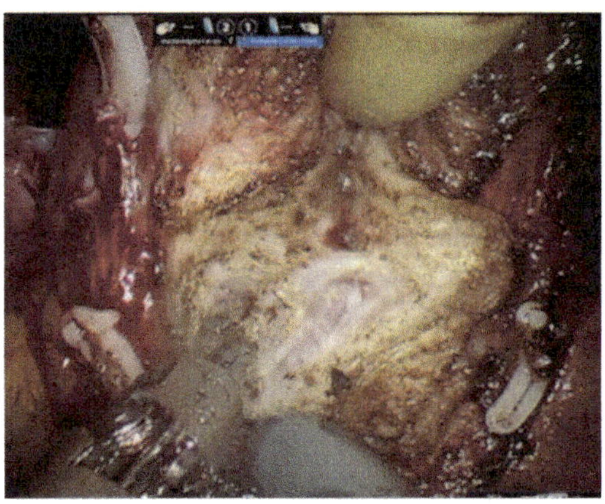

Fig. 1.19 In the anterior SV approach, the bladder neck is fully divided. The catheter is still held on traction towards the abdominal wall. Clips are seen laterally where lateral Santorini Plexus branches are controlled. These steps help open width to the space such that the SV's can be found without working in a tight ravine-like space

With either approach, once both pairs of vas/SV are freed, the structures can be lifted to the abdominal wall and expose the Dennonvillers fascia.

Posterior Planes: Creating a "High" Risk or "Low" Risk Plane

Although the Dennonvilliers fascia has a single label, it does have multiple layers [6, 7]. You can create a surgical plane in the higher layers posterior if risk of pT3 cancer in the area is not expected. The plane tends to but right under the base of the vas, and looks gray in shape. It is a nice plane to be in, as it will connect easier with the nerve sparing planes. For a high-risk plane you can go a full centimeter or so lower and

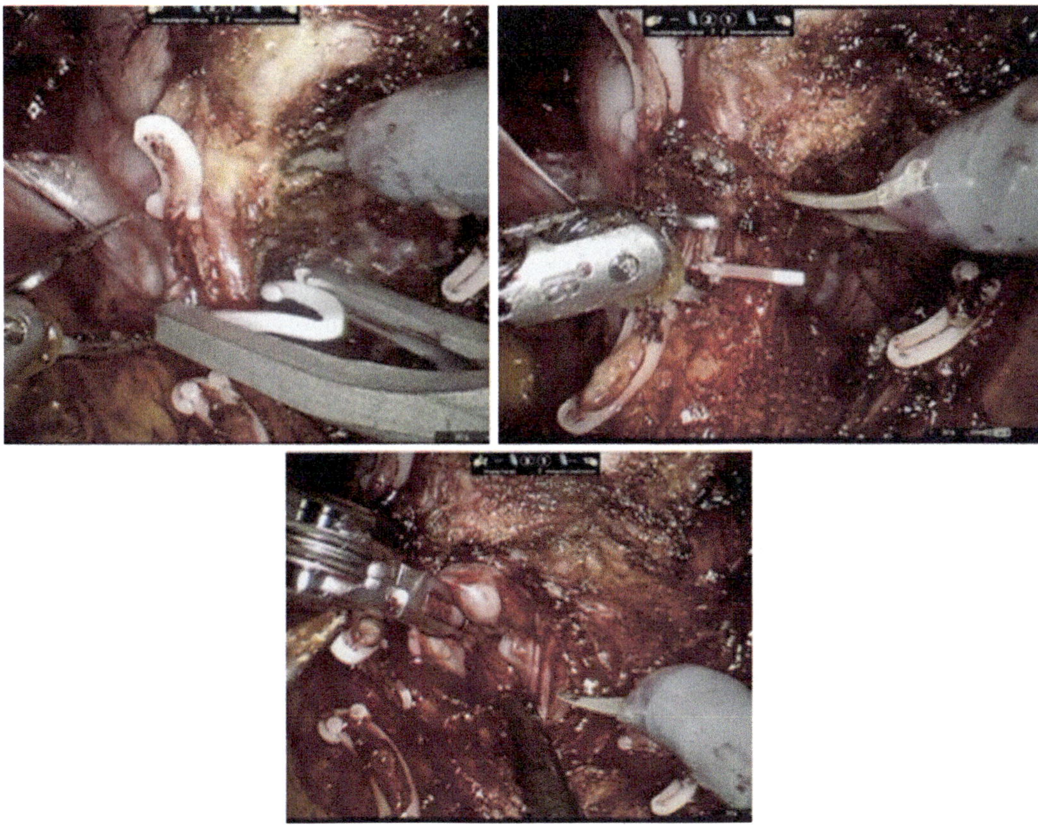

Fig. 1.20 If the space is still tight, additional bladder pedicle can be taken. Now the vas can be grasped and lifted to take the plane to the tip of the SV

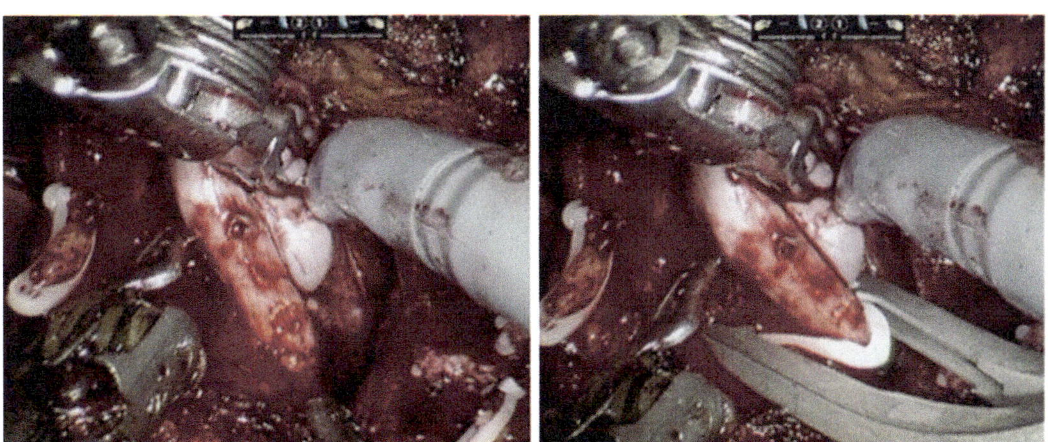

Fig. 1.21 If the tip of the SV can be determined and freed medially, the a Hemolock™ clip can seal the tip of the SV with the Vas

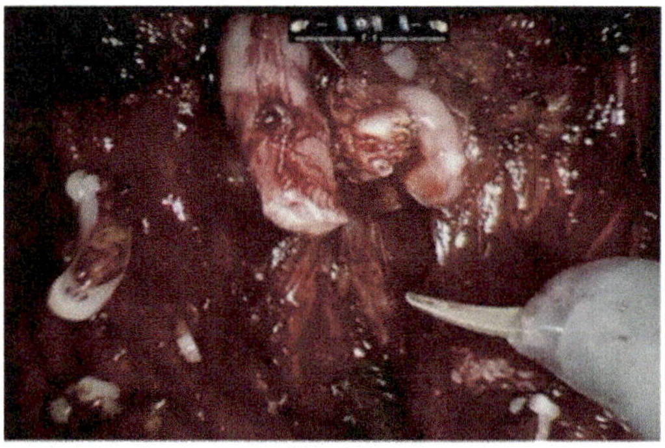

Fig. 1.22 After 2 or so clips, the SV pedicles are controlled and the step completed on each side. Efficiency is created by setting up the space properly

break into the more traditional peri-rectal plane, and that will have obvious peri-rectal fat as a signal. See Figs. 1.23, 1.24, and 1.25.

Troubleshooting Space

The later-generation robots have quite long instrumentation and sticking to standard port configurations described above and published elsewhere. It would be unusual to run out of instrument reach to the apex, as was encountered with the much shorter array of instruments used in pure laparo-

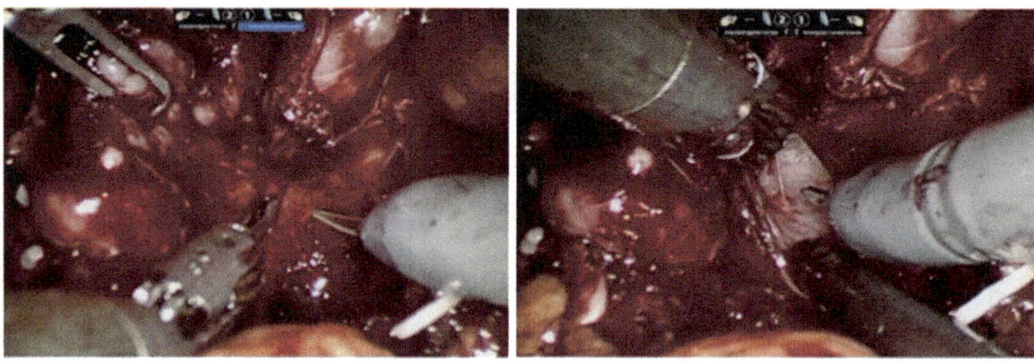

Fig. 1.23 The "low"-risk Dennonvilliers plane is just below the vasa, and has a characteristically gray appearance once entered

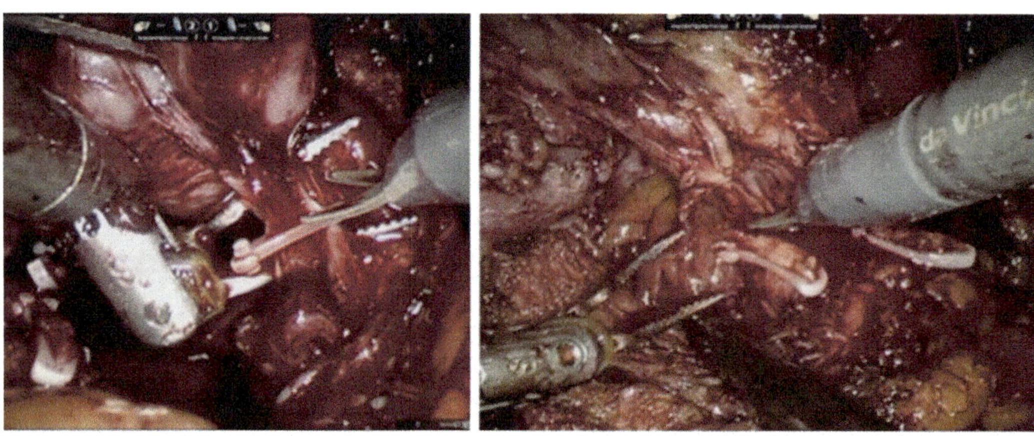

Fig. 1.24 From the posterior plane, find some of the pedicles in line with the posterior SV's. These run with Dennonvilliers fascia and are always there. They will bleed without proper clips. Dividing these creates additional "lift" on the prostate such that when you move to the nerve sparing step you are oriented on medial and lateral borders of the neurovascular bundles

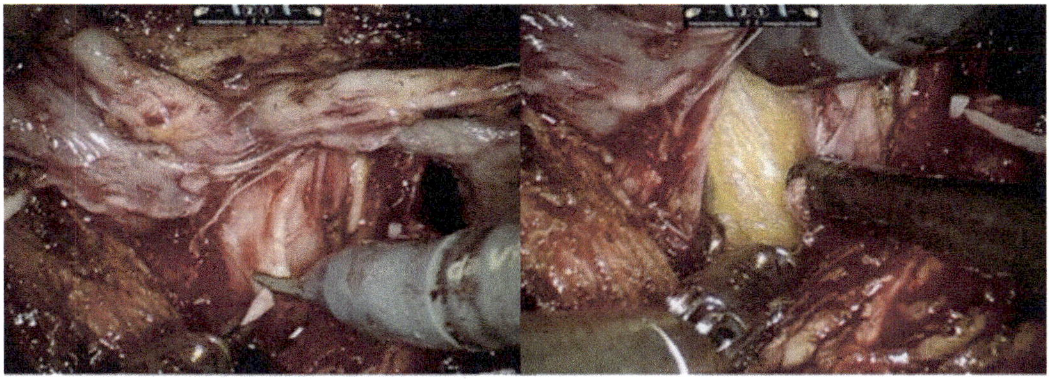

Fig. 1.25 By contrast, the "high"-risk plane is much lower through Dennonvilliers, and shows clear peri-rectal fat upon entry

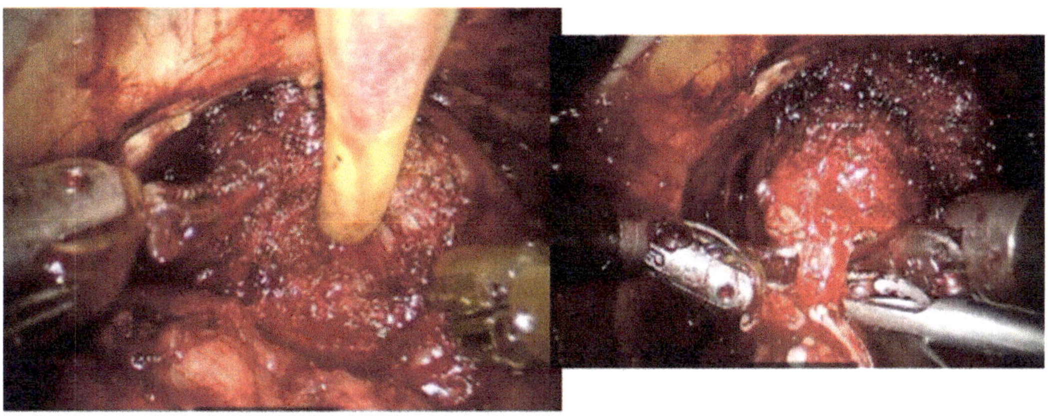

Fig. 1.26 Pubic arch interference. The prostate is mostly under the bone, and the lateral spaces very reduced. Standard maneuvers (*right*) such as pedicle division often lead to instrument collisions with the bone and the need to seal bleeders along the bone

scopic procedures. However some patients will challenge access due to gland size or pubic arch interference. In some cases, the entire base of the prostate can be under the pubic arch. There is no specific remedy for this, other than to remember that the robotic ports are held in a static position by the arm through which the instrument is rotated. That static position can be modified by pressing the set-up button and manually pushing the port down and into the abdomen. This will lower the angle of the instrument such that it can clear the pubic arch. If there is no pubic arch interference, we often pull the ports up and out to create more room for assistant instruments. See Figs. 1.26 and 1.27.

Accessory pudendal arteries are a 5–10 % variant, but higher rates are reported [8, 9]. They should be kept lateral with incision of the endopelvic fascia medial. The DVC stitch should be placed with care not to injure it at the apex—Fig. 1.28. In select cases, try the DVC cut without a suture and pneumoperitoneum to 19 briefly. Then selectively sew the DVC. Box et al. showed a 40 % rate of such arteries but no effect on potency return [8]. Given the controversy it is best to preserve what you can. What is not published as well but observed is that some vessels start out looking like accessories, but then insert into the prostate rather than course around it. These have to be taken.

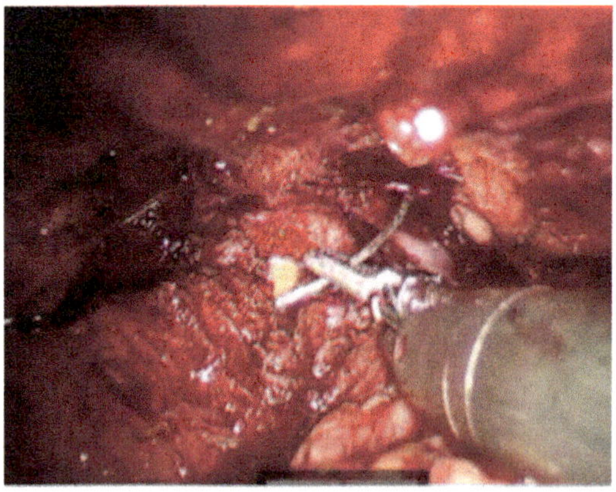

Fig. 1.27 With pubic arch interference, the apical spaces are reduced and the final sewing angles can be limited. The arms need to be adjusted up/down to give the straightest angle to the urethra and the assistant might need to provide additional retraction not needed in most cases

Occasionally, a patient with a pre-existing penile prosthesis subsequently needs RARP. The key is to leave the pseudocapsule intact and free of injury [10]. The reservoir should be full during initial exposure. Then drain the reservoir to create the space to the prostate. See Fig. 1.29.

Conclusions

The key steps of a successful RARP are the bladder neck division, neurovascular bundles, apex, and anastomosis. Yet to get to these steps, you need good exposure and an ability to adapt to hostile anatomy and variances. The concept of "space creation" is to access certain anatomic points in and around the key procedure steps that

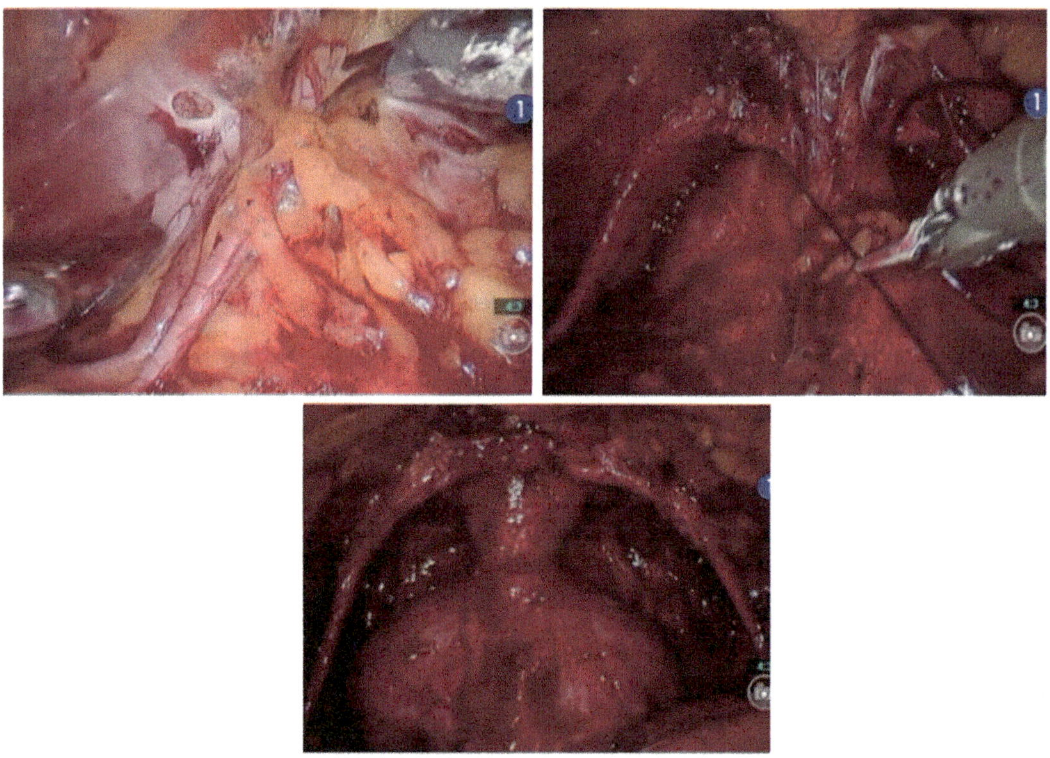

Fig. 1.28 Accessory pudendal arteries can be tricky. The endopelvic fascia should be incised medially and the artery pushed laterally. The challenge is then to place the DVC stitch without injury at the apex. Photo credit-Vipul Patel

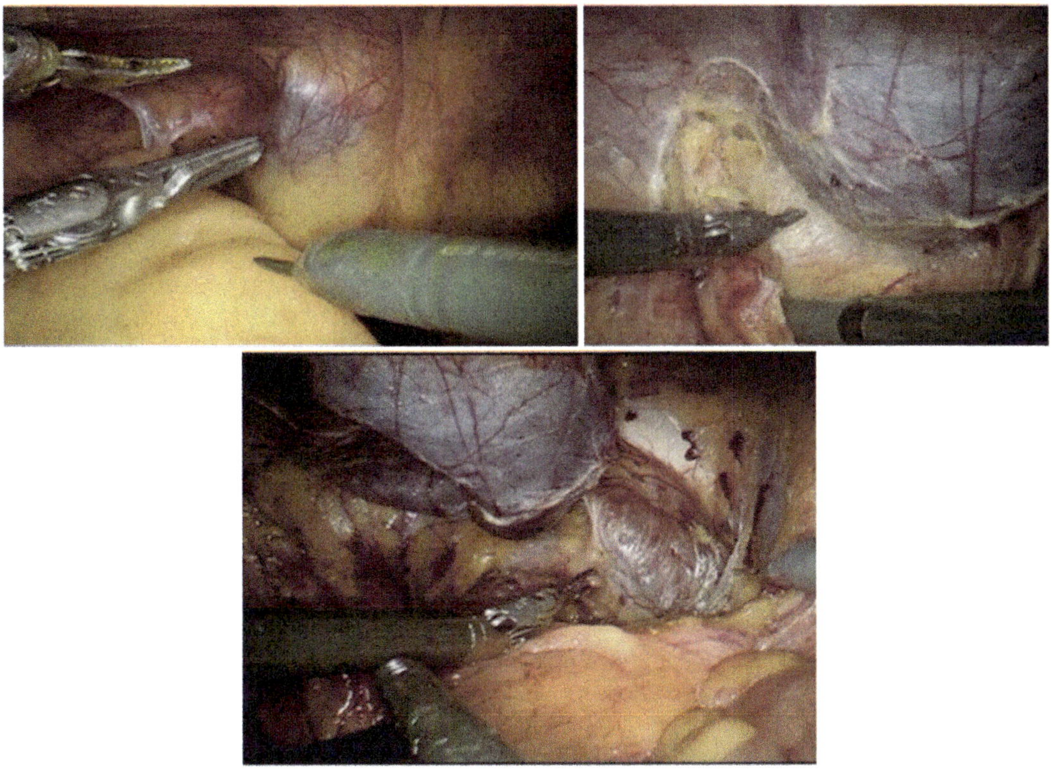

Fig. 1.29 Inflatable penile implant. Dissect out the reservoir without injuring the pseudocapsule and then empty the fluid (i.e. inflate the prosthesis) to create the space

optimize such performances. The choice of anterior or posterior seminal vesicle approach can be patient specific, and overall it is best for surgeons to learn both techniques. In my experience, transperitoneal is most efficient to set up, but extraperitoneal has its advantages and is worth adding to your repertoire.

Related concepts are involved in extended template pelvic lymph node dissection which will have its own chapter.

References

1. Shamiyeh A, Glaser K, Kratochwill H, et al. Lifting of the umbilicus for the installation of pneumoperitoneum with the Veress needle increases the distance to the retroperitoneal and intraperitoneal structures. Surg Endosc. 2009;23:313–7.
2. Ahmad G, O'Flynn H, Duffy JM, et al. Laparoscopic entry techniques. Cochrane Database Syst Rev. 2012;15:2.
3. Davis JW, Achim M, Munsell M, Matin SM. Effectiveness of postgraduate training for learning extraperitoneal access for robotic-assisted radical prostatectomy. J Endourol. 2011;25(8):1363–9.
4. Guru KA, Mansour AM, Nyquist J. Robot-assisted intracorporeal ileal conduit "Marionete" technique. BJU Int. 2010;106:1404–20.
5. Guillonneau B, Vallancien G. Laparoscopic radical prostatectomy: the Montsouris technique. J Urol. 2000;163:1643–9.
6. Muraoka K, Hinata N, Morizane S, et al. Site-dependent and interindividual variations in Denonvilliers' fasica: a histological study using donated elderly male cadavers. BMC Urol. 2015;15:42.
7. Hinata N, Sejima T, Takenaka A. Progress in pelvic anatomy from the viewpoint of radical prostatectomy. Int J Urol. 2013;20:260–70.
8. Box GN, Kaplan AG, Rodriguez Jr E, et al. Sacrifice of accessory pudendal arteries in normally potent men during robot-assisted radical prostatectomy does not impact potency. J Sex Med. 2010;7:298–303.
9. Secin FP, Touijer K, Mulhall J, et al. Anatomy and preservation of accessory pudendal arteries in laparoscopic radical prostatectomy. Eur Urol. 2006;2007:1229–35.
10. Erdeljan P, Brock G, Pautler SE. Robot-assisted laparoscopic prostatectomy in patients with preexisting three-piece inflatable penile prosthesis. J Sex Med. 2011;8:306–9.

Surgeon's Notebook: Beyond the Learning Curve: The Original Handouts from the American Urological Association Postgraduate Courses 2013–2015

2

John W. Davis, Fatih Atug, Koon Ho Rha, Kevin Zorn, Christopher Cheng, and Declan G. Murphy

Course Application

As with any CME related course, there are certain descriptors required for the application that the course director must submit. Here was our application:

J.W. Davis, M.D. (✉)
Department of Urology, Uro-surgical Prostate Cancer Program, The University of Texas M.D. Anderson Cancer Center,
Houston, TX, USA
e-mail: jdhdavis@aol.com

F. Atug, M.D.
Professor of Urology, Istanbul Bilim University School of Medicine, Instanbul, Turkey

K.H. Rha, M.D.
Department of Urology, Urological Science Institute, Yonsei University College of Medicine, 50 Yonsei-ro, Seodaemun-gu, Seoul 120-752, South Korea

K. Zorn, M.D.
Department of Urology–Director of Robotic Surgery, University of Montreal, Montreal, Canada

C. Cheng, M.D.
Professor and Senior Consultant, Singapore General Hospital, Singapore

D.G. Murphy, M.D.
Division of Cancer Surgery, Peter MacCallum Cancer Centre, University of Melbourne, East Melbourne, VIC 3002, Australia

Epworth Healthcare, Epworth Prostate Centre, Richmond, Melbourne, VIC, Australia

Course Description

This particular chapter and the text as a whole will focus on the advanced content of robot-assisted radical prostatectomy, for surgeons who have completed their first 100 cases. The course assumes that the learner has hands on experience with port placement, docking, and initial case performance in well-selected cases. For participants seeking advanced training, this course will provide video-based discussion, and literature-based didactic content for managing difficult/unexpected anatomy, advanced access techniques, extended lymphadenectomy, adjustments for high risk/locally advanced disease, radiation salvage, and complication management. The faculty will provide numerous techniques to improve time efficiency, and thoughts on how to perform the least traumatic dissection of the nerve bundles and apex. The faculty will provide international-based experience and evidenced based summaries of the risks and benefits of this procedure to aid in patient counseling.

Problems Assessment

We want to fix the problem of the learning curve of the surgeon who has learning the basics of robotic prostatectomy, but now needs to expand their practice to the broader range of case selection, and to improve their performance.

J.W. Davis (ed.), *Robot-Assisted Radical Prostatectomy*, DOI 10.1007/978-3-319-32641-2_2

Needs Assessment

Unless a surgeon has trained with a high volume robotic surgeon, they will not have sufficient experience with managing difficult case anatomy, and may still be experience longer operative times that may diminish the benefits of this approach. This course will seek to fill in the knowledge gaps so that the learning can apply their basic knowledge to advanced skills.

Learning Objective 1: to analyze a difficult anatomic variation in robotic prostatectomy and to apply the best solution to the problem.

Learning Objective 2: to select appropriate patients with high risk or recurrent disease for robotic surgery and to design and execute the most effective operation.

Learning Objective 3: To critique the best available evidence and to summarize the most up to date estimates of risk and benefit of robotic prostatectomy.

Learning Objective 4: To collect ten or more surgical tips/tricks that improve time efficiency, and the least traumatic dissection of the nerve bundles and apex.

Learning Objective 5: To Improve Functional Outcomes.

Difficult/Unexpected Anatomy

The learning curve for RARP is the topic of much debate and different findings. The initial 20 cases are important for basic port placement, time efficiency, step-by-step performance, etc. In many cases, the new robotic surgeon will have observed several cases and videos, and performed an animal lab for skills. Initial cases are very well selected and proctored, and therefore it is common that the first 3–5 cases are fairly smooth. However, somewhere between cases 5–20, an unexpected anatomic feature may be encountered that may lead to a lengthy case time and/or conversion to open. So let's think of three separate concepts to improve our training organization: (1) What is a "well selected case"? (2) What is an expected challenge? and (3) what cannot be predicted as a case challenge?

A well-selected case would include:

1. No obesity: BMI <30 for starters.
2. Reasonable prostate size of <40 g.
3. No prior abdominal/pelvic surgery.
4. No significant anesthesia risk for a prolonged case of 4–6 h.
5. Lower risk disease: this has changed with the need to avoid overtreatment, but at least try to exclude patients needing and extended PLND, and preferably no PLND.
6. No median lobe on TRUS.
7. No predictors for surgical plane scaring such as multiple biopsies, hormone use, pelvic radiation, prostatitis.

An expected challenge, therefore, would include patients who have one or more of the features excluded above.

That leaves us with the more troubling challenge—what constitutes an *unexpected challenge*. Lets compile a working list and propose some possible solutions that our faculty will discuss and demonstrate through video.

1. Narrow pelvis. You can tell you are in for a narrow pelvis at the bladder neck step if you observe that the bladder neck is still under and possibly distal to the pubic arch. To some extent, the severity of this problem is lessened with robotics compared to straight laparoscopy, because the robotic ports are placed much higher on the abdomen than laparoscopy. The 1 and 2 arms are generally at 15–17 cm from the pubic arch in robotics compared with 8–10 cm from laparoscopy. Therefore, the angle of entry in robotics is lower than laparoscopy and less likely to collide with the bone. Nevertheless, here are some tip descriptions:
   (a) The port alignment has some leeway in terms of anterior/posterior movement. Some call this "burping" the port. You

call hit the set-up joint and "pull" the port up to the ceiling. This is the common default move, as it allows greater separation between the working arms, camera, and assistant ports. In a narrow pelvis, however, the pulled-up position may exacerbate pubic arch collisions. During the PLND and most of the prostatectomy, this is not an issue, but when it is time for the anastomosis, you may need to "push" the port back down towards the floor, and this will allow a better collision free angle to the urethra.

(b) Suturing. With less angles and access, you may need to practice various one-handed maneuvers to get the sutures into their correct spots. The 4th arm can be useful in lowering the bladder neck out of the way, or the assistant does this. It will just take longer as each suture takes some setting up. Perineal pressure with a well placed sponge-stick may help push the urethra out further into a less collision prone spot.

2. Narrow Pelvis—*comments from Koon Rha.*
   (a) There is a paucity of anthroporphic studies comparing Asian pelvis to Caucasian pelvis. The last discourse on interracial pelvic variations was written by Turner [1] in 1885. He classified pelves into three types—platypellic (widest), mesatipellic, and dolichopelic (narrowest). However, his sample size of various races was limited and the Asian populations were heterogeneous by his classification (Mogolloid and Malayan peoples were classified as platypellic while Aino were dolichopellic).
   (b) There has been a recent revival in interest in pelvic dimensions with relation to outcome of radical prostatectomy. In a recent report by Hung [2] and colleagues, 190 men undergoing open radical prostatectomy were prospectively recruited and underwent MRI to obtain standard obstetric pelvimetric measurements of interspinous distance at the pelvic midplane, intertuberous distance at pelvic outlet and anteroposterior diameters of the midplane and outlet. Additionally, a new MRI-based parameter, apical depth, defined as the craniocaudal distance from the most proximal margin of the symphysis pubis to the level of the distal margin of the prostatic apex as measured on the mid-sagittal MRI image was developed. Using these parameters, a pelvic dimension index (PDI) was created where a wide, shallow pelvis would have a greater PDI and a narrow, deep pelvis would have a low PDI. However, at eventual multivariate analysis, only prostate size was a significant factor in predicting blood loss and none of the variables were significant in predicting positive margins.
   (c) In a follow-up study by Hung et al. [3] looking at 151 robot-assisted LRP only, he found that no pelvic dimensions were associated with prolonged operative time, estimated blood loss nor surgical margin status. Only prostate volume was positively correlated with longer operative duration ($p=0.015$) and estimated blood loss ($p=0.045$) on multivariate analysis.
   (d) Matikainen et al. [4] built on the PDI as described by Hung to retrospectively study 586 men with preoperative MRI prostate undergoing RRP or LRP to determine the risk factors for having an apical positive surgical margin (PSM). While limited by the small number of patients with apical PSMs (93), at logistic regression they found a positive correlation between apical depth and the occurrence of apical PSM.
   (e) Finally, Mason et al. [5] in a retrospective series of 76 patients undergoing robot-assisted LRP sought to combine pelvimetric indices measured using an endorectal coil MRI with prostate volume creating a prostate volume to prostate cavity index ratio. A ratio of <6 had significantly less blood loss (39 % less) and shorter operating time (12 % shorter) than those with a ratio >6. Indeed, it would be easier to perform a prostatectomy on a small gland in

a wide pelvis than a large gland in a narrow pelvis. In this study however, positive surgical margins were not associated with PCI or prostate volume.

3. Ureteral Position.
   (a) If the ureters are close, you have two common solutions:
      - 1 cm or so clearance to the cut edge. You can probably get away with a posterior reconstruction to push the ureters inward. This basically flows like open RP—posterior tennis racquet with interrupted 2-0 Vicryls. Doing a running anastomosis at this point is a bit tricky and we will demonstrate. The key is to get your two running strands very close to the posterior suture line so there is no gap. Place two suture lines on each side, and then parachute it down.
      - <1 cm clearance. Your call, but recommend trying to place JJ stents over a wire so you are not stuck with postoperative obstruction.
4. Median Lobe. Most can be predicted but not all. Many videos are available on this topic. Men with high IPSS score and voiding dysfunction should have preoperative assessment including ultrasound to look for intra-prostatic protrusion. Staging MRI often gives excellent definition of the anatomy. The bladder neck should be entered in a more cephalic position to avoid incising the prostate lobes. The bladder neck should be dissected away from the prostate keeping the median lobe on the prostate. Unusual asymmetrical prostate shapes can be suspected upon entering the bladder neck when the Foley balloon cannot be found in the usual median position.

   The key is to elevate the lobe, locate the ureters, and then truncate at the appropriate spot. Once you are full thickness bladder wall, you will hit the median lobe again. Follow this spot straight down to the vas. Either lift up on the lobe, or if it is huge, some have demonstrated placing a suture through it to elevate further. Once isolated the median lobe can be elevated by the fourth arm or using a Carter-Thomason device. Care should be taken to avoid enucleating the adenoma while dissecting along the median lobe. The vertical detrusor fibers and Denonvillier's fascia serve as the guide to the posterior bladder neck plane to the seminal vesicles.
5. *Obesity*.

   There are two main issues with obesity: (1) anesthetic and (2) access. For practical purposes specific to robotic surgery, we consider a BMI <30 as normal, BMI 30–40 as obese but not requiring specific changes in technique, and a BMI >40 as morbidly obese and at risk for complications/surgical challenge.

1. Anesthetic. Steep Trendelenburg position causes two problems:
   (a) Position sliding/compression injury. If a patient slides for any reason, the position of the legs may change, and cause a compartment syndrome, or additional injury to other pressure points such as a chest strap. At MDACC, we avoid these as follows:
      - Pelvis/gluteal area hands off the end of the table by a few centimeters.
      - Patient sits on an egg-crate cushion, which is taped to the bed.
      - Legs in Allen stirrups—legs weighted in alignment with the opposite shoulder.
      - For significant obesity with large arms, consider the "big boy" positioning. Keep the arm boards on the table and parallel such that the arms have full support rather than wrapped in sheets. In many of these cases, the arms would be off the bed otherwise. Wrap them with plenty of foam and sheets. Place the chest strap inside the arms equal to the nipples. Use pads and avoid the brachial plexus.
      - Consider a test Trendelenburg position before the draping so you can see if there is any movement.
      - Be especially careful with newer beds that have extreme Trendelenburg positioning. For most standard beds, the maximum is 40° and this is plenty.

(b) Increased ventilation pressure.
- For BMI's well over 40, there is the risk that there is excess pressure on the diaphragm that leads to increased ventilation pressures, and increased pCO2. One possible solution is to take the patient out of steep Trendelenburg. Exposure in the pelvis can be maintained with a simple externalized suture. Place a 2-0 Vicryl, full length into the field and suture around the urachus for several throws, pulling slack to the midpoint of the suture. Then use the Carter-Thomasen device to puncture just over the camera port to retrieve and externalize the suture. Use a hemostat pulled against the skin to now pull the urachus cephalad and place traction on the bladder so as to open the pelvis spaces. Of course, this suture needs to be taken down during the anastomosis. In general, this, move will act like a flap and keep the bowels out of the way.

2. Access.
(a) The suture trick helps with access as well as the Trendelenburg problem. After this, the pelvis may need to be defatted to create more space. In general, there is a flap of fat overlying bladder neck that splits down the middle and goes off to each side, wrapping around the superficial dorsal vein in parts. Aherling published a study showing the presence of lymph nodes in this area—same idea—just clear this plane to make the bladder neck look normal.

Previous Surgery

Adhesions from Previous Surgeries

Many minor procedures have fairly minor effects on access such as appendectomy, and laparoscopic cholecystectomy. However upper midline procedures (Nissen, spleenectomy) often leave scarring around the camera port. Colon surgery is fairly unpredictable. If the previous operation was performed mainly on one side of the abdomen (e.g., hemicolectomy), the Veress needle may be inserted in the opposite side for creation of pneumoperitoneum. The peritoneum could be entered under vision using a 5 mm clear tip port or a 10 mm Visiport (Covidien, Mansfield, MA). However, when in doubt, consider using open access over Veress needle. The balloon port from Applied medical is handy, as it can seal a defect made looking into the peritoneal cavity. With this knowledge, make an incision large enough to extract the prostate and probe around for the best access. Look further for the best areas to place 1–2 ports that would allow looking at any scarring and taking down adhesions. Using a standard 5 mm laparoscope, you can then look through any port to take down adhesions until low enough to proceed with robotic dissection.

In certain cases, adhesions may be so dense that only the camera port can be safely inserted. In such circumstances, a nephroscope with a working port can be inserted through the camera port (Siddiqui et al.). Adhesiolysis can then be performed to create space for insertion of additional ports.

In rare circumstances, if a first look shows too many adhesions, you can move the incision around the lower umbilicus and "convert" to extraperitoneal access—see below. In some cases, a lower midline scar from previous surgery may result in dense scarring, preventing vision or dilation of the pre-peritoneal space across the midline. In these situations, it may be helpful to move the infra-umbilical incision slightly off the midline (preferably towards the side where the larger diameter assistant port will be placed later). Using this incision, the pre-peritoneal space may be dilated on the ipsilateral side, allowing safe insertion of two ports on the ipsilateral side. The midline scarred tissues can then be taken down and additional trocars can be inserted on the contralateral side. In extreme cases, a combination of extraperitoneal and intraperitoneal trocars insertion could be performed and the robotic arms docked. Adhesiolysis and entry into the peritoneal cavity can then be more easily achieved with robotic assistance.

Previous Hernia Repairs

Bilateral hernia repairs especially laparoscopic extraperitoneal repairs can lead to the complete obliteration of the retropubic space. Studies have shown that patients with previous bilateral mesh repairs have the second highest rate of adhesions (Siddiqui et al.). It had been suggested by some authors that a transperitoneal approach to robotic prostatectomy might be easier than extraperitoneal or open approaches. Caution must be exercised when operating on patients with previous hernia repairs. If it is possible to identify the location of the edge of the mesh, then meticulous dissection may be possible to void disrupting the mesh repair. However, if extensive mesh and fibrosis are present, incising through the mesh might be necessary. This should be performed at the midline, with careful dissection of the obliterated space of Retzius, aiming for the inferior surface of the pubic symphysis.

Previous TURP

Radical prostatectomy after TURP is generally thought to be more difficult due to the resultant altered anatomy. Particularly, peri-prostatic fibrosis can lead to more difficult bladder neck dissection and nerve-sparing dissections. Studies have report worse erectile function, continence rates, positive margins and higher complication rates in such patients after radical prostatectomy (Jaffe et al.; Do et al.). Several points are to be noted during robotic prostatectomy in these patients.

- The prostatovesical junction will be difficult to identify due to the floppiness and fibrosis after TURP. A modified ultradissection of the bladder neck involving identification of the detrusor muscles and dissection of the lateral border of the bladder neck first before transection will help in preserving the bladder neck (Rha et al. Int J Urol. 2010 Mar;17(3):297–300). Changing to a 30° down lens would help.
- Because of cicatrization of the bladder neck after TURP, the ureteric orifices may be pulled closed to the bladder neck. Upmost care must be taken when dissecting the posterior bladder neck and the ureteric orifices should be visualized as far as possible, especially if the bladder neck is opened wide.
- There is a higher chance of a wide bladder neck and reconstruction of the bladder neck before vesicourethral anastomosis is often needed. A racket handle reconstruction can be performed to increase the distance of the ureteric orifices from the bladder neck before anastomosis. Intravenous Indigo carmine dye could help identify bilateral ureteric obstruction intraoperatively after vesicourethral anastomosis.
- Healing may be delayed due to inflammation and scarring after TURP, resulting in anastomotic urine leakage. It might be prudent to leave the catheter for 10–14 days before removal.

Extraperitoneal Access

I have learned this technique and published a learning process (Davis et al. J Endourology 25: 1–7, 2011). In summary, to learn this, you need to see a live demonstration, DVD instruction, and read through the technical diagrams. This is beyond the scope of this course, but we can outline a checklist to help you along.

Equipment additions include S retractors to find the fascia, a balloon (kidney shaped) dilator to start the extraperitoneal space dilation, sharp da Vinci obturators to place ports with less tension, a balloon port to seal the camera port, and xeroform gauze to seal further. Initial dissection is with a standard laparoscope.

The table position is similar with legs/arms tucked, but generally less Trendelenburg—20° vs. 40 for transperitoneal. The port comparisons are diagramed from the article—see Fig. 2.1, end of handout.

Troubleshooting is a major part of the learning curve. Specifically, you can run into gas leaking around the working ports, which is solved by making them very tight in size. Xeroform may be needed. The epigastric vessels are a major obstacles as this position puts you right on top of them. It is key to see and avoid at entry and also monitor the position as you change instruments. Peritonotomies are a problem is small, as they create a "wind-sock" budge that gets in the way. You have to either oversew, or just make larger so the gas exchanges. The 5 mm port is tricky—have to push enough peritoneum out of the way and use your finger to guide it in.

This is a reasonable thing to try, but in our learning curve, we found it longer to set up, frustrating to troubleshoot, and no major differences in outcomes. With the emphasis on more extended lymph nodes for intermediate to high risk disease, these are best done transperitoneal due to the lymphocele risk. Quite frankly, if there are adhesions from prior surgery, in most cases I

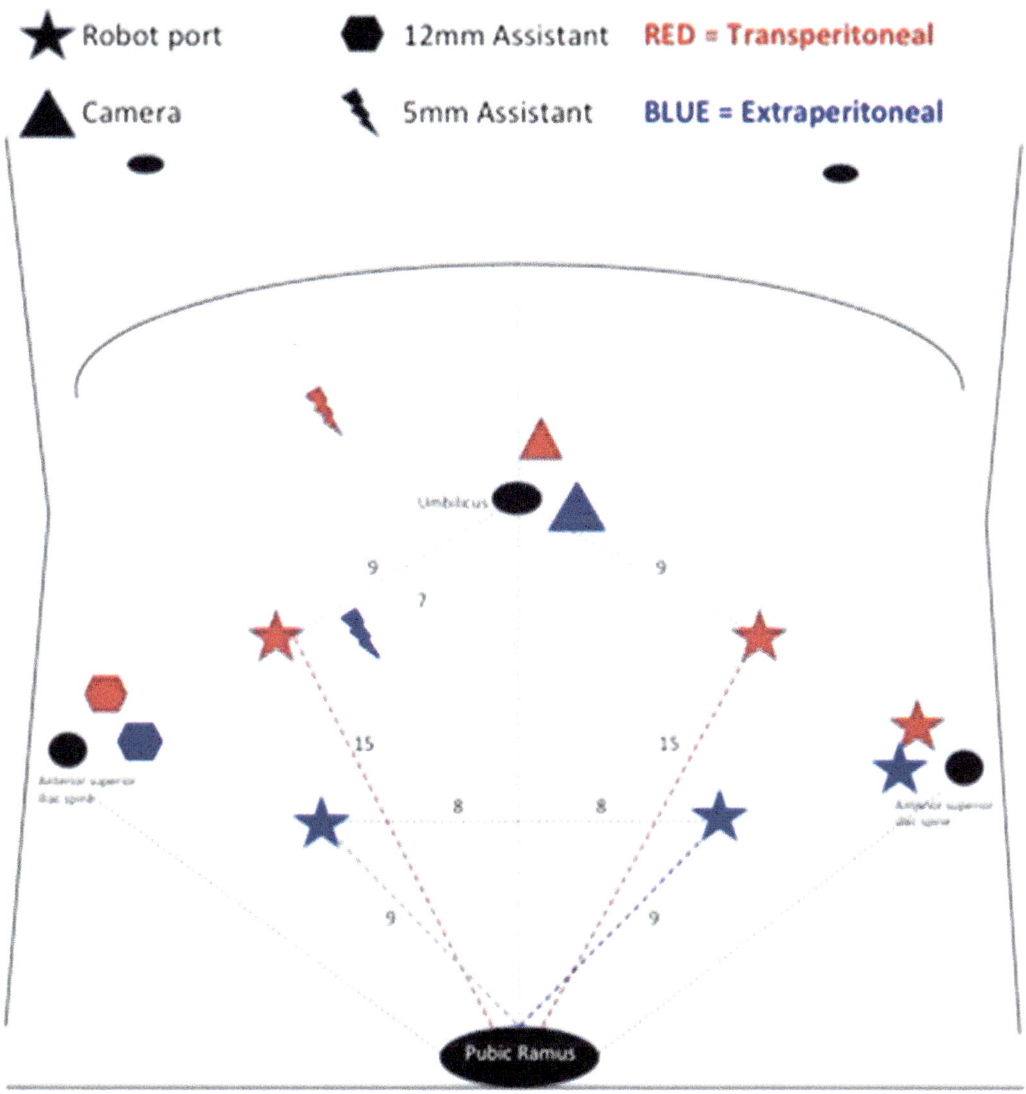

Fig. 2.1 Transperitoneal versus extraperitoneal access sites

would rather take them down in work in a larger transperitoneal space. Since abandoning this technique, I have gone back to the posterior approach to the SV's to reduce traction injury compared with the sharp angle/retraction needed for anterior exposure.

If adhesions are horrible, it is possible to "convert "to extraperitoneal, meaning move your incision around the inferior umbilicus, and reenter the extraperiteonal space and dilate it.

Extended Pelvic Lymph Node Dissection

In my experience, we doubled the lymph node count with extended templates, and consistently find 38–40 % positive nodes in high risk patients and 9–10 % in intermediate risk. We find effectively 0 % nodes in low risk disease, with the very rare exception of a major upgrade in the primary.

A longer-format article on learning extended nodes is published: Davis J, Shah, and Achim BJUI 108: 993–998, 2011. If you go to the BJUI website and search for the article and click "supporting information" there is a Web link to an attached video, but we will also show you updated video for this course. An obturator template is also called "standard" but there is also variation here, i.e., plucking a few nodes out, versus actually cleaning out the entire obturator fossa.

The major additions to the template are as follows:

1. Hypogastric.
   (a) The lateral part is a bit easier—going from the artery laterally and underneath the obturator nerve. So you really split/roll tissue around the nerve rather than stop there for a standard.
   (b) The medial part is much harder to do. You have to split right over the artery, and then get into a plane just under what looks like perivesical fat. It is tricky because the artery and vein trunks send off medial sub-branches at a right angle to your dissection, so you have to kind of tease off the tissue and watch for several branches underneath to avoid or seal.
   (c) The distal part is difficult to draw, i.e., from the Studer series of publications with dotted lines. However if you follow the hypogastric distally, you end up in a fat pad that sits over the endopelvic fascia. You can harvest this and then stop. Keep to bipolar for this entire step as you are very close to the nerve bundles. See *Sagalovich D* et al. *Assessment of required nodal yield in a high risk cohort undergoing extended pelvic lymphadenectomy in robotic-assisted radical prostatectomy and its impact on functional outcomes. BJU Int 111: 85–94, 2013.* They found reduced potency in extended PLND, and this zone is where the technique may matter.
2. External Iliac.
   (a) You actually do not harvest it all like a cystectomy. Go right down the junction of the artery and vein and distally, you migrate medially to the node of Cloquet.
3. The Triangle.
   (a) There is a triangle from the external iliac and internal iliac artery junction to the floor of the external iliac vein. The triangle is "sealed" by tissue as a default, but widens considerably as you dissect/mobilize this space. The idea is to get around the full triangle and clean it out, then move lateral to the external iliac vein within the triangle. From here you can mobilize to the most proximal extent of the obturator nerve. Once complete, when you get back to the obturator fossa, the proximal packet is loose and comes to you, whereas if you skip this step, at least 3–5 nodes are up in this corner.
4. Common iliac.
   (a) Depending upon time, risk and selected strategy, you can move up the common at least to the ureteral crossing, like a cystectomy template.

There are several other key concepts to discuss as an adjunct to seeing video:

1. Specimen packaging.
   (a) You can certainly do left versus right. I commonly would load the right nodes, then prostate, then left nodes so can separate after extraction.
   (b) If you use the Anchor Retrieval Bag product, you can reuse the bag for node subpackets. The key is judging how much will come out through the port. We currently try and send four specimens—right and left obturator/external iliac, and hypogastric (everything under the obturator nerve). The node counts increased by a mean of 5 with this, and we do see isolated hypogastric nodes positive as per Studer's work.
2. Sequencing.
   (a) More recently, we prefer the nodes to go first. After mobilizing the sigmoid colon, and then the SV/Vas through the pouch of Douglas, we leave the Urachus intact but mobilize everything else. This way the urachus becomes a site of traction to see the hypogastric planes well. This can be done after the prostatectomy, or even after prostate and anastomosis.
   (b) Once on a node dissection, try a sequence of mobilizing the tissue under the obturator nerve first and leave the bulk of the packet intact. The do the Triangle and external iliac line. Then finish in the obturator fossa and all of the extended nodes will come with you easily, and complete as you split/roll tissue over the obturator nerve.
3. Exposure.
   (a) You can use an externalized suture to improve exposure—sew to the medial umbilical ligaments and pull contralateral.
   (b) To harvest the higher nodes, you really need the sigmoid colon mobilized, the vasa cut, and cut a peritoneal flap down to the ureter to see it, move it medial, and find the hypogastric. This is fundamentally a larger dissection effort than the standard template move of just finding the external iliac vein and immediately jumping into the obturator fossa—as per above you will prefer to finish there.
4. Sealing lymphatics.
   (a) I'll be honest—I do not have the answer. If you place no clips, you have more JP output and more lymphoceles—often very delayed from surgery. But time is quick. If you place tons of clips, the time gets long, more cost of the clips, but fewer lymphoceles, less JP output. In rare cases, patients may have more nerve pains from all the metal in the area. So use a lot of bipolar, clip major proximal/distal lymphatics, and aim for a balance.
5. Time.
   (a) Early on this could take 45 min a side, but will eventually take 45 min for both, and sometimes 30 min for both when anatomy friendly and good assistance.
   (b) Time is significantly better with good assistance. The suction should be kept between the working arms on retraction or actually suction and the large assistant port always in use with a grasper or multi-fire titanium clip applier. Thus, unlike some steps, the assistant must be fully engaged as a laparoscopic surgical assistant rather than a spectator.
6. When to omit?
   (a) High risk—never.
   (b) Intermediate risk—consider for lower volume Gleason 3+4—will only rarely be positive unless upgrade. Factor in mismatches to tumor volume and/or MRI findings. Any significant risk of pT3 should prompt e-PLND consideration.
   (c) Low risk—can probably omit and hope for no major upgrade. You can go back and do a delayed—it is not too bad.

Adjustments for High Risk/Locally Advanced Disease

As per the previous session, the extended PLND is one consideration for high risk. AUA guidelines do not specify, but EAU guidelines recommend it.

Positive margins. In our hands, these remain <5 % for pT2 and approximately 25 % for pT3.

We use endorectal MRI for cases to evaluate the nerves. Incremental nerve sparing is utilized, which we will demonstrate.

Here is something to try: leave the higher risk side of the prostate for last. Do the bladder, lesser disease side, then DVC/apex. You can then take the pedicle on the high risk side and rotate the prostate vertical, seeing the entire line of the capsule versus NVB. Now you pick your plane and carve it around to the apex, where you see the gap from having taken this plane already. There is no precise science, but here are some examples:

- High volume Gleason 4+3, cT1c, normal MRI. Plan: nerve sparing plane with low fascia release.
- High volume Gleason 4+3, cT2a, capsular bulge on MRI. Plan: low release of fascia, partial nerve spare with 2–3 mm margin maintained.
- Gleason 9, cT1c, normal MRI: partial to complete nerve spare with low release.
- Bulky Gleason 8–9, suspicious MRI—take half the bundle.

For really bulky disease near the bladder, another technique is to leave the SV/Vas alone on that side initially, but free up the better side. Then get under Denonvilliers' fascia and work your way back to the pedicles. Start taking pedicles widely immediately after bladder division in that area. Now back from under Denonvilliers', you can connect that plane to the wide excision. You can do this so wide that you go right past the tip of the SV and leave all of that surrounding tissue with the specimen. Divide the vas and then start moving downhill. Continue to work laterally at push the rectum down at its lateral junction. You can really get wide planes doing this. Near the urethra, you do have to correct back after the apex and not go venturing into the rhapdosphincter.

Radiation/Salvage

As morbidities and complications of salvage prostatectomy are significant, it is essential to identify patients who would benefit most preoperatively. The ideal surgical candidate would be one with only local recurrence and of good anesthetic risks. Nguyen et al. published a nice review about patient selection for salvage prostatectomy (Cancer. 2007 Oct 1;110(7):1417–28).

In many ways, the case is no different, i.e., drop the bladder, endopelvic fascia, bladder neck. The DVC may be smaller/atrophied—especially with seeds. Several pointers would be shared.

Anterior or/and Posterior Approach

The key to the case is posterior, of course. Intuitive has an older instrument product called "Curved Scissors." These are cold, no cautery scissors. They are a little longer, stronger, and sharper than the hot scissors. I picked up this trick from Ash Tewari who uses it for the nerve sparing, and I'm addicted to this move also for the past 2–3 years—makes better packets and cuts better at times when you should not be using cautery. They are essential for radiation cases.

Orientation and sequencing—never the same. If you are more familiar with an anterior approach but is unsure if you are able to mobilize the seminal vesicle, then an initial posterior dissection might be the answer. The key is to work where the planes look friendly and be willing to go out of your usual sequence. If you get stuck or unsure in a location, then move somewhere else for a while. When you return, you will have more orientation and landmarks. This is key for parts of the posterior dissection, where the rectum interface is hard to locate. So work in as many friendly places as you can. At a certain point you will see the rectum in many places and then the stuck planes and can start making bold, sharp cuts to finish the dissection. However, if you are still unable to dissect the interface between the prostate apex and the rectum, changing to an anterior approach might help.

As mentioned, sequencing is never the same. Extensive apical dissection early in the surgery may lead to bleeding due to the distorted anatomy and fibrosis. If things are not going well, it might be easier to defer the apical dissection the later part of the surgery when the prostate is mobilized.

Avoiding Rectal Injuries

The pre-rectal fat separating the Denonvilliers' fascia and the rectal serosa may be absent due to desmoplastic changes after radiation. For this part of the surgery, use only 0° lens. Keeping close to the seminal vesicles, the prostatic apex and the midline are useful. Use sharp dissection with minimal cautery as far as possible to minimize inadvertent thermal injury to the rectum.

Always check for rectal injuries after dissection and before vesicourethral anastomosis. Intraoperative identification of rectal injury not only allows for primary repair (double layer closure of laceration) and is also associated with less postoperative complications. There are several ways to go about doing this.

- Have an assistant to do a digital rectal examination while the surgeon visually inspects the rectum.
- Fill up the pelvis around the rectum with normal saline and insert a flatus tube into the rectum. Compress the proximal rectum and have an assistant to push 50 ml of air into the flatus tube. Presence of bubbling suggests rectal perforation.
- Some groups used a flexible sigmoidoscope inserted into the rectum to transillumination which suggested thinning of rectal wall (Chauhan et al. J Endourology, June 2011;25:1013–1019).

Vesicourethral Anastomosis

Suturing—certainly a great indication to use posterior reconstruction/anterior reconstruction tricks to reinforce the primary anastomosis. Mucosa-to-mucosa apposition is essential and the anastomosis should be checked by injecting 150 ml of saline into the bladder to ensure watertight closure.

Least Traumatic Dissection of the NVB and Apex

Concepts to Discuss

- Closer planes to the prostate and less unnecessary apical dissection may improve continence. However, the radical nature of the operation shrinks to enucleation so patient selection is critical. Experienced surgeons mostly admit that they vary their technique back and forth as continence worsens or as positive margins increase.
- You have to seal vessels somehow!
  - We recognize that we cannot use electrocautery near/on the nerve bundles. But what about short bursts of bipolar? Clips?
  - Overall, large pedicles near the bladder need hemolock clips. I used to then clip everything else. But maybe that is too much clips. So now I blend bipolar with clips and pleased with the results—level 5 evidence for sure. But how would a surgeon quantitate all of these micro-decisions if they wanted to, and follow a sizeable cohort out for 12 months, controlling for patient age, nerve sparing on each side, and preoperative SHIM. So a lot of this is discussed more than published.
  - An insightful article is by Jim Hu—Alemozaffar et al. Eur Urol 61: 1222–1228, 2012. Gorgeous illustrations that we will show, but probably cannot paste into the handout. The key idea is to pay attention not only to cautery injury but also traction injury, and Dr. Hu demonstrates some dissection techniques that emphasize this point.
- A novel totally posterior, non-bladder dropping approach.
  - The anterior suspensory mechanism of the urethra and bladder comprises of the pubovesical complex (PVC), detrusor apron,

levator ani, and the soft tissue anterior fixation of the bladder to the abdominal wall and plays an important role in achieving postoperative continence.
- Dissection of the space of Reitz and dropping of the bladder during radical prostatectomy undoubtedly disrupt this suspensory mechanism.
- In a nutshell, this technique not only completely spares the anterior suspensory complexes but also allows for preservation of the bladder neck and neurovascular bundle.
- Preliminary continence rate is promising, probably as a result of reduced dissection trauma and retraction associated with this technique.

Summary of Risk/Benefits of the Procedure

The benefits of surgery are subject to the broader debate on localized prostate cancer. For lower risk disease, there are few deaths from disease, and more active surveillance needed. For intermediate risk disease, there is more solid understanding of 10–15 years progression to metastatic disease if untreated. For high risk disease, approximately 1/3 are fully localized, while many have EPE and/or nodes. The failure rate is high, but we have many systemic agents and clinical trials available. Local control in this population is favored by many experts for the young/fit patient, even if not curative by monotherapy.

There are three interesting articles that as a whole give the impression that there may be distinct benefits for surgery for high risk patients versus radiation—this may be driven by increased utilization of salvage radiation, but perhaps that is the point of emphasis.

- Cooperberg et al. Comparative risk-adjusted mortality outcomes after primary surgery, radiotherapy, or androgen-deprivation therapy for localized prostate cancer. Cancer, 116: 5226–34, 2010.
- Zelefsky MJ. Metastasis after radical prostatectomy or external beam radiotherapy for patients with clinically localized prostate cancer: a comparison of clinical cohorts adjusted for case mix. J Clin Oncol 28: 2010.
- Kibel AS. Survival among men with clinically localized prostate cancer treated with radical prostatectomy or radiation therapy in the prostate specific antigen era. J Urol 187: 1259–1265, 2012.

Noteworthy would be the Bill-Axelson paper in NEJM 2011—improved survival with surgery over surveillance in a clinically detected cohort, however the benefits disappear mostly for men > age 65.

The risks and complications merit some comment from insightful articles. The challenge for you personally is to know the range or complications reported, track your own, and constantly think about strategies to avoid them as you progress.

1. Di Pierro et al. A prospective trial comparing consecutive series of open retropubic and robot-assisted laparoscopic radical prostatectomy in a centre with limited caseload. Eur Urol 59: 1–6, 2011.
   (a) *Highlights: This is a learning curve paper from a lower volume center in Switzerland, where the surgeons underwent extended post-graduate robotics training. In the initial 75 RARP cases compared with 75 RRP, they were able to show lower positive margins (16 % vs. 32 %, continence 95 % vs. 83 % at 3 months as well has higher erectile function (55 % vs. 26 % at 12 months). Using Clavien criteria, major complications were 7 % vs. 28 %.*
   (b) *The attached editorial by Mani Menon provides an excellent history of the comparison of these techniques, controversies, marketing, and where we are now.*
2. Agarwal et al. Safety profile of robot-assisted radical prostatectomy: a standardized report of complications in 3317 patients. Eur Urol 59: 684–698, 2011.
   (a) *Highlights:*
      - Median hospitalization of 1 day.
      - 3317 consecutive cases at Henry Ford, five surgeons.
      - 368 complications in 326 patients (9.8 %).

- Transfusions 2.2 %.
- 2.4 % medical complications.
- 8.0 % surgical complications.
- Minor = 242, and major 126.
- 81.3 % complications within 30 days, 4.6 % 31–90 days, and 14.1 % after 90 days (mostly hernia, lymphocele).

3. Trinh et al. Perioperative outcomes of robot-assisted radical prostatectomy compared with open radical prostatectomy: results from the Nationwide Inpatient Sample. Eur Urol 61: 679–685, 2012.
   (a) *Highlights:*
   - Comparisons of RARP vs. ORP complications in inpatient dataset from the US—19, 462 RPs overall—61.1 % RARP.
   - RARP lower transfusions, complications, length of stay.
4. Tewari et al. Positive surgical margin and perioperative complication rates of primary surgical treatments for prostate cancer: a systematic review and meta-analysis comparing retropubic, laparoscopic, and robotic prostatectomy. Eur Urol 2012.
   (a) *Highlights:*
   (b) LRP and RARP had lower transfusions, shorter hospital stay.
   (c) RARP lower complications that LRP and ORP.
   (d) Positive margins—pT2 10.7 %, pT3 37.2 %.
   (e) Complications—7.8 % perioperative—all systems detailed.
   (f) EBL: 188 cc.
   (g) Transfusions 1.8 %.
   (h) Conversions 0.3 %.
   (i) LOS 1.4 days, U.S.
5. Ficarra et al. Systematic review and meta-analysis of studies reporting urinary continence recovery after robot-assisted radical prostatectomy. Eur. Urol. 2012; 62: 405–17.
   Highlights
   (a) Review of 51 studies comparing ORP or LRP to RARP
   (b) Twelve months urinary incontinence rate was 11.3 % after ORP and 7.5 % after RARP, with a 3.8 % absolute risk reduction in favor of RARP (OR 1.53; $p = 0.03$).
   (c) Similarly, the risk of urinary incontinence was 9.6 % after LRP and 5 % after RARP, showing an absolute risk reduction of 4.6 % in favor of RARP (OR 2.39; $p = 0.006$).
   (d) Age, body mass index, comorbidity index, lower urinary tract symptoms, and prostate volume were the most relevant preoperative predictors of urinary incontinence after RARP.
6. Ficarra et al. Systematic review and meta-analysis of studies reporting potency rates after robot-assisted radical prostatectomy. Eur. Urol. 2012; 62: 418–30.
   Highlights
   (a) Prevalence of ED at 12 months: ORP 47.8 %; RARP 24.2 % (OR 2.84, $p = 0.002$).
   (b) Non-statistical significant difference between LRP and RARP.
   (c) Age, baseline potency status, comorbidities index, and extension of the nerve-sparing procedure represent the most relevant preoperative and intraoperative predictors of potency recovery after RARP.
7. Davis et al. Learning curve assessment of robot-assisted radical prostatectomy compared with open-surgery controls from the Premier Perspective Database. J Endourology 2014; 28: 560–566.
   (a) In a community wide assessment of surgeons, RARP cases had consistently fewer complications during the inpatient recovery and these decreased further with surgeon experience.
   (b) From 2004 to 2010 years studied, the year of the procedure did not affect outcomes but surgeon experience did.
   (c) For RARP, hospital stay was shorter but OR times were longer.
   (d) This article is open access.

References

1. Turner W. The index of the pelvic brim as a basis of classification. J Anat Physiol. 1885;20(Pt 1):125–43.
2. Hong SK, Chang IH, Lee SE. Impact of variations in bony pelvic dimensions on performing radical retropubic prostatectomy. Urology. 2007;69:907–11.

3. Hong SK, Lee ST, Lee SE. Effect of bony pelvic dimensions measured by preoperative magnetic resonance imaging on performing robot-assisted laparoscopic prostatectomy. BJU Int. 2009;104:664–8.
4. Matikainan MP, Von Bodman C, Rabbani F. The depth of the prostatic apex is an independent predictor of positive apical margins at radical prostatectomy. BJU Int. 2010;106:622–6.
5. Mason BA, Hakimi AA, Ghavamian R. The role of preoperative endorectal coil magnetic resonance imaging in predicting surgical difficulty for robotic prostatectomy. J Urol. 2010;76:1130–5.

The Dorsal Vein Complex: Achieving Hemostasis and Proper Setup for Apical Division

3

Eric S. Wisenbaugh, Mark D. Tyson, and Erik P. Castle

Introduction

Management of the dorsal vein complex (DVC) and the setup for division of the apical urethra are critical aspects of the radical prostatectomy. Proper control and division of the DVC allows the procedure to be performed with minimal blood loss and provides excellent exposure of the prostatic apex and urethra, which is essential to avoiding positive surgical margins in this area. Multiple techniques have been described and are reviewed here, but the goals remain the same: to achieve negative apical margins, to maximize the length of the urethral stump, to preserve the external urinary sphincter, and to obtain reliable hemostasis.

E.S. Wisenbaugh, M.D. (✉)
E.P. Castle, M.D., F.A.C.S.
M.D. Tyson, M.D.
Department of Urology, Mayo Clinic Arizona, 5777 E Mayo Blvd, Phoenix, AZ 85054, USA
e-mail: wisenbaugh.eric@mayo.edu; castle.erik@mayo.edu; tyson.mark@mayo.edu

Relevant Anatomy

A thorough understanding of the periprostatic anatomy is vital to this portion of the procedure. Prior to the detailed anatomical studies of the DVC in the 1970s, excessive bleeding from this site was assumed to be a necessary complication of the radical prostatectomy [1], while today there is typically very minimal bleeding from this site, and transfusions are rare [2]. The deep dorsal vein of the penis travels underneath Buck's fascia and penetrates the urogenital diaphragm where it divides into a superficial and deep branch. The deep dorsal vein travels between and just deep to the puboprostatic ligaments and divides almost immediately into the lateral venous plexus of Santorini, which then travel lateral and posterolateral to the prostate (Fig. 2.1).

The striated external sphincteric muscle is the primary continence mechanism following radical prostatectomy. This lies just beyond the apex of the prostate and encircles the anterior and lateral portions of the membranous urethra. The lateral aspects of this muscle are often well visualized when the apex has been carefully dissected away from surrounding tissues. It is also closely associated with the DVC anteriorly, which underscores the importance of obtaining adequate control of the DVC, so that the urethra can be divided without injuring the sphincter.

J.W. Davis (ed.), *Robot-Assisted Radical Prostatectomy*, DOI 10.1007/978-3-319-32641-2_3

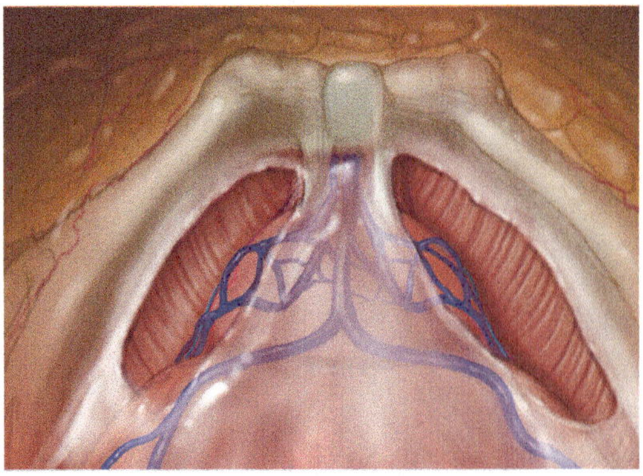

Fig. 2.1 Anatomy of the dorsal venous complex dividing early into the lateral plexus of Santorini

Exposure and Initial Apical Dissection

Following the takedown of the peritoneum and development of the space of Retzius, the superficial dorsal vein is divided with bipolar cautery and the periprostatic fat is swept away to expose the anterior surface of the prostate and bladder neck. The endopelvic fascia is opened lateral to the prostate to avoid injury to the lateral venous plexus, and then this incision is carried towards the apex to the level of the puboprostatic ligaments. If present, care must be taken to identify and spare the accessory pudendal arteries which travel on the anterolateral surface of the prostate and then perforate the genitourinary diaphragm at the prostatic apex [3]. Although these accessory arteries are rare, preservation may aid in postoperative erectile function or response to erectogenic medications [4]. At this point the lateral striated muscle fibers of the external sphincter can be visualized coursing around the urethra. While not necessary, some surgeons choose to divide the puboprostatic ligaments to maximize the apical exposure.

Ligation of the DVC

In the classic description of the anatomic open radical prostatectomy, the dorsal venous complex was isolated at the common trunk with a right angle clamp, then transected and ligated [1]. In the robotic era, multiple techniques have been described.

Early Ligation

The most commonly performed method involves suture ligation of the DVC once the apex of the prostate has been narrowed to the puboprostatic ligaments on either side. A 0-polyglactin suture on a ½ circle tapered needle is passed in a figure-of-eight fashion just underneath the DVC and anterior to the urethra, while staying distal to the apex, but proximal to the striated sphincter (Fig. 2.2). Some surgeons will place an additional suture more proximally, just anterior to the mid gland, which may help with identification of the bladder neck and is reminiscent of the open prostatectomy. Back bleeding is generally not the concern as pneumoperitoneum assists with venous bleeding and surgeons generally do not cut between the sutures. The DVC is then typically transected later in the case, after the bladder neck and posterior plane have been dissected and the vascular pedicles have been ligated and divided.

An additional technique for early ligation is the use of an endovascular stapler in place of the suture. With this technique the stapler is controlled by the bedside assistant and articulated downwards as needed to incorporate the DVC (Fig. 2.3). A metal urethral sound can be inserted before deploying the stapler to ensure that the urethra is not involved. Proponents of this technique theorize that it may lead to a faster and more secure ligation and that the positioning of the stapler between the pubis and prostate may leave a small layer of tissue at the apex between staple lines and lower the positive margin rate [5]. However, others feel that the stapler control of the DVC is somewhat blind and may cause urethral or sphincteral injury, and is an additional, unnecessary cost [6]. Comparative data is limited, but in a direct, retrospective comparison, there was no difference between suture and staple ligations in estimated blood loss, operative time, or positive margin rate [5].

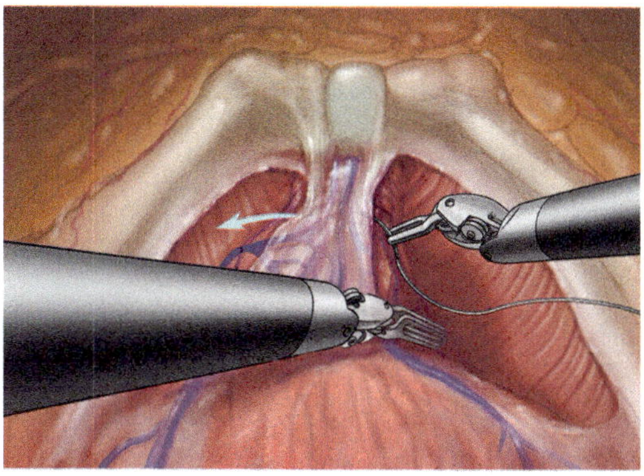

Fig. 2.2 The figure-of-eight suture is thrown just distal to the apex of the prostate, but proximal to the muscle fibers of the external sphincter, while also passing deep to the dorsal vein and superficial to the urethra

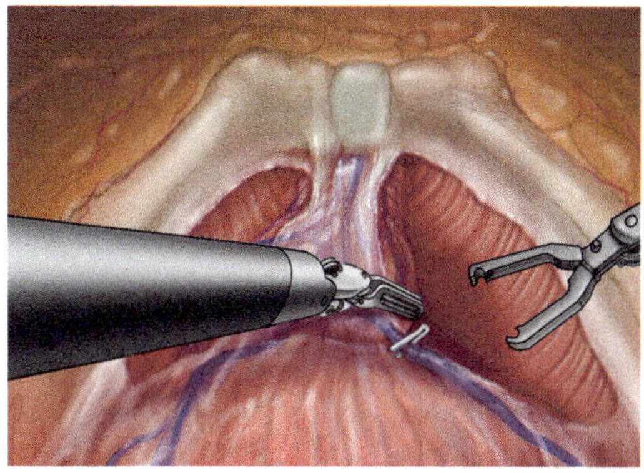

Fig. 2.4 Ligation of the lateral branches of the dorsal vein as they course over the bladder neck, providing hemostasis during dissection of the anterior bladder neck

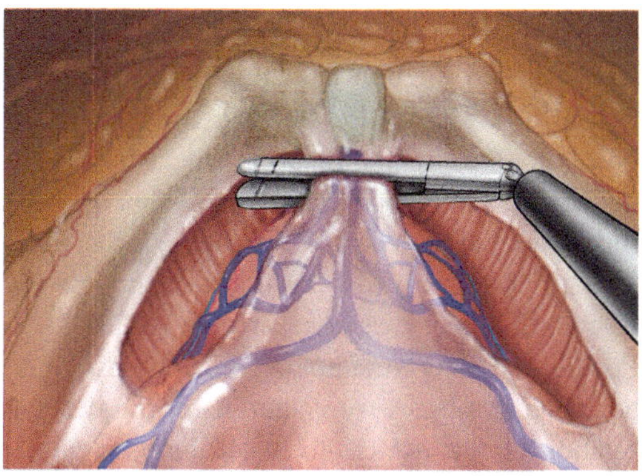

Fig. 2.3 Stapler ligation of the dorsal venous complex

Delayed Ligation

In this method, the DVC is left intact until the dissection of the bladder neck and posterior plane is complete and the pedicles have been ligated and divided. As the DVC remains patent, it is important to deliberately ligate its anterolateral branches over the bladder neck prior to the bladder neck dissection, which can be done with bipolar cautery or locking clips (Fig. 2.4). Once the posterior dissection is complete and the vascular pedicles have been taken, the DVC is pinched with the robotic grasper and divided with electrocautery prior to ligation. The pinching helps further identify the prostatic apex from the DVC to prevent inadvertent positive anterior apical margins. The pneumoperitoneum is increased to 20 mmHg prior to division, which we have found maintains excellent hemostasis even with the DVC left completely open [7]. If a vent is used through one of the accessory ports, it should be closed and it is critical that the bedside assistant employ only minimal suction in order to maintain this level of pneumoperitoneum and prevent venous bleeding. A similar technique has also been described that uses a bulldog clamp to control the DVC during division instead of increasing the pneumoperitoneum [6]. This may be cumbersome and unnecessary as the pneumoperitoneum is adequate to control the bleeding. Once the division is complete, the entire complex of veins is easily visualized separate from the anterior aspect of the urethra, and can now be oversewn with a running suture (Fig. 2.5). This same suture may then be used to perform an anterior urethropexy by throwing the needle through the periosteum of the pubic bone (Fig. 2.6), and then tying a slipknot to the tail of the original DVC suture. This last maneuver provides support to the urethra and DVC by recapitulating the puboprostatic ligaments, which may anecdotally hasten the recovery of continence [8].

Early vs. Delayed Ligation

While early ligation is more commonly performed and provides early control of potential venous bleeding from around the apex, delayed

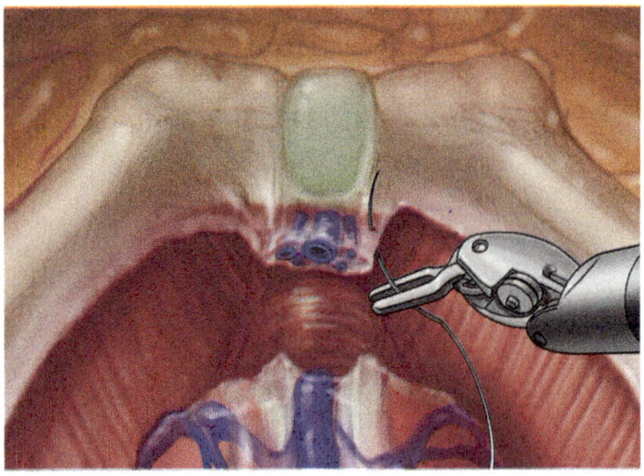

Fig. 2.5 Late suture ligation of the divided dorsal venous complex. This allows a secure closure in a running fashion with excellent visualization of the entire complex, the apex of the prostate, and the urethra

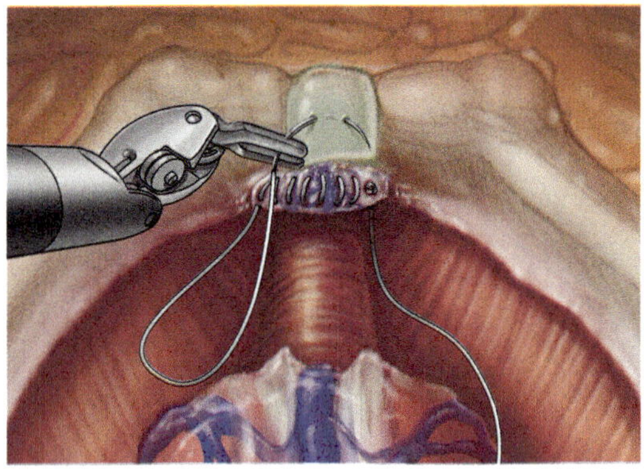

Fig. 2.6 A seamless anterior urethropexy suspension is performed by throwing the dorsal venous complex suture through the periosteum of the symphysis

ligation may have some potential benefits. One criticism of the early ligation method is that because the depth of the suture cannot always be seen clearly, it is less precise and may involve part of the sphincter or urethra. A misplaced suture can damage the sphincter or reduce the functional length of the urethra, which may increase the risk of urinary incontinence [9]. The delayed technique involves pinching the DVC at the time of transection without it being distorted by the figure-of-eight suture, which offers excellent exposure of the prostatic apex and it has been suggested to result in fewer positive margins. After transection, the entire DVC is exposed as a separate entity from the urethra, making it easier to avoid involving the urethra with this suture. Additionally, the running suture technique is likely to be more secure as there have been reports of the figure-of-eight suture loosening and causing postoperative hemorrhage. The authors agree that the running suture ligation under direct visualization may offer a more secure hemostatic closure of the plexus of veins and provide better control of the depth of the needle placement. Finally, this method also allows a seamless anterior urethropexy to the periosteum of the pubic bone to provide support to the DVC and urethra.

Several studies have compared these techniques and the results are somewhat variable. Lei et al. retrospectively compared 303 patients who underwent early ligation to 240 who underwent delayed ligation and found that those who underwent delayed ligation had slightly higher blood loss (184 vs. 175 mL), but had better 5-month postoperative urinary function (measured using the Expanded Prostate Cancer Index urinary function scale) and continence rates (61 vs. 40 %, defined as zero pads per day), although the 12-month urinary outcomes were similar [10]. Positive margins were not significantly different, but operative times were shorter for the delayed ligation group which they attribute to fewer instrument exchanges.

Guru et al. specifically evaluated positive apical margin rate in patients who had cancer located in the apex, and compared 158 patients who underwent early ligation to 145 patients who underwent delayed ligation and found that the delayed ligation group had significantly fewer apical positive margins (2 vs. 8 %, $p=0.02$) [11].

In contrast, however, Woldu et al. recently evaluated 244 patients who underwent either technique and found no differences in estimated blood loss, operative time, apical margin status, or continence rates at 3 months [12].

There are flaws in all of these studies, particularly with regard to their retrospective design and the learning curve biases that tend to occur as single surgeons change their technique. We believe that both techniques are acceptable and offer excellent hemostasis and good oncologic control, but the delayed ligation method likely offers better visualization.

References

1. Walsh PC. Anatomic radical prostatectomy: evolution of the surgical technique. J Urol. 1998;160(6 Pt 2):2418–24. Research Support, Non-U.S. Gov't.
2. Novara G, Ficarra V, Rosen RC, Artibani W, Costello A, Eastham JA, et al. Systematic review and meta-analysis of perioperative outcomes and complications after robot-assisted radical prostatectomy. Eur Urol. 2012;62(3):431–52. Meta-Analysis Review.
3. Breza J, Aboseif SR, Orvis BR, Lue TF, Tanagho EA. Detailed anatomy of penile neurovascular structures: surgical significance. J Urol. 1989;141(2):437–43.
4. Polascik TJ, Walsh PC. Radical retropubic prostatectomy: the influence of accessory pudendal arteries on the recovery of sexual function. J Urol. 1995;154(1):150–2.
5. Nguyen MM, Turna B, Santos BR, Frota R, Aron M, Stein RJ, et al. The use of an endoscopic stapler vs suture ligature for dorsal vein control in laparoscopic prostatectomy: operative outcomes. BJU Int. 2008; 101(4):463–6. Comparative Study.
6. Tufek I, Atug F, Argun B, Keskin S, Obek C, Coskuner E, et al. The use of a bulldog clamp to control the dorsal vein complex during robot-assisted radical prostatectomy. J Endourol. 2012;26(12):1605–8.
7. Wisenbaugh EW, Andrews PE, Castle EP. Ligation of the dorsal venous complex in a robot-assisted radical prostatectomy. J Endourol Part B Videourology. 2013, DOI: 10.1089/vid.2013.0079.
8. Patel VR, Coelho RF, Palmer KJ, Rocco B. Periurethral suspension stitch during robot-assisted laparoscopic radical prostatectomy: description of the technique and continence outcomes. Eur Urol. 2009;56(3):472–8.
9. NCCN Clinical practice guidelines in oncology: prostate cancer. Version 1; 2015.
10. Lei Y, Alemozaffar M, Williams SB, Hevelone N, Lipsitz SR, Plaster BA, et al. Athermal division and selective suture ligation of the dorsal vein complex during robot-assisted laparoscopic radical prostatectomy: description of technique and outcomes. Eur Urol. 2011;59(2):235–43.
11. Guru KA, Perlmutter AE, Sheldon MJ, Butt ZM, Zhang S, Tan W, et al. Apical margins after robot-assisted radical prostatectomy: does technique matter? J Endourol. 2009;23(1):123–7. Clinical Trial.
12. Woldu SL, Patel T, Shapiro EY, Bergman AM, Badani KK. Outcomes with delayed dorsal vein complex ligation during robotic assisted laparoscopic prostatectomy. Can J Urol. 2013;20(6):7079–83. Comparative Study.

4 The Simple Bladder Neck

John W. Davis

In the minimally invasive era, dissections were frequently described as antegrade, and the bladder neck division became a very early step of the resection [1, 2]. With laparoscopic or robotic technique, now the palpation component is taken away, and the surgeon must rely on visual cues. Furthermore, the anatomy can only be viewed at a fixed point that is essentially an angled coronal view that is flipped 180° from how it is usually illustrated or viewed on an MRI. Early on, my minimally invasive surgery mentors commented that they could spend 30–60 min trying to figure out how to get through a bladder neck in an anatomically correct plane. This was in part due to the limitations of nonarticulating laparoscopic instruments, but certainly the less-familiar antegrade approach played a role. Patients with large glands and median lobes were certainly excluded from early experience minimally invasive approaches. In this chapter, we will consider the simple bladder neck and discuss anatomic cues to turn this into a simple 5–10 min step.

J.W. Davis, M.D. (✉)
Department of Urology, Uro-surgical Prostate Cancer Program, The University of Texas M.D. Anderson Cancer Center, Houston, TX, USA
e-mail: jdhdavis@aol.com

Orientation Images

Figure 4.1 shows a typical size gland in the minimally invasive camera view. It is basically a coronal orientation but slightly angled from the bladder neck side due to the umbilical camera position. The head is image down and the legs image up. A common exposure trick is to switch to a 30° down camera angle to make the plan more truly coronal, and to see around the posterior lip of the bladder when moving on to the vas/SVs. However in some patient configurations, a zero lens is quick vertical and sufficient. If I have already performed the SV/Vas dissection from the posterior route, Pouch of Douglas, then I leave the camera on zero.

As a comparison, Fig. 4.2 shows an MRI image in the coronal plane. For a parallel orientation, the image was captured in the high slices just above where the prostate would be in view such as in Fig. 4.3. Figure 4.4 shows the lower slides just under the prostate where the vas/seminal vesicles are located. Our goal is to get from Figs. 4.2, 4.3, and 4.4 smoothly and without damaging the bladder neck funnel or getting too close to the prostate. Note that the images typically published by MRI software are with the head up—here they are flipped 180° to match the surgeon's viewpoint. Figure 4.4 also includes two images from Hinata et al. [3], that provide a very useful description of the posterior "longitudinal muscle."

J.W. Davis (ed.), *Robot-Assisted Radical Prostatectomy*, DOI 10.1007/978-3-319-32641-2_4

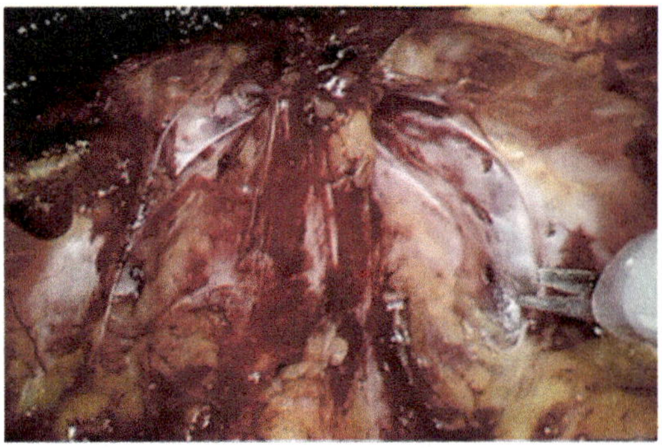

Fig. 4.1 The surgeon's view of the prostate—coronal orientation and slightly angled base to apex. The endopelvic fascia are mostly preserved by incising lateral/anterior prostatic fascia. The dorsal vein complex is oversewn and anchored to the pubic bone. Where is the bladder neck?

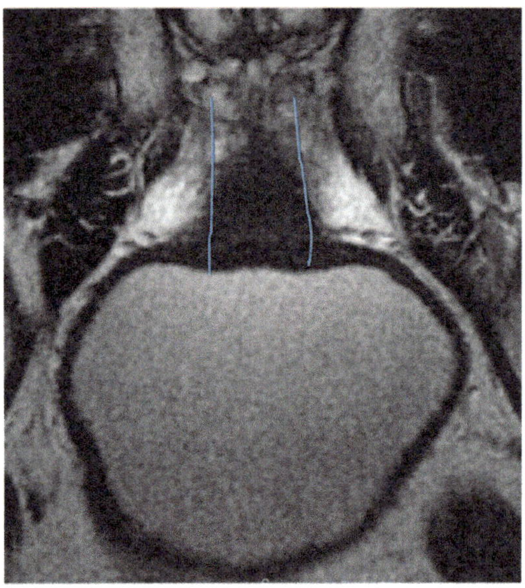

Fig. 4.2 This is a corresponding MRI in coronal orientation and then flipped 180° to match the surgeon view. The *blue lines* show the division of the "rule of thirds" in dissection—see text. At this far anterior cut that corresponds to the beginning of the dissection, the tissues encountered are mostly the detrusor apron in the midline, and the run-off branches of the Santorini plexus laterally

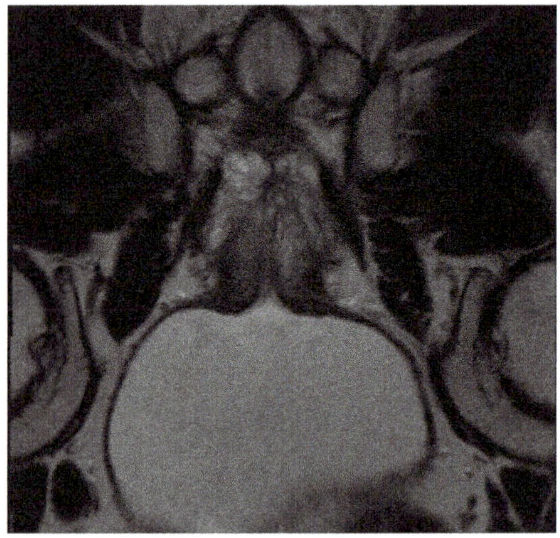

Fig. 4.3 At this mid-coronal view, the dissection will enter the bladder neck at a location depending upon how much of the "funnel" or bladder neck is selected to be spared versus resected to avoid a positive surgical margin

Walz et al. published a collaborative review for European Urology [4] that shows the better-illustrated sagittal view with the multiple anatomic landmarks and fascial layers denoted—Figs. 4.5 and 4.6. An MRI from our same patient is shown in Fig. 4.6. Structurally, it now looks straightforward to cut from one side of the bladder neck, through the urethra and pass it to the other side. The challenges remaining for a successful and efficient surgical division are: (1) what are the anatomic landmarks encountered, (2) what are the subtle cues that the dissection plane is on versus off target, (3) what are the rules for dissection, and (4) what are the anticipated hemostatic maneuvers.

Dissection Steps Linked to Anatomic Cues and Hemostasis

A common question asked by novices in the minimally invasive surgery training is "how do you know where the bladder neck is?" Therefore the first set of moves in dividing the simple bladder neck is to move the catheter around to look for the balloon movement. However in larger prostates, that motion can still be nondescript. The fat over the bladder neck needs to be stripped away, and then a two instrument "squeeze technique" will identify the midline detrusor apron layer—Fig. 4.7. This layer is cut with the monopolar scissors, and it may be helpful to turn down the cautery to 25 on a standard Valley lab setup. This layer of muscle tends to reflect very brightly to

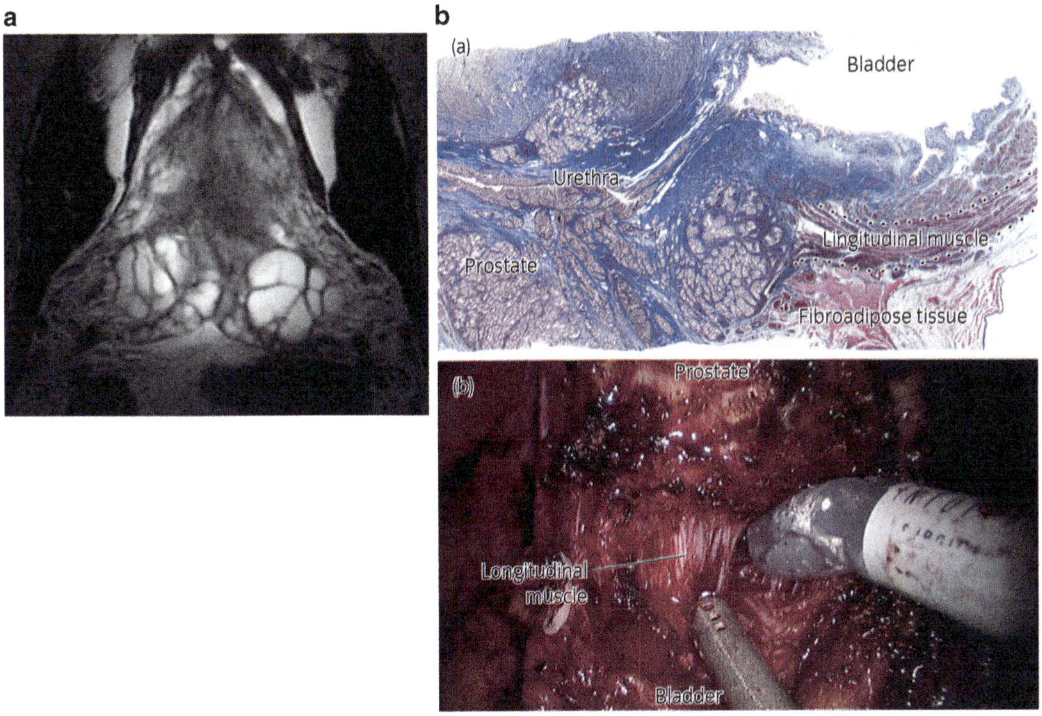

Fig. 4.4 At this more posterior coronal cut, the dissection is now behind the bladder neck and landing on the longitudinal muscle fibers (**a**) that Hinata refers to in (**b**) [4]

the camera compared to the surrounding tissues. On the console controls, you can manually turn down the light source and often see more tissue contrast—just remember to turn it back to default layer. Figure 4.8 shows the comparative images. At this point, a catheter balloon pull will show the plane better.

The "rule of thirds" can now be seen better—Fig. 4.8b. In the middle third between the blue lines, the dissection rules can allow for cautery. An under-appreciated technical issue by trainees is that the division in this plane is only half accomplished by the monopolar scissor cautery. The other half is from accurate retraction by the nondominant instrument (left sided grasper for a right-handed surgeon). Basically, if you are in the right plane, then these detrusor fibers will fly off the cautery quickly as counter traction is applied. In the lateral thirds (outside the blue lines), the predominant tissue initially encountered is run-off branches from Santorini (dorsal) vein plexus. In this area, I recommend avoiding cautery. Figure 4.9. These are some considerations:

1. Vein plexuses do not seal well with cautery.
2. The lateral neurovascular bundle is starting to get closer to the monopolar.
3. Vein plexuses do not seal well with cautery—even if they did, it would require an extended "burn." See #2 above.
4. In select cases, a short seal with bipolar is effective.
5. If you encounter continuous bleeding refractory to bipolar current and obstructing vision of the bladder neck planes, then consider changing out instruments and over sewing with 4-0 vicryl until dry.

You could leave these layers intact and deal with them later when it is time for clipping and dividing the neurovascular bundle. I have encountered cases where these veins can be brushed to

Fig. 4.5 From Walz et al. [3] the sagittal view of the bladder neck layers is very instructive, as are the specific anatomic landmarks seen in the abbreviation listings

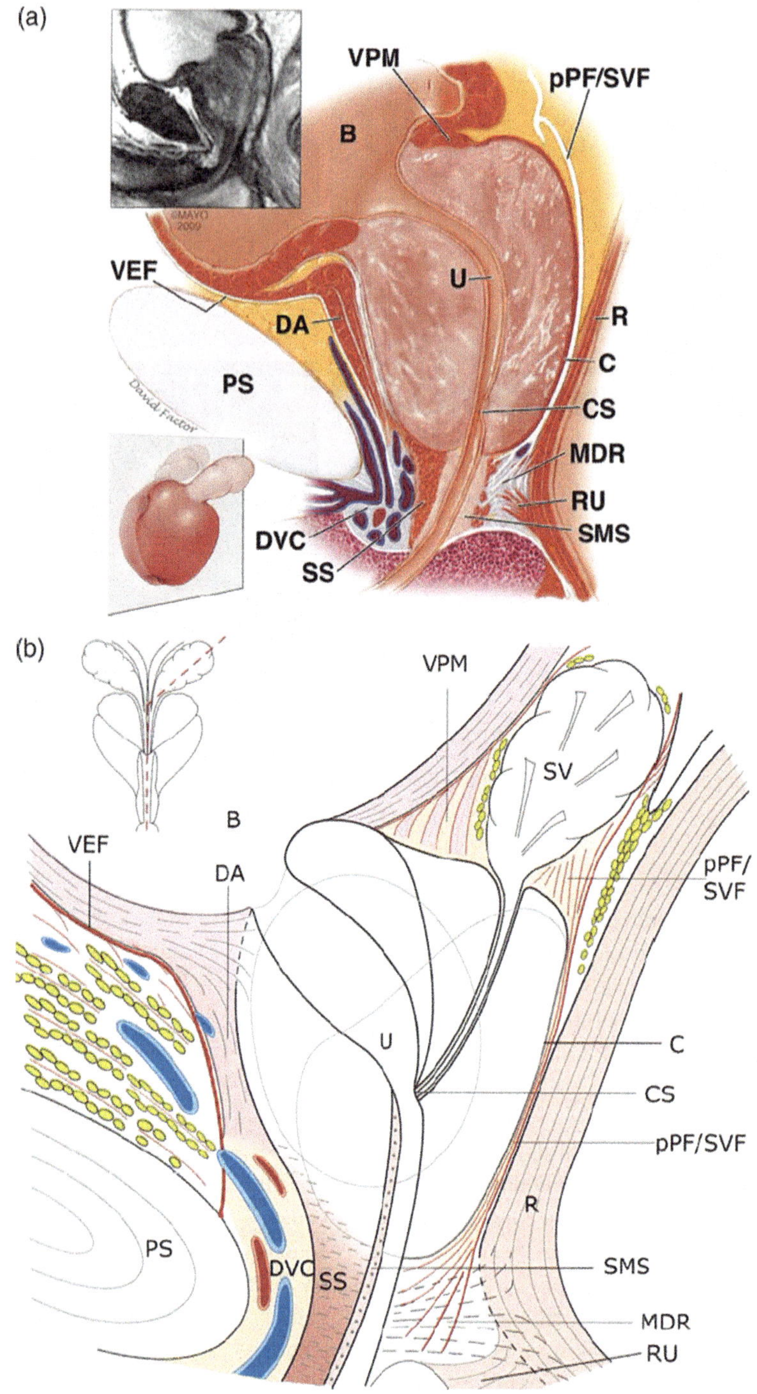

Fig. 2-Midline sagittal section of prostate. bladder, urethra, and striated sphincter; (a) anatomic (reprodused with permission from the mayo Clinic); (b) schematic. B - bladder; C - capsule of prostate; CS - colliculas seminalis (verumontanum); DA = detrusor apron; DVC = dorsal vascular complex; MDR = medial dorsal raphe; PS = pubic symphysis; pPF/SVF = posterior prostatic fascia/seminal veicle fascia (Denonvilliers fascia); R = rectum; RU = rectourethralis muscle; SMS = smooth muscle sphincter (lissosphincter); SS = striated sphincter (rhabdosphincter); U = urethra; VEF = visceral endopelvic fascia; VPM = vesicoprostatic muscle.

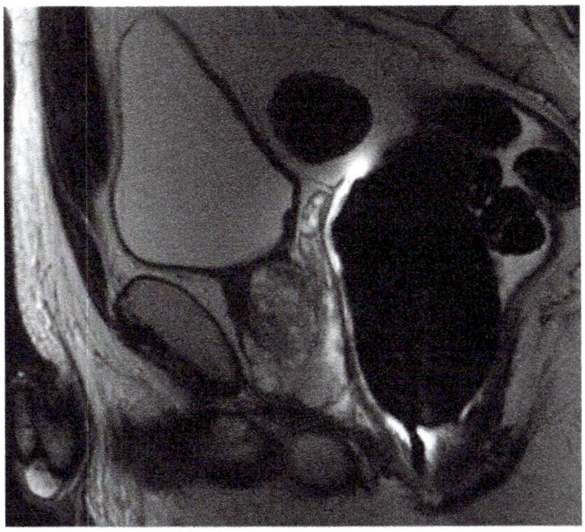

Fig. 4.6 The corresponding sagittal MRI view. In this case, the anatomy of the bladder neck appears simple: no median lobe, no TURP defect, no other hypertrophied lobes

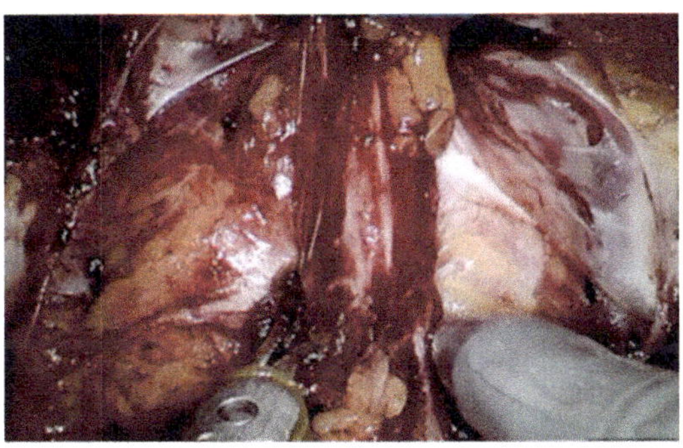

Fig. 4.7 The "two-handed squeeze technique." Using two active arms, the midline is pinched together showing the detrusor apron. The side structures are initially filled with run off vein plexuses from the dorsal vein

the side for later dissection. In many cases, however, leaving these veins keeps the bladder neck dissection narrow and you will have a smaller space to work in when working posterior to the bladder neck at the seminal vesical/vas deferens step. Figure 4.10a, b illustrate the near complete anterior dissection. Vertical fibers are encountered at the true bladder neck. Figure 4.10b shows the clipped lateral plexuses allowing greater lateral space for the subsequent steps.

Once the bladder is entered, the balloon is deflated and the Foley brought through the opening and grasped with the 3rd robotic arm or assistant arm and lifted up—Fig. 4.11. Anecdotally, I have encountered a few cases with meatal strictures postoperatively. A previous technique was to clamp the catheter with a padded hemostat externally at the meatus and then pull it on tension. I have avoided this for several years, and now just ask the nurse to hold the catheter on tension manually for the few minutes it takes to complete the posterior division.

The next moves are critical to success. The surgeon needs to see down the posterior bladder neck. With experience it is not necessary to see the full trigone, but at least some of it. If all you can see is prostatic urethra, you may be too close into the prostate and want to consider re-excising the plane back further. Otherwise you risk disoriented dissection and possibly into the prostate in front of the insertion of the vasa/SV's. This is truly a mess when encountered. Theoretically, if you persisted through such a false plane in front of the vas/SV insertion, you could keep going into the rectum. By staying in the correct plane, you have to see the vas/SV before the rectum. Furthermore, if you are in the correct plane behind the bladder and suddenly enter a new cavity that looks mucosal, this will almost certainly be a very low inserting Pouch of Douglas. You may be nervous for a few moments trying to confirm this.

My exposure tricks are seen in Fig. 4.12. The neck appears preserved and small and the catheter is on upward tension. The goal is for the left hand to enter the bladder neck just off center to the left, and with one blade fully inside of the bladder and one fully outside of the bladder. The tension is drawn down and left and this leaves room for the assistant with suction to retract inside the bladder neck down and right. Now the posterior wall is fully visualized. In other cases such as Fig. 4.12, the neck has just enough room that the bipolar alone can show down the neck. In Fig. 4.12b there is a space at 5 o'clock on the bladder neck—the assistant can retract here for more room.

Next, the posterior bladder neck mucosa can be incised as it curves. Cautery is acceptable and I have certainly tried using cutting current with the newer model daVinci systems—not sure it matters. A key concept is to maintain the integ-

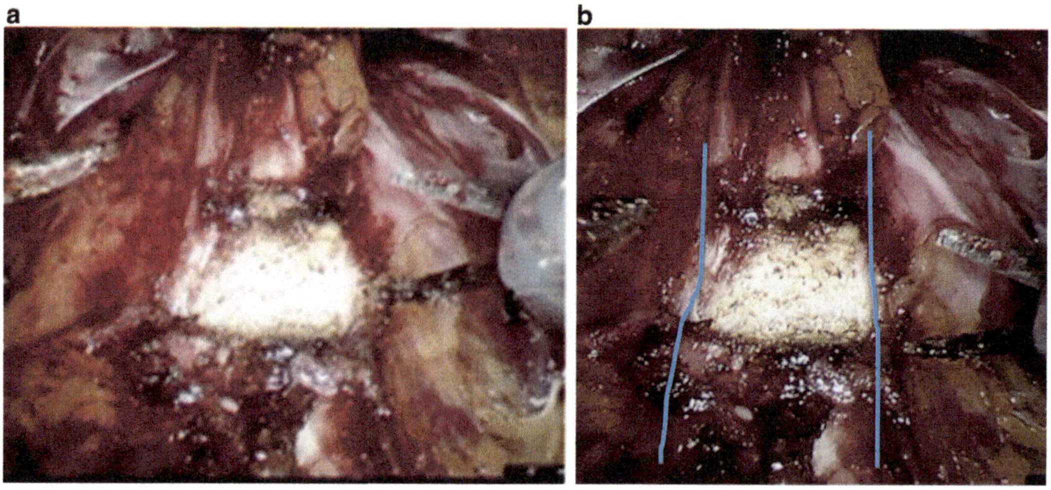

Fig. 4.8 (**a**, **b**) The detrusor apron is cut where the squeeze orientation (Fig. 4.7) was outlined in (**a**). The light is turned down to show more tissue contrast—(**b**) The *blue lines* show the "rule of thirds." See text

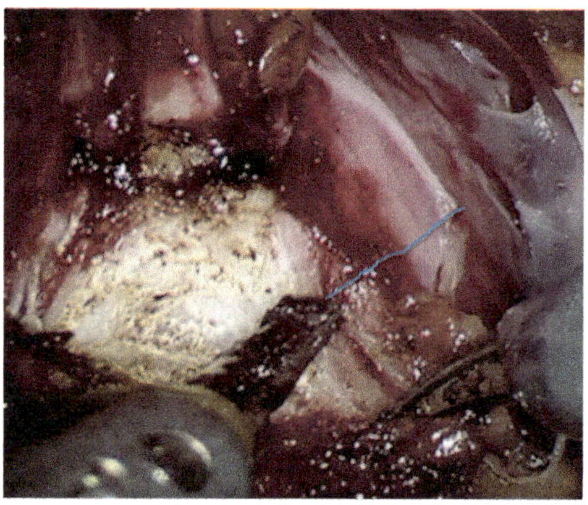

Fig. 4.9 The lateral third vein branches are targeted for bipolar or clip control—direction of the *blue line*

rity of the bladder neck layers—mucosa to detrusor. Thus, you must try and dissect behind the bladder and maintain its muscle. Figure 4.13 shows how the thickness of the bladder muscle rotates to the sides as you come across the circle. It's really a simple concept—the bladder is round and so the dissection stays round rather than a straight line down.

As discussed above, the lateral third layers are filled with veins, and if you have not divided them yet, you may need to at this point—Fig. 4.14a, b. Now the dissection can move down and behind the bladder—Fig. 4.15a, b. There should be a thin areolar layer behind the bladder. If you are still in really thick tissue behind the bladder then re-orient yourself. You might be into prostate. The final step involves the posterior longitudinal muscle described by Hinata et al. [3]. This layer can be very thin such as Fig. 4.16a, or thick such as Fig. 4.16b, or very thick—almost looking like peri-rectal fibers as shown in Fig. 4.4. Division of this layer puts you on the vasa in the midline and ready for the next step.

Backing up a bit, to finish the posterior plane, the Foley exposure starts the step but is not always ideal throughout. Once there are sufficient posterior layers on the specimen side, it may be more accurate to grasp these directly with the robotic 3rd arm—Fig. 4.17. The posterior bladder needs frequent checking and keeping in mind that sometimes the posterior bladder just past the trigone can jut forward into your dissection plane.

Troubleshooting Both Sides

Failure to diagnose a bladder neck variant anatomy can lead to a "button hole injury" where you are moving down to the vas but re-encouna b

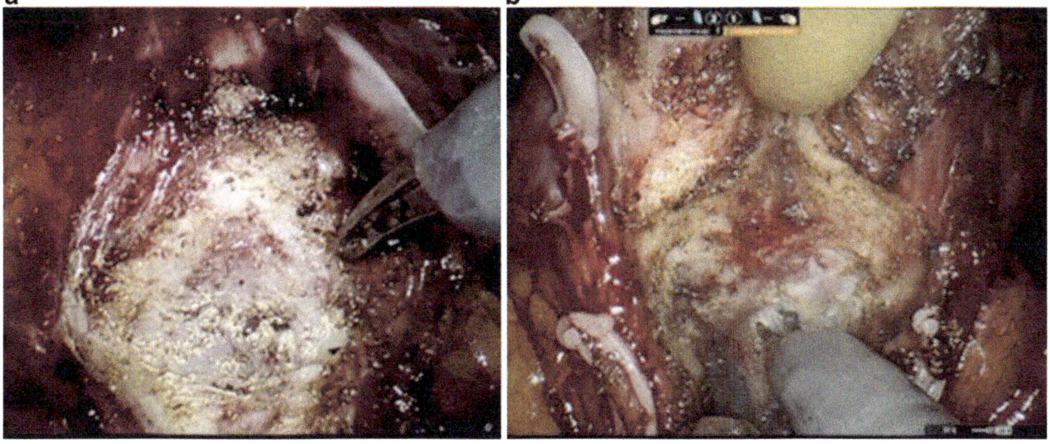

Fig. 4.10 (**a**, **b**) Two concepts are shown. In image (**a**), the anterior bladder neck is nearly complete, and there is a thin layer of vertical fibers encountered just before bladder entry. Dissecting veins in the lateral thirds is helpful in orienting these layers, and widening the left to right space that is helpful for the more posterior steps. In image (**b**), the clips show the lateral veins divided and controlled, and the poster space is improved (bladder neck divided at this step)

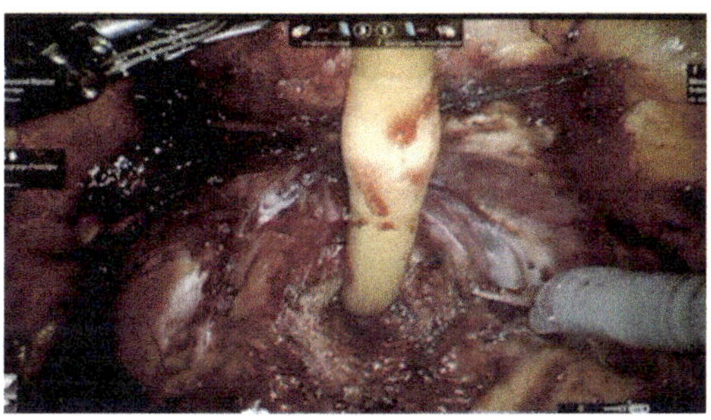

Fig. 4.11 The anterior bladder neck is entered, and the catheter lifted with assistant or robotic arm and gentle traction from scrubbed assistant helps create upward traction

ter bladder. Again, by frequently inspecting inside the bladder you can get a sense that the bladder is a straight funnel versus a variant that has another dependent portion jutting into the prostate plane. This point can be very subtle. In Fig. 4.18, the bladder is inspected during dissection and looks fine—nothing abnormal until you look a bit deeper and see the depending portion going more distal—Fig. 4.19. When the dissection reached the longitudinal muscle, a structure was grasped and divided, showing a bladder button hole Figs. 4.20 and 4.21. Again, the difference was very subtle and normal longitudinal muscle is seen just to the side. This hole was repaired post-resection by lifting up on the correct longitudinal muscle and placing interrupted 2-0 Vicryl sutures-Fig. 4.22. In general, these buttonhole injuries are on dependent bladder wall that is not part of the trigone. I have not seen a ureteral injury with these events nor the reconstructive sutures, but you should certainly re-inspect inside the bladder as well. A cautious management plan would be to leave the catheter for 10 days and perform a postoperative cystogram.

On the other extreme, if posterior dissection progresses but with resistance and failure to reach the loose areolar space and the longitudinal muscle, then consider the dissection is too distal. In Fig. 4.23, the 3rd arm retracts tissue upward and a dissection plane failed to progress. The 3rd arm was placed on the posterior bladder instead and the inside re-inspected. The plane was re-found closer to the bladder and the longitudinal muscle identified-Figs. 4.24, 4.25, and 4.26.

Matching Images to Anatomy

From the Walz et al. review and images, we have several structures to consider:

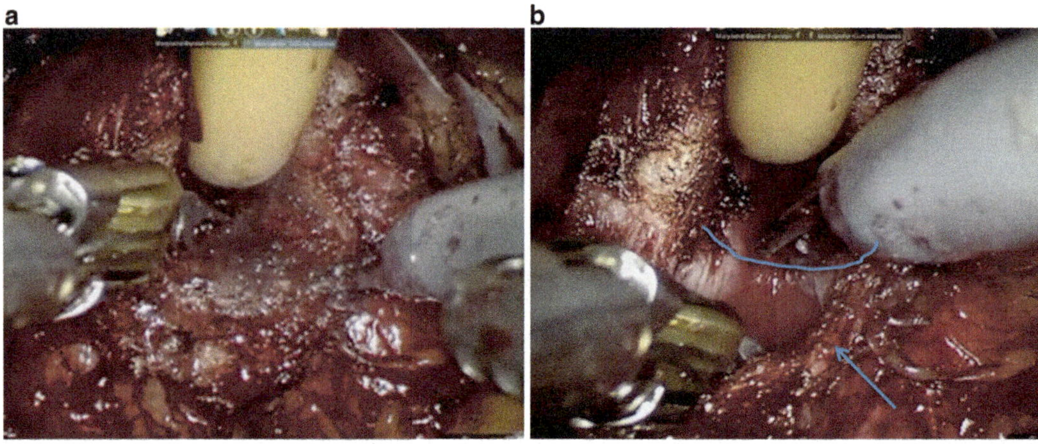

Fig. 4.12 (**a**, **b**) The catheter is lifted up—(**a**)—but the equally critical step is counter exposure with the instruments to see the full posterior bladder neck and plan the line of resection such as illustrated with the *blue line*. The *arrow* shows where an assistant can retract with the suction for a better view

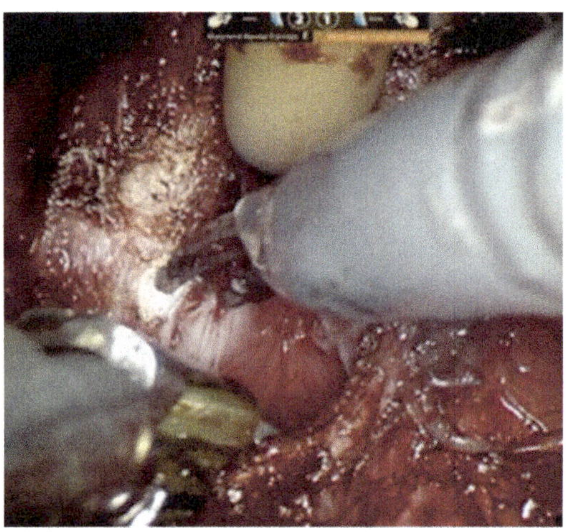

Fig. 4.13 Incise around the posterior bladder neck and keep full detrusor muscle layer intact. The *blue line* shows the likely thickness of the detrusor so the cautery line needs to preserve this for a strong reconstruction later

- Bladder-B.
- Visceral endopelvic fascia—VEF.
- Detrussor Apron—DA.
- Vesicoprostatic muscle—VPM.
- Posterior prostatic fascia/seminal vesicle fascia (Denonvilliers' fascia)—pPF/SVF.
- Urethra—U.

To match these terms, I would say that my middle thirds analogy puts you through the DA to the urethra. The lateral veins are not really illustrated in these sagittal views but you can see from the photos. The VPM is likely the same structure Hinata calls "Longitudinal muscle" in Fig. 4.4. Note that the well-known Denonvilliers fascia is posterior to vas/SV and is not truly related to the bladder neck division per se. It is, of course, a key landmark for the posterior dissection and leading into the neurovascular bundle planes as described elsewhere. Shimbo et al. demonstrate another nice sequence of steps to identify the anterior bladder neck accurately [5] including the anterior squeeze trick.

Summary

The simple bladder neck can be divided in approximately 10 min or less. The middle third is divided with low-setting monopolar cautery, and the lateral plexuses controlled with clips or bipolar. The bladder neck is then carved out posteriorly to the longitudinal muscle. The keys to success are recognizing the landmarks illustrated by Walz et al. [4] and reorienting when progress looks off-plane.

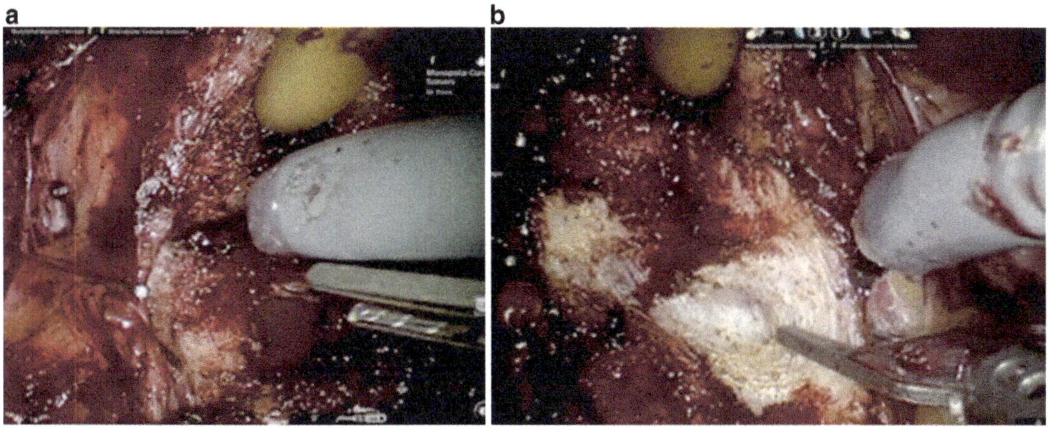

Fig. 4.14 (**a**, **b**) The lateral vein plexuses should be clipped and divided now, if not done previously. This shows the detrusor layers better and widens space for the next steps

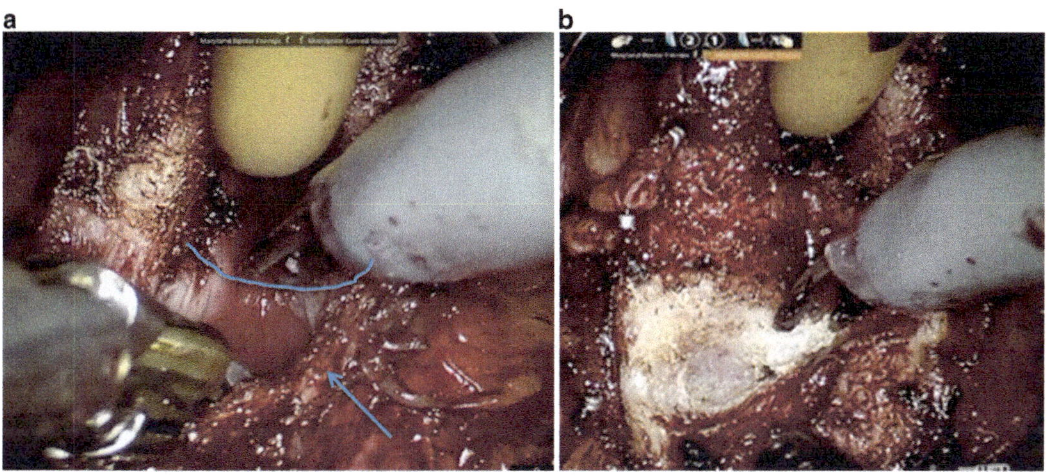

Fig. 4.15 (**a**, **b**) The layers are well seen and the dissection outlines the posterior bladder. Constant counter retraction is provided by the 2nd arm. An areolar layer is entered, and then the longitudinal muscle

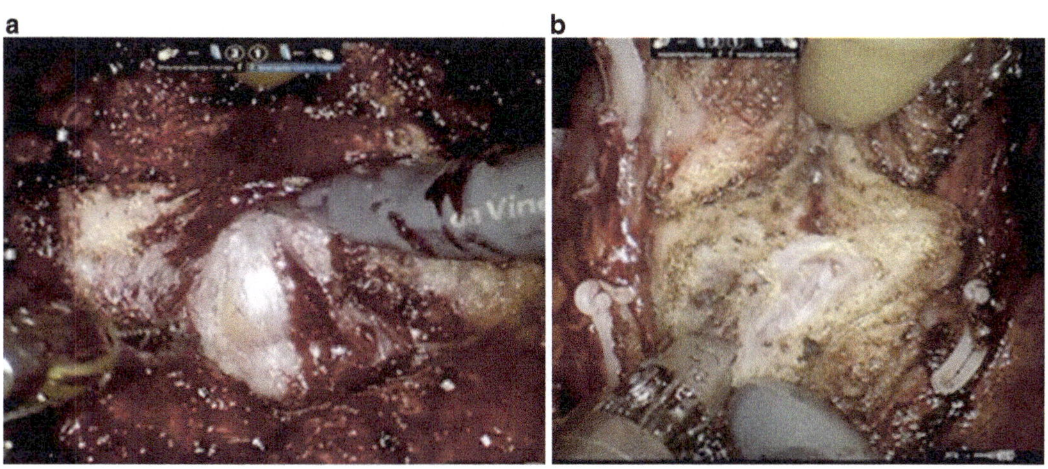

Fig. 4.16 (**a**, **b**) The longitudinal muscles can be almost absent, thick, or almost look like rectal wall such as in Fig. 4.4

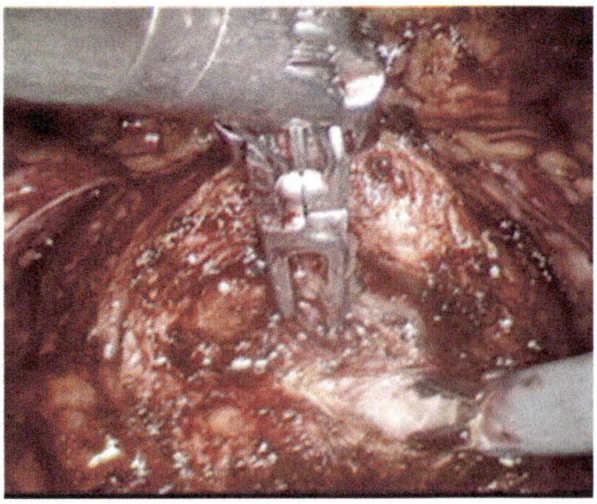

Fig. 4.17 The third arm can re-expose by grasping posterior prostatic urethra or tissue underneath. Keep the arm very vertical with up traction to assist and leave collision free space for the other arms

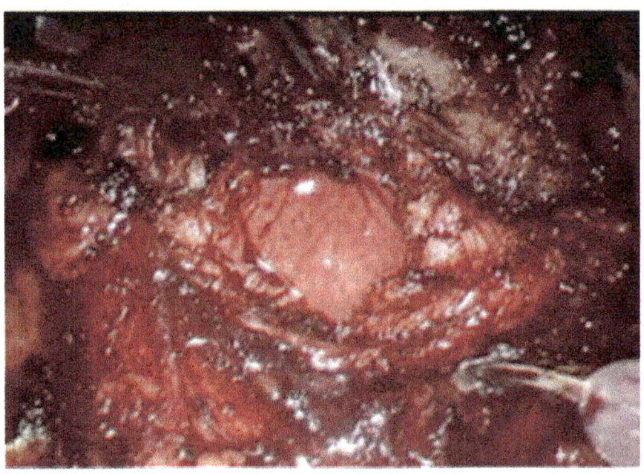

Fig. 4.18 The bladder is re-inspected several times to look for anomalies such as a dependent posterior wall that might migrate into the posterior dissection near the vas

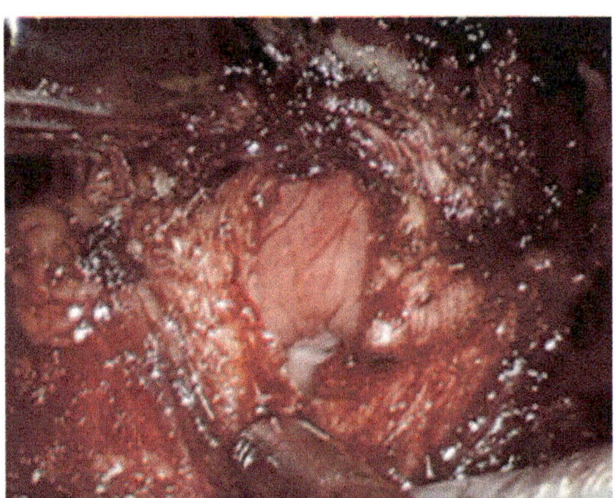

Fig. 4.19 The same patient as in Fig. 4.18 now shows there is a dependent portion of bladder "jutting" forward

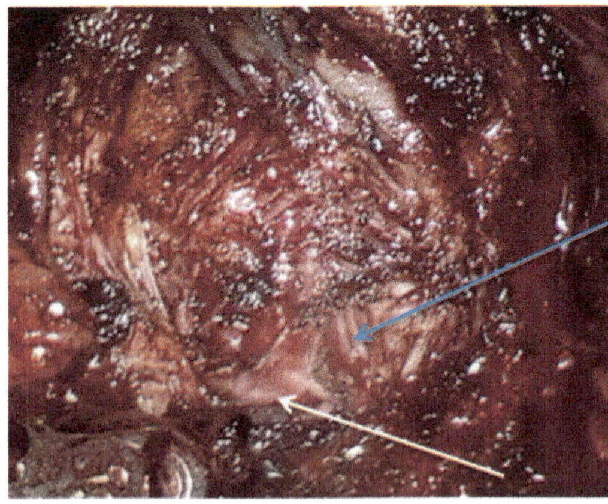

Fig. 4.20 The surgical plane looks correct with longitudinal muscle fibers seen on the right side (*blue arrow*). However the tissue at the *white arrow* was grasped and divided and turned out to be bladder

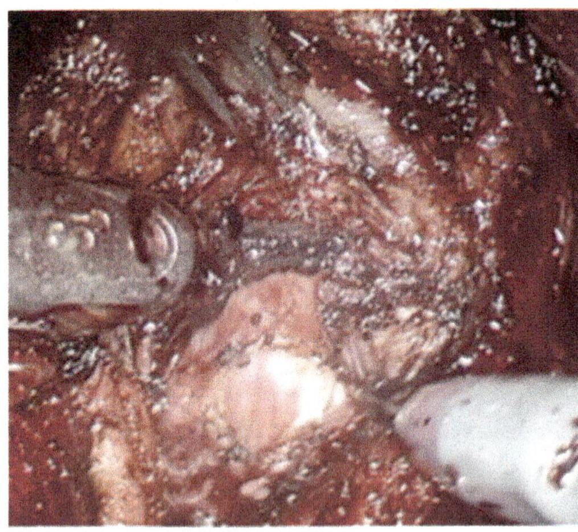

Fig. 4.21 The same patient from Fig. 4.20 a few frames later—the bladder has a "button hole" injury

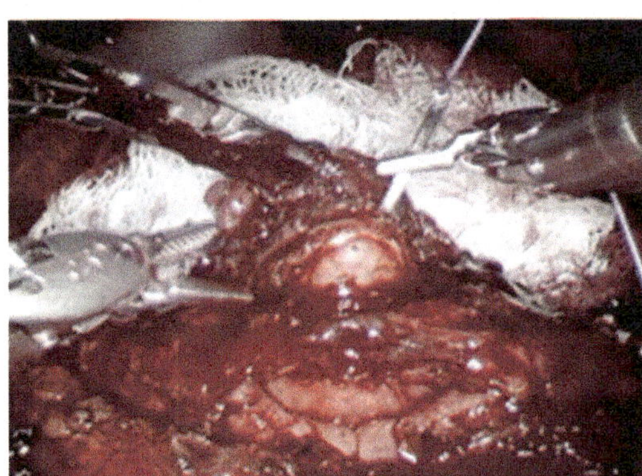

Fig. 4.22 The buttonhole injury is repaired post-resection

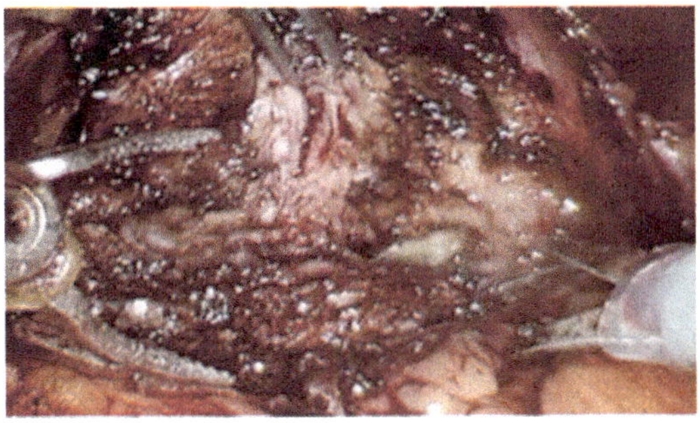

Fig. 4.23 Posterior tissue is grasped with the 3rd arm and lifted up. A plane is developed aimed at reaching the longitudinal muscle. However, the plane never made adequate progress

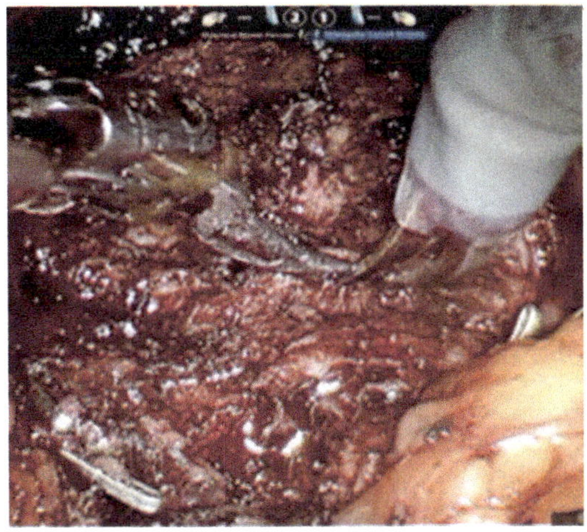

Fig. 4.25 A new plane was found closer to the bladder and lifted up—several inside inspections along the way

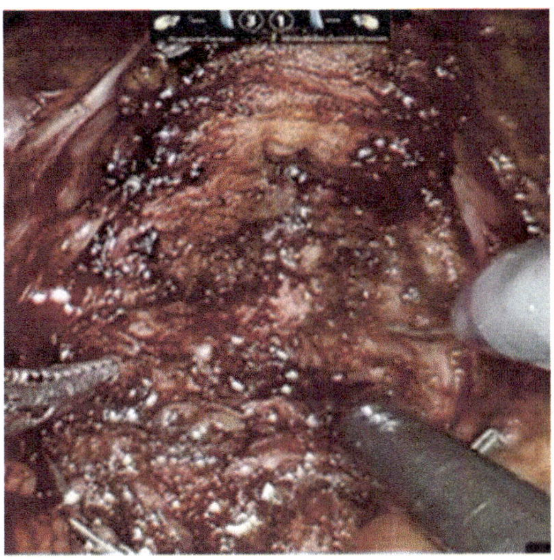

Fig. 4.24 The 3rd arm is switched to the bladder and the planes re-inspected

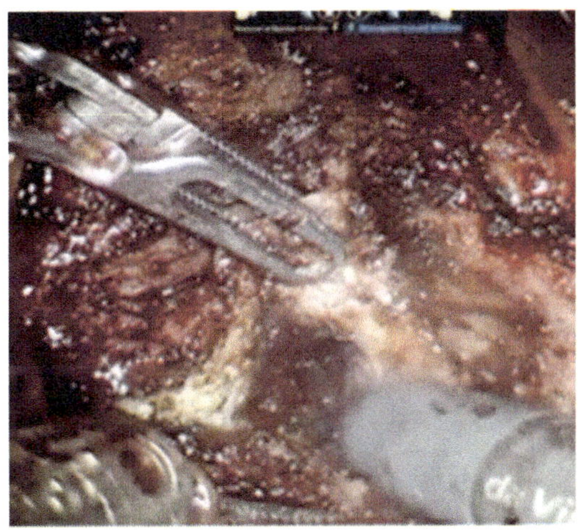

Fig. 4.26 This corrected plane opened up as expected to the longitudinal muscle and the vas were seen next

References

1. Türk I, Deger S, Winkelmann B, et al. Laparoscopic radical prostatectomy. Technical aspects and experience with 125 cases. Eur Urol. 2001;40:46–52.
2. Guillonneau B, Vallancien G. Laparoscopic radical prostatectomy: the Montsouris technique. J Urol. 2000;163:1643–9.
3. Hinata N, Sejima T, Takenaka A. Progress in pelvic anatomy from the viewpoint of radical prostatectomy. Int J Urol. 2013;20:260–70.
4. Walz J, Burnett AL, Costello AJ, et al. A criticawwl analysis of the current knowledge of surgical anatomy related to optimization of cancer control and preservation of continence and erection in candidates for radical prostatectomy. Eur Urol. 2010; 57:179–92.
5. Shimbo M, Hattori K, Endo F, et al. Modified anterior approach to the bladder neck: simple and reproducible procedure for anterior bladder neck transection during robot-assisted radical prostatectomy. Int J Urol. 2014;21:946–8.

Bladder Neck: Anatomic Variants, Prior TUR, Locally Advanced Tumours

5

Declan G. Murphy, Daniel A. Moon, and Bernardo Rocco

Some Principles for Bladder Neck Dissection

The previous chapter has already described a standardised technique for dissection of the straightforward bladder neck. It cannot be overemphasised how important it is to have a standardised approach to bladder neck dissection. Adhering to a standardised technique will not just ensure good results for standard RARPs, but will be of particular value in managing the more difficult anatomical variants we discuss in this chapter. It is therefore of upmost importance to develop a standardised approach to bladder neck dissection, so that this can be applied to more difficult cases. Before we describe the management of challenging bladder neck anatomy, we will briefly revisit our standard technique [1]. This includes the following steps:

1. *Division of the anterior bladder neck:* This step is performed following mobilisation of the bladder, opening of the endopelvic fascia, and ligation of the dorsal vascular complex. The bladder is retracted to help tent up the prostato-vesical junction, and the catheter is then pulled in and out so that the catheter balloon demonstrates the bladder neck. This is then incised in a horizontal plane where the detrusor fibres decussate over the prostato-vesical junction, with the bladder under cepahlad tension, until the catheter is visualised (Fig. 5.1). The catheter is delivered into the operative field and is retracted anteriorly using the EndoCatch™ technique as previously described [2].
2. *Incision of the posterior bladder neck*: Prior to incising the posterior bladder neck, the bladder lumen is first inspected to ensure that the standard "drop-off" of the posterior bladder is as expected, and that there is no unexpected median lobe. The lateral horns of the bladder are then mobilised. In smaller sized prostates, this is not difficult. The lateral wings of the bladder are dissected off the prostate, typically leaving a thin layer of detrusor muscle on the prostate. The posterior bladder neck is then incised, ensuring that a reasonable bladder thickness is established (usually about 5 mm) (Fig. 5.2). The incision is progressed laterally to continue the mobilisation of the bladder, ensuring that an even bladder thickness is established.

D.G. Murphy, M.B., F.R.A.C.S., F.R.C.S. (✉)
D.A. Moon, M.D.
Division of Cancer Surgery, Peter MacCallum Cancer Centre, University of Melbourne, East Melbourne, VIC 3002, Australia

Epworth Healthcare, Epworth Prostate Centre, Richmond, Melbourne, VIC, Australia
e-mail: declan.murphy@petermac.org

B. Rocco
Clinica Urologica I, Ospedale Maggiore Policlinico, Fondazione IRCCS Ca' Granda, Universita degli Studi di Milano, Milan, Italy

J.W. Davis (ed.), *Robot-Assisted Radical Prostatectomy*, DOI 10.1007/978-3-319-32641-2_5

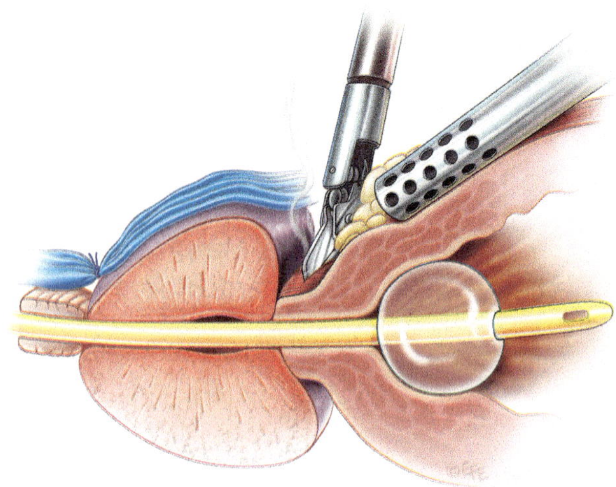

Fig. 5.1 In a normal, small prostate, the anterior bladder neck is divided using monopolar cautery. Reproduced from Murphy et al. with permission [1]

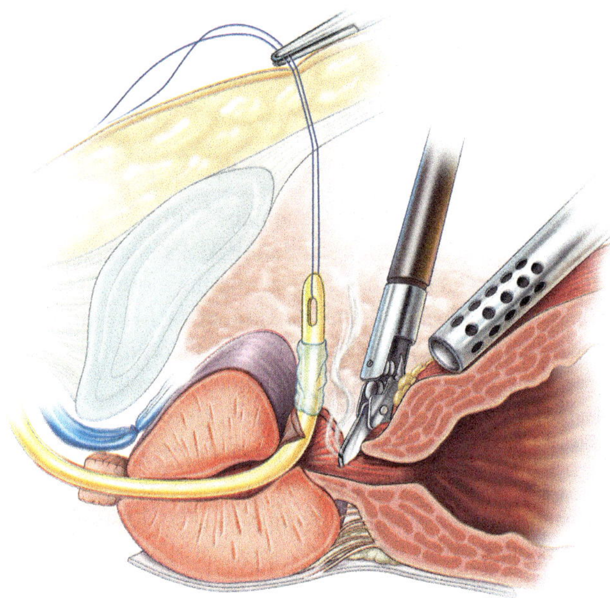

Fig. 5.2 In a normal, small prostate, the posterior bladder neck is divided in the midline. The vasa and seminal vesicles are identified once the longitudinal fibres of the detrusor fascia have been divided. Reproduced from Murphy et al. with permission [1]

3. *Further mobilisation of the posterior bladder neck*: Once an appropriate bladder neck thickness is established, the mobilisation is continued posteriorly, ensuring that the same thickness is maintained until the vasa and seminal vesicles are reached. To ensure that the same thickness is maintained, it is useful to look in the bladder periodically to ensure that the dissection does not drift either too close to or too far from the bladder.

A most important principle to adhere to during posterior bladder neck dissection is *to maintain the thickness of the posterior bladder neck* as dissection proceeds from the initial incision in the posterior bladder neck, and more posteriorly as the bladder is dissected off the prostate. If the bladder thickness is evenly maintained during this step, then complications such as button-holing of the bladder (caused by dissecting too close to the bladder), intra-prostatic incision (dissecting too close to the prostate), and amputation of the seminal vesicles (dissecting too far off the bladder and entering an incorrect plane) can be avoided. In addition, while adhering to this principle during cases with a straightforward bladder neck will ensure a good anatomical plane, the same principle is even more important to maintain during the more difficult scenarios detailed below.

Outcomes for Patients Undergoing RARP with Difficult Bladder Neck Anatomy

Invariably, added difficulty in dissecting the posterior bladder neck, already a difficult step, may have an impact on certain outcomes of RARP. In particular, there may be somewhat adverse outcomes in terms of operative time, blood loss, and positive surgical margins. While there is no high-level evidence to quantify this, some observations can be made based on published data.

Regarding l*arge prostates including those with a median lobe*, Huang et al. [3] reported that men with larger prostates and median lobes experienced higher estimated blood loss (EBL) (213.5 vs. 176.5 ml; $p<0.001$ and 236.4 vs. 193.3 ml; $p=0.002$), and larger prostates were associated with more transfusions (4 vs. 1; $p=0.037$). Total operative times were longer for men with larger prostates (164.2 vs. 149.1 min; $p=0.002$), and median lobes (185.8 vs. 155.0 min; $p=0.004$). In another series comparing prostates with final weight greater or less than 75 g, Bishara et al. reported that larger prostate size was associated with lower Gleason score on final pathology ($p=0.004$) and lower pathological stage ($p=0.02$) but an increased length of hospital stay ($p=0.05$) [4]. In addition, PSA density independently predicted biochemical recurrence (BCR) on binary logistic regression when defined as postoperative PSA >0.1 ($p=0.001$). In a study looking at men with very large prostates (>100 g), Labanaris et al. demonstrated a significant increase in blood loss, operative time, increased need for bladder neck reconstruction, as well as an increase in intraoperative complications in these very large prostates compared with smaller glands [5]. Nevertheless, patients with large glands exhibited less aggressive tumours, less positive surgical margins, and a lower incidence of biochemical recurrence. Regarding functional outcomes, patients with larger glands had no difference regarding continence rates when compared to patients with smaller glands but exhibited significantly lower potency rates. Furthermore, a Japanese study examining health-related quality-of-life (QoL) scores demonstrated significant improvements in urinary QoL for patients with larger prostates (defined as >50 g) [6]. At follow-up ranging from 18 to 36 months, patients in group 3 had improved EPIC urinary domain summary and subscale scores, including scores for urinary irritation and obstruction and urinary bother subscale scores, compared with their baseline scores ($p<0.05$).

There is no consensus on whether *previous surgery for bladder outlet obstruction* has a negative impact on outcomes following radical prostatectomy. Although some authors have demonstrated longer operative times, increased complications, and higher rates of PSMs in patients undergoing ORP [7] or LRP [8] following prior surgery for bladder outlet obstruction, others have shown that outcomes are equivalent following ORP in patients who had previously undergone TURP [9]. Hampton et al. reported on 51 of 1768 patients who underwent RARP having previously undergone TURP [10]. Compared to patients who had not undergone previous TURP, post-TURP patients had a significantly higher PSM rate (35.3% vs. 17.6%, $p<0.015$) and these PSMs were more likely to be located at the bladder neck. Huang et al. also reported that patients with prior BPH interventions experienced more prostate base PSM (5.1% vs. 1.2%; $p=0.018$) but similar overall PSM in adjusted analysis [3]. While these outcomes may not be exclusive to the RARP approach, it should be borne in mind when counselling such patients for this procedure [11].

Regarding locally advanced and other high-risk localised prostate cancers, there is now quite convincing data regarding the oncological safety of RARP for such tumours, at least in the hands of experienced surgeons [12–14]. In a systematic review of 1360 cases of high-risk prostate cancer, Yuh et al. reported that 65% of patients had at least T3 disease with a PSM rate of 35 % and a 3-year biochemical recurrence-free survival which ranged from 45 to 86 % [13]. Overall, the complication rates were low in this review, although there are little data on the specific complications which might be experienced with such cases.

Step by Step: Dealing with Difficult Anatomy

1. *Median lobe*: These vary in size from modest intravesical protrusions to extremely large, irregular masses, and the level of difficulty generally correlates with size. Apart from the extra bulk and distortion which a large median lobe adds to the posterior bladder dissection, there are particular issues around maintaining the correct plane, and avoiding injury to the ureteric orifices. While these do not have to routinely be visualised during the dissection of small prostates, it is imperative to identify the trigone in median lobe cases as the intravesical protrusion can extend close to the ureteric orifices. This usually means that the bladder neck will be wider than usual and will require reconstruction.

   Incise under the lobe or across the lobe? In smaller median lobes, it is possible to elevate the median lobe and make the incision into the posterior bladder *underneath the lobe*. The posterior dissection can then continue as usual, with the median lobe being continually elevated using the fourth arm or perhaps using a suture [15, 16]. Our recommendation in this case is to use a 1/0 Vicryl® suture on a CT needle which can be passed horizontally through the median lobe, and this suture can then be elevated with the fourth arm, or passed through the eye of the urethral catheter if using the anterior retraction technique [2]. However, in larger lobes, there may be issues with this approach as it will bring the incision very close to the ureteric orifices, and the bulk of the lobe may be difficult to retract due to its size.

   Therefore the preferred approach for most median lobes is to incise the mucosa *across the lobe*, and enucleate the median lobe while preserving the bladder neck. The challenge here is in maintaining the correct anatomical plane in what can be a challenging operative field with a large adenoma and a variable amount of bleeding. The surgeon should use the monopolar shears (single blade) to make a confident incision into the mucosa until the enucleation plane is established. The depth of this incision will correspond with the bladder neck thickness. Once the correct plane is identified, the dissection can usually proceed with a combination of sharp and blunt dissect the adenoma off the bladder (Fig. 5.3). As stated above, the most important principle here is to maintain the bladder neck thickness as the dissection proceeds as this will lead to the correct plane for identification of the vasa. This is often quite deep dissection and it is recommended that the console surgeon frequently inspects the inside of the bladder to ensure that the correct bladder thickness is maintained and a buttonhole is avoided (Fig. 5.4). As the dissection proceeds, the fourth arm (or retracting suture) can be adjusted to continually elevate the median lobe (Fig. 5.5).
2. *Previous bladder outlet surgery:* The degree of difficulty associated with this step depends on the extent of previous bladder neck surgery, and perhaps the type of technique employed (TURP vs. various types of laser surgery). Regardless, the difficulty is usually characterised by difficulty in identifying the true posterior bladder neck due to previous surgery, and occasionally difficulty in identifying the ureteric orifices. Prior to opening the anterior bladder neck, it is possible to identify the extent of the TUR defect by pulling down on the catheter balloon and observing how much the balloon travels into the intra-prostatic fossa. Consequently, it can be difficult to identify the correct location to incise the anterior bladder neck. This can partly be overcome by mobilising the detrusor apron off the lateral aspect of the prostate to better identify the curvature of the base of the prostate as it curves towards the bladder neck. However, if in any doubt, it is better to remain closer to the bladder than to the prostate, even if this

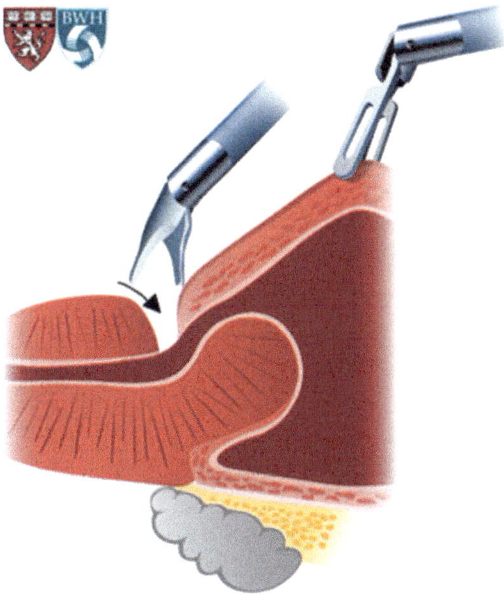

Fig. 5.3 In a case with a large median lobe, the fourth arm tents up the bladder for antero-cephalad retraction. Monopolar dissection is used to open the anterior bladder neck, and the bladder is peeled off of the prostate in the direction of the *arrow*. Reproduced from Huang et al. with permission [3]

means leaving a wider bladder neck requiring reconstruction, rather than risk entering into the gland.

Once the bladder has been opened, a careful inspection of the lumen must be undertaken to identify the probable location of the true posterior bladder neck, and the ureteric orifices. It is often necessary to open the bladder neck wider than usual in order to fully identify this anatomy. As the midline of the prostate has usually been extensively resected or ablated, it is helpful to inspect the more lateral aspects of the luminal bladder first, to get a better appreciation of where the true posterior bladder neck is located. The bladder neck is then incised as usual, taking care to ensure that the ureteric orifices are well clear. There can be considerable deep scarring in the posterior bladder neck due to the previous energy, but as long as the principle of *maintaining bladder thickness* is observed, then this should allow the dissection to continue in the correct plane until the posterior structures are reached.

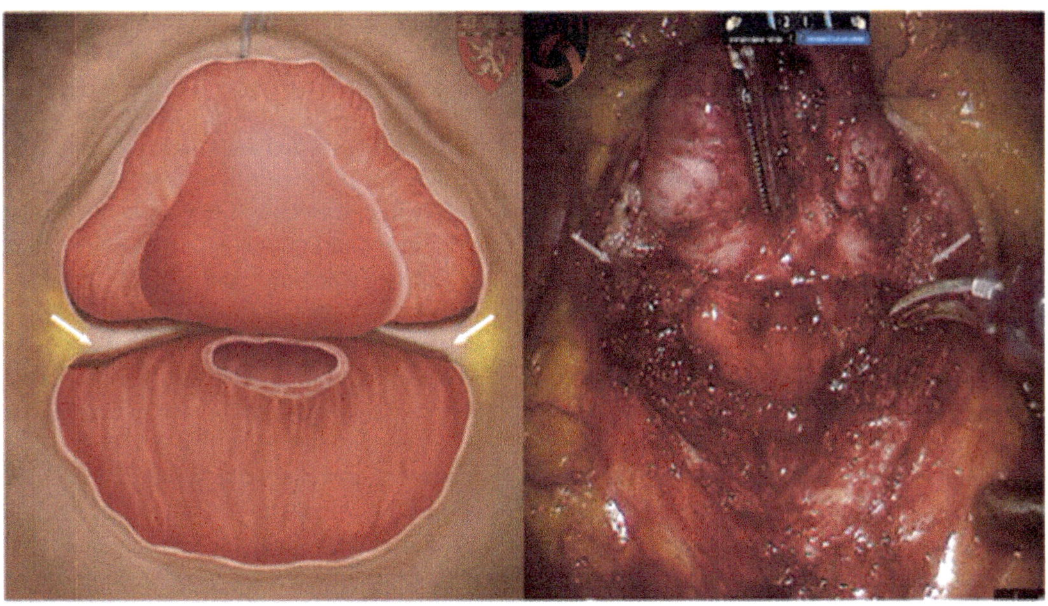

Fig. 5.4 Prior to bladder entry, bladder attachments are dissected off of the prostate until reaching the prostatovesical junction (*arrows*). Releasing these attachments posterolaterally until encountering the lateral pedicle fat pad minimizes subsequent tearing of the bladder neck; tearing may occur with traction to facilitate dissection. The posterior bladder neck is peeled off of the median lobe to allow grasping with the Prograsp forceps for anterocaudal retraction (*right*). Reproduced from Huang et al. with permission [3]

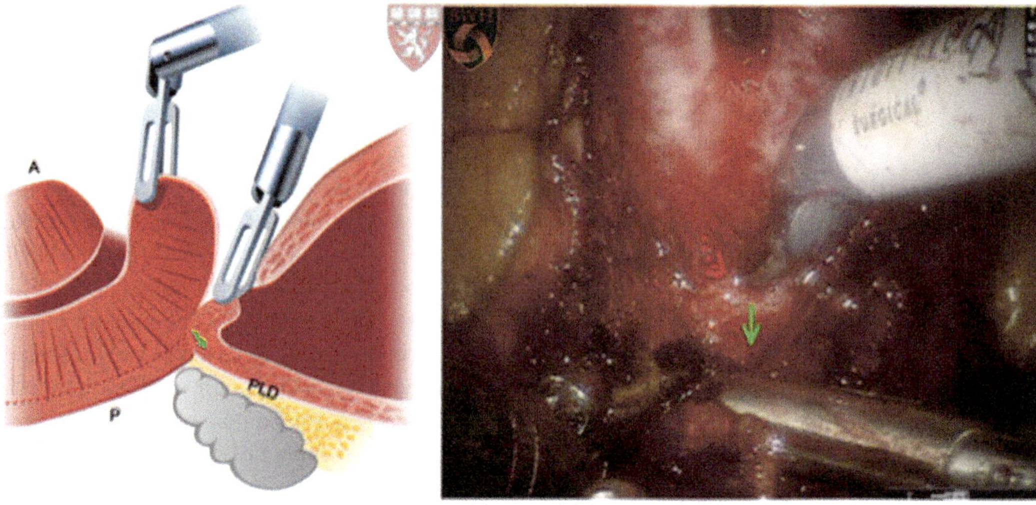

Fig. 5.5 The fourth arm is used to retract the median lobe anteriorly, while the assistant retracts posteriorly to help open up the correct dissection plane. The assistant intermittently releases the posterior bladder neck to allow the surgeon to index the bladder mucosa contour to avoid dissecting too proximally and "button-holing". Care must be taken not to follow the curve of the median lobe (*dotted red line/arrow*), as the correct posterior plane lies in a postero-cephalad direction (*green arrow*) and the posterior (P) versus anterior (A) prostate distance is always greater. Reproduced from Huang et al. with permission [3]

If a bladder neck reconstruction is required (and it frequently is in these situations), we prefer a lateral reconstruction using a fish-mouth technique at the 3 and 9 o'clock positions.

Some authors advocate a cystoscopy and possibly placement of ureteric stents to help identify and protect the ureteric orifices. Our practice is not to do this, although a cystoscopy can certainly be helpful (especially early in the surgeon's experience), in appreciating the endoscopic anatomy prior to the RARP.

3. *Large prostate size:* Similar to the discussion on median lobes above, these cases provide challenges related to maintaining the correct anatomical plane when proceeding with mobilisation of the bladder as the posterior dissection proceeds. Even in the absence of a median lobe, large prostates tend to protrude into the bladder which can lead to the bladder being "draped" around the lateral lobes of the prostate. Care must therefore be taken not to inadvertently enter the bladder during lateral mobilisation (a "lateral buttonhole"). Large prostates (certainly those over 75 g) add time to the procedure and more blood loss is typical. There is always a balance to be achieved between tolerating some venous ooze and continuing to make progression. Once the correct plane has been reached and the vasa are exposed, anterior retraction of these will usually help any venous ooze to settle.

   The posterior dissection often takes place in a somewhat deep abyss as the bladder is excavated from the large adenoma and the posterior structures often seem to be very deep within the pelvis. Once again, the key to avoiding complications here is to maintain the bladder thickness as the dissection proceeds. Regular reinspection of the bladder will help ensure that the surgical plane is not too close to or too far from the bladder. This will therefore lead into the correct plane in front of the vasa and seminal vesicles. As the bulk of the prostate is mobilised, the fourth arm can aid with anterior retraction of the prostate, while the assistant uses both the suction device and grasper to retract posteriorly. An experienced assistant is very helpful in such cases.
4. *Locally advanced tumour:* There are specific technical challenges associated with cT3 cases due to the lack of tactile sensation during RARP. Therefore great care must be taken to

adequately mobilise the prostate well away from the bulk of the tumour. For example, for cases which are cT3 at the base, the periprostatic fascia must be mobilised outside the extrafascial plane to allow adequate mobilisation of the base. Typically, the incision through the endopelvic fascia is continued so that the peri-rectal fat is exposed. This plane can then be developed back towards the base of prostate. More medially, the posterior plane is also developed such that the Denonvilliers' fascia remains on the prostate and the perirectal fat is exposed. The combination of this medial mobilisation and the lateral mobilisation previously described will allow the base of prostate to be mobilised and retracted adequately so that the base pedicles can be controlled with haemostatic clips. As with all aspects of robotic surgery, the superior visualisation more than makes up for the loss of tactile sensation, and hence PSMs can be minimised.

For cases with suspicion of bladder neck invasion, the bladder must be adequately visualised following division of the anterior bladder neck. The bladder may be opened with a wider bladder neck than usual so that a thicker layer of detrusor may be left on the specimen. For patients with seminal vesicle invasion, the seminal vesicles should be left inside their surrounding fascia as much as possible, with wider mobilisation and the use of clips and cautery to control the surrounding vasculature.

Avoiding Complications

As with most surgical dissection, there are pitfalls which can be avoided by having a detailed understanding of the anatomy and employing meticulous surgical technique. For bladder neck dissection, some of the pitfalls include:

- "Button-holing" the bladder
- Intra-prostatic incision
- Ureteric injury
- Amputation of the seminal vesicles
- Excessive bladder neck excision

None of these are insurmountable, but obviously all are best avoided if possible. Hopefully the tips provided here will go some way towards avoiding these.

Conclusion

Overall, it appears that the issues outlined above are no longer a limitation to a robotic-assisted approach to radical prostatectomy. These more complex cases are best avoided within the early robotic experience of any centre and patients must be adequately counselled regarding the increased morbidity when compared to more straightforward RARPs. Patients in these circumstances should understand that a robotic approach does not negate the increased likelihood of morbidity which they are at risk of developing compared to patients without such confounding factors.

References

1. Murphy DG, Kerger M, Crowe H, Peters JS, Costello AJ. Operative details and oncological and functional outcome of robotic-assisted laparoscopic radical prostatectomy: 400 cases with a minimum of 12 months follow-up. Eur Urol. 2009;55:1358–67.
2. Murphy DG, Agarwal D, Costello AJ. Anterior retraction of the prostate during robotic-assisted laparoscopic radical prostatectomy using the EndoClose device. BJU Int. 2009;103:558–62.
3. Huang AC, Kowalczyk KJ, Hevelone ND, Lipsitz SR, Yu HY, Plaster BA, et al. The impact of prostate size, median lobe, and prior benign prostatic hyperplasia intervention on robot-assisted laparoscopic prostatectomy: technique and outcomes. Eur Urol. 2011;59:595–603.
4. Bishara S, Vasdev N, Lane T, Boustead G, Adshead J. Robotic prostatectomy has a superior outcome in larger prostates and PSA density is a strong predictor of biochemical recurrence. Prostate Cancer. 2014; 2014:763863.
5. Labanaris AP, Zugor V, Witt JH. Robot-assisted radical prostatectomy in patients with a pathologic prostate specimen weight ≥100 grams versus ≤50 grams: surgical, oncologic and short-term functional outcomes. Urol Int. 2013;90:24–30.
6. Miyazato M, Kaiho Y, Mitsuzuka K, Yamada S, Namiki S, Saito H, et al. Impact of prostate size on urinary quality of life scores after open radical prostatectomy: a single-center experience. Scand J Urol. 2014;48:146–52.

7. Colombo R, Naspro R, Salonia A, Montorsi F, Raber M, Suardi N, et al. Radical prostatectomy after previous prostate surgery: clinical and functional outcomes. J Urol. 2006;176:2459–63.
8. Jaffe J, Stakhovsky O, Cathelineau X, Barret E, Vallancien G, Rozet F. Surgical outcomes for men undergoing laparoscopic radical prostatectomy after transurethral resection of the prostate. J Urol. 2007;178:483–7.
9. Palisaar JR, Wenske S, Sommerer F, Hinkel A, Noldus J. Open radical retropubic prostatectomy gives favourable surgical and functional outcomes after transurethral resection of the prostate. BJU Int. 2009;104:611–5.
10. Hampton L, Nelson RA, Satterthwaite R, Wilson T, Crocitto L. Patients with prior TURP undergoing robot-assisted laparoscopic radical prostatectomy have higher positive surgical margin rates. J Robotic Surg. 2008;2:213–6.
11. Murphy DG, Bjartell A, Ficarra V, Graefen M, Haese A, Montironi R, et al. Downsides of robot-assisted laparoscopic radical prostatectomy: limitations and complications. Eur Urol. 2009;57:735–46.
12. Connolly SS, Cathcart PJ, Gilmore P, Kerger M, Crowe H, Peters JS, et al. Robotic radical prostatectomy as the initial step in multimodal therapy for men with high-risk localised prostate cancer: initial experience of 160 men. BJU Int. 2012;109:752–9.
13. Yuh B, Artibani W, Heidenreich A, Kimm S, Menon M, Novara G, et al. The role of robot-assisted radical prostatectomy and pelvic lymph node dissection in the management of high-risk prostate cancer: a systematic review. Eur Urol. 2014;65:918–27.
14. Yuh BE, Ruel NH, Mejia R, Wilson CM, Wilson TG. Robotic extended pelvic lymphadenectomy for intermediate- and high-risk prostate cancer. Eur Urol. 2012;61:1004–10.
15. Patel SR, Kaplon DM, Jarrard D. A technique for the management of a large median lobe in robot-assisted laparoscopic radical prostatectomy. J Endourol. 2010;24:1899–901.
16. Abreu AL, Chopra S, Berger AK, Leslie S, Desai MM, Gill IS, et al. Management of large median and lateral intravesical lobes during robot-assisted radical prostatectomy. J Endourol. 2013;27:1389–92.

Neurovascular Bundle Preservation: Anatomic and Technical Considerations

6

Anup Kumar, Srinivas Samavedi,
and Vipul R. Patel

Introduction

In the United States of America (USA) prostate cancer is the most common noncutaneous malignancy affecting men and the second most common cause of cancer death in men [1–3]. With the use of prostate specific antigen (PSA) screening and increased public awareness about prostate cancer, the number of cases being diagnosed yearly has been increasing. According to American Cancer Society in 2014, approximately 233,000 new cases of prostate cancer will be diagnosed [4]. Every year younger and healthier men are being diagnosed with localized prostate cancer, with an annual percentage increase of approximately 9.5 %,as per data from the Surveillance, Epidemiology and End Results (SEER) registry [4]. Radical prostatectomy, a standard of care for localized prostate cancer, has evolved from open through laparoscopic to robot-assisted radical prostatectomy (RARP) over the last few decades [5, 6]. This subset of younger and healthier patients is a challenge for treating urologists, who has to meet the expectations of not only cancer control but also excellent postoperative functional outcomes (potency and continence). With advances in robotic techniques and the increase in the experience using the robotic platform, RARP has shown improved functional outcomes and at least comparable oncological outcomes as compared to open and laparoscopic radical prostatectomy [7–14]. This is possible because of 3-D vision, improved magnification, tremor reduction with motion scaling, and improved ergonomics of da Vinci robotic surgical system resulting in six degrees of freedom of movement and reduction of fatigue [7–10]. Despite these advances, the incidence of 1 year and 2 year erectile dysfunction (ED) ranges from 10 to 46 % and 6 to 37 % respectively after a nerve sparing RARP [15–23]. This wide range of ED in various reported series may be attributed to different definitions/measures of ED, difference in nerve sparing (NS) techniques/patients selection, and different postsurgical rehabilitation programs in these centers. Probably one of the key elements in the outcomes is the experience of the surgeon and the surgical volume. The various predictors of ED after RARP include age at surgery, preoperative potency status, comorbidity (diabetes, hypertension, neurological disorder), and type/extent of NS [15, 24].

Erectile dysfunction after RARP is certainly multifactorial including vasculogenic and neurogenic causes. The direct mechanical injury to NVBs during RARP can occur due to the use of thermal energy, traction, direct transaction, and incorporation into hemostatic sutures or clips [24, 25].

A. Kumar (✉) • S. Samavedi • V.R. Patel
Global Robotics Institute, Florida Hospital-Celebration Health, University of Central Florida College of Medicine, Orlando, FL, USA
e-mail: anup_14k@yahoo.com

J.W. Davis (ed.), *Robot-Assisted Radical Prostatectomy*, DOI 10.1007/978-3-319-32641-2_6

Table 6.1 Sir Herbert Seddon's classification of peripheral nerve injuries

Categories of peripheral nerve injury	Features	Recovery	Duration of recovery
Neurapraxia	Mild compression, stretch injury with no structural damage leading to transient conduction block	Full	Hours to weeks
Axonotmesis	Moderately severe injury: axonal disruption and Wallerian degeneration	Nerve regeneration/growth from point of injury to end organ at 1 in./month	8–24 Months
Neurotmesis	Severe permanent injury/ laceration: complete nerve transaction	– No capacity for regrowth – A neuroma/scar formation: potential for partial recovery	Months–years

This causes various grades of pelvic autonomic nerve injury ranging from neurapraxia, axonotmesis and neurotmesis as well as muscle degeneration/damage, thus contributing to postoperative ED and urinary incontinence (Table 6.1) [25, 26].

The association between NS and postoperative continence is multifactorial. It has been proposed that both afferent and efferent nerves of NVBs play a role in urinary continence restoration. The intraoperative stimulation of NVBs causes increased urethral pressure, thus demonstrating the potential impact of autonomic innervation on the external urinary sphincter. Urine entering membranous urethra in presence of intact proximal sensations leads to a spinal reflex of voluntary contraction of urethral sphincter (increasing tone of sphincter and pelvic floor), improving continence [27–29].

It has been proven in various series that bilateral NS RARP results in improved ability to regain some level of postoperative sexual function [7–14, 27–29]. The road map for nerve sparing RP was laid down by the pioneering work of Walsh and Donker on the surgical anatomy of the prostate documenting the concept of neurovascular bundles (NVB in relation to the prostate [30]. Based on these findings, Walsh et al. proposed the first nerve sparing RARP. Since then, a plethora of NS techniques with variable outcomes during RP have been reported, so as to further improve the postoperative potency and continence, considered as surrogates of functional outcomes of RP. In this chapter, we will discuss the applied neuroanatomy of the prostate, various techniques of NS including our technique, along with recent innovations and potency outcomes after RARP.

Applied Neuroanatomy of the Prostate

Eckhard introduced the concept of nerves having a role in potency and defined them as nervi erigentes in 1863 in animal models [31]. However, the detailed anatomy of cavernosal nerves and current concept of NVBs were introduced by Walsh and Donker [30]. They traced the autonomic innervations of the corpora cavernosa in a male fetus and newborn, and then in a 60-year-old human cadaver. They demonstrated that the pelvic plexus is formed by the parasympathetic fibers (S2-S4 anterior sacral roots) and sympathetic fibers from the hypogastric nerve. This plexus is situated on the anterolateral wall of the rectum retroperitoneally, at the tips of seminal vesicles. The superior part of the plexus is called the vesical plexus an inferior part as prostatic plexus. The prostatic plexus unites with several vessels to form the NVB of Walsh, described as a tubular structure running along the posterolateral aspect of prostate gland enclosed in fascial sheaths, in close relation to the capsular vessels of the prostate. As the branches of the inferior vesical artery and vein supplying the bladder and prostate perforate the pelvic plexus, ligation of lateral prostatic pedicles in its midportion can damage the nerves innervating the prostate, urethra, and corpora cavernosa. Based upon these findings, Walsh reported the first RP with nerve preservation, in which incision in lateral pelvic fascia anterior to NVBs was given and the lateral pedicles were divided close to the prostate, avoiding injury to NVBs, traveling along capsular vessels of the prostate [32, 33]. This was a new landmark era in treatment of prostate cancer, where benefits outweighed the risks for then highly invasive RP.

Costello et al. further modified this concept in 2004, working on human cadavers [34]. They demonstrated that the majority of the NVB descends as posterior nerves distally and dorsolaterally to seminal vesicles (SV), while the remaining portion (anterior nerves) courses along the posterolateral border of SV. The anterior and posterior nerves of NVB, separated by a distance of 3 cm at the base of the prostate, run distally towards the apex, converge at midprostatic level, and then diverge again as they approach the prostate apex, where its course and architecture is most variable. They proposed a functional organization of NVB—posterior portion (fibers supplying rectum), midportion (true cavernosal nerves), and anterior portion (fibers supplying prostate).

Tewari et al. proposed the concept of a trizonal neural architecture in relevance to RARP, working on ten fresh and two fixed male cadavers [35]. They divided the neural architecture into three surgically important zones. The proximal zone (zone 1) contains the proximal neurovascular plate (PNP),which covers a significant portion of proximal prostate on its lateral aspect, and is related to bladder neck and seminal vesicles. The PNP is located 5–10 mm lateral to SV and is at risk of thermally damaged, or crushed in clips/bull dog clamps, thus affecting postoperative recovery of potency. The mid-zone (zone 2) contains the predominant neurovascular bundles (PNB), located on the side of the prostate gland, in a posterolateral groove. This bundle is well formed in 50 % of the patients and is spread widely in periprostatic space in the other 50 %. This is closely related to prostate pedicles and fascia; thus there is difficulty in identification and risk of injury in periprostatic inflammation and extracapsular extension. The distal zone (zone 3) contains the accessory pathways and periapical nerves. Accessory nerves can be found around the prostate, between prostate and lateral prostatic fascia, between prostate and Denonvilliers' fascia, and between the layers of periprostatic fascia. In apical dissection, retroapical nerves can be damaged during urethral transaction and anastomosis.

Role of Fascial Planes in Nerve Sparing RARP

One of the key steps during NVB dissection is the development of appropriate periprostatic fascial planes, to prevent mechanical and thermal injury. This requires a thorough knowledge of anatomy of pelvic fascial structures. This is facilitated by 3-D vision and 10× magnification of robotic platform during RARP. The prostate capsule is not a true capsule but fibromuscular band located between glandular units and periprostatic connective tissue. The endopelvic fascia is a multilayer fascia, covering the prostate and bladder, and is linked to the prostate capsule by collagen fibers. This finally inserts into pubic bone as pubourethral ligaments [36]. The part of endopelvic fascia that covers the prostate is called the prostatic fascia and the outer layer of endopelvic fascia is called lateral pelvic fascia/levator fascia. Denonvilliers' fascia is the fascia covering the rectum posterior to prostate. It has an anterior extension which fuses laterally with the endopelvic fascia. The layers of the periprostatic fascia fuse with the anterior layer of Denonvilliers' fascia lateral to the prostate, forming a potential triangular space containing NVBs. The various walls of this triangle are: medial vertical wall—prostatic fascia; lateral wall—lateral pelvic fascia; posterior wall—anterior layer of Denonvilliers' fascia. The triangular space is wide near the base of the prostate and narrow at apex. Thus, the autonomic fibers (cavernosal nerves) arising from the caudal portion of pelvic plexus, close to the tips of seminal vesicles, travel towards posterolateral base of the prostate. They coalesce into more organized bundles, approximately 6 mm wide at the level of the prostate. Then these branches course along the posterolateral aspect of the prostate towards the apex and membranous urethra, embedded in between different layers of periprostatic fascia [37].

Kiyoshima et al. reported that NVB was localized near posterolateral region in only 48 % cases, and in remaining 52 %; these nerves were spread without bundle formation, on the entire lateral surface of the prostate [38]. Further, the site and localization of NVB was related to the degree of fusion between the lateral pelvic fascia and the prostate capsule. There are various series reporting NS techniques with reference to these periprostatic fascial planes as intrafascial, interfascial, and extrafascial. The extrafascial plane dissection is right through the NVBs and might enable some preservation of neural tissue or none. The interfascial plane is the plane between lateral pelvic and prostatic fascia. This plane exists as avascular plane between the prostatic fascia and the Denonvilliers' fascia/anterior extension of Denonvilliers' fascia. Most of NVBs lie between the lateral pelvic fascia and anterior extension of Denonvilliers' fascia. The intrafascial plane is the plane between the prostate capsule and the prostatic fascia. The endopelvic fascia is incised only anteriorly, medial to puboprostatic ligaments. Thus, complete preservation of NVBs can be achieved through either intrafascial or interfascial dissection [22, 23, 39, 40].

Surgical Techniques of NS During RARP

The NVB preservation during RARP is vital for improved postoperative potency and continence. Therefore, the surgical technique plays a very important role. However, there is a significant learning curve associated with NS [7]. Further, there is an increased chance of positive surgical margins (PSM: surrogate marker of oncological outcome) with NS especially for a novice surgeon [7, 8, 18]. The association of nerve sparing with PSM has been controversial. Some series have reported significant positive association between NS and PSM; however, others have denied their association [16, 20, 21, 50]. There is no doubt that attempt for NS brings plane of posterolateral dissection very close to the prostate and tumor. Thus the surgeon has the challenge of reducing PSM along with maintaining quality of life in terms of postoperative erectile function and continence.

Categorization of Approaches to NS in RARP

The approach to NS can be antegrade (from the prostate base to apex) or retrograde (from the apex to the base) or a combination of two. The retrograde approach has advantages of earlier identification and release of NVB from the prostate before ligating the prostatic pedicle, thus avoiding a misplaced clip on pedicle and reduced neuropraxia [16, 41]. The NS can also be divided as thermal (monopolar, bipolar, harmonics) and athermal. Since cavernosal nerves are unmyelinated axons and prone to thermal damage, a lot of importance has been given to avoid possible thermal damage to NVBs in different techniques [42–44]. Ahlering et al. compared potency outcomes in patients undergoing NS RARP using a cautery versus noncautery group [42]. The potency rates were significantly higher in noncautery bilateral NS group (72.8 % vs. 16.7 % at 9 months and 92 % vs. 67.9 % at 24 months respectively). There is another way of categorization of NS—intrafascial, interfascial, and extrafascial (already described above) [22, 23, 39, 40]. Earlier, NS used to be reported as all or none phenomenon (complete, partial, and none). However, recently it has been reported that NS can be graded anatomically and thus NS can be tailored individually as per patient's tumor characteristics [45–48].

Our Technique of Nerve Sparing During Robotic Radical Prostatectomy

General Considerations

Our preferred technique of NS is an athermal early retrograde release of NVB with minimization of traction [16]. The optimal technique of achieving this is with the use of delicate surgical technique and identification of the "landmark prostatic artery" (LA) [49]. We have reported earlier the role of this LA as an anatomic marker for the plane of dissection of the full neurovascular bundle for nerve sparing during RARP [49]. The LA is a capsular branch of the prostatic artery and originates from vesico-prostatic trunk of internal iliac artery. It reaches the prostate on its anterolateral aspect at the base. It then continues distally down to the perineum or gives origin to a network of capsular arteries (CA), running along lateral border of the prostate. The landmark artery represents the most anterio-medial aspect of the NVB guiding the surgeon into the optimal surgical plane for NVB preservation, medial to it. These LA and CA are related closely to cavernosal nerves (CN) and provide a scaffold to the nerves at their course along the prostate. Therefore, the LA can provide a macroscopic landmark for identifying and preserving the CN during RARP. There are some important considerations which help in identifying LA. First, the dorsal vein complex and bladder attachments to the prostate must be secured to decompress venous flow to the prostate. Second, the posterior plane must be widely developed between the prostate and rectum, especially laterally, until the medial aspect of the NVB is identified by the presence of fatty tissue under the lateral lobes of the prostate as this will give the prostate mobility along its longitudinal axis. Third, it is very important to rotate the prostate, sharply open prostatic fascia, and approach the NVB from above. Fourth, there is a bifurcation of the arterial supply at the edge of the pedicle, about 2–3 mm from the prostate, with LA running alongside the prostate and the perforating urethral vessels penetrating the prostate at the base. It is vital to identify this bifurcation before clipping the prostate pedicle, as this 2–3 mm window is the only place where the pedicle can be safely clipped without injury to NVB. This is important especially in cases with history of prostatitis or bleeding after prostate biopsy, in which NVB is stuck to the prostate. Recently, we have reported that NS during RARP can be graded anatomically as per patients' tumor characteristics, rather than all or none phenomenon [45, 48]. The goal of NS is to preserve the greatest possible amount of nerve tissue without compromising surgical margins. Thus, a very fine tailoring is required to achieve precise amount of NS needed for an individual patient. Thus, we report NS during RARP as—no NS, <50 % NS, 50 % NS, 75 % NS, and ≥95 % NS [45, 48].

Technique

The seminal vesicles are dissected athermally and lifted upward (Fig. 6.1a). Then, the posterior plane between the rectum and the prostate is developed through the layers of Denonvilliers' fascia. This plane is further extended anteriorly towards the apex and laterally until the medial aspect of the NVB is recognized bilaterally, by the presence of fatty tissue under the lateral lobes (Fig. 6.1b). The prostate is then rotated contralaterally on its axis; prostatic fascia is opened sharply, with the NVB being approached from above.

For a left retrograde release of the NVB, the assistant grasps the lateral edge of the prostate base and rotates it contralaterally. The fourth arm is used to gently pull cephalad on the bladder and align the prostate pedicle with the NVB. With the help of the assistant that keeps the prostate rotated medially and stable, the lateral pelvic fascia is identified and incised on the lateral aspect of the prostate. A distinctive LA can often be found between the midprostate and base, as a variably sized tortuous vessel over anterolateral aspect of the prostate (Fig. 6.2a–c). A plane of dissection is then developed between the LA and prostate (prostatic fascia and lateral pelvic fascia) at the level of midprostate, with the combined use of a

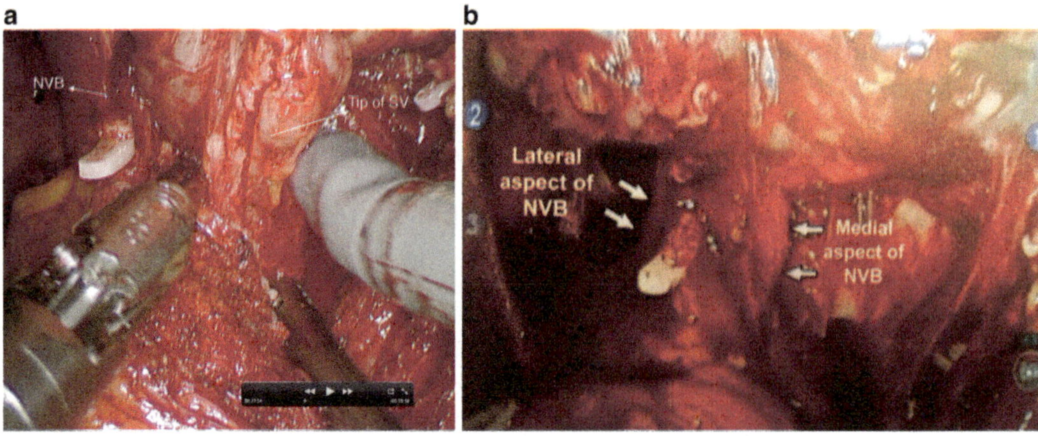

Fig. 6.1 (**a**) The relation of NVB with tip of seminal vesicle during posterior dissection. (**b**) After development of posterior plane, the medial and lateral aspect of NVB become apparent

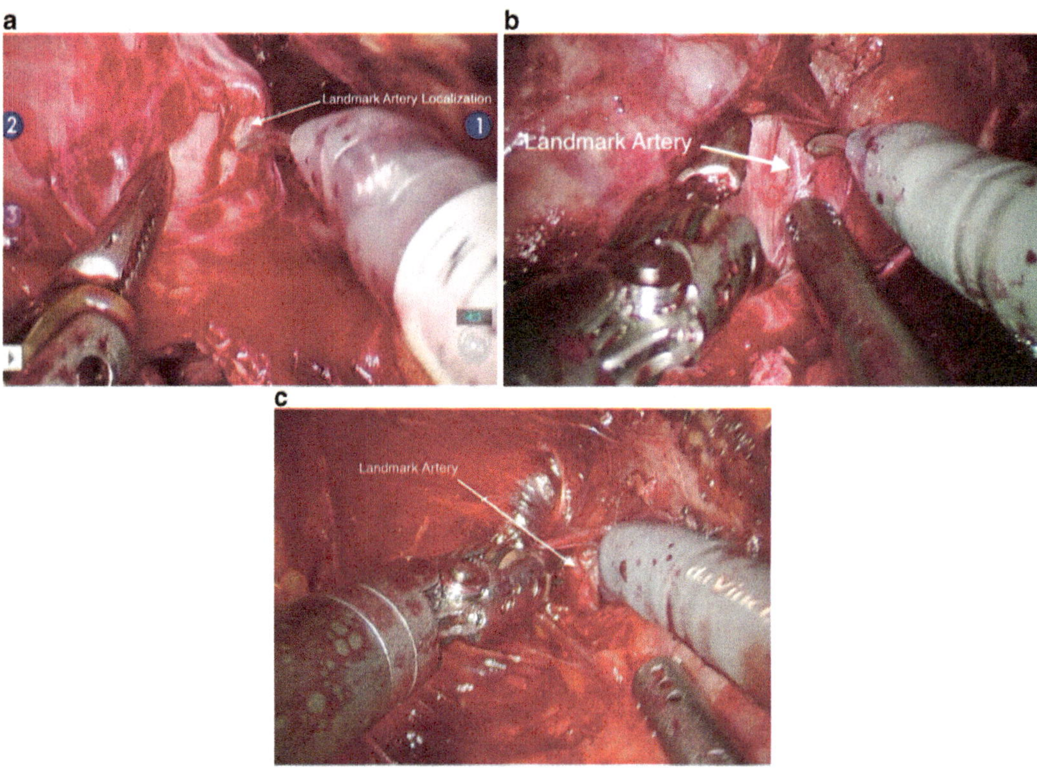

Fig. 6.2 (**a**–**c**) Landmark artery on anterolateral aspect of prostate

Maryland dissector on the left robotic arm and scissors on the right. This results in a natural detachment of the NVB from the prostate, as LA occupies most medial aspect of the NVB. The correct plane of dissection should be fairly avascular, as prostatic vessels stay attached to the NVB that is peeled off the prostatic fascia. In the correct plane the dissection is simple as the natural surgical plane between the fascial layers protecting the prostatic capsule is divided from the fascia surrounding the NVB. This plane is continued posteriorly, until the previously created posterior plane is reached. The plane is then continued retrogradely towards the base of the prostate to completely detach the NVB from the prostatic pedicle (Fig. 6.3). It is vital to keep the field clean and bloodless during dissection, especially when the posterolateral edge of the prostate is reached, as clear visualization of the contour of the prostate will allow the surgeon to stay in the correct plane. The prostatic pedicles can now be safely clipped using Hem-o-lok® clips, without injuring NVB (Fig. 6.4). The dissection is then carried in an antegrade manner towards the apex. The Maryland dissector is used continuously to stabilize the NVB avoiding excessive traction and the prostate is stroked away with the scissors (Fig. 6.5).It is very important to completely release the NVB as distal as possible, so as to avoid injury during apical dissection. For right release of NVB, the same principles are followed, as on left side (Figs. 6.6 and 6.7). We now describe the finer details of our technique of anatomic grading of NS [45, 48].

1. Grade 5, a complete NS (≥95 % NS): The LA is identified and used to delineate the course of the NVB in a retrograde manner up to the prostatic pedicle. The NS is performed medial to LA, just outside the prostatic fascia at the

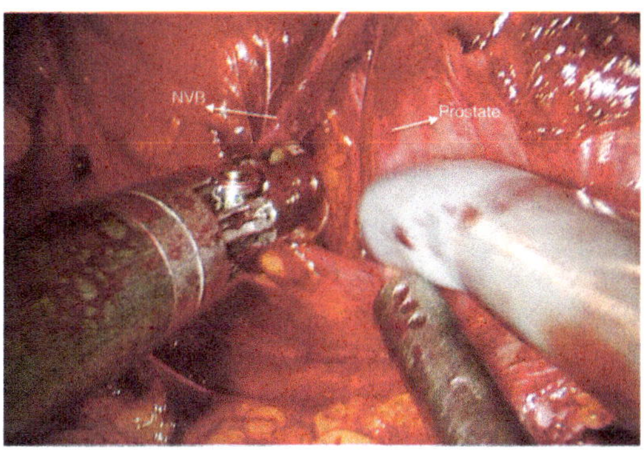

Fig. 6.3 Left retrograde dissection towards the base of the prostate to completely detach the NVB from the prostatic pedicle

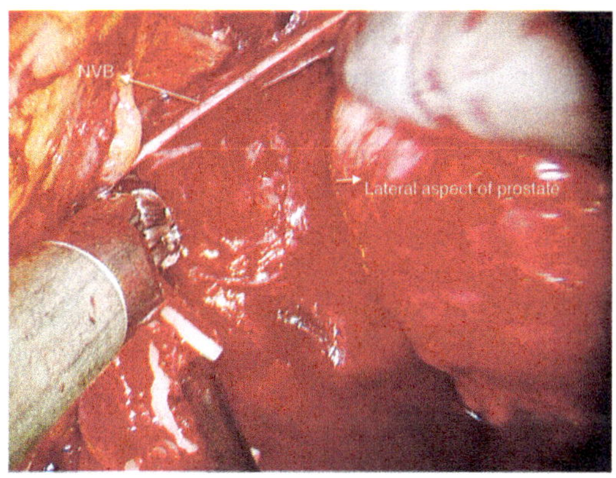

Fig. 6.5 Left antegrade dissection towards apex of prostate with minimized traction on NVB

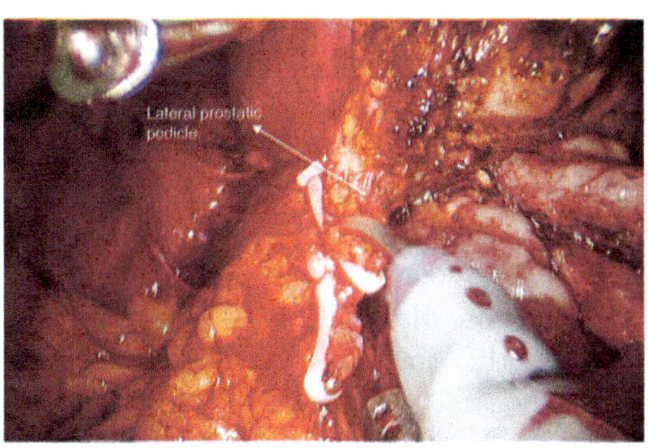

Fig. 6.4 Clipping and cutting of prostate pedicles without injury to NVB

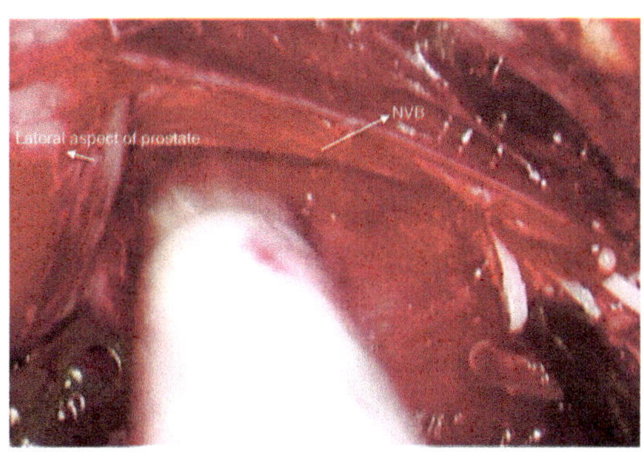

Fig. 6.6 Right antegrade dissection towards apex of prostate with assistant's suction stabilizing NVB

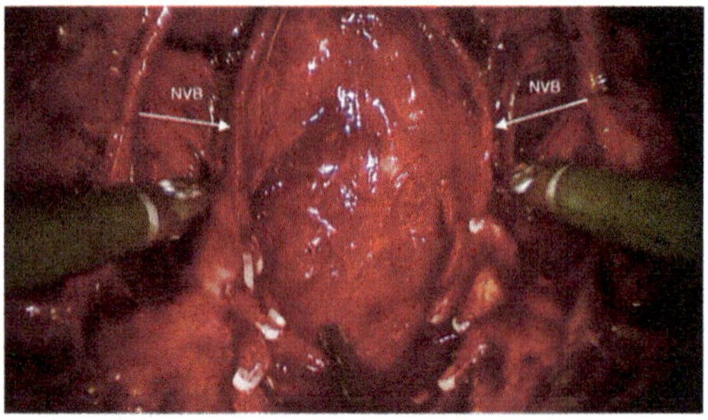

Fig. 6.7 Bilateral preserved NVB coursing towards perineum

pearly areolar tissue between the prostate and the NVB. Thus, the prostate and the NVB can be gently and bloodlessly detached from each other, without the need for sharp dissection. Intraoperatively, the right plane of dissection is confirmed by the presence of a pink coloration on the prostate [45, 48].

2. Grade 4, near complete NS (75 %): After identification of LA, NS is performed using sharp dissection at a plane between the LA and the prostatic capsule across the NVB—not at the pearly areolar plane (as in complete NS). Intraoperatively, the right plane of dissection is confirmed by the presence of a strip of fat over the prostate with an absence of arterial vessels [45, 48].
3. Grade 3, partial NS (50 %): After identification of LA, the plane of NS is created at the artery's lateral aspect. Therefore, the LA is clipped at the level of the prostatic pedicle. Intraoperatively, the right plane of dissection is identified by the presence of a fat strip over the prostate, with the LA on the top [45, 48].
4. Grade 2, <50 %: After identification of LA, NS is performed several millimeters lateral to the artery, following the prostatic contour. Intraoperatively, the right plane of dissection is identified by the presence of a thick fat strip over the prostate, with arteries embedded [45, 48].
5. Grade 1, non-NS (0 %): A wide resection of the NVB is performed by sequentially clipping below the prostate across the NVB. The prostate is lifted up and only rotated when approximating the apex as the pelvis gets narrow and the NVB travels in the direction of perineum. Intraoperatively, the right plane of dissection is confirmed by the presence of the levator fascia, which is not incised [45, 48].

Recent Findings

In 133 consecutive patients undergoing RARP, we could identify LA in 73.3 % of the operated sides. The area of residual nerve tissue on the prostate specimen, when examined microscopically, was significantly lesser when the NS was performed medial to LA in comparison to lateral dissection (0 vs. 14 mm, $p<0.001$). Thus, we concluded that fine tailoring on the medial border of an LA could consistently result in complete or near complete NS [49].

In 133 consecutive patients undergoing RARP, we performed a standardized NS grading system based on intraoperative visual cues and the area of residual nerve tissue on prostatectomy specimen was compared with the intraoperative nerve sparing score (NSS). A higher NSS was significantly associated with a decreasing area of residual nerve tissue on prostatectomy specimens ($p<0.001$). Overall 9.02 % patients had a positive surgical margin (PSM). Side specific PSMs as per NSS were: NSS 5–3.6 %; NSS 4–7.5 %; NSS 3–16.7 %; NSS 2–5.7 %; NSS 1–0 % [45].

In 1111 consecutive patients (preoperatively Sexual Health Inventory score for Men, SHIM >21 and potent, undergoing bilateral full NS, with at least 12 months follow-up) after RARP, we reported our pentafecta outcomes (continence, potency, cancer cure, negative surgical margins, and no postoperative complications). Potency was defined as the ability to achieve and maintain satisfactory erections firm enough for sexual intercourse in >50 % attempts, with or without the use of PDE5 (score ≥4 on questions 2, 3, 5). Potency rates were evaluated using the SHIM questionnaire. We found pentafecta rate at 12 months was 70.8 % (continence—96.4 %, potency—89.8 %, biochemical recurrence free survival—96.4 %,no postoperative complications—93.4 %,negative surgical margins—90.7 %) [20].

In another series, 172 patients with antegrade NS RARP were compared with a propensity matched group of 172 with retrograde NS. All patients had preoperative SHIM score >21 and underwent bilateral NS. We used same criteria to evaluate potency rates as described above. We found that PSMs were similar in two groups (11.1 % vs. 6.9 % respectively, $p=0.19$). At 3.6 and 9 months, the potency rate was significantly higher in retrograde group (65 % vs. 80.8 % and 72.1 % vs. 90.1 %, and 85.3 % vs. 92.9 % respectively). Both groups had similar continence outcomes [16].

In recent series, we analyzed preoperative or intraoperative factors responsible for the early return of continence after RARP in 1229 patients. A self-administered validated questionnaire (Expanded Prostate Cancer Index Composite) was used for the assessment of continence status and time to recovery. The continence was found in 86.6 % of patients at 3 months after surgery. On multivariable Cox regression analysis, age and performance of NS were significant predictors of postoperative continence. The median time to recovery of continence was prolonged in the non-nerve sparing group compared to nerve sparing counterparts at 6 (5.12–6.88), 4 (3.60–4.40), and 5 weeks (4.70–5.30) in the no nerve sparing, partial nerve sparing, and bilateral nerve sparing groups, respectively, with log rank $p<0.01$. Thus, we concluded that likelihood of postoperative urinary control was significantly higher in younger patients and when a NS procedure was performed [50].

Our Recent Innovations in NS RARP

Dehydrated Human Amniotic Membrane Allograft Nerve Wrap Around the Prostatic Neurovascular Bundle

Even in the most well-preserved neurovascular bundles (NVBs), there remains a convalescent period which is characterized by incontinence and impotency [51–53]. This delay is likely due to inflammatory response secondary traction related injury to NVB [54]. The physical traction that is placed on the NVB can be minimized by surgeon but it cannot be eliminated during mobilization of the prostate. We have been awaiting the next step of innovation that would go beyond the technical aspect of nerve sparing by reducing the inflammatory response produced by the nerve dissection. Dehydrated human amniotic membrane (dHAM) is a potential source of growth factors and cytokines that can be locally applied to facilitate neural recovery and reduce inflammation following surgical trauma. Amniotic tissue is harvested from eligible amnion donors, whom are subjected to screening processes approved by the FDA and American Association of Tissue Banks (AATB) standards to reduce the risk of serological cross infections [55–57]. We performed the first study involving 58 preoperatively potent (Sexual Health Inventory for Men (SHIM) score >19) and continent patients, who underwent full nerve sparing RALP, followed by intraoperative dHAM placement at our institution. They were propensity matched using our prospective database in matched, nongrafted patients from the same time period. Full nerve sparing surgery was performed as previously described using the retrograde athermal technique, with fully preserved neurovascular bundles. The dHAM allograft (Fig. 6.8) was cut into two longitudinal pieces and placed over each NVB as a "nerve wrap" (Fig. 6.9). The wrap was placed after the procedure was fully circumferential around the NVB, post-anastomosis (Fig. 6.10). At mean

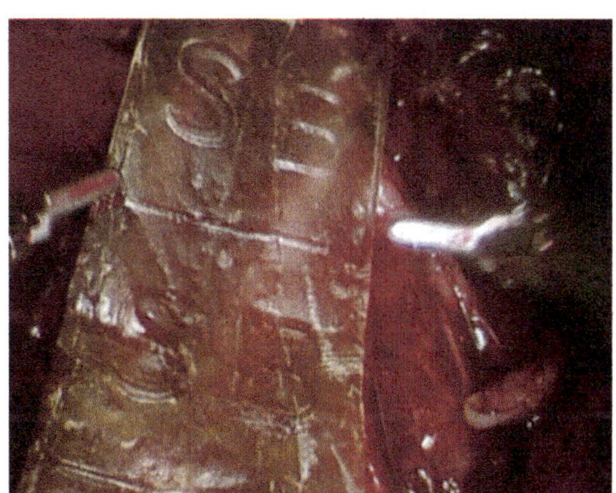

Fig. 6.8 DHAM allograft (AmnioFix®)

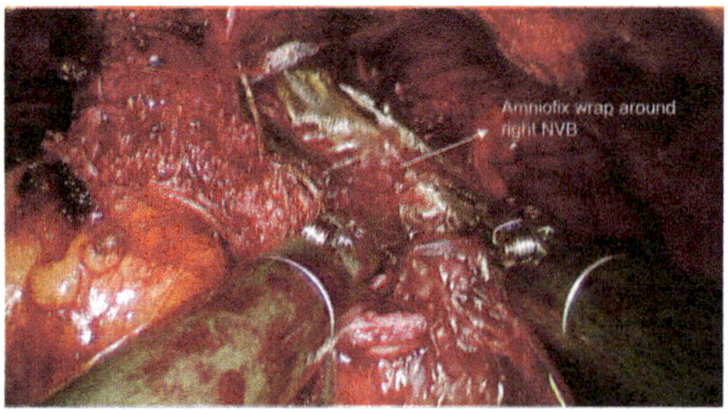

Fig. 6.9 AmnioFix placed over as right-sided nerve wrap on NVB

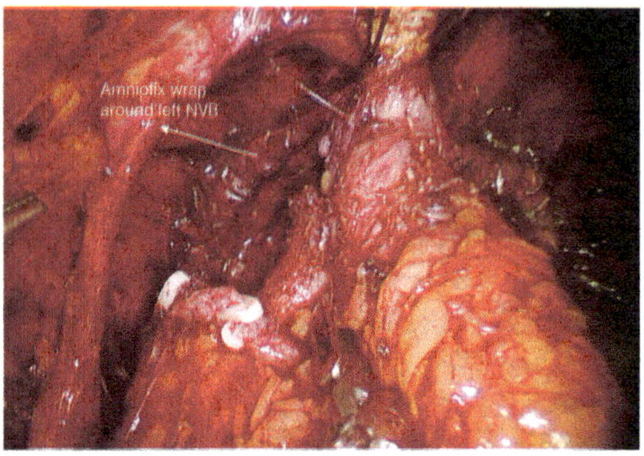

Fig. 6.10 AmnioFix placed over as left-sided nerve wrap on NVB

follow-up of 4 months, the mean time to potency and continence was significantly faster in the dHAM group in comparison to the non-dHAM group (1.21 months vs. 1.83 months, $p=0.03$ and 1.34 months vs. 3.39 months, $p=0.007$ respectively), with no adverse effects related to graft. Thus, we concluded that the use of dehydrated human amniotic membrane allograft appears to hasten the early return of continence and potency in patients following RARP (unpublished data).

Role of Indocyanine Green (ICG) Fluorescence in Visualization of the Prostatic Neurovasculature During RARP

We have earlier reported the role of LA in NS RARP [49]. However, identification of LA might be difficult for a novice surgeon and in patients with adverse anatomy. Here, the innovative intraoperative imaging like Firefly® fluorescence technology uses a new illuminator integrated with infrared laser, a new camera and endoscope compatible with fluorescence and enhanced user interface at console.

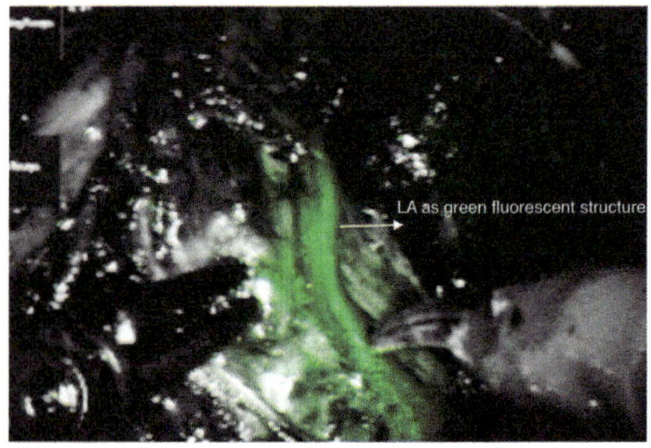

Fig. 6.11 Landmark artery seen as green fluorescent structure over lateral surface of prostate in firefly mode

We performed the first ever prospective case series examining the effectiveness of ICG fluorescence and Firefly® technology in identifying the prostatic artery during ten cases of NS RARP. First, indocyanine green dye is injected intravenously in patient, which is carried by albumin in blood to target vascular site. Then, the infrared laser from illuminator causes indocyanine green dye to emit fluorescence, picked up by endoscope and carried to console, where the surgeon visualizes that structure as green fluorescent structure. During nerve sparing, 0.75 ml of ICG was given initially by the anesthetist intravenously, with additional fixed doses directed into the intravenous catheter until optimal intraoperative fluorescence was achieved. Once indocyanine green dye was given intravenously and firefly mode was activated, we could appreciate the location and pathway of artery as green fluorescent vessel over lateral surface of the prostate (Fig. 6.11). Once LA and course of NVB (Fig. 6.12) were identified, NS was performed as described earlier. In some patients, this technology helped us in revising our plane of NVB dissection (Fig. 6.13a, b). We could identify landmark artery and its pathway in 85 % cases. In three patients, the artery was present underneath large veins and could not be identified. The use of indocyanine green dye resulted in neither an increase in operating time nor any immediate and long-term complications. Therefore, we concluded that indocyanine green and firefly technology during nerve sparing robotic radical prostatectomy has potential to identify landmark artery accurately and frequently. Identification of this artery and its pathway helps both experienced and novice surgeons in neurovascular bundle preservation, thus improving the quality of nerve sparing. However, further prospective studies are required to validate this novel technology.

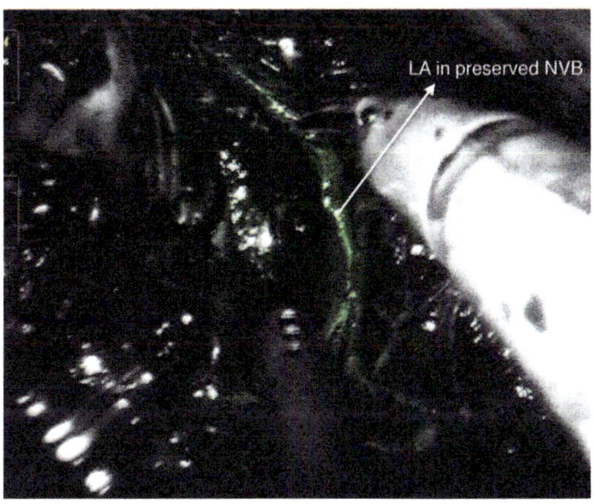

Fig. 6.12 LA in medial aspect of preserved NVB

Other Innovations to Improve Identification of the Landmark Artery or Prevent the Neuropraxia

Hypothermic NS Robot-Assisted Laparoscopic Prostatectomy (hRLP)

Finley and Ahlering et al. reported the first application of preemptive local hypothermia during RARP [25]. They hypothesized that inflammation of the bladder and sphincter mechanism secondary to dissection of the prostate and bladder (surgically induced acute injury to nerves and muscles) can cause transient incontinence. Therefore, local hypothermia to the pelvis prepares tissue for damage by lowering their metabolic rate and oxygen demands. As a result, less lactate formation occurs, protein synthesis is preserved and thus blunting the inflammatory response of surgery to surrounding nerves and muscles. Local hypothermia was achieved by devising an endorectal cooling balloon system (ECB), extending from the membranous urethra to the SV. A 40 cm, 24 Fr, three way latex urethral catheter was placed inside an elliptic latex balloon. The lubricated ECB was inserted inside the anus and anchored by inflating the catheter balloon to 20 ml. Pelvic cooling was achieved using cold irrigation and an ECB cycled with 4 °C. The intracorporeal temperatures were measured using a 9 Fr esophageal probe directly along the anterior surface of rectum/NVB.

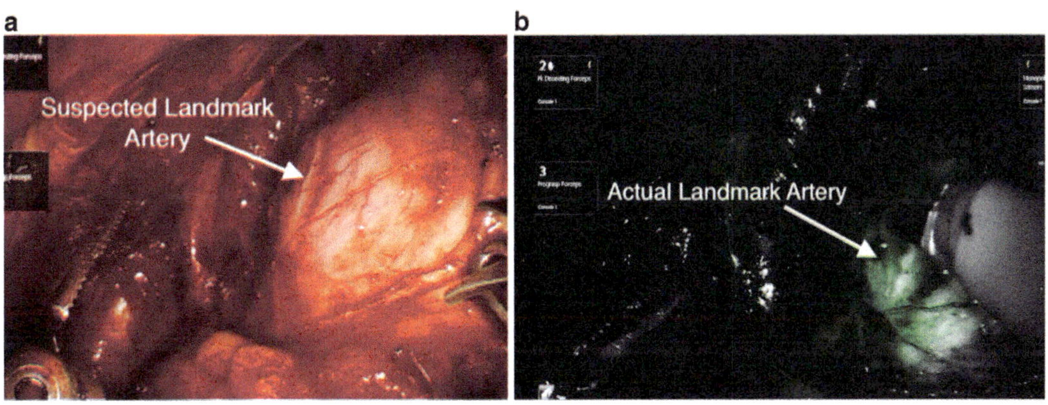

Fig. 6.13 (**a**) Suspected landmark artery in normal mode. (**b**) Actual LA in firefly mode, thus helping in revision of plane of NVB dissection

The 50 consecutive patients undergoing hRLP when compared with standard RARP showed statistically significant increase in the early postoperative continence ($p = 0.002$). However, the potency outcomes are still awaited.

Laparoscopic Doppler Ultrasound (LDU) Probe in NS RARP

A 20 mHz LDU probe was introduced into the pelvis through the 12 mm assistant port, and it was then manipulated by the console surgeon using a robot needle driver. The probe was placed upon six prespecified locations of NVB—the base, mid-gland, and apex of the prostate bilaterally, in order to trace its course along posterolateral aspects of the prostate. The arterial flow at 6 locations was measured and four independent reviewers evaluated signal intensity. Measurements were made before and after NVB dissection. In nine patients undergoing NSRARP using LDU, the plane of NVB dissection was altered in five patients (56 %) on the left and in four patients (44 %) on the right. At 8 months follow-up, seven (78 %) patients had recovery of erections. Badani et al. concluded that LDU was a safe, easy to use and effective method to identify NVB during RARP, and can potentially be used to achieve greater nerve preservation [58].

Potency Outcomes in Noncomparative and Comparative Series of RARP

Table 6.2 summarizes the potency outcomes of various series of RARP. Table 6.3 summarizes the potency outcomes in various series comparing RARP with open radical prostatectomy (ORP) and laparoscopic radical prostatectomy (LRP). These series have different inclusion criteria of patients, methods of evaluation of potency, NS techniques, surgeon's experience, and follow-up [6, 16, 17, 19–23, 59]. Although there is no standardized definition of potency but most of high volume centers series have defined potency as "Adequate erection sufficient for intercourse, with or without use of PDE 5 inhibitors." Various series, including meta-analysis studies, have shown better potency rates in RARP as compared to ORP and LRP [7, 10–13, 60–62].

Conclusions

RARP has become a standardized treatment for localized prostate cancer providing better functional outcomes and at least comparable oncological outcomes, in comparison to open and laparoscopic approaches. The patient's age, preoperative potency status, and extent of NS are the important predictors of postoperative functional outcomes. Surgeon experience and surgical volume also play a large role. Bilateral NVB preservation is essential for providing better postoperative continence and potency outcomes, without compromising oncological outcomes. Although there are different NS techniques reported for RARP, careful patient selection, use of intraoperative clinical judgment, and tailored "customized" approach for each patient are required, when decision for nerve sparing is made. The next step is to further define the anatomy and to use imaging to allow us to better see the relationship between the cancers and the neurovascular structures. This will allow a better quantitative and qualitative NVB preservation. The use of anti-inflammatory and neuroregenerative agents is exciting as it attacks the problem of NVB injury at the cellular level. Future innovations hold the key to further improvements in the recovery of sexual function post-prostatectomy.

Table 6.2 Potency outcomes in noncomparative series of RARP

Study	*N*	Inclusion criteria	Definition of potency	NS technique	Mean age (years)	Follow-up	Potency rate (unilateral NS)	Potency rate (bilateral NS)	Potency rate (overall)
Ko et al. [16]	344	Preoperative SHIM >21, bilateral NS, minimum of 1 year follow-up	Adequate erection for intercourse in >50 % of attempts ± PDE 5 inhibitors	Antegrade NS:172 vs. retrograde NS:172	57.9 vs. 57.2	Minimum 1 year	–	3 Months—65 % vs. 80.8 % 6 Months—72.1 % vs. 90.1 % 9 Months—85.3 % vs. 92.9 %	–
Patel et al. [20]	332	Preoperative SHIM >21, bilateral NS, minimum of 1 year follow-up	Adequate erection for intercourse in >50 % of attempts ± PDE 5 inhibitors	Retrograde	58.5	Minimum 1 year	–	53.9 %—6 Weeks 68 %—3 Months 86.1 %—6 Months 89.8 %—1 Year	–
Patel et al. [21]	404	Preoperative SHIM >21, bilateral NS, minimum of 1 year follow-up	Adequate erection for intercourse in >50 % of attempts ± PDE 5 inhibitors	Retrograde	58	18 Months	–	53.5 %—6 Weeks 68.8 %—3 Months 91.5 %—6 Months 97.4 %—12 Months 96.6 %—18 Months	–
Ficarra et al. [6]	183	Consecutive patients with minimum follow-up of 5 years	Adequate erection for intercourse ± PDE 5 inhibitors	–	62.3	81.3 Months	–	–	10 %—3 Months 53 %—6 Months 82 %—12 Months
Kowalczyk et al. [19]	342-NS 0C Vs 268—NS C	Consecutive patients undergoing NS RARP	Adequate erection for intercourse ± PDE 5 inhibitors	Antegrade	59.6 vs. 57.9	12 Months	–	5 Months—45 % vs. 28.4 % 12 months—50 % vs. 54.1 %	–
Potdevin et al. [22]	147	Patients with bilateral NS and preoperative SHIM ≥20	Adequate erection for intercourse ± PDE 5 inhibitors	Retrograde (interfascial—77 vs. intrafascial—70)	58.5 vs. 58.7	9 Months	–	–	3 Months—16.67 % vs. 24.24 % 6 Months—43.75 % vs. 81.81 % 9 Months—66.67 % vs. 90.9 %
Alemozaffar et al. [17]	400	Consecutive patients undergoing RARP	Adequate erection for intercourse ± PDE 5 inhibitors	Retrograde	59.8	12 Months	–	–	5 Months—33.3 % 12 Months—59.3 %
Shikanov et al. [23]	813	Patients undergoing bilateral NS RARP	Adequate erection for intercourse ± PDE 5 inhibitors	Antegrade (extrafascial—110 vs. interfascial—703)	60 vs. 58.5	8 vs. 13 months	–	–	3 Months—22 % vs. 42 % 6 Months—34 % vs. 47 % 12 Months—40 % vs. 64 %
Menon et al. [59]	721	Preop SHIM > 17, with minimum 12 months follow-up	Adequate erection for intercourse ± PDE 5 inhibitors	Antegrade	60.2	12	–	79.2 %	79.2 %

NS-0C nerve sparing without assistant's countertraction, *NS-C* nerve sparing with assistant's countertraction, *PDE-5* phosphodiesterase-5

Table 6.3 Potency outcomes in comparative series of open (RRP), laparoscopic (LRP), and robotic (RARP) radical prostatectomy

Study	Comparison	*N*	Inclusion criteria	Definition of potency	NS technique	Mean age (years)	Follow-up	Potency rate (unilateral NS)	Potency rate (bilateral NS)	Potency rate (overall)
Porpiglia et al. [13]	RARP vs. LRP (RCT)	60 vs. 60	Consecutive patients with localized prostate cancer	IIEF-5 score >17	Antegrade	63.9 vs. 64.7	12 Months	–	–	80 % vs. 54.2 % (12 months)
Berge et al. [12]	LRP vs. RARP	210 vs. 210	Consecutive patients with localized prostate cancer	Adequate erection for intercourse ± PDE 5 inhibitors	Antegrade	61.7 vs. 61.7	36 Months	40.2 % vs. 45.9 % (at 36 months)	57.3 % vs. 61.3 % (at 36 months)	–
Willis et al. [10]	RARP vs. LRP	174 vs. 175	Consecutive patients with localized prostate cancer	Adequate erection for intercourse in last 4 weeks ± PDE 5 inhibitors	Antegrade	58.1 vs. 58.2	12 Months	–	–	3 Months—59.8 % vs. 42.2 % 6 Months—71.2 % vs. 51.3 % 12 Months—73.7 % vs. 66.2 %
Asimakopoulos et al. [11]	LRP vs. RARP	91 vs. 136	Age ≤70 years, clinically localized prostate cancer, preoperative potent, with bilateral NS	Adequate erection for intercourse in last 4 weeks ± PDE 5 inhibitors	Antegrade	63 vs. 60	18 Months vs. 21 months	–	–	66.2 % vs. 39.6 %
Ficarra et al. [60]	RRP vs. RARP	588 vs. 294	Consecutive patients with bilateral NS	11EF>17	Antegrade	61 vs. 61	12	–	49 % vs. 81 %	
Rocco et al. [61]	RRP vs. RARP	105 vs. 103	All patients	Adequate erection for intercourse in last 4 weeks ± PDE 5 inhibitors	Retrograde	63 vs. 63	12	–	–	41 % vs. 61 %
Krambeck et al. [62]	RRP vs. RARP	588 vs. 294		Adequate erection for intercourse in last 4 weeks ± PDE 5 inhibitors	–	61 vs. 61	12			62.8 % vs. 70 %

RRP open radical prostatectomy, *LRP* laparoscopic radical prostatectomy, *RARP* Robot-assisted radical prostatectomy, *IIEF* international index of erectile function, *PDE 5* phosphodiesterase-5

References

1. Minino AM, Smith BL. Deaths: preliminary data for 2000. Natl Vital Stat Rep. 2001;49:1–40.
2. Crawford ED. Epidemiology of prostate cancer. Urology. 2003;62:3–12.
3. Jani AB, Johnstone PA, Liauw SL, Master VA, Brawley OW. Age and grade trends in prostate cancer (1974–2003): a surveillance, epidemiology, and end results registry analysis. Am J Clin Oncol. 2008;31:375–8.
4. Edwards BK, Noone AM, Mariotto AB, et al. Annual report to the nation on the status of cancer, 1975-2010, featuring prevalence of comorbidity and impact on survival among persons with lung, colorectal, breast, or prostate cancer. Cancer. 2014;120(9):1290–314.
5. Ficarra V, Cavalleri S, Novara G, Aragona M, Artibani W. Evidence from robot-assisted laparoscopic radical prostatectomy: a systematic review. Eur Urol. 2007;51:45–56.
6. Ficarra V, Borghesi M, Suardi N, et al. Long-term evaluation of survival, continence and potency (SCP) outcomes after robot-assisted radical prostatectomy (RARP). BJU Int. 2013;112(3):338–45.
7. Ficarra V, Novara G, Artibani W, Cestari A, Galfano A, Graefen M, Guazzoni G, Guillonneau B, Menon M, Montorsi F, Patel V, Rassweiler J, Van Poppel H. Retropubic, laparoscopic, and robot-assisted radical prostatectomy: a systematic review and cumulative analysis of comparative studies. Eur Urol. 2009;55:1037–63.
8. Coelho RF, Rocco B, Patel MB. Retropubic, laparoscopic, and robot-assisted radical prostatectomy: a critical review of outcomes reported by high-volume centers. J Endourol. 2010;24(12):2003–15.
9. Park B, Kim W, Jeong BC, et al. Comparison of oncological and functional outcomes of pure versus robotic-assisted laparoscopic radical prostatectomy performed by a single surgeon. Scand J Urol. 2013;47(1):10–8.
10. Willis DL, Gonzalgo ML, Brotzman M, et al. Comparison of outcomes between pure laparoscopic vs robot-assisted laparoscopic radical prostatectomy: a study of comparative effectiveness based upon validated quality of life outcomes. BJU Int. 2012;109(6):898–905.
11. Asimakopoulos AD, Miano R, Di Lorenzo N, et al. Laparoscopic versus robot-assisted bilateral nerve-sparing radical prostatectomy comparison of pentafecta rates for a single surgeon. Surg Endosc. 2013;27(11):4297–304.
12. Berge V, Berg RE, Hoff JR, et al. A prospective study of transition from laparoscopic to robot-assisted radical prostatectomy: quality of life outcomes after 36-month follow-up. Urology. 2013;81(4):781–6.
13. Porpiglia F, Morra I, Lucci Chiarissi M, et al. Randomised controlled trial comparing laparoscopic and robot-assisted radical prostatectomy. Eur Urol. 2013;63(4):606–14.
14. Asimakopoulos AD, Pereira Fraga CT, Annino F, et al. Randomized comparison between laparoscopic and robot-assisted nerve-sparing radical prostatectomy. J Sex Med. 2011;8(5):1503–12.
15. Ficarra V, Novara G, Ahlering TE, et al. Systematic review and meta-analysis of studies reporting potency rates after robot-assisted radical prostatectomy. Eur Urol. 2012;62(3):418–30.
16. Ko YH, Coelho RF, Sivaraman A, et al. Retrograde versus antegrade nerve sparing during robot-assisted radical prostatectomy: which is better for achieving early functional recovery? Eur Urol. 2013;63(1):169–77.
17. Alemozaffar M, Duclos A, Hevelone ND, et al. Technical refinement and learning curve for attenuating neurapraxia during robotic-assisted radical prostatectomy to improve sexual function. Eur Urol. 2012;61(6):1222–8.
18. Ficarra V, Sooriakumaran P, Novara G, et al. Systematic review of methods for reporting combined outcomes after radical prostatectomy and proposal of a novel system: the survival, continence, and potency (SCP) classification. Eur Urol. 2012;61(3):541–8.
19. Kowalczyk KJ, Huang AC, Hevelone ND, et al. Stepwise approach for nerve sparing without countertraction during robot-assisted radical prostatectomy: technique and outcomes. Eur Urol. 2011;60(3):536–47.
20. Patel VR, Sivaraman A, Coelho RF, et al. Pentafecta: a new concept for reporting outcomes of robot-assisted laparoscopic radical prostatectomy. Eur Urol. 2011;59(5):702–7.
21. Patel VR, Coelho RF, Chauhan S, et al. Continence, potency and oncological outcomes after robotic-assisted radical prostatectomy: early trifecta results of a high-volume surgeon. BJU Int. 2010;106(5):696–702.
22. Potdevin L, Ercolani M, Jeong J, et al. Functional and oncologic outcomes comparing interfascial and intrafascial nerve sparing in robot-assisted laparoscopic radical prostatectomies. J Endourol. 2009;23(9):1479–84.
23. Shikanov S, Woo J, Al-Ahmadie H, et al. Extrafascial versus interfascial nerve-sparing technique for robotic-assisted laparoscopic prostatectomy: comparison of functional outcomes and positive surgical margins characteristics. Urology. 2009;74(3):611–6.
24. Orvieto MA, Coelho RF, Chauhan S, et al. Erectile dysfunction after robot-assisted radical prostatectomy. Expert Rev Anticancer Ther. 2010;10(5):747–54.
25. Finley DS, Osann K, Skarecky D, Ahlering TE. Hypothermic nerve-sparing radical prostatectomy: rationale, feasibility, and effect on early continence. Urology. 2009;73(4):691–6.
26. Seddon HJA. review of work on peripheral nerve injuries in Great Britain during World War II. J Nerv Ment Dis. 1948;108:160–8.
27. Takenaka A, Leung RA, Fujisawa M, Tewari AK. Anatomy of autonomic nerve component in the male pelvis: the new concept from a perspective for robotic nerve sparing radical prostatectomy. World J Urol. 2006;24(2):136–43.
28. Srivastava A, Chopra S, Pham A. Effect of a risk-stratified grade of nerve-sparing technique on early

return of continence after robot-assisted laparoscopic radical prostatectomy. Eur Urol. 2013;63(3):438–44.
29. Ludovico GM, Dachille G, Pagliarulo G, et al. Bilateral nerve sparing robotic-assisted radical prostatectomy is associated with faster continence recovery but not with erectile function recovery compared with retropubic open prostatectomy: the need for accurate selection of patients. Oncol Rep. 2013;29(6):2445–50.
30. Walsh PC, Donker PJ. Impotence following radical prostatectomy: insight into etiology and prevention. J Urol. 1982;128:492–7.
31. Eckhard C. Untersuchungen uber die Erection des beim Hunde. Anat Physiol. 1863;3:123–66.
32. Lepor H, Gregerman M, Crosby R, Mostofi FK, Walsh PC. Precise localization of the autonomic nerves from the pelvic plexus to the corpora cavernosa: a detailed anatomical study of the adult male pelvis. J Urol. 1985;133(2):207–12.
33. Quinlan DM, Epstein JI, Carter BS, Walsh PC. Sexual function following radical prostatectomy: influence of preservation of neurovascular bundles. J Urol. 1991;145(5):998–1002.
34. Costello AJ, Brooks M, Cole OJ. Anatomical studies of the neurovascular bundles and cavernosal nerves. BJU Int. 2004;94(7):1071–6.
35. Tewari A, Takenaka A, Mtui E, et al. The proximal neurovascular plate and the tri-zonal neural architecture around the prostate gland: importance in athermal robotic technique of nerve sparing prostatectomy. BJU Int. 2006;98(2):314–23.
36. Martinez-Pineiro L, Cansino JR, Sanchez C, et al. Laparoscopic radical prostatectomy. Differences between interfascial and intrafascial techniques. Eur Urol. 2006;5(suppl):331.
37. Stolzenburg JU, Schwalenberg T, Horn LC, et al. Anatomical landmarks of radical prostatectomy. Eur Urol. 2007;51(3):629–39.
38. Kiyoshima K, Yokomizo A, Yoshida T, et al. Anatomical features of peri-prostatic tissue and its surroundings: a histological analysis of 79 radical retropubic prostatectomy specimens. Jpn J Clin Oncol. 2004;34(8):463–8.
39. Martinez-Salamanca JI, Ramanathan R, Rao S. Second prize: pelvic neuroanatomy and innovative approaches to minimize nerve damage and maximize cancer control in patients undergoing robot-assisted radical prostatectomy. J Endourol. 2008;22(6):1137–46.
40. Carter S, Le JD, Hu JC. Anatomic and technical considerations for optimizing recovery of sexual function during robotic-assisted radical prostatectomy. Curr Opin Urol. 2013;23(1):88–94.
41. Chauhan S, Coelho RF, Rocco B, et al. Techniques of nerve sparing and potency outcomes following robot assisted laparoscopic prostatectomy. Int Braz J Urol. 2010;36:259–72.
42. Aherling TE, Eichel L, Chou D, et al. Feasibility study for robotic radical prostatectomy cautery free neurovascular bundle preservation. Urology. 2005;65(5):994–7.
43. Ahlering TE, Eichel L, Skarecky D, et al. Evaluation of long-term thermal injury using cautery during nerve sparing robotic prostatectomy. Urology. 2008;72(6):1371–4.
44. Gill IS, Ukimura O. Thermal energy-free laparoscopic nerve-sparing radical prostatectomy: one-year potency outcomes. Urology. 2007;70(2):309–14.
45. Schatloff O, Chauhan S, Sivaraman A, et al. Anatomic grading of nerve sparing during robot-assisted radical prostatectomy. Eur Urol. 2012;61(4):796–802.
46. Tewari AK, Srivastava A, Huang MW. Anatomical grades of nerve sparing: a risk-stratified approach to neural-hammock sparing during robot-assisted radical prostatectomy (RARP). BJU Int. 2011;108(6 Pt 2):984–92.
47. Tewari AK, Ali A, Metgud S, et al. Functional outcomes following robotic prostatectomy using athermal, traction free risk-stratified grades of nerve sparing. World J Urol. 2013;31(3):471–80.
48. Schatloff O, Chauhan S, Kameh D, et al. Cavernosal nerve preservation during robot assisted radical prostatectomy is a graded rather than all or none phenomenon: objective demonstration by assessment of residual nerve tissue on surgical specimens. Urology. 2012;79(3):596–600.
49. Patel VR, Schatloff O, Chauhan C, et al. The role of the prostatic vasculature as a landmark for nerve sparing during robot assisted radical prostatectomy. Eur Urol. 2012;61:571–6.
50. Ko YH, Coelho RF, Chauhan S, et al. Factors affecting return of continence 3 months after robot-assisted radical prostatectomy: analysis from a large, prospective data by a single surgeon. J Urol. 2012;187(1):190–4.
51. Steineck G, Helgesen F, Adolfsson J, Dickman PW, Johansson JE, Norlén BJ, Holmberg L. Quality of life after radical prostatectomy or watchful waiting. Scandinavian Prostatic Cancer Group Study Number 4.
52. Tewari A, Peabody JO, Fischer M, Sarle R, Vallancien G, Delmas V, Hassan M, Bansal A, Hemal AK, Guillonneau B, Menon M. An operative and anatomic study to help in nerve sparing during laparoscopic and robotic radical prostatectomy. Eur Urol. 2003;43(5):444–54.
53. Menon M, Kaul S, Bhandari A, Shrivastava A, Tewari A, Hemal A. Potency following robotic radical prostatectomy: a questionnaire based analysis of outcomes after conventional nerve sparing and prostatic fascia sparing techniques. J Urol. 2005;174(6):2291–6.
54. Liang H, Liang P, Xu Y, Wu J, Liang T, Xu X. DHAM-BMSC matrix promotes axonal regeneration and functional recovery after spinal cord injury in adult rats. J Neurotrauma. 2009;26(10):1745–57.
55. Fairbairn NG, Randolph MA, Redmond RW. The clinical applications of human amnion in plastic surgery. J Plast Reconstr Aesthet Surg. 2014;67(5):662–75.
56. Seo JH, Kim YH, Kim JS. Properties of the amniotic membrane may be applicable in cancer therapy. Med Hypotheses. 2008;70(4):812–4.

57. Amniofix® Dehydrated Human Amniotic Membrane Allograft. MiMedx. [Online]. www.mimedx.com/products. Accessed 10th Nov 2014.
58. Badani KK, Shapiro EY, Berg WT, et al. A pilot study of laparoscopic Doppler ultrasound probe to map arterial vascular flow within the neurovascular bundle during robot-assisted radical prostatectomy. Prostate Cancer. 2013;2013:810715.
59. Badani KK, Kaul S, Menon M. Evolution of robotic radical prostatectomy: assessment after 2766 procedures. Cancer. 2007;110:1951–8.
60. Ficcara V, Novara G, Fracalanza S, et al. A prospective non randomized trial comparing robot assisted laparoscopic and retropubic radical prostatectomy in one European institution. BJU Int. 2009;104:534–9.
61. Rocco B, Matel DV, Melegari S, et al. Robotic vs open prostatectomy in a laparoscopic naïve centre: a matched pair analysis. BJU Int. 2009;104(7):991–5.
62. Krambeck AE, DiMarco DS, Rangel LJ, et al. Radical prostatectomy for prostate adenocarcinoma: a matched comparison of open retropubic and robot assisted techniques. BJU Int. 2009;103:448–53.

7 Partial Neurovascular Bundle Sparing During Robot-Assisted Radical Prostatectomy

Marcelo A. Orvieto and Surena F. Matin

Introduction

Since the studies of Walsh et al. [1] on surgical anatomy of the prostate and his description of nerve sparing (NS) radical prostatectomy (RP), the purpose of the urologist has been to perform an oncologically effective surgical procedure while maintaining functional outcomes in the patient. Large series have reported adequate cancer control and urinary continence rates after RP [2, 3]. However, erectile dysfunction (ED) after RP is an ongoing challenge with well-recognized high incidence rates [4, 5].

The etiology of post-prostatectomy ED is multifactorial. Local changes to the vascular supply of the penis and neurovascular bundles are inherent to removal of the prostate. Additionally, direct injury to the neurovascular bundles (NVBs) may occur during RP due to several factors such as undue traction [6], damage from thermal energy [7], or direct transection of neural tissue during prostate excision [8]. The latter may occur due to unintentional damage of the NVB owed to the inherent difficulty recognizing its pathway. Conversely, the surgeon may deem unsafe to spare the NVB depending on the oncologic status of the patient. It is well accepted that a positive surgical margin (PSM) during RP increases the risk of biochemical recurrence [9] and NS surgery has in some cases been associated with an increased risk to develop a PSM, even in patients with organ-confined disease [10].

With the development of minimally invasive technology to perform RP coupled with a better understanding of surgical anatomy, urologic surgeons have now recognized that dissection and excision of the NVB is not an "all or nothing" condition. Instead, the unique layered-based organization of the NVB allows the surgeon gradation of NS based on patient's preoperative sexual function, location and extension of cancer as well as intraoperative findings during dissection of the NVB. This could provide the patient an increased possibility of return of sexual function without compromising oncologic efficacy. Moreover, even in patients with high-risk features of disease, the 15-year prostate cancer-specific mortality is only in the range of 15–25 % [11]. As such, high-risk patients who received a wide excision of their NVBs will likely have a long life probability to live with post RP ED.

In spite of the widespread acceptance amongst urologic surgeons performing robotic-assisted radical prostatectomy (RARP) procedures regarding the actual feasibility and potential benefits to performing incremental levels of dissection of the

M.A. Orvieto
Department of Urology, Clinica Alemana, Santiago, Chile
e-mail: morvieto@alemana.cl

S.F. Matin (✉)
MD Anderson Cancer Center, The University of Texas, Houston, TX, USA
e-mail: surmatin@mdanderson.org

J.W. Davis (ed.), *Robot-Assisted Radical Prostatectomy*, DOI 10.1007/978-3-319-32641-2_7

NVB, there is a paucity of well-designed studies assessing this subject. The aim of this chapter is to analyze the available literature regarding relevant anatomical background, technical aspects, and sexual outcomes after partial NS.

Materials and Methods

A MEDLINE search was performed between 2000 and 2015 using the keywords "radical prostatectomy," "neurovascular bundle," nerve sparing," "interfascial nerve sparing," "partial nerve sparing," "robot-assisted," "potency," and "outcomes." Additional hand search on landmark manuscripts and review articles concerning the topic was performed. Only studies published in English language were included.

Anatomic Landmarks of the NVB

The milestone studies from Walsh and Donker [1] using male fetuses and newborn cadavers, combined with a follow-up study form Lepor et al. on a male adult cadaver [12], paved the way to our current understanding of the course of the NVB, running on the dorsolateral aspect of the prostate. Moreover, these studies established that the corpora cavernosa of the penis were innervated by autonomic nerve branches arising from the hypogastric plexus that negotiate through the urogenital diaphragm in a posterolateral aspect to the urethra [1, 12].

Despite the dramatic improvement in postoperative recovery of EF since the reports from Walsh et al. post RP ED results remain highly variable and often unsatisfactory. This has led several authors to reassess and challenge the classic concept of the NVB as a tubular structure running on the dorsolateral aspect of the prostate [13–15]. Recent studies have recognized the presence of nerve packets within the NVB, some of them innervating structures other than the cavernosal tissue, as well as a more variable course (spray-like distribution) of these nerves along the prostatic capsule.

Studies from Costello et al. on human cadavers [15] demonstrated a dual configuration of nerves within the NVB (i.e., anterior and posterior branches). While the posterior aspect of the NVB closely courses in the dorsolateral aspect of the SVs, the anterior branches emerge from the hypogastric plexus to run along the posterolateral aspect of the SVs. Additionally, Costello proposed a "three-compartment" functional organization of the NVB: (1) An anterior portion (closest to the prostate) including mostly fibers innervating the prostate. (2) A posterior portion with mostly fibers supplying the rectum. (3) An in-between portion, comprising true cavernosal nerves. Thus, the nerve branches in charge of the erectile function are layered by neurovascular tissue, which may not be related to sexual function. These extraordinary results provide strong anatomical evidence to explain how patients undergoing partial NS are able to recover adequate erectile function after RALP. Similarly, Tewari et al. [13] provided further knowledge on the anatomic distribution of the NVB tissue from cadaveric studies and video analysis from 200 surgical procedures. In their studies, the authors described a "tri-zonal" configuration of the erectogenic neural tissue. In addition to the standard NVB (so-called predominant NVB by the authors), they described two additional areas where neural tissue for erection could be identified. A proximal neural plate (PNP), running posterolaterally to the bladder neck and the lateral to the tip of the seminal vesicles and accessory neural pathways (ANP), located both on the anterior/anterolateral and posterior aspect of the prostate. Furthermore, the authors recognized the presence of fatty tissue between the layers of the NVB. This landmark would provide the surgeon cues to develop planes with "incremental" levels of preservation of the NVB according the risk for ECE and location of cancer in each individual patient. Similarly, Ganzer et al. reported a highly variable distribution of the NVBs. However, the authors did not find a correlation between prostate size and distribution of the periprostatic nerves [16].

Prostatic Fascial Layers

The idea of dissecting the NVB at different fascial planes (i.e., intrafascial, interfascial, and extrafascial dissection) is not new and was first introduced by Weiss et al. three decades ago [17]. However, the introduction of laparoscopic and robotic prostatectomy has provided the urologic surgeon with excellent magnified vision in a rather bloodless surgical field, leading to improved ability to recognize different tissue planes and structures. Consequently, over the last decade there has been a bolstering interest among urologist to better understand the surgical anatomy of these tissue planes and develop technical modifications to the procedure in order to improve surgical outcomes. In order to fully understand these concepts, one must have a deep understanding of the distribution of the fascial layers investing the prostate.

The endopelvic fascia (EPF) refers to covering layers of connective tissue located in the intermediate area between the pelvic wall and pelvic viscera. The EPF is composed of multiple layers that fold around contiguous organs and attach laterally to the pelvic wall and musculature. Distally, at the level of the dorsal venous complex, a condensation of the fascial layers form the puboprostatic ligaments, providing connective tissue support to the membranous urethra. Laterally, the EPF condenses as it meets the fascia of the levators' ani muscles, (i.e., tendinous arch of the pelvis). At this level, the EPF divides into two layers; one to fold back and follow the prostate posteriorly, intimately bounded with the true prostatic capsule (i.e., prostatic fascia). A second layer also travels posteriorly remaining as an outer layer, in close proximity to muscle fibers of the levator ani. This outer layer (i.e., lateral pelvic fascia) runs adjacent to tips of the seminal vesicles and the autonomic fibers forming the NVB [18]. As such, an intrafascial plane of dissection would require developing a space between the prostatic capsule and prostatic fascia, allowing for maximal preservation of NVB tissue. An interfascial dissection entails developing a plane between the prostatic fascia and the lateral pelvic fascia. Posteriorly, this plane can be recognized as the avascular space between the prostatic fascia and the Denonvilliers' fascia. On the posterolateral aspect, Denonvilliers' fascia extends anteriorly, medial to most neural tissue encompassing the NVB. Hence full preservation of NVBs is accomplished with either intrafascial or interfascial dissection. Finally, an extrafascial plane of dissection will occur lateral to the lateral pelvic fascia, thus compromising the totality of the dorsolateral portion of the NVB.

The concept of partial NS is also debatable. Some authors have paralleled this to an interfascial dissection, while others have described it as a partial extrafascial dissection of the NVB [19]. Herein, the surgeon sharply dissects along the thickness of the NVB. In these cases, the NVB is partly damaged, as the lateral aspect of the prostate remains covered with a portion of neurovascular tissue. Whether the erectogenic nerves and thus erectile function is preserved in these cases will require functional, patient self-reported outcomes from controlled studies.

Nerve Sparing and Cancer Control

It seems reasonable to consider that wider excision of tissue around the prostate specimen will correlate with a decreased risk of a PSM. However, the literature shows conflicting results regarding this matter. Shikanov et al. compared their oncologic and functional outcomes between patients who underwent interfascial (IF) NVB dissection and extrafascial (EF) dissection. As expected, patients who were offered IF dissection had statistically significantly lower PSA level, preoperative Gleason score and clinical stage. In this setting, the authors found that the PSM rates between the groups were comparable. Moreover, the PSM rate in patients with ECE on final pathology was 23 % lower amongst patients who received an EF dissection compared to those who received IF dissection [20]. Previously, in a different report from the same group, Zorn et al. had shown a 52 % reduction in the incidence of posterolateral PSMs for those patients who received an EF dissection compared to those who did not [19].

Lavery et al. performing NS dissection in high-risk patients reported opposing results. The authors retrospectively reviewed the data from 146 patients with high-risk features according to D'Amico risk group stratification. Patients with biopsy-proven seminal vesicle invasion or clear ECE of tumor on MRI had wide excision of the neurovascular bundle on the affected side while the remaining patients underwent full NS (unilateral or bilateral). Intriguingly, they found a lower incidence of PSMs among patients who underwent a NS procedure (20 % for bilateral NS, 41 % for unilateral, 51 % for non-NS). The authors attributed these results to surgeon's experience performing the procedure, allowing accurate recognition of abnormally adherent tissue planes between the NVB and the prostate or the presence of a bulging prostatic capsule suggesting ECE of disease, leading to wider excision [21]. Similarly, Ward and colleagues reported a higher PSM rate for patients who underwent wide excision than for NS (42 % vs. 34 %), underscoring that tumor biology may play a more important role than the technical aspect of the procedure [22].

Technical Aspects to Perform Partial NS

Despite the advantages provided by the robotic platform with regard to improved visualization during RARP, coupled with better understanding on the anatomical distribution of the NVB, it is unclear whether the surgeon is able to perform the intended NS procedure according to his/her preoperative planning. Some groups have reported no correlation between their intent to perform a NS procedure and NVB thickness [23]. Conversely, an expert robotic surgeon recently reported a high correlation between his intended NS type during RARP and the histologic findings of residual neural tissue on the pathologic prostate specimen [24]. Still, the authors found more variability on the left (nondominant) side compared with the right. Similar findings regarding handedness of the surgeon and disparity with the amount of neural tissue resected were reported by Andino et al. [25]. These findings highlight the challenges associated with NS techniques, even in expert hands. A novice robotic surgeon should consider this variability when performing RARP as it may have implications on oncologic and potency results.

Several authors have reported points of technique during NVB dissection in an effort to help recognize landmark structures to aid the surgeon achieve the intended type of NS. Recently, Patel et al. described a novel method to perform partial or full NS based on the visual recognition of a landmark artery (LA) running on the course of the NVB [26, 27]. The authors analyzed 133 video cases of patients undergoing RARP with various types of NS procedures. They identified a reasonably consistent presence (73 %) of the LA. Further, the authors recognized that when dissection of the NVB was performed medial to this LA, the amount of residual nerve tissue left with the specimen was significantly less than when dissection was performed lateral to this LA (median (interquartile range) of 0 (0–3) mm^2 vs. 14 (9–25) mm^2; $p<0.001$, respectively). Utilizing this landmark artery, the authors developed a grading system (1–5) based on the location of dissection (medial vs. lateral to the LA) and the distance (in mm.) from the LA. This study did not assess the association between postoperative ED and the grade of NVB dissection. In a follow-up study utilizing the same grading system, the authors found that the intraoperative perception of the amount of nerve tissue spared by the surgeon correlated significantly with the amount of neural tissue found on the prostatectomy specimens as determined by the pathologist [28]. In a similar study, Tewari et al. [29] described a four-point grading scale of NVB dissection based on different anatomical landmarks (i.e., the posterolateral venous distribution and the periprostatic fascial planes).

These studies highlight that different degree of partial NS procedures can be achieved without negatively impacting on cancer control outcomes, when selected properly based on patients' individual oncologic status. Sohayda et al. recognized that, while approximately 50 % of the extracapsular extension (ECE) sites are located posterolaterally where dissection of the NVB takes place, the median amount of ECE was 1.1 mm., and the extent of ECE was <3 mm in 90 % of patients [30].

Nerve Sparing and Potency Outcomes

The lack of standardization when reporting potency outcomes by different institutions makes the results extremely challenging to compare. Some series utilize validated and others nonvalidated questionnaires while others present surgeon's reported data. Moreover, it is well recognized that sexual function outcomes may be affected by a myriad of variables other than the type of NS [31]. Finally, a consistent definition of potency recovery after RP is also lacking. As stated by Mulhall, a consensus panel is required to develop guidelines for defining and reporting EF outcomes after RP. Until then, available data reports have to be carefully analyzed understanding their deficiencies [32]. Table 7.1 summarizes available literature comparing potency outcomes between complete, partial, and non-NS procedures.

Conclusion

The development of minimally invasive technology to perform RP coupled with a better understanding of surgical anatomy has allowed urologists to develop a gradation of NS based on patient's preoperative sexual function, location and extension of cancer. This could provide the patient an increased probability of return of sexual function without compromising oncologic efficacy. This becomes particularly important considering that even in patients with high-risk features of disease, long-term prostate cancer-specific mortality is low, severely impacting on quality of life in this patient population. The surgeon performing RARP should be aware of the visual cues and points of technique than can allow him/her to deliver an oncologically safe surgical procedure with the least impairment on sexual function. Additional studies are needed to determine the true benefit of partial NS on preserving erectile function.

Table 7.1 A summary of available literature comparing potency outcomes between complete, partial, and non-NS procedures

Author	No. pts.	Comparison	Potency outcomes				Potency assessment
			Preop.	3 Months	6 Months	112 Months	
Shikanov et al. [20]	883	Interfascial Extrafascial	– –	42 % 22 %	47 % 34 %	64 % 40 %	Objective (UCLA-PCI)
Bradford et al. [23]	60	Bilateral Unilateral no NS		36.3 22.7 16	– – –	43.7 35 20.4	Objective EPIC (means)
Levinson et al. [33] (Lap)	313	Bilateral Unilateral no NS	75.3	30.9	38.6 – –	47.4 (64.3 %) – 10 %	Objective EPIC
Ko et al. [34]	122	Intrafascial Interfascial Wide resect	– – –	– – –	– – –	88.9 % 65.6 % 0 %	Subjective (Surgeon's assessed)
Zorn et al. [19]	92	Interfascial Partial EF Wide EF	– – –	47 % 35 % 11 %	65 % 53 % 11 %	80 % 67 % 11 %	Objective SHIM
Tewari [35]	1380	Grade 1 Grade 2 Grade 3 Grade 4	– –	– –	– –	92.4 % 81.4 % 66.3 % 58.7 %	Objective SHIM

Editor's Comments—Matin and Orvieto

In the 1990s, Christopher Wood designed a single center study at MD Anderson Cancer center to evaluate the sural nerve graft concept as a phase II randomized trial. Patients received unilateral nerve sparing plus contralateral non-nerve sparing with or without a sural nerve graft. Ultimately, the trial was reported as a negative result at the time of an interim analysis [36]. If you look at the details of the report, a number of patients were selected for unilateral nerve sparing surgery on the basis of three cores of cancer on one side—even if they were Gleason 3+3 to 3+4 range. In modern times, these are all performed with attempted bilateral nerve sparing, and the higher volume tumors are now imaged with endorectal coil MRI and also selected for bilateral nerve sparing if the images are normal or partial nerve sparing as reported by Matin and Orvieto if the images, clinical staging, or intraoperative findings are concerning for extra prostatic extension. Pugh et al. [37] looked at our MD Anderson Cancer Center experience with MRI imaging in intermediate risk and found that with an organ confined result on MRI and clinical T1c staging, then >95 % of cases were either pathologically organ confined or had at most 2 mm of extraprostatic extension from the capsule. Thus, the concept of incremental/partial nerve sparing with imaging has been popular in our center, and described by other authors as reviewed by Matin/Orvieto in the context of "graded" nerve sparing.

As a case example, a 74 year old presented to our center with a cT2a exam, PSA of 5.6, and 12 core biopsy showing eight cores of cancer, including two cores of Gleason 8 at the left mid and left apex biopsies. An MRI is shown in Fig. 7.1 supporting apical disease but organ confined. He had a SHIM score of 21 and AUA score of 8. He elected robotic surgery and was selected for right nerve sparing and left partial nerve sparing. The following Figs. 7.1, 7.2, 7.3, 7.4,

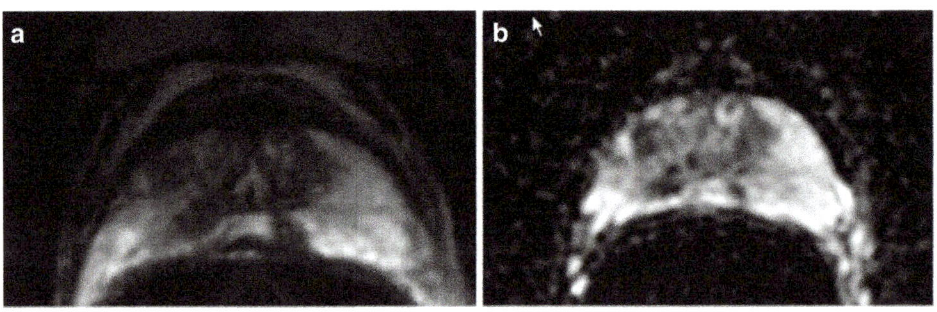

Fig. 7.1 (**a**, **b**) A T2 weighted endorectal coil MRI image shows an apical lesion (**a**) with restricted diffusion on the map (**b**). The image turned out to be a false negative with the finding of pT3a disease, but the margins were not compromised with partial excision planed based upon the cT2a exam and multi-core Gleason 8 biopsies

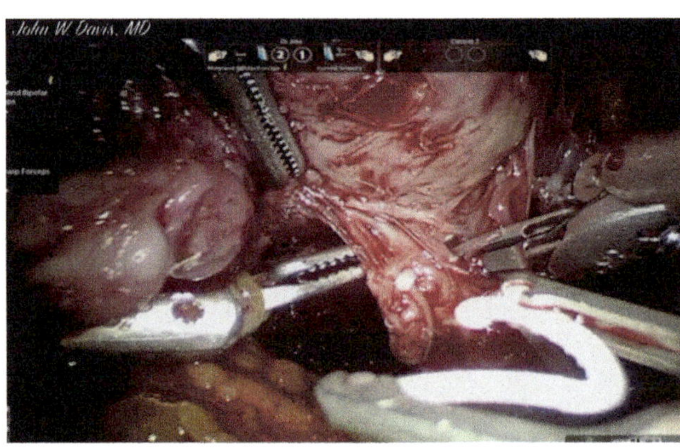

Fig. 7.2 The right nerve was spared and you can see the base capsular surface well defined as the pedicle is being clipped and divided

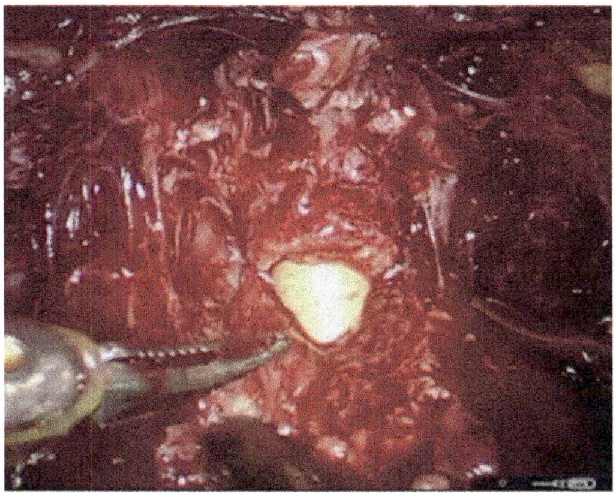

Fig. 7.3 In this case, we used a method of full mobilization of the prostate with the diseased side sequenced last. The DVC was divided and the urethra divided. This allows additional rotation and orientation to plan and execute the partial nerve spare on the left

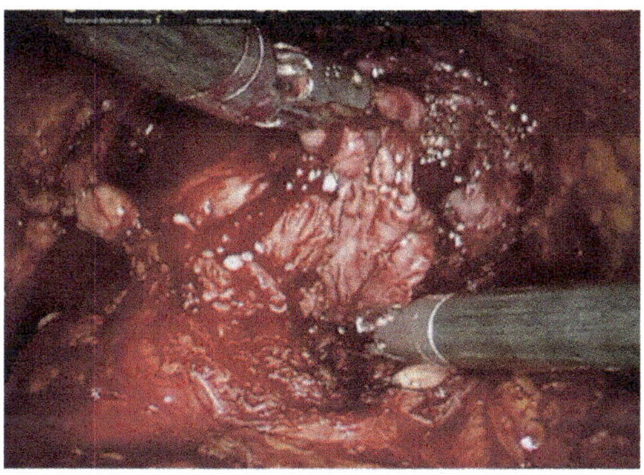

Fig. 7.4 The prostate can be rotated right and the left nerve spare setup

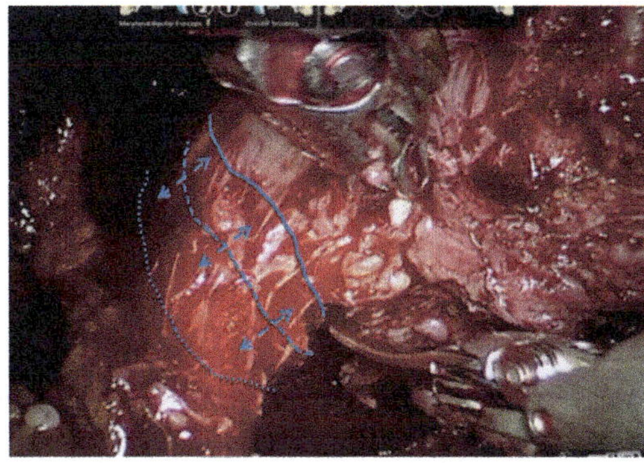

Fig. 7.5 The left partial nerve spare is exposed. The solid line would be a nerve sparing plane. The *dashed line* would be an incremental nerve spare with the *arrows* showing the discretionary amount of tissue that could be spared or taken depending upon imaging and surgeon judgment. The dotted line would the a non-nerve sparing plane

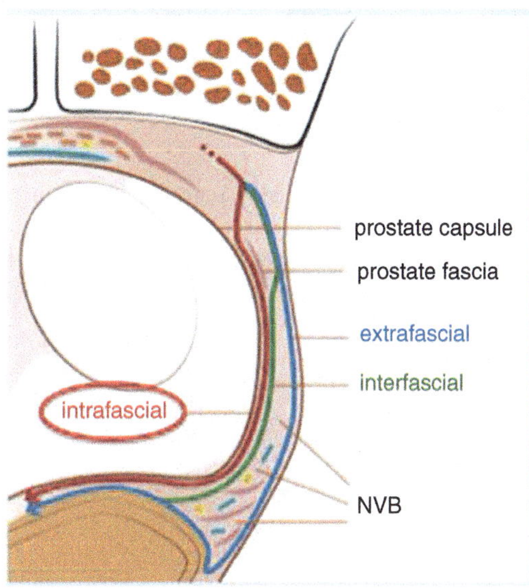

Fig. 7.6 Planes of nerve sparing from Salonia et al. [38]

7.5, 7.6, 7.7, 7.8, 7.9, and 7.10 demonstrate the surgical technique, imaging, and pathology. His surgical pathology showed pT3a Gleason 4+3, negative margins and nodes (22 total). He reached an undetectable PSA but by 9 months it rose to 0.5 at which time he elected salvage radiation therapy. He had recovered urinary continence prior to salvage radiation and maintained it but had not regained potency. He is disease free with additional 2 years of follow-up.

In summary, the modern approach to radical prostatectomy continues to emphasize maximal feasible nerve sparing to improve quality of life. Incremental nerve sparing is an option and imaging can assist. Full wide excision of a nerve bundle is less common than in the 1990s. An alternate approach is illustrated by the Martini group that uses near universal nerve sparing with frozen section analysis rather than imaging or nomograms with planed incremental nerve excision.

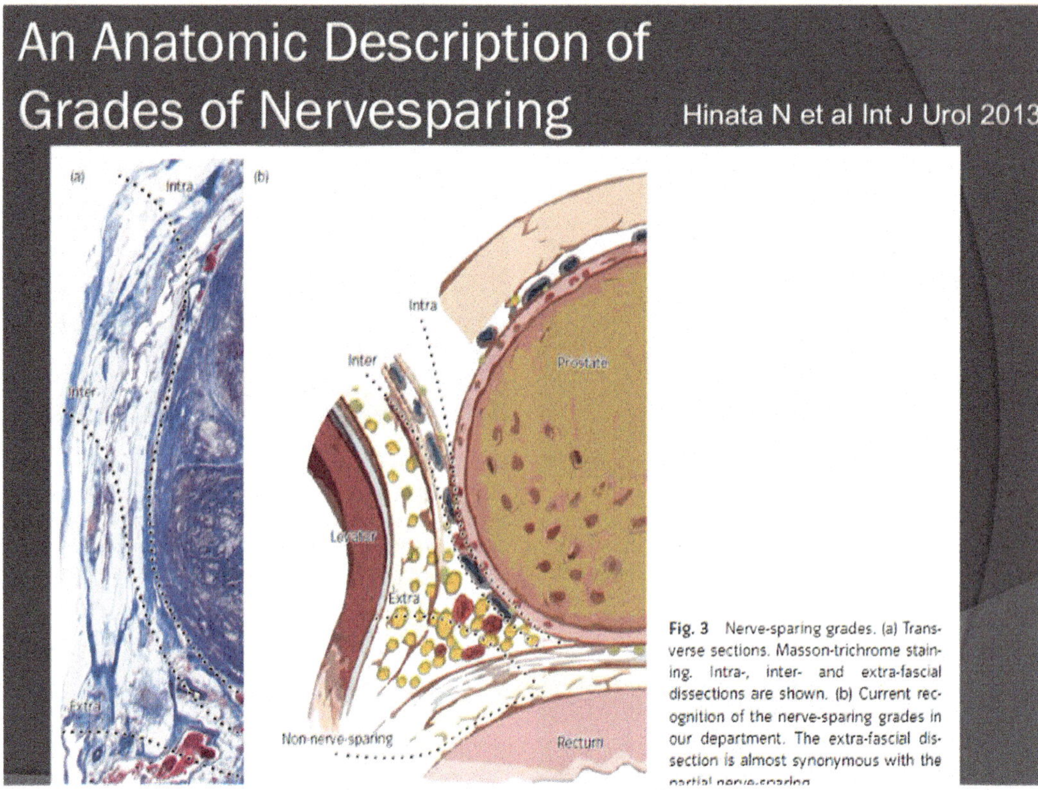

Fig. 7.7 Planes of nerve sparing as depicted by Hinata et al. [39]

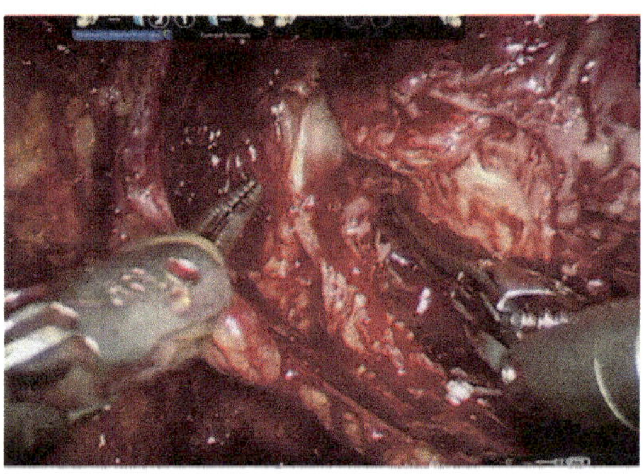

Fig. 7.8 The partial nerve sparing plane is sharply cut down and bleeders later oversewn or briefly sealed with the bipolar tip

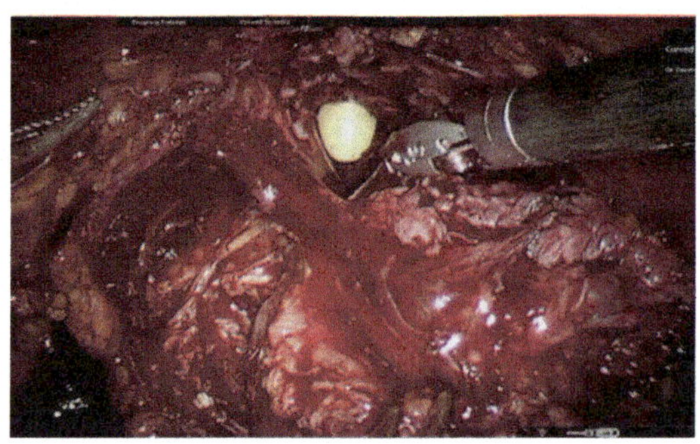

Fig. 7.9 With the DVC and urethra previously cut, the apex can rotate nicely and the partial plane maintained around the apical corner. The bundle of tissue at the tip of the scissor remains the last division before the gland is freed

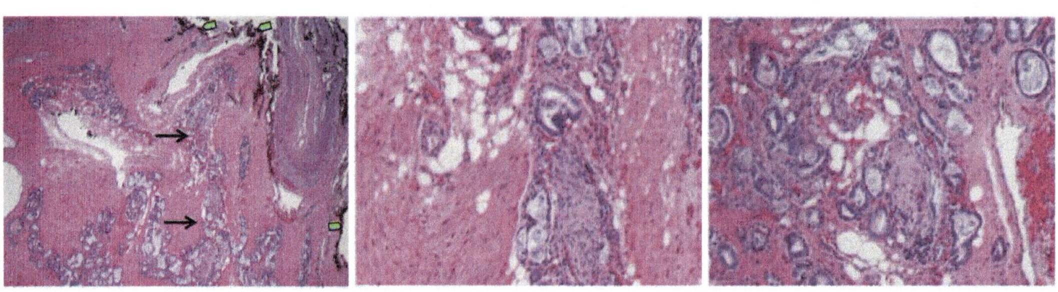

Fig. 7.10 The histopathology shows extraprostatic extension (*black arrows*) but not touching the inked margin (*green arrows*). Below—tumor cells touching fat are indicative of pT3a stage. Images courtesy Patricia Troncoso

References

1. Walsh PC, Donker PJ. Impotence following radical prostatectomy: insight into etiology and prevention. J Urol. 1982;128:492–7.
2. Han M, Partin AW, Pound CR, Epstein JI, Walsh PC. Long-term biochemical disease-free and cancer-specific survival following anatomic radical retropubic prostatectomy. The 15-year Johns Hopkins experience. Urol Clin North Am. 2001;28(3):555–65.
3. Bianco Jr FJ, Scardino PT, Eastham JA. Radical prostatectomy: long-term cancer control and recovery of sexual and urinary function ("trifecta"). Urology. 2005;66(5 Suppl):83–94.
4. Carlsson S, Drevin L, Loeb S, Widmark A, Franck Lissbrant I, Robinson D, Johansson E, Stattin P, Fransson P. Population-based study of long-term functional outcomes after prostate cancer treatment. BJU Int. 2015. Ahead of Print.
5. Montorsi F, McCullough A. Efficacy of sildenafil citrate in men with erectile dysfunction following radical prostatectomy: a systematic review of clinical data. J Sex Med. 2005;2(5):658–67.
6. Tewari A, Srivastava A, Sooriakumaran P, Grover S, Dorsey P, Leung R. Technique of traction-free nerve-sparing robotic prostatectomy: delicate tissue handling by real-time penile oxygen monitoring. Int J Impot Res. 2012;24(1):11–9.
7. Ahlering TE, Skarecky DW. Reserving sexual function after robotic radical prostatectomy: avoiding thermal energy near nerves. BJU Int. 2014;114(1):131–2.
8. Orvieto MA, Patel VR. Evolution of robot-assisted radical prostatectomy. Scand J Surg. 2009;98(2):76–88.
9. Orvieto MA, Alsikafi NF, Shalhav AL, et al. Impact of surgical margin status on long-term cancer control after radical prostatectomy. BJU Int. 2006;98:1199–203.
10. Preston MA, Breau RH, Lantz AG, Morash C, Gerridzen RG, Doucette S, Mallick R, Eastham JA, Cagiannos I. The association between nerve sparing and a positive surgical margin during radical prostatectomy. Urol Oncol. 2015;33(1):1810.
11. Eggener SE, Scardino PT, Walsh PC, Han M, Partin AW, Trock BJ, Feng Z, Wood DP, Eastham JA, Yossepowitch O, Rabah DM, Kattan MW, Yu C, Klein EA, Stephenson AJ. Predicting 15-year prostate cancer specific mortality after radical prostatectomy. J Urol. 2011;185(3):869–75.
12. Lepor H, Gregerman M, Crosby R, Mostofi FK, Walsh PC. Precise localization of the autonomic nerves from the pelvic plexus to the corpora cavernosa: a detailed anatomical study of the adult male pelvis. J Urol. 1985;133(2):207–12.
13. Tewari A, Takenaka A, Mtui E, et al. The proximal neurovascular plate and the tri-zonal neural architecture around the prostate gland: importance in the athermal robotic technique of nerve-sparing prostatectomy. BJU Int. 2006;98(2):314–23.
14. Takenaka A, Murakami G, Soga H, Han SH, Arai Y, Fujisawa M. Anatomical analysis of the neurovascular bundle supplying penile cavernous tissue to ensure a reliable nerve graft after radical prostatectomy. J Urol. 2004;172(3):1032–5.
15. Costello AJ, Brooks M, Cole OJ. Anatomical studies of the neurovascular bundle and cavernosal nerves. BJU Int. 2004;94(7):1071–6.
16. Ganzer R, Blana A, Stolzenburg JU, Rabenalt R, Fritsche HM, Wieland WF, Denzinger S. Nerve quantification and computerized planimetry to evaluate periprostatic nerve distribution-does size matter? Urology. 2009;74(2):398–403.
17. Weiss JP, Schlecker BA, Wein AJ, Hanno PM. Preservation of periprostatic autonomic nerves during total perineal prostatectomy by intrafascial dissection. Urology. 1985;26(2):160–3.
18. Stolzenburg JU, Schwalenberg T, Horn LC, Neuhaus J, Constantinides C, Liatsikos EN. Anatomical landmarks of radical prostatecomy. Eur Urol. 2007;51(3):629–39.
19. Zorn KC, Gofrit ON, Steinberg GP, Taxy JB, Zagaja GP, Shalhav AL. Planned nerve preservation to reduce positive surgical margins during robot-assisted laparoscopic radical prostatectomy. J Endourol. 2008;22(6):1303–9.
20. Shikanov S, Woo J, Al-Ahmadie H, Katz MH, Zagaja GP, Shalhav AL, Zorn KC. Extrafascial versus interfascial nerve-sparing technique for robotic-assisted laparoscopic prostatectomy: comparison of functional outcomes and positive surgical margins characteristics. Urology. 2009;74(3):611–6.
21. Lavery HJ, Nabizada-Pace F, Carlucci JR, Brajtbord JS, Samadi DB. Nerve-sparing robotic prostatectomy in preoperatively high-risk patients is safe and efficacious. Urol Oncol. 2012;30(1):26–32.
22. Ward JF, Zincke H, Bergstralh EJ, Slezak JM, Myers RP, Blute ML. The impact of surgical approach (nerve bundle preservation versus wide local excision) on surgical margins and biochemical recurrence following radical prostatectomy. J Urol. 2004;172(4 Pt 1):1328–32.
23. Bradford TJ, Weizer AZ, Gilbert SM, Dunn RL, Wojno K, Shah R, Wood DP. Is residual neurovascular tissue on prostatectomy specimens associated with surgeon intent at nerve-sparing and postoperative quality of life measures? Urol Oncol. 2010;28(5):487–91.
24. Kim KH, Rha KH. Pathological confirmation of nerve-sparing types performed during robot-assisted radical prostatectomy (RARP). BJU Int. 2013;111(3):367–8.
25. Andino L, Davis JW, Wei W, Prokhorova I, Troncoso P, Matin SF. Correlation of histomorphologic findings and partial neurovascular bundle preservation during laparoscopic and robotic radical prostatectomy. J R Soc. 2011. Online
26. Patel VR, Schatloff O, Chauhan S, Sivaraman A, Valero R, Coelho RF, Rocco B, Palmer KJ, Kameh D. The role of the prostatic vasculature as a landmark for nerve sparing during robot-assisted radical prostatectomy. Eur Urol. 2012;61(3):571–6.
27. Schatloff O, Chauhan S, Sivaraman A, Kameh D, Palmer KJ, Patel VR. Anatomic grading of nerve sparing during robot-assisted radical prostatectomy. Eur Urol. 2012;61(4):796–802.

28. Schatloff O, Chauhan S, Kameh D, Valero R, Ko YH, Sivaraman A, Coelho RF, Marquinez J, Palmer KJ, Patel VR. Cavernosal nerve preservation during robot-assisted radical prostatectomy is a graded rather than an all-or-none phenomenon: objective demonstration by assessment of residual nerve tissue on surgical specimens. Urology. 2012;79(3):596–600.
29. Tewari AK, Srivastava A, Huang MW, Robinson BD, Shevchuk MM, Durand M, Sooriakumaran P, Grover S, Yadav R, Mishra N, Mohan S, Brooks DC, Shaikh N, Khanna A, Leung R. Anatomical grades of nerve sparing: a risk-stratified approach to neural-hammock sparing during robot-assisted radical prostatectomy (RARP). BJU Int. 2011;108(6 Pt 2):984–92.
30. Sohayda C, Kupelian PA, Levin HS, Klein EA. Extent of extracapsular extension in localized prostate cancer. Urology. 2006;55(3):382–6.
31. Ayyathurai R, Manoharan M, Nieder AM, Kava B, Soloway MS. Factors affecting erectile function after radical retropubic prostatectomy: results from 1620 consecutive patients. BJU Int. 2008;101(7):833–6.
32. Mulhall JP. Defining and reporting erectile function outcomes after radical prostatectomy: challenges and misconceptions. J Urol. 2009;181(2):462–71.
33. Levinson AW, Pavlovich CP, Ward NT, Link RE, Mettee LZ, Su LM. Association of surgeon subjective characterization of nerve sparing quality with potency following laparoscopic radical prostatectomy. J Urol. 2008;179(4):1510–4.
34. Ko WJ, Hruby GW, Turk AT, Landman J, Badani KK. Pathological confirmation of nerve-sparing types performed during robot-assisted radical prostatectomy (RARP). BJU Int. 2013;111(3):451–8.
35. Tewari AK, Srivastava A, Huang MW, Robinson BD, Shevchuk MM, Durand M, et al. Anatomical grades of nerve sparing: a risk-stratified approach to neural-hammock sparing during robot-assisted radical prostatectomy (RARP). BJU Int. 2011;108(6 Pt 2):984–92
36. Davis JW, Chang DW, Chevray P, Wang R, Shen Y, Wen S, Pettaway CA, Pisters LL, Swanson DA, Madsen LT, Huber N, Troncoso P, Babaian RJ, Wood CG. Randomized phase II trial evaluation of erectile function after attempted unilateral cavernous nerve-sparing retropubic radical prostatectomy with versus without unilateral sural nerve grafting for clinically localized prostate cancer. Eur Urol. 2008;55(5):1135–43.
37. Pugh TJ, Frank SJ, Achim M, Kuban DA, Lee AK, Hoffman KE, McGuire SE, Swanson DA, Kudchadker R, Davis JW. Endorectal magnetic resonance imaging for predicting pathologic T3 disease in Gleason score 7 prostate cancer: Implications for prostate brachytherapy. Brachytherapy. 2013;12(3):204–9.
38. Salonia A, Burnett AL, Graefen M, et al. Prevention and management of postprostatectomy sexual dysfunction part 1: choosing the right patient at the right time for the right surgery. Eur Urol. 2012;62:261–72.
39. Hinata N, Sejima T, Takenaka A. Progress in pelvic anatomy from the viewpoint of radical prostatectomy. Int J Urol. 2013;20:260–70.

Neurovascular Structure-Adjacent Frozen-Section Examination (NeuroSAFE) in Robot-Assisted Radical Prostatectomy

8

Burkhard Beyer, Alexander Haese, and Markus Graefen

Frozen Sections in Radical Prostatectomy

The indication for a nerve-sparing modification at radical prostatectomy (NS-RP) remains under debate. The judgments on the quality of selection criteria for NS-RP are mainly based on the positive surgical margin rate. However, the efficacy of selection criteria are another important criteria in the way that as many patients as possible should be considered for an NS-RP as long as the margin rates are not compromised. Men with a preoperative low-risk constellation might present upgrading and upstaging in the final pathology, whereas patients with a clinically high-risk cancer might harbor pathologically organ-confined disease. Latter patients would have been eligible for a preservation of the neurovascular tissue.

Intraoperative performed frozen-section (IFS) analysis allows a histological assessment of surgical margins and enables the surgeon to decide to spare or to resect the neurovascular bundles during radical prostatectomy. In the current absence of adequate imagining techniques to identify microscopically positive margins, IFS are the only tools to unambiguously clarify the tumor status at the dissection plane. Commonly used in Urology as well as in other surgical specialties, they are available in most clinics. In prostate cancer surgery frozen sections are still not the general rule and are often not considered to be beneficial. Reasons behind the discordance in studies supporting frozen sections are small sample sizes, different indications for IFS, and the technique of collecting the IFS-samples itself.

Ye and coworkers investigated the role of IFS in prostatectomy on the urethral margin with snap biopsies of the urethral soft tissue on the resected prostate. They concluded that in a high volume center with respective cancer selection RPs are associated with a small rate of positive surgical margins and underline the limited value of IFS performed routinely [1]. Another study with 196 consecutive patients treated with laparoscopic radical prostatectomy recommends a snap biopsy based IFS only at the apical region of the prostate, but not at the neurovascular bundles or the bladder neck due to a low predictive value of this technique [2]. More recently, Kakiuchi and colleagues confirmed the lack of accuracy of small and randomly snap based IFS [3]. Without an adequate adjustment for these confounding factors, outcome analyses on occasional IFS are inherently biased.

In summary, studies that question the role of IFS are either based on snap-biopsies from the prostate surface suspicious for a positive margin or random samples from the prostatic bed. Considering the large area of the prostate adjacent

B. Beyer • A. Haese • M. Graefen (✉)
Martini-Clinic, Prostate Cancer Center, University Medical Center Hamburg-Eppendorf, Hamburg, Germany
e-mail: graefen@uke.de

J.W. Davis (ed.), *Robot-Assisted Radical Prostatectomy*, DOI 10.1007/978-3-319-32641-2_8

to the neurovascular bundle—frequently several square centimeters—it is evident, that random snap-biopsies in millimeter-dimensions are inadequate to assess the resection plane in its entity.

Studies that support IFS are those in whom large areas of the prostate were examined. Goharderakhshan et al. recommended wedge sections of the prostate in high-risk patients as they were able to show that it was possible to accurately predict the final surgical margin status [4]. Subsequently, wedge resection based IFS was also feasible and predictive in laparoscopic radical prostatectomy [5]. These results are now verified by newer studies analyzing IFS [6, 7].

The NeuroSAFE Approach

Schlomm and colleagues first introduced the complete neurovascular structure-adjacent frozen-section examination (NeuroSAFE) approach in 2012. In a chort of 11,069 consecutive patients who underwent radical prostatectomy between 2002 and 2011 was shown, that NeuroSAFE is an oncological safe technique and results in a significant increase in the rate of a nerve-sparing procedure and a reduction in the positive surgical margin rate (Fig. 8.1).

With the information received by the pathologist it is possible to convert a positive surgical margin during the procedure into a prognostic more favorable negative surgical margin by a secondary resection of the corresponding neurovascular bundle. In 2014 we introduced the NeuroSAFE-technique adaption for the robot-assisted approach [8].

Technique of NeuroSAFE in Robot-Assisted Radical Prostatectomy

Step 1: The Control of the Dorsal Vein Complex and Apical Dissection

Following the complete mobilization of the prostate and the preservation of the neurovascular tissue the intra-abdominal pressure is set up from 10 to 20 mmHg.

This largely prevents an increased blood loss from the dorsal vein complex. The bedside surgeon may use a small spongestick to additionally compress larger bleeding vessels and water irrigation via laparoscopic suction to keep a clear vision of the operative field.

After a urethral sphincter preparation in its full functional length, the prostate is separated from the sphincter. The anterior part of the urethra is transsected first to the transurethral catheter. The blocking balloon is deflated and the catheter is retracted until the tip becomes visible. Than the Maryland forceps in robotic arm number 2 picks up the catheter and lifts it towards the symphysis pubis. In addition the scrub nurse applies exterior traction to the catheter. With this maneuver the compression of the dorsal vein complex is maintained during the complete harvesting process when the intraabdominal pressure is zero.

Thereafter the dorsal part of the urethra is transsected using the scissors in arm #1 and the needleholder in arm #3.

Step 2: Removing the Prostatectomy Specimen

After complete separation of the prostate, the specimen is put into an endocatch bag, which is applied through a 12 mm assistant trocar and secured. The scissors (arm #1) and the needleholder (arm #3) are removed creating more freedom to act in the abdomen. Then the camera is also removed and the robotic arm is disconnected from the camera trocar.

All other arms from the patient cart stay connected to the trocars throughout the whole harvesting process. The Maryland forceps in arm #2 keeps its upward traction on the transurethral catheter. The thread of the endocatch bag is passed though to the 12 mm camera trocar in the umbilical region using a laparoscopic grasper. During this procedure the freehand-guided camera provides a clear vision.

The camera trocar is removed and the skin incision is extended semi-circularly around the umbilicus. This extension has to be adapted according to the size of the prostate specimen in the preoperative

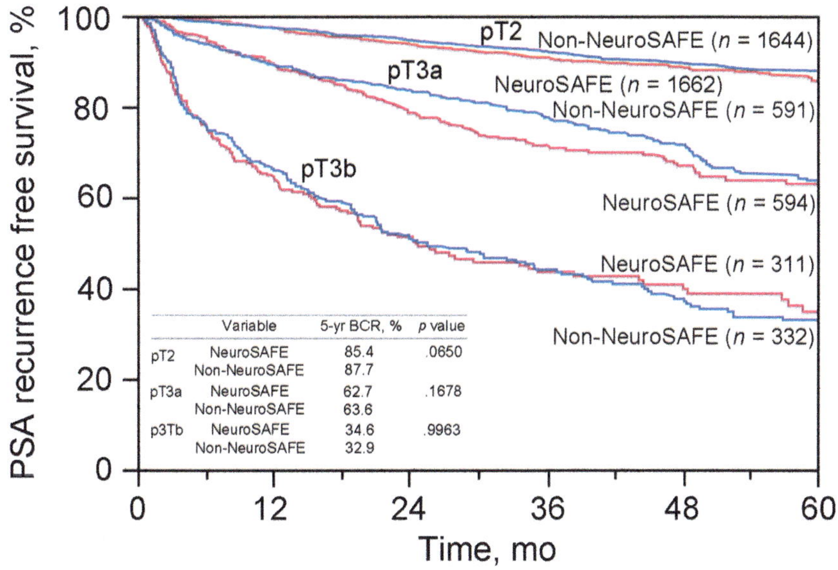

pT2	BCR NeuroSAFE	0	41	83	107	119	128
	BCR Non-NeuroSAFE	0	45	84	117	148	163
	At risk NeuroSAFE	1662	1358	989	667	427	253
	At risk Non-NeuroSAFE	1644	1492	1330	1171	1003	795
pT3a	BCR NeuroSAFE	0	61	111	136	145	150
	BCR Non-NeuroSAFE	0	62	90	116	137	158
	At risk NeuroSAFE	594	469	340	225	133	73
	At risk Non-NeuroSAFE	591	479	403	321	240	161
pT3b	BCR NeuroSAFE	0	101	130	142	146	150
	BCR Non-NeuroSAFE	0	108	150	166	178	186
	At risk NeuroSAFE	311	165	104	61	42	26
	At risk Non-NeuroSAFE	332	200	130	101	69	53

Fig. 8.1 Oncologic outcome of neurovascular structure-adjacent frozen-section examination (NeuroSAFE) and non-NeuroSAFE patients

assessment. Afterwards subcutaneous tissue and the transversal fascia are divided under direct vision and digital control to prevent intestinal injuries. The bedside surgeon lifts up the abdominal wall with Langenbeck retractors. Then the prostatectomy specimen is securely removed.

Institutions that use trocar devices like Alexis™ Port or GelPort® can extend the incision as a first step of surgery when placing the trocars. It was shown that these systems could make the harvesting process much easier and faster [9] (Fig. 8.2).

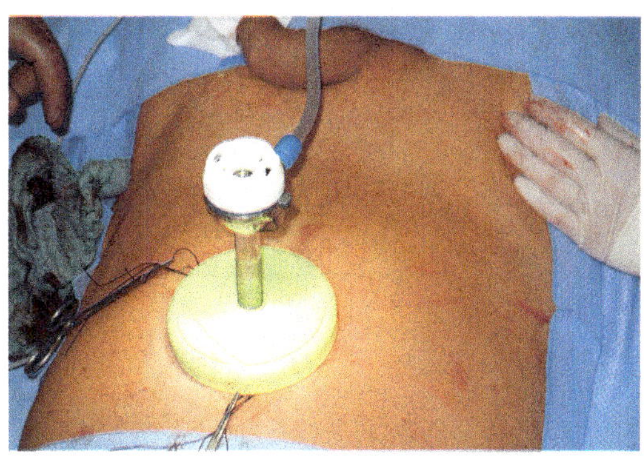

Fig. 8.2 Alexis™ Port for an easy intraoperative removal of the prostate

Step 3: Replacement of the Trocars and Reestablishing Pneumoperitoneum

After removal of the specimen a vicryl CT 1 running suture closes the transversal fascia under visual and digital guidance. The 12 mm camera trocar is replaced and the pneumoperitoneum is reestablished at 20 mmHg. To keep the trocar airtight traction is continued by placing Pean clamps on both sides of the suture. If a gas leakage occurs, the edges of the incision may be closed additionally with sharp towel clamps. When the camera trocar is in place the robotic arm can be re-docked.

Users of the previously described port systems can easily replace the cap and the trocar and reconnect the camera arm. To keep this process most effectively, it is preferable to prepare the fascial sutures when the port system is set in place at the beginning of surgery.

Step 4: NeuroSAFE Frozen-Section Analysis

While the pneumoperitoneum is reestablished, the surgeon performs a generous resection of the complete neurovascular structure-adjacent prostatic tissue as a wedge reaching from the apex to the base of the prostate on both sides. For a perfect anatomical orientation, the wedges are inked in different colors. The inner surface of the specimen is marked yellow and the apical site is marked with a red dot to facilitate the correct anatomical orientation. The outer surfaces on each side are inked in different colors as well. After sending the frozen sections to the department of pathology the hemostasis, dorsal reconstruction, and lymph node dissection is performed (Figs. 8.3 and 8.4).

According to the Stanford protocol, the wedges are processed in the department of pathology by cutting the specimen into thin slices of 3–4 mm. As a result all these tissue blocks are embedded in freezing media on top of a cryostamp and frozen at −25 °C. From each block two 6-mm cryosections are hemotoxylin and eosin stained, and reviewed by a genitourinary pathologist. After a processing time of 35–40 min the surgeon receives the results and details of the analysis. By definition a positive surgical margin is present if at least one malignant cell reaches the color inked resection plane.

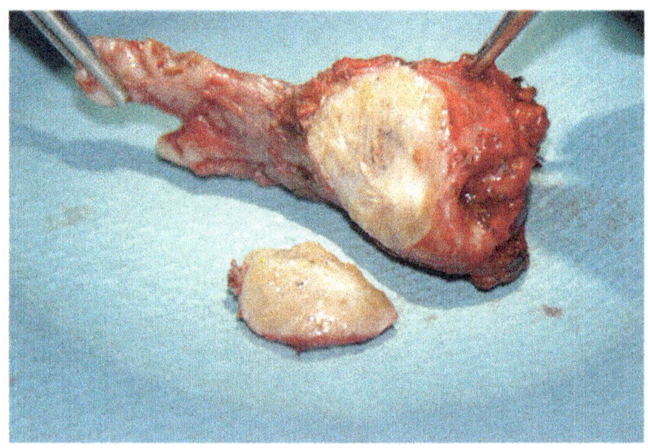

Fig. 8.3 Intraoperative view of neurovascular structure-adjacent frozen section examination section (whole wedge, apex to posterolateral)

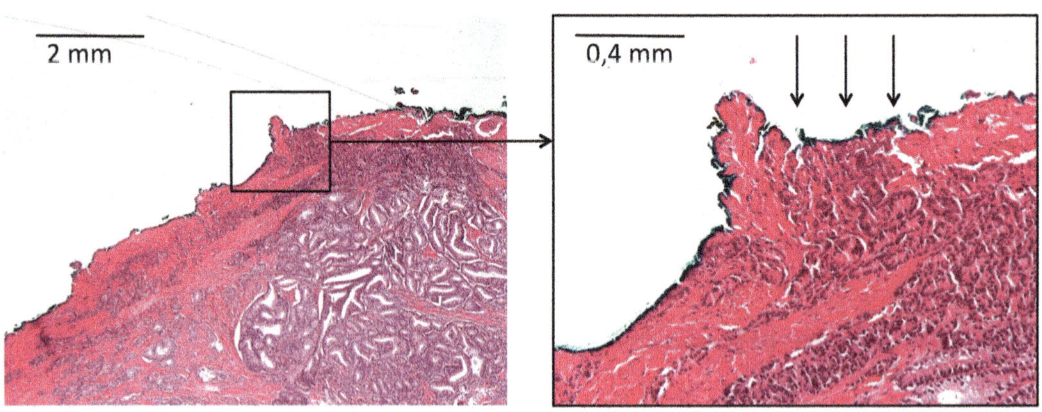

Fig. 8.4 Microscopic view of a hematoxylin and eosin-stained intraoperative frozen section prostate specimen, Gleason 3+4 with tumor contact at the inked surface

Step 5: Hemostasis, Dorsal Reconstruction, Lymph Node Dissection, and Anastomosis

When all instruments are in place again, the bedside surgeon cleans the surgical field with irrigation-suction device. If there is no such a system an alternative may be irrigation with a bladder syringe via the transurethral catheter.

Hemostasis of the dorsal vein complex (Santorinis plexus) is achieved by an interlocking 4/0 Vicryl suture. The preservation of the sphincteric muscle is of the utmost importance in this step. By reducing the intraabdominal pressure down to 5 mmHg, it becomes possible to check for persistent bleedings.

The decision to perform or to omit a lymph node dissection is based on a preoperative risk stratification (D'Amico) and the intraoperative findings when resecting the prostate. In general in patients with intermediate- and high-risk tumors an extended lymph node dissection is performed. Only in a low-risk situation (minimal tumor volume, PSA below 10 ng/ml and Gleason Score 3 + 3) a lymph node dissection can be omitted. The resected material can be collected via a 12 mm assistant trocar.

Furthermore the dorsal reconstruction of Denonvilliers Fascia according Rocco et al. [10] and the anastomosis of the bladder in van Velthovens technique [11] are performed.

The procedure is finished, if the pathological results reveal no tumor in the frozen sections. The instruments and trocars are removed under visual control and the closure of the wound is performed.

Secondary Resection of the Neurovascular Bundle

In those cases NeuroSAFE procedure uncovers a positive surgical margin, a secondary resection of the corresponding neurovascular bundle and the Denonvilliers fascia is performed on the respective side. If the anastomosis is already in place, the inflated catheter is pulled caudally to protect the anastomosis. Robotic arm number 3 is used to pull the urinary bladder away from the respective neurovascular bundle. The caudal and cranial aspects of the neurovascular bundles are identified and separated over Hem-o-lok® or small 5 mm titanium clips. Then the neurovascular bundle is completely released and removed.

Evaluation of NeuroSAFE-Technique

To evaluate the oncological impact of this technique it is crucial to compare the rate of nerve sparing procedures and positive surgical margins. In a cohort of 1040 patients it was possible to increase the rate of nerve sparing from 81.1 to 97.3 % ($p<0.0001$) independent of the tumor stage. Stratified into the different tumor stages the nerve-sparing rate was raised from 89.7 % up to 99.0 % in organ-confined tumors (pT2), from 74.2 to 94.1 % in pT3a tumors ($p<0.0005$). And even in pT3b tumors it was possible to increase the nerve-sparing rate from 30.2 to 90.9 % ($p<0.0001$).

A positive surgical margin is defined a contact of at least one single tumor cell with the inked surface of the surgical margin. In the same cohort it was possible to reduce the rate by 7.8–16.1 % ($p=0.0037$) across all tumor stages and in particular in pT2 tumors to 8.2 % (−6.7 %; $p=0.0068$) and in pT3a tumors to 22.0 % (−16.7 %; $p=0.0191$). In pT3b cancers the positive surgical margin rate was reduced by 18.5 % from 67.4 to 48.9 % ($p=0.0429$).

Looking at the secondary resected neurovascular tissue only in a small amount of cases (14–33 %) tumor cells were found in the resected specimen [6, 12]. Despite the fact that more neurovascular bundles are removed without revealing tumor involvement, this may be an additional safety gain for the patient as otherwise we would leave a positive surgical margin. In addition, the number of neurovascular bundles preserved exceeds the number of bundles resected substantially.

The NeuroSAFE procedure was not associated with an increased blood loss prolonged OR-time due to the harvesting of the prostate [8].

Possible Alternatives to NeuroSAFE

Preoperative Nomograms

Nomograms are easy-to-use methods for a statistical evaluation of posttreatment outcomes. Numerous preoperative models are known to predict an extracapsular extension of a tumor.

Most widely used are the Partin tables, in which biopsy Gleason grade, preoperative PSA, and clinical stage are used to predict the histological stage after prostatectomy [13]. One drawback of this method was the lack of a side-specific prediction of an extracapsular extension. As a result Graefen et al. introduced a model to predict a probability of a non-organ-confined tumor for each side by generating regression tree analysis [14]. Based on this work Steuber et al. generated a logistic regression based nomogram to predict a side-specific extracapsular extension [15].

Limitations of these calculations are impaired clinical practicability. On one hand, these nomograms give a realistic estimate what the surgeon or the patient can expect after surgery. On the other hand, nomograms evaluate only probabilities. This isn't feasible to perform an oncologic safe procedure with superior functional outcome. The true benefit of NeuroSAFE technique lies in the useful supplement of preoperative nomograms.

Multiparametric MRI of the Prostate

Several studies tried to predict an extracapsular extension with diverse imaging techniques preoperatively. Especially multiparametric MRI has emerged to improve the prediction most. Main problem of this technique is the lack of satisfying resolution of the images. Therefore it is often only possible to predict an established contact to the neurovascular bundle but not for a focal infiltration [16].

A new approach to combine intraoperative frozen sections with preoperative MRI findings was published by Petralia et al. By using a multiparametric MRI-directed frozen section, it was possible to reduce the risk of positive surgical margins after prostatectomy compared to control patients [17].

In 2011 Tewari et al. published a new risk-adapted technique for an anatomic optimal preservation of the neurovascular bundles, also using MRI findings.

Based on PSA value, biopsy Gleason grade, percentage of tumor in the biopsy, number of positive cores, presence of unilateral or bilateral positive cores, clinical stage, and multiparametric MRI (tumor location and volume, possible extracapsular extension) patients are selected to one out of five grades of an anatomical nerve sparing [18]. This resulted in higher potency rates without compromising cancer control.

Conclusion

Adapting NeuroSAFE-technique to robot-assisted radical prostatectomy is a cornerstone to oncological safety and minimal patient harm during surgery. Concerns regarding feasibility and OR-time should be a thing of the past. NeuroSAFE-technique enables histologic monitoring of the oncologic safety of nerve-sparing in real-time. It can significantly increase nerve-sparing frequency and decrease positive surgical margin rates (Fig. 8.5).

Nomograms and new imaging techniques have emerged the field of preoperative surgical planning. The multiparametric MRI for example starts to show a benefit for the evaluation of extracapsular extension or seminal vesicle infiltration. But as these techniques will always have a certain degree of uncertainty for the prediction of such adverse pathologic features intraoperative frozen section remain the only certain method to exclude avoidable positive margins.

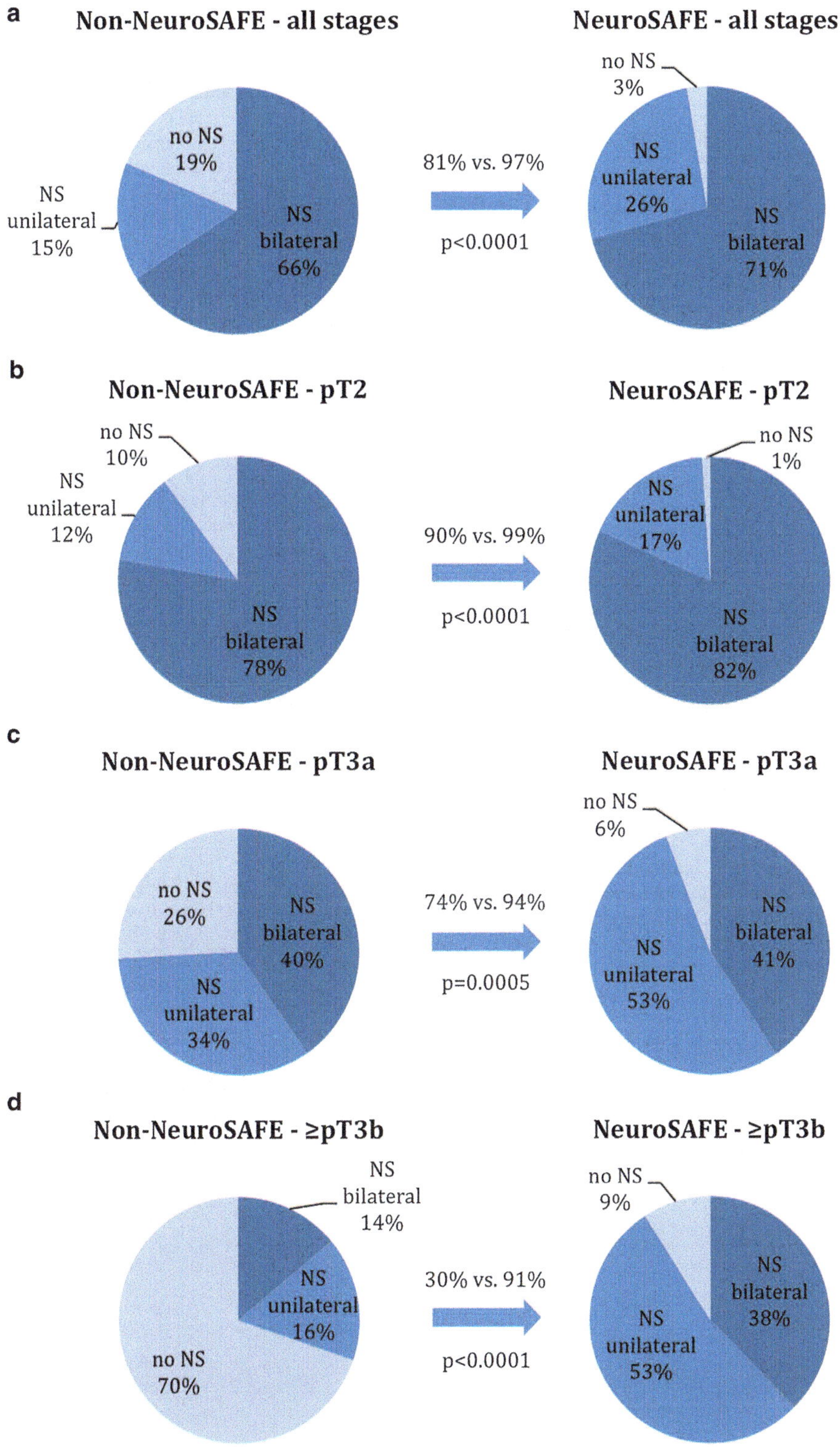

Fig. 8.5 Nerve-sparing (NS) rates with and without neurovascular structure-adjacent frozen section examination (NeuroSAFE) in (**a**) all stages, (**b**) pT2, (**c**) pT3a, and (**d**) IpT3b tumors

References

1. Ye H, Kong X, He TW, et al. Intraoperative frozen section analysis of urethral margin biopsies during radical prostatectomy. Urology. 2011;78(2):399–404.
2. Dillenburg W, Poulakis V, Witzsch U, et al. Laparoscopic radical prostatectomy: the value of intraoperative frozen sections. Eur Urol. 2005;48(4):614–21.
3. Kakiuchi Y, Choy B, Gordetsky J, et al. Role of frozen section analysis of surgical margins during robot-assisted laparoscopic radical prostatectomy: a 2608-case experience. Hum Pathol. 2013;44(8):1556–62.
4. Goharderakhshan RZ, Sudilovsky D, Carroll LA, Grossfeld GD, Marn R, Carroll PR. Utility of intraoperative frozen section analysis of surgical margins in region of neurovascular bundles at radical prostatectomy. Urology. 2002;59(5):709–14.
5. Fromont G, Baumert H, Cathelineau X, Rozet F, Validire P, Vallancien G. Intraoperative frozen section analysis during nerve sparing laparoscopic radical prostatectomy: feasibility study. J Urol. 2003;170(5):1843–6.
6. Schlomm T, Tennstedt P, Huxhold C, et al. Neurovascular structure-adjacent frozen-section examination (NeuroSAFE) increases nerve-sparing frequency and reduces positive surgical margins in open and robot-assisted laparoscopic radical prostatectomy: experience after 11,069 consecutive patients. Eur Urol. 2012;62(2):333–40. Epub 2012/05/18.
7. von Bodman C, Brock M, Roghmann F, et al. Intraoperative frozen section of the prostate decreases positive margin rate while ensuring nerve sparing procedure during radical prostatectomy. J Urol. 2013;190(2):515–20.
8. Beyer B, Schlomm T, Tennstedt P, et al. A feasible and time-efficient adaptation of NeuroSAFE for da Vinci Robot-assisted radical prostatectomy. Eur Urol. 2013. Epub 2014/01/15.
9. Almeida GL, Musi G, Mazzoleni F, et al. Intraoperative frozen pathology during robot-assisted laparoscopic radical prostatectomy: can ALEXIS trocar make it easy and fast? J Endourol. 2013;27(10):1213–7. Epub 2013/07/03.
10. Rocco B, Gregori A, Stener S, et al. Posterior reconstruction of the rhabdosphincter allows a rapid recovery of continence after transperitoneal videolaparoscopic radical prostatectomy. Eur Urol. 2007;51(4):996–1003.
11. Van Velthoven RF, Ahlering TE, Peltier A, Skarecky DW, Clayman RV. Technique for laparoscopic running urethrovesical anastomosis: the single knot method. Urology. 2003;61(4):699–702.
12. Eichelberg C, Erbersdobler A, Haese A, et al. Frozen section for the management of intraoperatively detected palpable tumor lesions during nerve-sparing scheduled radical prostatectomy. Eur Urol. 2006;49(6):1011–6. discussion 6-8.
13. Partin AW, Kattan MW, Subong EN, et al. Combination of prostate-specific antigen, clinical stage, and Gleason score to predict pathological stage of localized prostate cancer. A multi-institutional update. JAMA. 1997;277(18):1445–51. Epub 1997/05/14.
14. Graefen M, Haese A, Pichlmeier U, et al. A validated strategy for side specific prediction of organ confined prostate cancer: a tool to select for nerve sparing radical prostatectomy. J Urol. 2001;165(3):857–63. Epub 2001/02/15.
15. Steuber T, Graefen M, Haese A, et al. Validation of a nomogram for prediction of side specific extracapsular extension at radical prostatectomy. J Urol. 2006;175(3 Pt 1):939–44. discussion 44.
16. Feng TS, Sharif-Afshar AR, Smith SC, et al. Multiparametric magnetic resonance imaging localizes established extracapsular extension of prostate cancer. Urol Oncol. 2015;33(3):109 e15–22. Epub 2014/12/17.
17. Petralia G, Musi G, Padhani AR, et al. Robot-assisted radical prostatectomy: multiparametric MR imaging-directed intraoperative frozen-section analysis to reduce the rate of positive surgical margins. Radiology. 2015;274(2):434–44.
18. Tewari AK, Srivastava A, Huang MW, et al. Anatomical grades of nerve sparing: a risk-stratified approach to neural-hammock sparing during robot-assisted radical prostatectomy (RARP). BJU Int. 2011;108(6b):984–92.

The Neurovascular Bundle: Wide Excision

9

Kristen R. Scarpato and Joseph A. Smith Jr.

Introduction

The neurovascular bundle (NVB) is the subject of much discussion and debate in the urologic literature, instigated with the development of radical retropubic prostatectomy (RRP). There has been renewed interest in the NVB with the development of robotic-assisted radical prostatectomy (RARP), especially in low-to-intermediate risk disease, as urologists continue to strive for improved postoperative potency and urinary continence. However, in men with higher risk prostate cancer, preservation of the NVB is often not an option. This chapter will review the indications and complications of wide excisions of the NVB during RARP, relevant prostate anatomy, as well as discuss some of the potential advantages of a robot-assisted approach. As robotic technology advances and training improves, familiarity and skill with RARP have resulted in outcomes equal to and sometimes better than those seen with RRP.

Indications for Wide Excision of NVB

Not all men are candidates for nerve sparing procedures. Although the primary goal of RARP is complete cancer removal, positive margins may occur and are predictive of disease recurrence. Wide excision of the NVB to achieve negative margins is often appropriate for more advanced or high-grade tumors. In fact, urologists are more commonly performing RARP on high-risk patients while low-risk patients are often observed. Up to 20 % of those patients with high-risk features may experience a significant survival benefit following RARP [1].

For men who have already undergone treatment with either brachytherapy or external beam radiotherapy, salvage prostatectomy, in experienced hands, has been shown to be feasible in both open and robotic series [2–4]. Although the surgical technique for post-radiation surgery does not differ from that of the standard approach, the resultant destruction of tissue planes following radiation often necessitates wide excision of the NVB.

There are no existent guidelines for which patients require wide surgical excision. For many surgeons performing open RRP, the decision is based upon preoperative parameters and intraoperative haptic feedback while robotic surgeons often rely on preoperative parameters alone and more recently MRI findings. The National Comprehensive Cancer Network (NCCN) 2015 Prostate Cancer Guidelines comment on operative technique and adverse events noting that recovery of erectile function is dependent in part upon the degree of cavernosal nerve preservation but do not recommend for or against nerve sparing or wide excision in any particular patient populations [5].

There are various tools available to aid the surgeon with the decision between a nerve sparing procedure or wide excision of the neurovascular

K.R. Scarpato, M.D., M.P.H. (✉) • J.A. Smith Jr., M.D.
Urologic Surgery, Vanderbilt University Medical Center, 1161 21st Avenue South, Nashville, TN 37232, USA
e-mail: kristen.r.scarpato@vanderbilt.edu

J.W. Davis (ed.), *Robot-Assisted Radical Prostatectomy*, DOI 10.1007/978-3-319-32641-2_9

bundle. Tsuzuki et al. developed a predictive model for determining the probability of extracapsular extension (ECE) into the NVB based upon the following preoperative features: PSA, side-specific biopsy Gleason score and DRE, percent involvement of each positive core and percentage of side-specific cores positive for tumor [6]. This model was able to identify patients with a 10 % or greater probability of tumor extension into the neurovascular bundle and thus provides a parameter for preoperative surgical planning.

Increasingly, MRI is being used to predict the presence of extracapsular extension for surgical planning purposes, specifically in regards to the necessity of wide excision of the NVB. Park et al. assessed the accuracy of pre-RARP multiparametric 3.0T MRI in 353 patients and found a sensitivity of 55.9 % and specificity of 82.2 % for ECE [7]. Based on the author's findings, the initial surgical plan was altered after MRI review in 26 % of patients with accuracy above 90 %.

Complications of Wide Excision During RARP

Resecting widely around the prostate impacts disease recurrence, postoperative potency, and urinary continence. Several studies have examined the impact of wide excision of the NVB on prostate cancer outcomes [7, 8]. The oncologic benefit of wide NVB excision in the radical retropubic prostatectomy population was demonstrated in 221 consecutive patients who underwent wide excision on the side of positive biopsy [7]. Pathologic review revealed that overall 39 % of patients had extracapsular extension and 20 % had a positive surgical margin (PSM) involving the NVB, suggesting that optimal cancer control may require wide excision. Contrary to that, Ward et al. examined outcomes in 7268 men following radical prostatectomy over 10 years and found a positive surgical margin rate of 38 % overall, 42 % in nerve sparing procedures and 34 % after wide excision ($p \leq 0.001$). Disease extension into the region of the NVB does not necessarily translate into positive surgical margins, however. Hernandez et al. retrospectively reviewed 204 pathologic specimens with ECE around the NVB and found an overall PSM rate of 5.9 %. This rate was identical between two surgeons—one who widely excised the NVB in 16 % of patients and the other in 63 % [9]. Sofer further exemplified this in a study where he found the frequency of PSM is the same in nerve sparing (24 %) and non-nerve sparing (31 %) procedures ($p = 0.06$) [10]. More research regarding the impact of wide excision on cancer outcomes in needed.

The effect of both bilateral and unilateral non-nerve sparing procedures on potency has been extensively studied since Walsh's original description where he reported a potency rate of 83 % in patients with bilateral NVB preservation [11]. Prior to this, men undergoing RP were almost universally rendered impotent. Menon evaluated functional results following nerve sparing RARP with preservation of a veil of prostatic fascia in 2652 patients and found that 100 % of men with no preoperative erectile dysfunction who underwent bilateral veils were able to have intercourse at 48 months of follow-up [12]. This was further demonstrated in a feasibility study where preservation of the prostatic fascia in RARP resulted in 97 % potency at 12 months with 86 % of men reporting normal erections [13].

The degree to which preservation of the neurovascular bundle impacts urinary continence is not well described and the etiology of incontinence following wide excision is not clearly understood. Two recent studies sought to better elucidate this relationship. Steineck et al. prospectively evaluated data from 3379 men who had robotic or open radical prostatectomy and correlated degree of nerve preservation with urinary continence at 1 year as measured by patient-reported pad use [14]. A strong association was found between NVB preservation and urinary control, which held true in the elderly and impotent men. The relative risk (RR) of developing urinary incontinence after wide excision of the NVB was 2.4 with a 95 % CI 1.52–3.69 compared to bilateral intrafascial dissection with a RR 1.0. In a systematic review and meta-analysis including over 13,000 patients, bilateral nerve preservation was found to improve early urinary continence rates in the first 6 months following surgery but did not show a significant difference beyond that time frame [15].

Anatomy

It is critical for urologists to possess an excellent understanding of the peri-prostatic anatomic relationships and furthermore the potential implications of wide excision as discussed above. Walsh et al first described the surgical anatomy of the NVB and its relationship to sexual function following RRP in 1986 [11]. Since that time, numerous studies have tried to further elucidate the anatomy of the peri-prostatic tissues and their role in erectile function.

The prostate gland is an encapsulated, ovoid structure covered in a complex layer of endopelvic fascia containing nerves, vessels, and smooth muscle. The overlying fascia is contiguous with the prostatic capsule and covers the anterior and lateral surfaces. The lateral pelvic, or parietal layer of the endopelvic fascia houses the cavernosal nerves that run posterolaterally and are thought to be important for penile erections. The neurovascular bundle is located between the levator fascia and prostatic fascia—layers of the lateral pelvic fascia. Posteriorly, an extension of the peritoneum known as Denonvilliers fascia covers the prostate (Fig. 9.1).

Attempts at preservation of the prostatic fascia have furthered our understanding these complex fascial relationships, although there is still not uniform agreement on either the terminology or the anatomy of the periprostatic fascia [16]. Kaul et al. examined the feasibility of preserving the prostatic fascia in 35 RARP patients and found that this layer stains positive for smooth muscle and neural tissue but negative for PSA and therefore is indeed separate from the prostate [13]. In an effort to determine the nerve distribution along the prostatic capsule Eichelberg et al. evaluated permanent sections of 31 non-nerve sparing patients [17]. The authors found the majority of the NVB to be at the rectolateral side of the prostate between the 4 O'clock and 7 O'clock position while up to 25 % of the nerves were in a more ventral location. The neurovascular plate, as described by Tewari et al. via anatomical cadaveric studies and close attention to video-recorded procedures, can be found at a distance of 0–15 mm from the prostate depending on proximal to distal location [18].

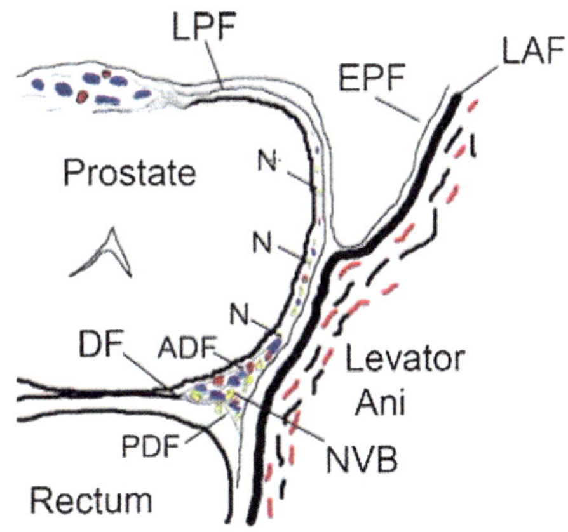

Fig. 9.1 Periprostatic tissue on the left aspect of the prostate—seen as transverse cut through the center of the prostate. *ADF* anterior lamina of Denonvilliers' fascia, *DF* Denonvilliers' fascia, *EPF* endopelvic fascia, *LAF* levator ani fascia, *LPF* lateral pelvic fascia, *N* nerves, *NVB* neurovascular bundle, *PDF* posterior lamina of Denonvilliers' fascia. World J Urol (2007) 25:31–38

Description of Procedure

The decision to proceed with wide excision during RARP is typically made preoperatively based on clinical parameters and more recently, prostatic MRI findings. Clear identification of the neurovascular bundle along the lateral prostate, even in non-nerve sparing procedures, can be beneficial. Generally, this occurs after the seminal vesicles are dissected and surgeon begins defining the posterior plane and developing the lateral pedicles.

The initial bladder neck incision should be wide to allow an adequate margin. The surgeon must then identify and secure the ureteral orifices to avoid unwanted injury. If they are not readily visible, anesthesia may administer methylene blue or indigo carmine to aid with identification.

For wide excision, the surgeon remains extrafascial, meaning posterior to Denonvilliers fascia along the perirectal fat while the lateral dissection incorporates the entire lateral pelvic fascia with its vascular and neural tissue from the apex to the seminal vesicle. Posteriorly, the fascia should be sharply incised, exposing the perirectal fat (Figs. 9.2 and 9.3). In the absence of tumor extension, this plane typically develops quite easily. As the lateral pedicles are being developed and the dissection proceeds apically, it is not

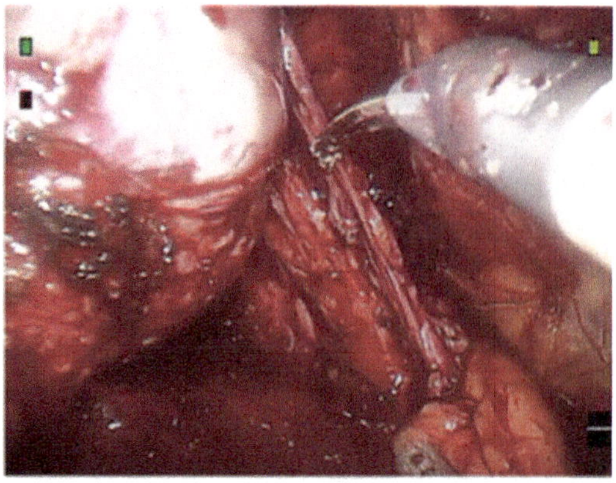

Fig. 9.2 Relationship of the right prostatic pedicle and neurovascular bundle. From Smith JA Jr, Howards SS, Preminger GM. (2012) Hinman's Atlas of Urologic Surgery 3rd Edition. Philadelphia: Saunders

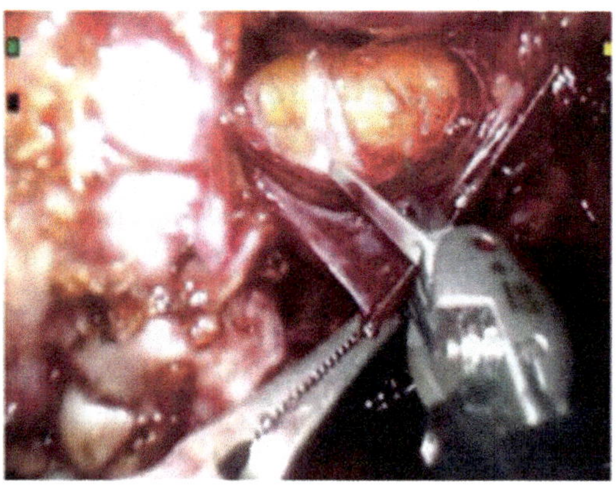

Fig. 9.3 Extrafascial dissection with incision through Denonvilliers fascia exposing perirectal fat. From Smith JA Jr, Tewari A. (2008). Robotics in urologic surgery. Philadelphia: Saunders

always necessary to use clips to control bleeding. In some settings, these pedicles may be taken down with bipolar or bovie electrocautery.

Often the two sides of the prostate are treated independently regarding their risk for ECE and therefore the need for wide excision. In patients undergoing unilateral nerve sparing procedures, the surgeon should adhere to the well-described principles of nerve sparing on the contralateral side. This includes meticulous anatomic dissection of the fascial layers with an attempt to remain intrafascial, limited or no electrocautery in the area of the NVB, and avoidance of excessive tension on the neural tissues.

Is There Value in Nerve Grafting Following with Wide Excision of NVB?

Sural nerve interposition grafting at the time of radical prostatectomy was introduced as a potential strategy for improving erectile function and urinary control following wide bilateral and unilateral NVB resection [19, 20]. Results in the literature regarding success of this procedure have been conflicting. Namiki et al. conducted a 3-year longitudinal study of 113 patients undergoing RRP with variable degrees of nerve sparing and found that interposition grafting can provide some benefit in recovery of erectile function and urinary continence [21]. However, a randomized phase II trial from MD Anderson evaluating erectile function using sural nerve grafting after unilateral cavernous nerve resection was stopped early for futility [22]. There are limited data regarding robotic sural nerve grafting at the time of RARP although early reports note that it is technically feasible [23, 24]. More studies are needed to elucidate whether or not reconstruction of these nerves is beneficial and what materials and techniques work best.

Conclusion

Wide excision of the neurovascular bundle is often warranted in patients undergoing RARP. The decision to remove this neural tissue is based on preoperative patient factors including findings on DRE, PSA value, Gleason grade, and more recently MRI findings. The urologist must be well versed in the complex fascial layers encasing the prostate and their relationship to the NVB. Attaining negative margins and achieving good oncologic outcomes remain the primary objective of RARP and patients must be adequately counseled on the known risks of wide excision on potency and continence as well as the risks of *not* proceeding with aggressive excision.

References

1. Pierorazio PM, Ross AE, Lin BM, et al. Preoperative characteristics of high-Gleason disease predictive of favourable pathological and clinical outcomes at radical prostatectomy. BJU Int. 2012;110:1122–8.
2. Chade DC, Shariat SF, Cronin AM, et al. Salvage radical prostatectomy for radiation-recurrent prostate cancer: a multi-institutional collaboration. Eur Urol. 2011;60:205–10.
3. Sanderson KM, Penson DF, Cai J, et al. Salvage radical prostatectomy: quality of life outcomes and long-term oncological control of radiorecurrent prostate cancer. J Urol. 2006;176:2025–32.
4. Eandi JA, Link BA, Nelson RA, et al. Robotic assisted laparoscopic salvage prostatectomy for radiation resistant prostate cancer. J Urol. 2010;183:133–7.
5. NCCN Clinical Practice Guidelines in Oncology: Prostate Cancer. www.nccn.org/professionals/physician_gls/pdf/prostate.pdf. Accessed 15 Dec 2014.
6. Tsuzuki T, Hernandez DJ, Aydin H, Trock B, Walsh PC, Epstein JI. Prediction of extraprostatic extension in the neurovascular bundle based on prostate needle biopsy pathology, serum prostate specific antigen and digital rectal examination. J Urol. 2005;173:450–3.
7. Park BH, Jeong HG, Jeong BC, et al. Influence of magnetic resonance imaging in the decision to preserve or resect neurovascular bundles at robotic assisted laparoscopic radical prostatectomy. J Urol. 2014;192:82–8.
8. Park EL, Dalkin B, Escobar C, Nagle RB. Site-specific positive margins at radical prostatectomy: assessing cancer-control benefits of wide excision of the neurovascular bundle on a side with cancer on biopsy. BJU Int. 2002;91:219–22.
9. Ward JF, Zincke H, Bergstralh EJ, et al. The impact of surgical approach (nerve bundle preservation versus wide local excision) on surgical margins and biochemical recurrence following radical prostatectomy. J Urol. 2004;172:1328–32.
10. Hernandez DJ, Epstein JI, Trock BJ, Tsuzuki T, Carter HB, Walsh PC. Radical retropubic prostatectomy. How often do experienced surgeons have positive surgical margins when there is extraprostatic extension in the region of the neurovascular bundle? J Urol. 2005;173:446–9.
11. Sofer M, Hamilton-Nelson KL, Schlesselman JJ, Soloway MS. Risk of positive surgical margins and biochemical recurrence in relation to nerve-sparing radical prostatectomy. J Clin Oncol. 2002;20:1853–8.
12. Walsh PC, Lepor H, Eggleston JC. Radical prostatectomy with preservation of sexual function: anatomical and pathological considerations. Prostate. 1983;4:473–85.
13. Menon M, Shrivastava A, Kaul S, et al. Vattikuti Institute Prostatectomy: contemporary technique and analysis of results. Eur Urol. 2007;51:648–58.
14. Kaul S, Bhandari A, Hemal A, et al. Robotic radical prostatectomy with preservation of the prostatic fascia: a feasibility study. Urology. 2005;66:1261–5.
15. Steineck G, Bjartell A, Hugosson J, et al. Degree of preservation of the neurovascular bundle during radical prostatectomy and urinary continence 1 year after surgery. Eur Urol. 2015;67:559–68.
16. Reeves F, Preece P, Kapoor J, et al. Preservation of the neurovascular bundles is associated with improved time to continence after radical prostatectomy but not long-term continence rates: results of a systematic review and meta-analysis. Eur Urol. 2014. http://dx.doi.org/10.1016/j.eururo.2014.10.020.
17. Stolzenburg J, Schwalenberg T, Horn L, Neuhaus J, Constantinides C, Liatsikos EN. Anatomical landmarks of radical prostatectomy. Eur Urol. 2007;51:629–39.
18. Eichelberg C, Erbersdobler A, Michl U, et al. Nerve distribution along the prostatic capsule. Eur Urol. 2007;51:105–11.
19. Tewari A, Takenaka A, Mtui E, et al. The proximal neurovascular plate and the trizonal neural architecture around the prostate gland: importance in the athermal robotic technique of nerve-sparing prostatectomy. BJU Int. 2006;98:314–23.
20. Kim ED, Nath R, Sawin KM, et al. Bilateral nerve grafting during radical retropubic prostatectomy: extended follow up. Urology. 2001;58:983–7.
21. Singh H, Karakiewicz P, Shariat SF, et al. Impact of unilateral interposition sural nerve grafting on recovery of urinary function after radical prostatectomy. Urology. 2004;63:1122–7.
22. Namiki S, Saito S, Nakagawa H, Sanada T, Yamada A, Arai Y. Impact of unilateral sural nerve graft on recovery of potency and continence following radical prostatectomy: a 3-year longitudinal study. J Urol. 2007;178:212–6.
23. Davis JW, Chang DW, Chevray P. Randomized phase II evaluation of erectile function after attempted unilateral cavernous nerve-sparing retropubic radical prostatectomy with vs. without unilateral sural nerve grafting for clinically localized prostate cancer. Eur Urol. 2009;55:1135–44.
24. Kaouk JH, Desai MM, Abreu SC, Papay F, Gill IS. Robotic assisted laparoscopic sural nerve grafting during radical prostatectomy: initial experience. J Urol. 2003;170:909–12.

Apex: The Crossroads of Functional Recovery and Oncologic Control

10

Fatih Atug

Introduction

Prostate cancer is the most common non-dermatologic cancer in men and radical prostatectomy is the standard treatment now [1]. In order to reduce the morbidity of open procedure, new techniques have been developed such as laparoscopic radical prostatectomy and recently robotic surgery. Robotic surgery with 3-D view, optical magnification, and 7° moving instruments has developed very rapidly. And today, robot-assisted radical prostatectomy (RARP) is the most popular radical prostatectomy technique with more than 100,000 cases/year in the USA [2]. The utilization of robotic technology to radical prostatectomy operations led surgeons to make more careful, precise, and accurate dissections to see important anatomic structures in order to achieve a negative surgical margin, full continence, and recovery of erectile function.

Apex is the most different and unique part of the prostate, which is the crossroad of functional recovery and oncological control in radical prostatectomy operations. However, there are significant anatomic variations of prostate apex from one individual to another (Fig. 10.1). Every robotic surgeon should know and realize these anatomic variations and their relationship to urethra, distal sphincter, and neurovascular bundles. An appropriate and careful apical dissection of prostate should include three important steps:

(a) The last step of prostate removal: cutting the prostate apex at the most precise point to achieve a negative surgical margin.
(b) Preserving the maximum length of urethra for protecting the urethral sphincter as much as possible.
(c) If a nerve-sparing procedure was performed, to protect neurovascular bundles by gently dissecting out from apex and the cutting point of urethra.

Anatomic Considerations

All men created equal ***but not all prostates are***.

The shape of the prostate differs from one individual to another. The majority of these differences originate from the apical part of the prostate. At puberty, prostate starts to grow and incorporates urethral sphincter. Specifically at the level of prostatic apex, the fibers of the urethral sphincter are partly overlapped by the prostate and covered with it [3–5]. Anatomic and functional studies demonstrated that the length of the functional urethra changes between 1.5 and 2.4 cm and a significant part was located intraprostatically

F. Atug (✉)
Professor of Urology, Istanbul Bilim University School of Medicine, Istanbul, Turkey
e-mail: fatihatug@hotmail.com

J.W. Davis (ed.), *Robot-Assisted Radical Prostatectomy*, DOI 10.1007/978-3-319-32641-2_10

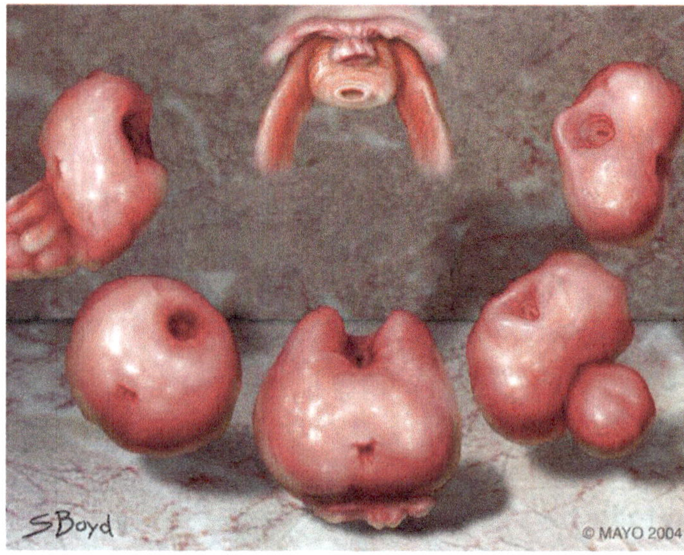

Fig. 10.1 Different apical shapes of prostates overlapping the urethral sphincter

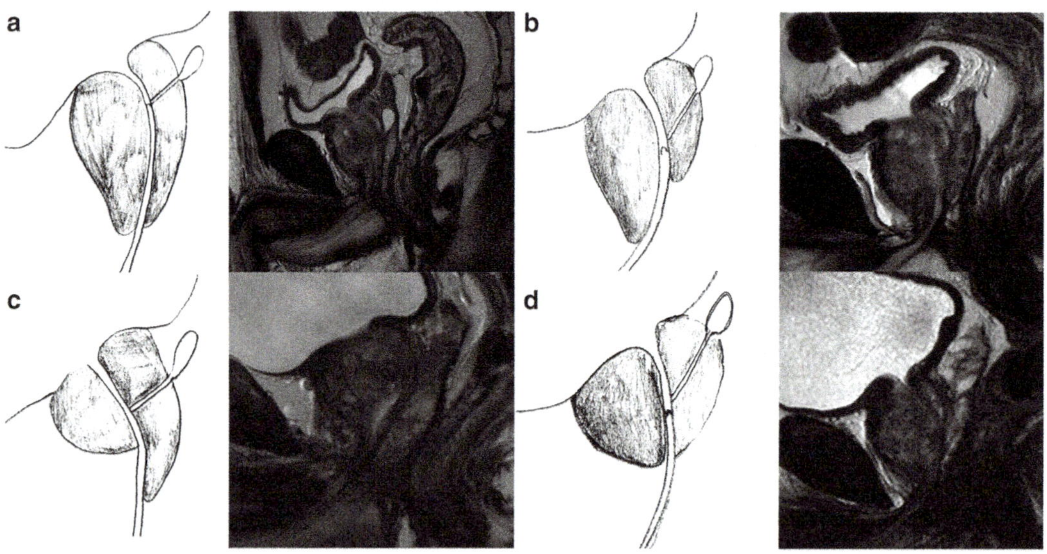

Fig. 10.2 Different shapes of prostatic apex by MRI. (**a**) Apex overlapping the membranous urethra both anteriorly and posteriorly. (**b**) Apex overlapping membranous urethra anteriorly. (**c**) Apex overlapping membranous urethra posteriorly. (**d**) Apex overlapping membranous urethra (Lee et al.)

between the prostatic apex and the verumontanum [6–12].

The apex may overlap the urethral sphincter circumferentially, symmetrically bilaterally, asymmetrically unilaterally, anteriorly only, and posteriorly only, or can bluntly end above the sphincter (Fig. 10.1) [12, 13]. The shape of the prostate at the apex may vary substantially, directly influencing the length of the urethra after emerging from the apex [14].

Lee et al. reported that circumferential overlap is observed in 38 % of all cases, anterior overlap in 25 %, posterior overlap in 22%, and no overlap in 15 %. Which means that apical overlap or variations can be seen in nearly 85 % of patients (Fig. 10.2) [15].

Moreover, significant overlap makes the preservation of urethral sphincter difficult and should be considered during dissection and appropriate transection of the urethra at the apex (Fig. 10.3). When the prostatic parenchyma was covered by

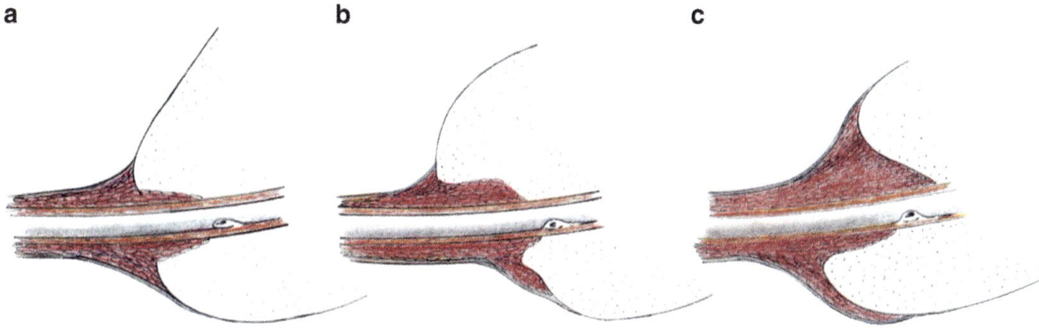

Fig. 10.3 (**a**, **b**) The functional urethra is covered by parenchymal apex tissue. (**c**) The prostatic apex is covered by urethral sphincter on the ventral and rectal sides

the muscular urethra, there is greater risk of urethral shortening and urinary incontinence [15].

Identifying the exact border of the sphincter overlapped by the prostate intraoperatively is the main surgical difficulty for the surgeon. In addition, preserving the urethral sphincter during apical dissection of the prostate must be balanced with minimizing positive surgical margins.

Surgical Technique

The apical dissection of prostate is the most difficult part of the radical prostatectomy operation due to several reasons:

- The prostate is located in the deep part of the narrow bony pelvis; moreover the apex of the prostate is located at the deepest and narrowest part of the pelvis.
- There is no real capsule at the level of prostatic apex.
- Prostatic overlap over the urethra exists in majority of patients.
- The ventral part of the apex is covered by the dorsal vascular complex.
- The lateral aspect of the apex is surrounded by neurovascular bundles.

Surgical Technique

Before starting the apical dissection, the prostate should be free from the bladder neck and neurovascular bundles. Bleeding from neurovascular should be minimal to obtain the ideal visualization. Increasing pneumoperitoneum to 18–20 mmHg prior to transection of the dorsal venous complex may help to obtain a bloodless clear field. After division of DVC, the apex of the prostate and urethra should be inspected very carefully to see the anatomic variations. The apical prostate shape varies significantly from one patient to another; apical overlap or variations can be seen in nearly 85 % of patients [16].

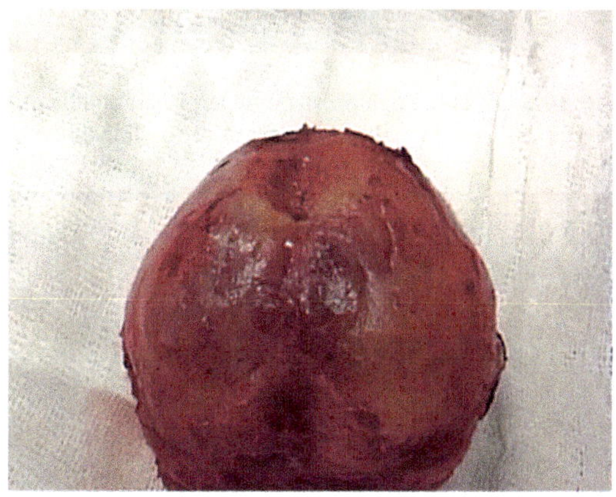

Fig. 10.4 Prostate apex in a circumferential shape

Some different shapes of prostate and variations are given below:

The prostate apex may be in a circumferential shape and end bluntly above the sphincter. There is no overlap of prostate tissue in such patients (Fig. 10.4).

The apex may be asymmetrical unilaterally and protrude over the urethra because of a BPH nodule on one side. In such kind of patients surgeons should be very careful not to leave an apical prostate tissue behind (Fig. 10.5).

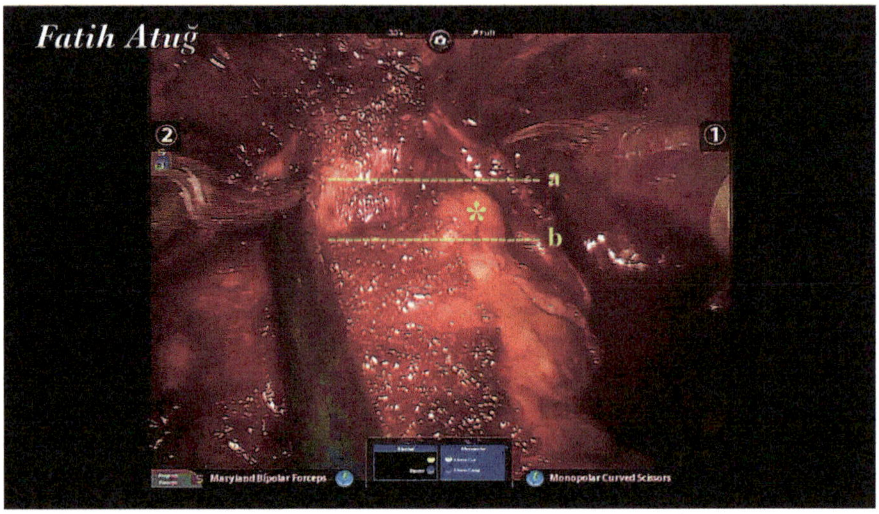

Fig. 10.5 BPH (benign prostatic hyperplasia) nodule on right side of the prostate. (**a**) Transection of the urethra at the level of BPH nodule. (**b**) Correct transection line of the urethra. (*) BPH nodule

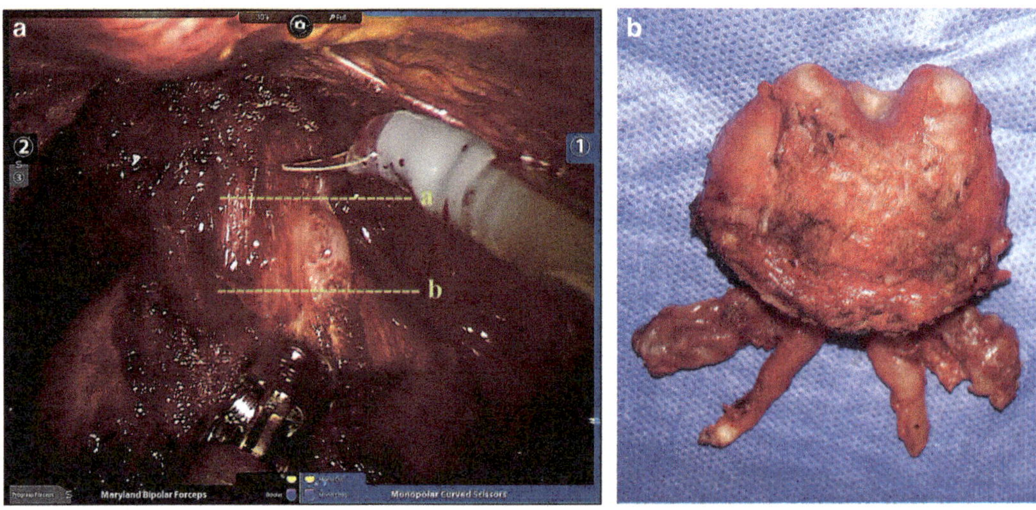

Fig. 10.6 (**a**) Prostate apex in a horn shape. Transection of the urethra at the level of the prostate horn. (**b**) Border of proximal urethra. Prostate specimen of the same patient after the RARP operation

The apical tissue may be in a horn shape on one side or both sides and protrude over the urethra. If the transection is performed at or beyond the horn of the prostate, the residual length of urethra will be short and this may result in delayed return of continence in these patients (Fig. 10.6a, b).

It has been demonstrated by several anatomical studies that an important functional part of the urethral sphincter is located intraprostatically between the apex and verumontanum [3, 7, 8, 12, 15]. With the growth of the prostate at puberty, the prostate starts to occupy the sphincteric muscle with covering some part of the sphincter and integrating it within the prostatic tissue [17]. Consequently, depending on the individual apex shape, between 10 and 40 % of the functional urethra is covered by parenchymal apex tissue among different patients [10–14, 18].

Moreover, in some patients the prostatic parenchyma may be covered by the muscular urethral sphincter on the anterior side of prostate. Such anatomic variations will cause extra technical difficulty in preservation of distal sphincteric mechanism, Fig. 10.7.

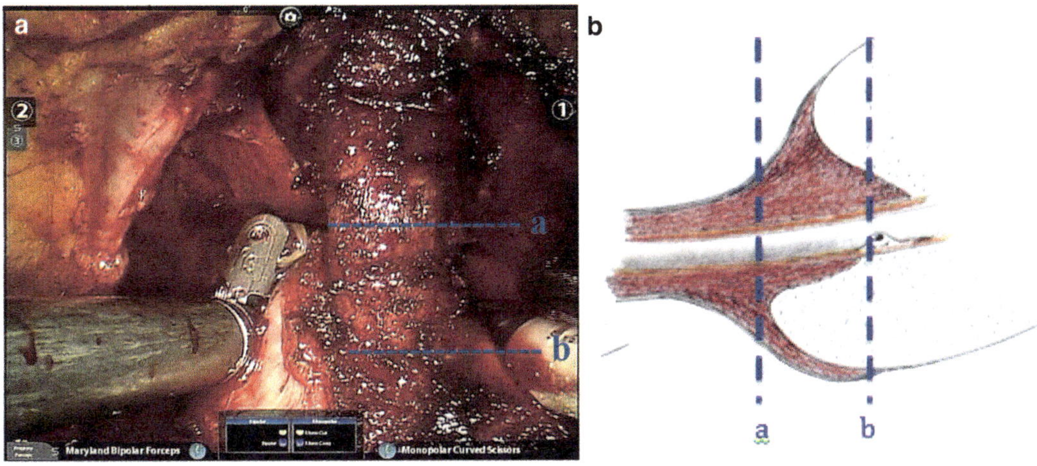

Fig. 10.7 Prostatic apex is covered by muscular urethral sphincter. (**a**) Edge of the prostatic apex. (**b**) Intraprostatic part of the urethra

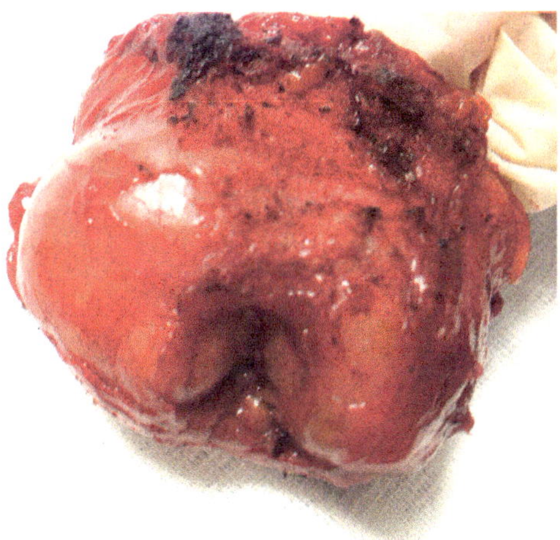

Fig. 10.8 The prostate specimen. After removing the intraprostatic part of the urethra, the lateral lobes and veru are clearly seen

The intraprostatically located structures of the sphincter should be appropriately and safely separated from the surrounding prostatic tissue in order to achieve maximum urethral length. After removing the intraprostatically located urethra from the prostate, the lateral lobes of the prostate and verumontanum should be seen clearly, Fig. 10.8.

Conclusion

Apical dissection of prostate during RARP is the most critical and important part of the radical prostatectomy operations. Dissection of apex will have an intense effect on three important parameters: surgical margin status (apical margin), continence, and sexual function (neurovascular bundles). As every surgeon would agree and know, understanding the complex anatomy of male pelvis and prostate is certainly vital for achieving these goals in RRP operations.

References

1. Center MM, Jemal A, Lortet-Tieulent J, et al. International variation in prostate cancer incidence and mortality rates. Eur Urol. 2012;61:1079–92.
2. In: Howlader N, Noone AM, Krapcho M, Garshell J, Miller D, Altekruse SF, Kosary CL, Yu M, Ruhl J, Tatalovich Z, Mariotto A, Lewis DR, Chen HS, Feuer EJ, Cronin KA, editors. SEER Cancer statistics review. National Cancer Institute; 1975–2012.
3. Oelrich TM. The urethral sphincter muscle in the male. Am J Anat. 1980;158:229–46.
4. Koraitim MM. The male urethral sphincter complex revisited: an anatomical concept and its physiological correlate. J Urol. 2008;179:1683–9.

5. Light JK, Rapoll E, Wheeler TM. The striated urethral sphincter: muscle fibre types and distribution in the prostatic capsule. Br J Urol. 1997;79:539–42.
6. Groutz A, Blaivas JG, Chaikin DC, et al. The pathophysiology of postradical prostatectomy incontinence: a clinical and video urodynamic study. J Urol. 2000;163:1767–70.
7. Hammerer P, Huland H. Urodynamic evaluation of changes in urinary control after radical retropubic prostatectomy. J Urol. 1997;157:233–6.
8. Myers RP, Cahill DR, Devine RM, King BF. Anatomy of radical prostatectomy as defined by magnetic resonance imaging. J Urol. 1998;159:2148–58.
9. Nguyen L, Jhaveri J, Tewari A. Surgical technique to overcome anatomical shortcoming: balancing post-prostatectomy continence outcomes of urethral sphincter lengths on preoperative magnetic resonance imaging. J Urol. 2008;179:1907–11.
10. Paparel P, Akin O, Sandhu JS, et al. Recovery of urinary continence after radical prostatectomy: association with urethral length and urethral fibrosis measured by preoperative and postoperative endorectal magnetic resonance imaging. Eur Urol. 2009;55:629–39.
11. Walz J, Burnett AL, Costello AJ, et al. A critical analysis of the current knowledge of surgical anatomy related to optimization of cancer control and preservation of continence and erection in candidates for radical prostatectomy. Eur Urol. 2010;57:179–92.
12. Myers RP. Practical surgical anatomy for radical prostatectomy. Urol Clin North Am. 2001;28:473–90.
13. Myers RP. Male urethral sphincteric anatomy and radical prostatectomy. Urol Clin North Am. 1991;18:211–27.
14. Myers RP, Villers A. Anatomic considerations in radical prostatectomy. In: Kirby RS, Partin AW, Feneley M, Parsons JK, editors. Prostate cancer; principles and practice, vol. 1. Abingdon, UK: Taylor & Francis; 2006. p. 701–13.
15. Lee SE, Byun SS, Lee HJ, et al. Impact of variations in prostatic apex shape on early recovery of urinary continence after radical retropubic prostatectomy. Urology. 2006;68:137–41.
16. Lee H, Kim K, Hwang SI, Lee HJ, Byun SS, Lee SE, Hong SK. Impact of prostatic apical shape and protrusion on early recovery of continence after robot-assisted radical prostatectomy. Urology. 2014;84(4):844–9.
17. Wallner C, Dabhoiwala NF, DeRuiter MC, Lamers WH. The anatomical components of urinary continence. Eur Urol. 2009;55:932–44.
18. Schlomm T, Heinzer H, Steuber T, Salomon G, Engel O, Michl U, Haese A, Graefen M, Huland H. Full functional-length urethral sphincter preservation during radical prostatectomy. Eur Urol. 2011;60(2):320–9.

Post-resection: Hemostasis, Checking for Rectal Injury, and Anastomotic Leaks

11

Dylan Stoy, Bernardo Rocco, Giancarlo Albo, Francesco Alessandro Mistretta, Maria Chiara Clementi, Vladimir Mourviev, and David M. Albala

Hemostasis

Meticulous hemostasis during prostate surgery is accomplished by the use of a magnifying robotic lens and can be performed with mechanical devices, several energy sources, and/or chemical substances. In their systematic review of 110 papers evaluating oncological outcomes following robot-assisted radical prostatectomy (RARP), Ficarra et al. [1] demonstrated that blood loss (weighted mean difference 582.77; $p<0.00001$) and transfusion rate (odds ratio [OR] 7.55; $p<0.00001$) were lower in RARP than in retropubic radical prostatectomy (RRP), although all other features were similar regardless of the surgical approach. However, for many reasons, hemostasis remains a crucial topic. First, a bloodless field is necessary for the surgeon to perform a perfect dissection. Second, more often than not, these procedures are performed on older patients with several comorbidities and taking anticoagulant and antiplatelet therapy [2].

D. Stoy (✉)
Associated Medical Professionals,
Syracuse, NY 13210, USA
e-mail: datoy@ampofny.com

B. Rocco
Clinica Urologica I, Ospedale Maggiore Policlinico, Fondazione IRCCS Ca' Granda, Università degli Studi di Milano, Via Commenda, 15, Milan 20122, Italy
e-mail: bernardo.rocco@gmail.com

G. Albo • M.C. Clementi V. Mourviev
Department of Urology, University Vita-Salute, Milan, Italy
e-mail: albo.giancarlo@gmail.com; maria.clementi@gmail.com; vladimir.mouraviev@flhosp.org

F.A. Mistretta
Department of Urology, Fondazione IRCCS Ca, GrandaOspedale Maggiore Policlinico, University of Milan, Italy
e-mail: francesco.mistretta@gmail.com

D.M. Albala, M.D.
Department of Urology, Crouse Hospital, Syracuse, NY, USA
e-mail: dalbala@ampofny.com

Mechanical Hemostasis

Mechanical means of hemostasis, such as suture ligation or the use of an endovascular stapler, are the most common techniques used to control the dorsal venous complex (DVC). Guru et al. [3] demonstrated that cold incision of the DVC without ligation was followed by significantly shorter operative times, a lower apical positive surgical margin rate and more successful earlier continence rates compared with incision after suture ligation [4]. However, blood loss was higher in those cases in which ligation was not used. Wu et al. [5] found that staple ligation was associated with significantly lower blood loss compared with suture ligation of the DVC. The benefit associated with stapling might have been attributable to clearing off the fat overlying the DVC

J.W. Davis (ed.), *Robot-Assisted Radical Prostatectomy*, DOI 10.1007/978-3-319-32641-2_11

before stapling, thus providing better visualization before ligation. Since suture ligation of the DVC may injure the urethra and external sphincter and decrease the functional urethral length, Tufek and associates [6] described a novel technique based on the use of a laparoscopic bulldog clamp. According to the authors, this technique provides clear visualization during the apical dissection and urethral division while potentially minimizing external sphincter trauma. However, with the evidence from their study, it cannot be stated that this new technique is better than conventional suture ligation.

Energy-Based Hemostasis

With the recent advances in surgical technology for laparoscopic (and robotic) surgery, efficient and reliable energy-based vascular sealing instruments have rapidly become an integral tool for most urologists. As a result of their mode of action, traditional monopolar and bipolar cautery devices generate significant heat, with substantial thermal spread [7].

For this reason, energy-based hemostasis of the prostatic vascular pedicles (PVP) during RARP may cause collateral thermal injury to adjacent neural tissue and has shown to negatively impact in the recovery of sexual function [8–10]. Various athermal cautery-free techniques have been described for PVP control during RARP. For example, permanent hemostatic clips, such as the Weck Hem-o-lok clips (Teleflex Medical, Triangle Park, NC) or titanium clips, are successfully used, but carry a risk of migration, erosion, and stone formation [11–13].

The aforementioned drawbacks have prompted the development of more advanced feedback-monitored bipolar forceps, such as Ligasure (Valleylab, Inc, Boulder, CO) and EnSeal (Ethicon, Cincinnati, OH). Ligasure uses high-power, low-voltage bipolar radiofrequency energy in combination with a feedback-controlled response system that automatically delivers and disrupts the power according to the composition and impedance of the tissue between the jaws. EnSeal, a newer device, is a bipolar instrument that combines a high-compression jaw with a tissue-dynamic energy delivery mechanism. The instrument has a blade that is advanced as the tissue is being sealed and simultaneously cuts the sealed tissue. EnSeal produces the least amount of lateral thermal tissue damage of any bipolar advanced energy modality: 1 mm lateral thermal tissue damage [14].

Induced local hypothermia represents another route to reduce inflammation and tissue trauma at supraphysiologic temperatures [15]. Rat models have shown that irrigation performed simultaneously with bipolar cautery plays a significant role in thermo protection [9, 16].

Finely and coworkers [17] described this phenomenon in RARP, applying both an endorectal cooling balloon and cold irrigation during RARP to mitigate collateral thermal damage. These methods proved to result in faster and higher rates of postoperative continence. Zorn et al. [18] also reported that a combination of EnSeal tissue sealant and cool saline irrigation resulted in a significantly lower quantity of thermal damage.

Chemical Hemostasis

Chemical hemostasis is based on the use of several substances that act on the coagulation cascade. These topical hemostatic agents are either flowable or non-flowable. The first group, fibrin and synthetic sealants, can be combinations of gelatin and thrombin, or stand-alone thrombin. The second group includes collagen pads, gelatin sponges, fibrinogen-coated collagen and oxidized cellulose. While flowable hemostats have their utility in deep wounds, hemostatic pads and fleeces are widely used to stop bleeding in superficial surgical application (i.e., suture lines and broad areas of bleeding).

The oxidized regenerated cellulose (i.e., Surgicel, Ethicon, Cincinnati, OH) is derived from plant fibers, and swells upon contact with fluids. Although the exact mechanism of action is unclear, it appears to promote coagulation by providing mesh for platelets to start adhesion and aggregation. When wet, these materials can be easily shaped and applied on wounds that are difficult to reach; resulting in good adhesion properties and relatively immediate hemostasis. Biodegradation starts within 24 h, and depending on the amount used and the tissue bed, giant cells may appear within 1 week, resulting in complete absorption in 4–8 weeks.

Fibrin glues are fibrinogen and thrombin blends, either flowable or non-flowable. When applied to the bleeding site, they facilitate the conversion of fibrinogen to fibrin. Additionally, cross-linking of soluble fibrin monomers creates an insoluble fibrin clot that acts as a vessel sealant [19]. Flowable fibrin glues (i.e., Tisseal, Baxter Healthcare, Deerfield, Il; Tachosil, Baxter Heathcare, Deerfield, Il and Evicel, Ethicon, Sommerville, NJ) can be applied in more limited bleeding sites, such as at the anastomatic site and in parenchymal lacerations.

First introduced for use in cardiothoracic surgery in 1988 [20], the use of fibrin and other tissue sealants and hemostatic products has expanded across surgical disciplines. In urology, fibrin sealants are the most commonly employed means of hemostasis, and though many applications are off-label uses, there has been mounting evidence for its usefulness [21–26]. Diner et al. [26] report that fibrin sealant utilization in RRP decreases perioperative drain output. However, they also suggest that in some patients undergoing traditional open RRP, the application of a fibrin sealant could accelerate discharge. Morey et al. have successfully used a fibrin sealant in simple RRP, and have observed that those patients required no perioperative drain. Additionally [27], Evans et al. [23] reported success with the use of fibrin sealants in trauma and fistula repair. To further broaden their range of uses, fibrin sealants are also used in partial nephrectomy, renal trauma, hypospadias, ureteral anastomoses, urethroplasty, pyeloplasty, ureteral anastomoses, and open RRP. Flury et al. [28] expanded the potential use to include reinforcing the suture line the urethrovescical anastomosis in RARP—this specific application seemed to facilitate sealing, thereby allowing earlier removal of the drain by 0.8 days and the Foley catheter by 2.35 days in patients undergoing RARP.

Conversely, there are several disadvantages of biologic sealant technology. These include allergic reaction and the potential transmission of prior diseases due to its bovine derivation, to name a few. As such, the manufacturers have now initiated the use of human thrombin in all sealants to eliminate the chance of this problem. The need to mix two components and/or sequentially apply them, as well as the cost of the products have also proven to be problematic in the use of biological sealants, and should be taken into consideration.

Rectal Injuries

A rectal injury is a rare but severe complication of radical prostatectomy. This type of event has the potential to convert the surgical procedure from clean-contaminated to contaminated and can also lead to other complications such as rectourinary fistula, pelvic abscess, wound infection, sepsis, and even death [29].

During the last few decades, the series published regarding open retropubic radical prostatectomy reported a significant decrease in the rate of occurrence of rectal injuries. The frequency typically ranges anywhere from 0.5 %, for the newest data, to 9 % for the oldest [30–32]. During standard laparoscopic prostatectomy, rectal injuries occur at a different rate, especialy when taking in to consideration multiple large series (incidence 0.7–2 %), or the smaller series (incidence as high as 8 %) [33–36]. Recently Ficarra et al. in a systematic review of the literature described the specific complication of rectal injuries after RALP with a mean of 0.2 % (range 0–1.5 %) [1].

The most common predisposing factors for rectal injury described in literature seem to be associated with a desmoplastic reaction and periprostatic fibrosis, which tend to lead to a more difficult dissection. Prostatitis, previous prostate or rectal surgery, previous hormonal or radiotherapy and locally advanced tumors can also be included in this list [36, 37]. However, the aforementioned predisposing factors are still debated. Despite the small series, Yee and Ornstein reported that none of their patients had a history of radiotherapy, prostate surgery, or prostatitis [38].

To our knowledge, Wedmid et al. published the largest series to date of rectal injury which occurred during robotic radical prostatectomy [39]. They demonstrated that no preoperative patient characteristics such as age or BMI, intraoperative events such as limiting visualization due to blood loss, or differences in parameter like prostate size, correlated with the occurrence of rectal injuries. Even the pathological findings appeared to show no association with rectal injuries. In particular, the authors have described that two-thirds of the positive surgical margins had no correlation with the portion of cases where rectal injury occurred.

At any rate, no significant association has been found with the learning curve. Kheterpal et al. described their experience of 4400 cases of a single surgeon perforing the RALPs. They reported that out of ten rectal injuries, three occurred after 1700 cases, and the last one after case 2789. This denounced any association between the surgeon experience and the rectal injury occurrence [33].

Diagnosis of Rectal Injuries

Most rectal injuries are usually identified by intraoperative direct visualization during the prostatectomy procedure. In a multi-institutional review of rectal injuries in which 6650 patients subjected to RALP, Wedmid et al. reported that out of 11 rectal injuries, 8 (72.7 %) were diagnosed during the procedure. Most of the injuries occurred during the posterior dissection of the prostate (45 %), with a small portion occurring during the dissection of the prostatic gland apex or the seminal vesicles [39].

Similar data could be found in a previous but smaller series in which Yee et al. reported the occurrence of rectal injuries during the posterior plane dissection occurring between prostate and rectum, near the prostatic gland apex and the division of the rectourethral muscle [38]. The importance of an adequate and careful dissection of the posterior plane is emphasized by Katz et al. in a study conducted on laparoscopic radical prostatectomies [36].

Contrarily, rectal injuries not identified intraoperatively usually develop a clinical relevance 2–3 weeks after the surgical procedure [40, 41]. The development of a rectourethral fistula is characterized by signs and symptoms such as pneumaturia, fecaluria, anal urinary discharge, bloody stool, rectal bleeding, or could be associated with septic complications. At least one of these occurs in every patient with a rectourethral fistula. Furthermore, in the diagnostic process, urethrocystoscopy, retrograde urethrography, and Gastrografin enemas provide additional information such as the size and localization of the fistula.

Management of Rectal Injuries

If small rectal injuries are intraoperatively diagnosed, they can be immediately repaired.

In the aforementioned multi-institutional review, Wedmid et al. described several intraoperative techniques used to close the wound, such as 2- and 3-layer closure or 2-layer closure with an additional peritoneum free graft over the rectal injury followed by a final air insufflation test via the rectum in a fluid-filled pelvis, to check the integrity of the suture. Moreover, these authors suggested a longitudinal closure with respect to a Heineke-Mikulicz or transverse technique to minimize anastomotic tension [39].

Conversely from the past, nowadays it is a common practice to recommend a diverting colostomy in cases characterized by a tense suture line, previous radiotherapy or massive fecal spillage.

Also worth mentioning is the use of preoperative bowel preparation [30] or the addition of an omental interposition to the primary rectal closure [31, 32, 38]. This may increase the success rate of the primary repair, avoiding the burden of a diverting ileostomy.

Another common practice is to delay the catheter removal from 14 to 21 days from the standard 7 to 10 days, [39] and use a postoperative antibiotic prophylaxis for 1–2 weeks [31, 34]. On the other hand, if a rectal injury is intraoperatively misdiagnosed, the management usually consists of a colonic diversion, a prolonged catheter drainage and, if a rectourethral fistula develops, a delayed closure using a rectal mucosal advancement flap [38, 39].

However, despite the effort produced to codify a clear algorithm, the management of rectal injuries is under debate, and the goal, as emphasized in literature, remains as the production of a watertight vesicourethral anastomosis to avoid the severity of a rectourethral fistula development [42].

Anastomotic Leakage

Anastomotic urinary leakage is one of the most common short-term complications of radical prostatectomy. Until recently, there has been no consensus on its definition. However, current literature defines an anastomotic urinary leakage as a persistent cystographic contrast extravasation between postoperative days 3 and 14 [43].

Among the causes that lead to an anastomotic urinary leakage that Ramsden and Chodak identified, the most common is the presence of an intraoperative leak. This is most often caused by an imprecise suture placement and poor hemostasis [44].

In addition, ischemic heart disease [44], urinary tract infection [45], previous pelvic radiation [46] and specific technical details in the performance of the anastomosis are potential predictive factors [47].

Rebuck et al. showed that patients with postoperative urinary leakage after robot-assisted radical prostatectomy typically presented with a higher BMI, lower proportions of clinical stage T2 disease, and an increased rate of blood transfusion; all while showing that the presence of a median lobe does not increase the risk anastomotic urine leaks [48].

The use of the endowrist technology, the 3D vision and tenfold magnification of robotic surgery have aided in the facilitation of the most complex reconstructive steps of standard laparoscopic surgery, such as the vesico-urethral anastomosis. On the other hand, the intraperitoneal approach, which is typical both of laparoscopic and robotic procedures, may cause anastomotic intraperitoneal leakage that is often avoided with open extraperitoneal surgery.

Diagnosis

Over the last three decades, surgeons have struggled with the will to improve the patients' quality of life, reducing the bladder catheterization time, and the necessity to avoid the increasing of anastomotic urinary leakage and acute urinary retention rate at the catheter removal. Moreover, there is no consensus on the reliability of the preoperative, intraoperative, and postoperative parameters routinely used to predict urinary extravasation [49].

Typically in best clinical practices, a routine cystographic exam is not performed. In fact, the most common approach in detecting an anastomotic leak is to assess the presence of urine in the perivesical drain fluid, where a high creatinine level in the drain output is key when discriminating urine from lymph (if a lymphadenectomy was performed).

However, when the cystogram is performed after retropubic radical prostatectomy, anastomotic leaks are described in a range from 3 to 33 % of cases [45, 50], in the 10–17 % of patients undergoing laparoscopic radical prostatectomy [35, 51], and in 8.6–13.6 % of robotic cases [52, 53].

Lee et al. reported that CT cystography is more sensitive for detecting an anastomatic leak than conventional cystography after radical retropubic prostatectomy. In a study where CT and fluoroscopic cystography studies were compared, CT cystography had a significantly better detection rate of leakage (80.4 % vs. 54.3 %) and detected a significantly smaller volume of leakage (2.2 ± 2.1 mL vs. 19.3 ± 14.1 mL) [54]. Moreover, in a recent systematic review and metanalysis of the literature describing the specific complications of the RALP, Ficarra et al. reported the urine leak mean as 1.8 % (range 0.1–6.7 %) [1]. Although it is refuted that the clinical detection method alone underestimates the real prevalence of postoperative urinary leakage, the data described may suggest that the urinary leaks discovered only by cystography, and not found in the perivesical drain, are not of high clinical relevance [48, 55].

We agree to define an anastomotic urinary leak as clinically significant when it dictates interventional drainage. This is often associated with fever, signs of sepsis, and extends intraperitoneally resulting in ileus, leading to conditions which require readmission and/or adjunctive treatments [56].

Management

The first step in the management of an anastomotic leak is utilizing an intraoperative sterile water flush to check the integrity of the anastomosis. Leakage seen by the extravasation of the sterile water through the anastomosis may indicate the need for additional sutures or even complete revision of the anastomosis. In the first large study performed to evaluate the anastomotic leak rate, Williams et al. described how the majority of leaks were of modest occurance and were most often confined to the surgical bed. Conversely, the larger and more severe leaks which required a prolonged catheterization were less common [52].

Usually, patients were clinically followed maintaining the bladder catheter in place and repeating imaging after 6–7-day intervals until the leak resolved. The less common intraperitoneal leaks required a CT guided pigtail catheter placement to drain the postoperative urinomas [52].

Several conservative measures have been proposed for these occurrences, such as the correct replacement of the bladder catheter or the application of gentle traction. In regard to the drain, pulling back or withdrawing it and switching from an active to passive drainage, are maneuvers that may help proper urine drainage [49, 57]. The aspiration of a postoperative urinoma can be accomplished by the placement of a pelvic drain under the aid of CT guidance [53, 55]. Additionally, at the very least ureteral stenting or a nephrostomy placement should be used before a reoperation [58]. Surgical intervention should be considered the last choice. The decision to pursue this treatment option depends primarily on the amount of urine drainage. The surgical repair itself may vary from a partial anastomotic repair to a complete reconstruction of the anastomosis [57, 59].

Complications

The short-term complications of urine leakage are well described and include the formation of an urinoma, infections, ileus, metabolic abnormalities, and possibly a prolonged hospital stay. On the other hand, little is known about the long-term effects on continence and potency. To our knowledge, only Rebuck et al. demonstrated that anastomotic urinary leakage after RALP may not have significant long-term morbidity in terms of bladder neck contracture, incontinence, and erectile function [48].

Editorial Comments—John W. Davis

This is an important chapter, as many aspects of finishing up a resection go unreported compared to the traditional oncologic and functional outcomes. Team Albala has put together a very nice narrative with key citations to navigate this step of the operation. Every surgeon struggles with these steps of the operation and gains various preferences over time and as experience develops. Here are a few additional tips from my toolbox:

- I have tried every hemostatic trick in this book and eventually have settled on the old fashion 4-0 Vicryl stitch. These cost under $2 USD each compared to hundreds spent on fibrin products. Occasionally I resort to Fibrular—a fluffier substance that Surgiceal—to pack small vein channels. However, I have often heard that these products can be acidic and possibly nerve damaging. So I do my best to just sew.
- Check for hemostasis twice: first at the end of resection, and a final time after the anastomosis. If blood is welling from the nerve bundle and spilling downhill, it will likely continue postoperatively, and you may be left with an excellent estimated blood loss intraoperative but a discharge hemoglobin <10 or possibly need to transfuse or take-back.
- The rate of rectal injury was definitely higher in the laparoscopic prostatectomy era. In part this was mechanical as with the fixed instruments it was harder to aim your tips up when

going uphill to the apex. Articulation definitely helps. We used the air leak test routinely—fill the pelvis with water and then instill air in the rectum with a foley. If you see microbubbles then track those down and oversew. In the robotic era, I only do this for wide excision of nerve bundle cases where you are much closer to the rectum.

- The tips and citations on anastomotic leaks are excellent. In addition, you can reference my previous group's work on using a Lapra-Ty clip (Ball et al.). Prior to the Rocco stitch, this was our method of keeping tension on a running anastomosis to prevent leaks. When I see an occasional leak, there are two main possibilities—(1) gaps, and (2) inadequate tension. If there is a gap, then try and sneak another interrupted 3-0 Vicryl to close. If the running line is loose, then pull it tight, and slide a Lapra-Ty clip or two to hold the tension—much less traumatic than starting over. Of course, surgeons using barbed suture will have different circumstances to handle leaks.

References

1. Novara G, et al. Systematic review and meta-analysis of perioperative outcomes and complications after robot-assisted radical prostatectomy. Eur Urol. 2012;62(3):431–52.
2. Nowfar S, et al. Initial experience with aspirin use during robotic radical prostatectomy. J Laparoendosc Adv Surg Tech A. 2012;22(3):225–9.
3. Guru KA, et al. Apical margins after robot-assisted radical prostatectomy: does technique matter? J Endourol. 2009;23(1):123–7.
4. Lei Y, et al. Athermal division and selective suture ligation of the dorsal vein complex during robot-assisted laparoscopic radical prostatectomy: description of technique and outcomes. Eur Urol. 2011;59(2):235–43.
5. Wu SD, et al. Suture versus staple ligation of the dorsal venous complex during robot-assisted laparoscopic radical prostatectomy. BJU Int. 2010;106(3):385–90.
6. Tufek I, et al. The use of a laparoscopic bulldog clamp to control the dorsal vein complex during robot-assisted radical prostatectomy: a novel technique. J Endourol. 2013;27(1):29–33.
7. Khan F, et al. Spread of thermal energy and heat sinks: implications for nerve-sparing robotic prostatectomy. J Endourol. 2007;21(10):1195–8.
8. Smith TL, Smith JM. Electrosurgery in otolaryngology-head and neck surgery: principles, advances, and complications. Laryngoscope. 2001;111(5):769–80.
9. Donzelli J, et al. Neuroprotection due to irrigation during bipolar cautery. Arch Otolaryngol Head Neck Surg. 2000;126(2):149–53.
10. Kumar N, et al. Functional anatomy of the deer spine: an appropriate biomechanical model for the human spine? Anat Rec. 2002;266(2):108–17.
11. Tugcu V, et al. Stone formation from intravesical Hem-o-lok clip migration after laparoscopic radical prostatectomy. J Endourol. 2009;23(7):1111–3.
12. Tunnard GJ, Biyani CS. An unusual complication of a Hem-o-Lok clip following laparoscopic radical prostatectomy. J Laparoendosc Adv Surg Tech A. 2009;19(5):649–51.
13. Blumenthal KB, et al. Bladder neck contractures related to the use of Hem-o-lok clips in robot-assisted laparoscopic radical prostatectomy. Urology. 2008;72(1):158–61.
14. Person B, et al. Comparison of four energy-based vascular sealing and cutting instruments: a porcine model. Surg Endosc. 2008;22(2):534–8.
15. Phillips JM, et al. Histological evaluation of cold versus hot cutting: clinical impact on margin status for laparoscopic partial nephrectomy. J Urol. 2008;180(6):2348–52.
16. Donzelli J, et al. Thermoprotective mechanisms of irrigation during bipolar cautery. Otolaryngol Head Neck Surg. 1998;119(3):153–8.
17. Finley DS, et al. Hypothermic robotic radical prostatectomy: impact on continence. J Endourol. 2009;23(9):1443–50.
18. Zorn KC, et al. Application of ice cold irrigation during vascular pedicle control of robot-assisted radical prostatectomy: EnSeal instrument cooling to reduce collateral thermal tissue damage. J Endourol. 2010;24(12):1991–6.
19. Gill IS, et al. Improved hemostasis during laparoscopic partial nephrectomy using gelatin matrix thrombin sealant. Urology. 2005;65(3):463–6.
20. US Department of Health and Human Services. New fibrin sealant approved to help control bleeding in surgery. FDA Talk Paper T98-22 May 1988.
21. Evans LA, Morey AF. Current applications of fibrin sealant in urologic surgery. Int Braz J Urol. 2006;32(2):131–41.
22. Kumar U, Albala DM. Fibrin glue applications in urology. Curr Urol Rep. 2001;2(1):79–82.
23. Evans LA, et al. Fibrin sealant for the management of genitourinary injuries, fistulas and surgical complications. J Urol. 2003;169(4):1360–2.
24. MacDonald MF, Santucci RA. Adjunctive use of fibrin sealant in urethroplasty for early catheter removal. Issues Urol. 2006;36–40.
25. Hick EJ, Morey AF. Initial experience with fibrin sealant in pendulous urethral reconstruction. Is early catheter removal possible? J Urol. 2004;171(4):1547–9.

26. Diner EK, Patel SV, Kwart AM. Does fibrin sealant decrease immediate urinary leakage following radical retropubic prostatectomy? J Urol. 2005;173(4):1147–9.
27. Morey AF, et al. Drain-free simple retropubic prostatectomy with fibrin sealant. J Urol. 2002;168(2):627–9.
28. Flury SC, Starnes DN, Steers WD. Application of fibrin sealant at the urethrovesical anastomosis in robotic assisted radical prostatectomy: does it enable earlier Foley catheter and Jackson-Pratt drain removal? J Robot Surg. 2008;1(4):303–6.
29. Sabiston, DC. Jr. Antisepsis, technique, sutures and drains. In: Principles of Operative Surgery, 11th edition. W. B. Saunders Co., Philadelphia; 1977. p. 323–339.
30. Smith AM, Veenema RJ. Management of rectal injury and rectourethral fistulas following radical retropubic prostatectomy. J Urol. 1972;108(5):778–9.
31. Borland RN, Walsh PC. The management of rectal injury during radical retropubic prostatectomy. J Urol. 1992;147(3 Pt 2):905–7.
32. Lepor H, Nieder AM, Ferrandino MN. Intraoperative and postoperative complications of radical retropubic prostatectomy in a consecutive series of 1,000 cases. J Urol. 2001;166(5):1729–33.
33. Castillo OA, Bodden E, Vitagliano G. Management of rectal injury during laparoscopic radical prostatectomy. Int Braz J Urol. 2006;32(4):428–33.
34. Guillonneau B, et al. Laparoscopic [correction of laproscopic] management of rectal injury during laparoscopic [correction of laproscopic] radical prostatectomy. J Urol. 2003;169(5):1694–6.
35. Rassweiler J, et al. Laparoscopic versus open radical prostatectomy: a comparative study at a single institution. J Urol. 2003;169(5):1689–93.
36. Katz R, et al. Operative management of rectal injuries during laparoscopic radical prostatectomy. Urology. 2003;62(2):310–3.
37. McLaren RH, Barrett DM, Zincke H. Rectal injury occurring at radical retropubic prostatectomy for prostate cancer: etiology and treatment. Urology. 1993;42(4):401–5.
38. Yee DS, Ornstein DK. Repair of rectal injury during robotic-assisted laparoscopic prostatectomy. Urology. 2008;72(2):428–31.
39. Wedmid A, et al. Rectal injury during robot-assisted radical prostatectomy: incidence and management. J Urol. 2011;186(5):1928–33.
40. Thomas C, et al. Incidence, clinical symptoms and management of rectourethral fistulas after radical prostatectomy. J Urol. 2010;183(2):608–12.
41. Dal Moro F, et al. Successful repair of iatrogenic rectourinary fistulas using the posterior sagittal transrectal approach (York-Mason): 15-year experience. World J Surg. 2006;30(1):107–13.
42. Kheterpal E, et al. Management of rectal injury during robotic radical prostatectomy. Urology. 2011;77(4):976–9.
43. Hakimi AA, et al. Assessment of complication and functional outcome reporting in the minimally invasive prostatectomy literature from 2006 to the present. BJU Int. 2012;109(1):26–30. discussion 30.
44. Ramsden AR, Chodak GW. Can leakage at the vesicourethral anastomosis be predicted after radical retropubic prostatectomy? BJU Int. 2004;93(4):503–6.
45. Gnanapragasam VJ, et al. Identification and validation of risk factors for vesicourethral leaks following radical retropubic prostatectomy. Int J Urol. 2005;12(11):948–52.
46. Eandi JA, et al. Robotic assisted laparoscopic salvage prostatectomy for radiation resistant prostate cancer. J Urol. 2010;183(1):133–7.
47. Tyritzis SI, Katafigiotis I, Constantinides CA. All you need to know about urethrovesical anastomotic urinary leakage following radical prostatectomy. J Urol. 2012;188(2):369–76.
48. Rebuck DA, et al. What is the long-term relevance of clinically detected postoperative anastomotic urine leakage after robotic-assisted laparoscopic prostatectomy? BJU Int. 2011;108(5):733–8.
49. Fenig DM, Slova D, Lepor H. Postoperative blood loss predicts the development of urinary extravasation on cystogram following radical retropubic prostatectomy. J Urol. 2006;175(1):146–50. discussion 150.
50. Noguchi M, et al. Early catheter removal 3 days after radical retropubic prostatectomy. Int J Urol. 2004;11(11):983–8.
51. Guillonneau B, et al. Perioperative complications of laparoscopic radical prostatectomy: the Montsouris 3-year experience. J Urol. 2002;167(1):51–6.
52. Williams TR, et al. Incidence and imaging appearance of urethrovesical anastomotic urinary leaks following da Vinci robotic prostatectomy. Abdom Imaging. 2008;33(3):367–70.
53. Patil N, et al. Evaluating and grading cystographic leakage: correlation with clinical outcomes in patients undergoing robotic prostatectomy. BJU Int. 2009;103(8):1108–10.
54. Lee HJ, et al. MDCT cystography for detection of vesicourethral leak after prostatectomy. AJR Am J Roentgenol. 2008;191(6):1847–51.
55. Guru KA, et al. Is a cystogram necessary after robot-assisted radical prostatectomy? Urol Oncol. 2007;25(6):465–7.
56. Tan G, et al. Optimizing vesicourethral anastomosis healing after robot-assisted laparoscopic radical prostatectomy: lessons learned from three techniques in 1900 patients. J Endourol. 2010;24(12):1975–83.
57. Shah G, Vogel F, Moinzadeh A. Nephroureteral stent on suction for urethrovesical anastomotic leak after robot-assisted laparoscopic radical prostatectomy. Urology. 2009;73(6):1375–6.
58. Mochtar CA, et al. Urinary leakage after laparoscopic radical prostatectomy: a systematic review. J Endourol. 2007;21(11):1371–9.
59. Moinzadeh A, et al. Continuous needle vented foley catheter suction for urinary leak after radical prostatectomy. J Urol. 2004;171(6 Pt 1):2366–7.

12 Denonvilliers' Fascia: Anatomy, Surgical Planes, Use in Reconstruction

Bernardo Rocco and Gabriele Cozzi

Denonvilliers' Fascia: Embryology, Anatomy, and Surgical Planes

Traditionally, the first description of a "prostato-peritoneal membranous layer" is supposed to have been provided by Charles-Pierre Denonvilliers in 1836, even if already in 1820 Granville Sharp Pattison had described the "fascia of the prostate gland" as a structure to be preserved during perineal lithotomy.

The embryological origin of the Denonvilliers' fascia is matter of a debate which began in 1899 and is still ongoing. Although conventionally thought to develop by obliteration of the rectovesical peritoneal pouch, some studies suggested that it may actually represent a condensation of mesenchymal tissue.

Denonvilliers' fascia lies at the posterior and lateral angle of the prostate and covers the posterior aspect of the seminal vesicles. It relates to the prostate and seminal vesicles anteriorly, and to the rectal wall, the thin anterior mesorectum and the fascia propria posteriorly (Fig. 12.1). This fascia has no defined lateral edge: it widens and becomes continuous with the extensions of the endopelvic fascia.

Histologically, Denonvilliers' fascia is composed of dense collagen, smooth muscle fibers, and coarse elastic fibers. The fascia is more densely applied to the prostate than to the rectum, and the references to a posterior layer actually describe the fascia propria of the rectum.

Denonvilliers' fascia fuses with prostatic fascia anteriorly, and Hong et al. suggested in a histological study that the periprostatic fascias were not clearly limited and that they could fuse.

After seminal vesicles dissection, we tend to dissect the Denonvilliers' fascia from the posterior aspect of the prostate, unless the clinical staging is highly suggestive for extracapsular extension of the disease (T3a). This plane provides a safe surface for the detachment of the prostate from the rectum and allows Denonvilliers' fascia preservation for reconstruction purposes.

In case of locally advanced disease, we leave Denonvilliers' fascia on the prostate and we develop the plane on the rectal fascia propria.

Reconstruction of the Posterior Musculofascial Plate: The Original Technique

In 2006, F Rocco et al. proposed a technique for restoration of the posterior musculofascial plate, which demonstrated to shorten time to continence in patients undergoing open radical retropubic

B. Rocco (✉) • G. Cozzi
Clinica Urologica I, Ospedale Maggiore Policlinico, Fondazione IRCCS Ca' Granda, Università degli Studi di Milano, Via Commenda, 15, Milan 20122, Italy
e-mail: bernardo.rocco@gmail.com; cozzi.gabriele@gmail.com

J.W. Davis (ed.), *Robot-Assisted Radical Prostatectomy*, DOI 10.1007/978-3-319-32641-2_12

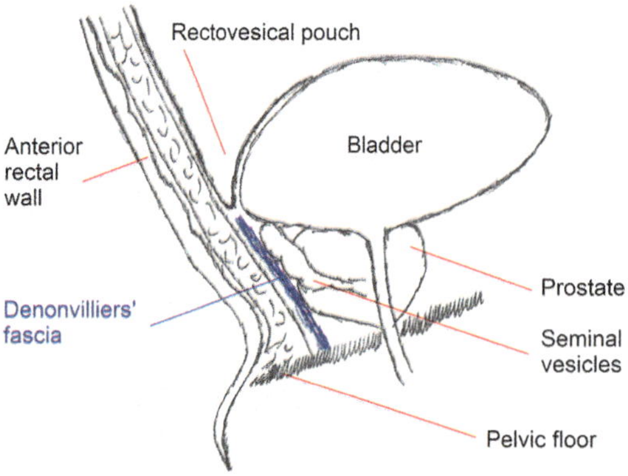

Fig. 12.1 Schematic representation of the anatomy of the Denonvilliers fascia

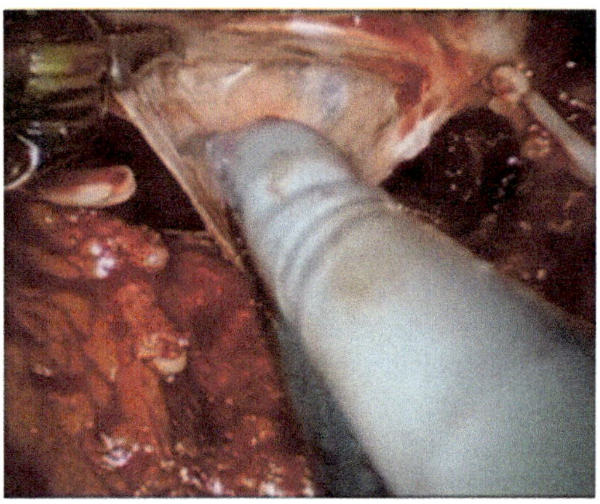

Fig. 12.2 Dissection of the Denonvilliers' fascia from the posterior aspect of the prostate

prostatectomy (RRP). Two modifications to the standard Walsh procedure were introduced: the reconstruction of the posterior musculofascial plate, and the suspension of the urethral sphincteric complex from the bladder.

Before freeing the prostatic apex, the posterior median raphe is carefully prepared and preserved, separating it from the neurovascular bundles and rectal fascia. The raphe is then sectioned and marked with two sutures. The apex of the prostate is then freed, and the prostatovesiculectomy is completed.

Before proceeding to vesicourethral anastomosis, the posterior median raphe is fixed to the residual Denonvilliers' fascia using the two previously placed marking sutures. This way, the posterior wall of the sphincter is elongated cranially.

The posterior median raphe joined to the Denonvilliers' fascia is then attached to the posterior bladder wall with two sutures applied about 1–2 cm cranial and dorsal the new bladder neck: thus the urethral sphinteric complex is suspended from the bladder neck. The dorsal aspect of the bladder becomes the new cranial insertion of the sphincter and posterior median raphe, fixing the sphincter. The anastomosis is then performed.

Application of the Reconstruction to Robotic-Assisted Radical Prostatectomy

In 2007, B Rocco et al. described the application of the posterior reconstruction technique to transperitoneal laparoscopic radical prostatectomy (LRP). In 2008, G Coughlin et al. described the application of the posterior reconstruction of the rhabdosphincter to robotic-assisted radical prostatectomy (RARP) with some minor technical modifications. Later, VR Patel et al. further modified the technique, as described in this paragraph.

The first, essential step is careful dissection of Denonvilliers' fascia underneath the prostate (Fig. 12.2). In this step the assistant can provide helpful counter traction with the sucker.

After the completion of the prostatectomy, the reconstruction is performed using a continuous suture of two 12 cm long 3/0 poliglecaprone 25 sutures (RB1 needle) of different colors, tied together. Ten knots are placed when tying the sutures together to provide a bolster.

The free edge of the remaining Denonvilliers' fascia is identified anterior to the rectum, just caudal to the bladder and seminal vesicle dissection (Fig. 12.3). This edge is approximated to the posterior aspect of the rhabdosphincter and the posterior median raphe by means of one arm of the continuous poliglecaprone 25 suture (Fig. 12.4). The Denonvilliers' fascia and the rhabdosphincter/median raphe are passed four times, approximating the edge in a tension-free manner (Fig. 12.5). The suture is then tied.

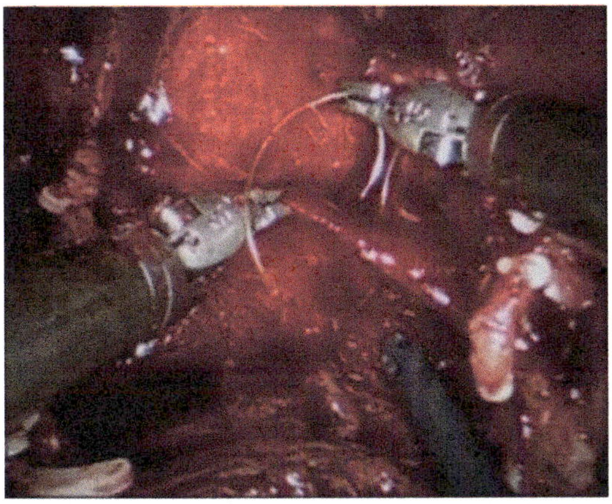

Fig. 12.3 The posterior musculofascial plate reconstruction begins from the remnant of the Denonvilliers' fascia

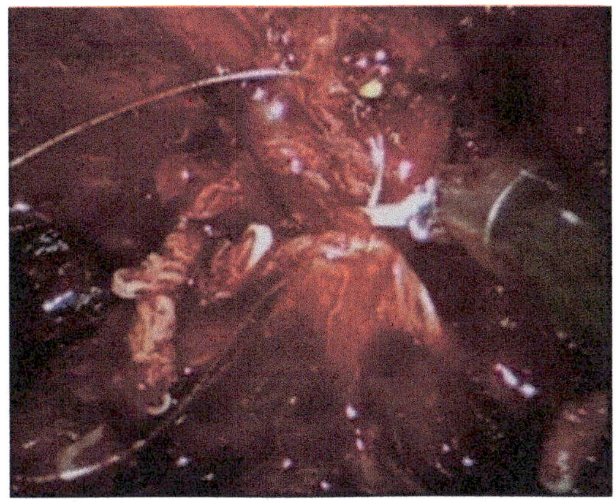

Fig. 12.5 The first layer of the reconstruction is completed

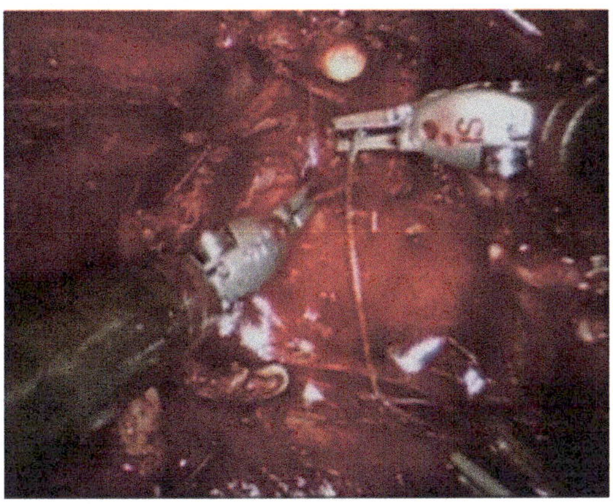

Fig. 12.4 The remnant of the Denonvilliers' fascia is joined to the rhabdosphincter/median raphe

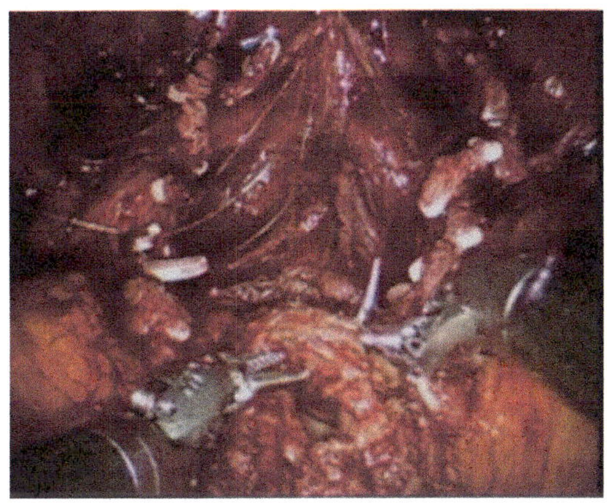

Fig. 12.6 The second layer of the reconstruction begins from the bladder neck

The second layer of the reconstruction is performed with the other arm of the poliglecaprone 25 suture. The bladder neck is approximated to the urethra (Figs. 12.6 and 12.7). The running suture passes three times each, and the suture is tied (Fig. 12.8). Anastomosis is conducted with a running suture according to the modified Van Velthoven technique.

The Role of the Posterior Musculofascial Plate Reconstruction in RARP

The role of posterior reconstruction in early return to continence after radical prostatectomy has been widely debated and investigated by many authors.

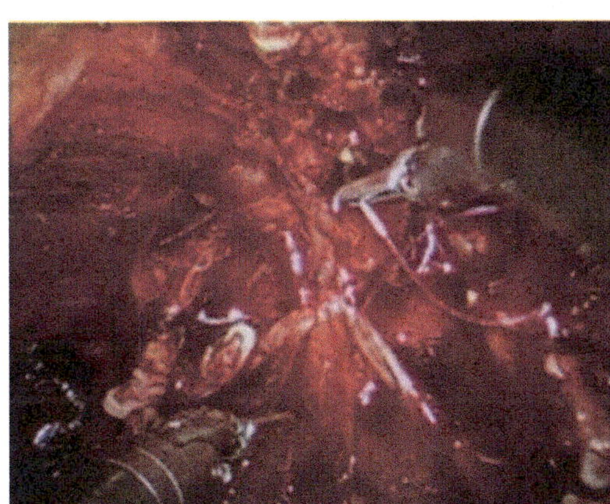

Fig. 12.7 The bladder neck is joined to the urethra

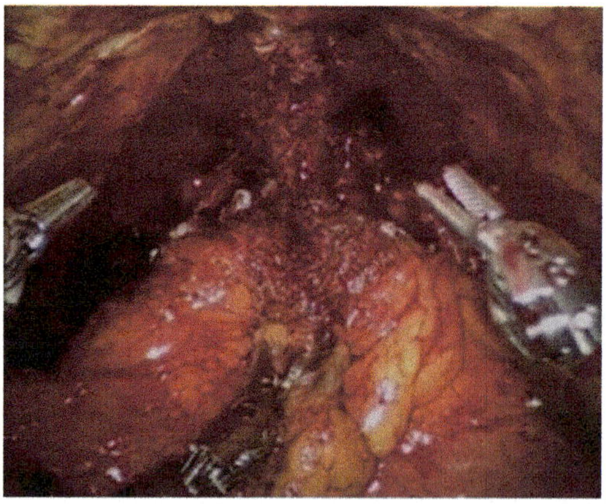

Fig. 12.8 The posterior musculofascial plate reconstruction is completed

A meta-analysis published by our group in 2012 showed a statistically significant advantage for reconstruction within the first 30 days from catheter removal and no associated complications. Ficarra et al. independently obtained the same results in a meta-analysis of studies reporting urinary continence recovery after RARP.

Since then, four new studies have been published, showing earlier return to continence after RARP with posterior reconstruction (Table 12.1). Among them, particularly remarkable is the randomized trial conducted by Hurtes et al.

In 2013, in the European Association of Urology Robotic Urology Section (ERUS) survey of RARP, it was reported that PR is "always" performed by 51.7 % of RARP surgeons, and "sometimes" by 19.8 % of them.

Apart from improving early continence, posterior reconstruction can also play a role in other functional aspects of RARP. Menon et al. and Coelho et al. observed less anastomotic leakages in patients receiving the reconstruction. Furthermore, Bernie et al. evaluated the influence of posterior reconstruction on anastomotic time, finding that the reconstruction decreases anastomosis time for robotic surgeons in training.

Table 12.1 Continence outcomes at 3–7, 45–75, 90, 180 days, and 1 year in patients who underwent robotic assisted radical prostatectomy with or without posterior reconstruction of the rhabdosphincter (PR)

Author	Type of study	Number of patients		Continence at catheter removal (3-7 days)		Continence at 30 days		Continece at 45–75 days		Continence at 90 days		Continence at 180 days		Continence at 1 year	
		PR	No PR	PR	No PR	PR	No PR	PR	No PR	PR	No PR	PR	No PR	PR	No PR
Tewari A et al. 2008	Retrospective	182	214	38.37 %	13.5 %	82.56 %	35.21 %			91.30 %	50.23 %	97.14 %	61.97 %		
				($p<0.01$)		($p<0.01$)				($p<0.01$)		($p<0.01$)			
Menon M et al.2008	Randomized trial	59	57	1 Day	1 Day	80.0 %	74.0 %								
				34.0 %	26.0 %										
				2 Days	2 Days										
				46.0 %	49.0 %										
				7 Days	7 Days										
				54.0 %	51.0 %										
				($p>0.1$)		($p>0.1$)									
Nguyen MM et al. 2008	Retrospective	32	30	34.0 %	3.0 %	56.0 %	17.0 %								
				($p=0.007$)		($p=0.006$)									
Krane LS et al. 2009	Retrospective	34	37					85.0 %	86.0 %						
Kim IY et al. 2010	Retrospective	25	25	19.0 %	38.1 %	72.6 %	71.4 %			88.0 %	80.0 %	96.0 %	96.0 %		
				($p=0.306$)		($p=1$)				($p=0.718$)					
Joshi N et al. 2010	Prospective	53	54							75.0 %	69.0 %	51.0 %	43.0 %		
										($p=0.391$)		($p=0.686$)			
Coelho RF et al. 2010	Prospective	473	330	28.7 %	22.7 %	51.6 %	42.7 %			91.1 %	91.8 %	97.0 %	96.3 %		
				($p=0.045$)		($p=0.016$)				($p=0.908$)		($p=0.741$)			
Sutherland DE et al. 2011	Randomized trial	47	47							63 %	81 %				
										($p=0.07$)					
Brien JC et al. 2011	Retrospective	31	58							64.0 %	50.0 %	69.0 %	62.0 %		
										($p=0.05$)		($p=0.27$)			

(continued)

Table 12.1 (continued)

Author	Type of study	Number of patients		Continence at catheter removal (3-7 days)		Continence at 30 days		Continenece at 45–75 days		Continence at 90 days		Continence at 180 days		Continence at 1 year	
		PR	No PR	PR	No PR	PR	No PR	PR	No PR	PR	No PR	PR	No PR	PR	No PR
Atug F et al. 2012	Retrospective	125	120	71.2 %	23.33 %	72.8 %	49.1 %			80.8 %	76.6 %	84.8 %	80.8 %	91.2 %	88.33 %
				($p<0.0001$)		($p=0.0002$)				($p=0.5176$)		($p=0.5088$)		($p=0.5956$)	
Hurtes X et al. 2012	Randomized trial	39	33			26.5 %	7.1 %			45.2 %	15.4 %	65.4 %	57.9 %		
						($p=0.047$)				($p=0.016$)		($p>0.5$)			
Gondo T et al. 2012	Retrospective	160	39	48.7 %	15.4 %	75.0 %	20.5 %	86.9 %	53.9 %	91.2 %	71.8 %	95.6 %	79.5 %	96.3 %	87.2 %
You YC et al. 2012	Retrospective	28	31			57.2 %	35.5 %			89.2 %	71 %	92.8 %	87.5 %	94.5 %	92.1 %

Green background highlights studies finding a significant advantage for PR, while orange background highlights studies finding no significant advantage

Vesicourethral Anastomosis: Putting It Back Together

13

Côme Tholomier, Roger Valdivieso, Abdullah M. Alenizi, and Kevin Zorn

Introduction

Robot-assisted radical prostatectomy (RARP) has progressively gained popularity amongst urologists and is now the dominant surgical approach for localized prostate cancer [1]. Despite the advantages of the da Vinci surgical system (high 3-D definition, magnified vision, movement scaling, tremor filtration, and wristed instruments with 7-degrees of freedom [2]), the watertight vesicourethral anastomosis (VUA) remains one of the challenging aspects of this procedure, particularly in the early learning curve. Compared to open radical prostatectomy (ORP), where 4–6 simple stitches are placed along with bladder mucosa eversion during VUA, well over 15–20 continuous Van Velthoven suture passages are performed during RARP [3].The key elements in the vesicourethral anastomosis are the following: tension-free, well-vascularized, mucosal apposition, sparing of the neurovascular bundles and water-tightness. A suboptimal VUA may result in urinary leak and prolonged urethral catheterization, along with secondary ileus, prolonged hospitalization, bladder neck contracture, as well as urinary incontinence [4, 5]; all of which affect patient short and long-term quality of life. In order to achieve optimal functional outcomes and optimal VUA, various techniques have been developed over the years to reinforce the sphincter mechanism. These include optimization of the urethral length [6], anterior suspension to the pubic bone [7], hemostasis verification [8], bladder neck preservation [9], special considerations in obese patients [10], posterior floor reconstruction (Rocco) [11], and puboprostatic ligament preservation [12].Overview of the Traditional and the New Types of Sutures. The standard of care to perform the VUA during RARP is the use of a continuous monofilament Van Velthoven suture. However, its use can lead to loss of tension due to suture loosening. Modifications or additional techniques have been used in order to improve continence outcomes, such as the posterior rhabdosphincter reconstruction, usage of Lapra-Ty (Ethicon Endo-Surgery, Cincinnati, OH) clips to secure tension [13], or asking the bedside assistant to follow the suture-line with a laparoscopic needle-driver. Although helpful, these techniques are associated with some disadvantages such as tissue tearing, suture breakage and juxta-anastomosis foreign body application.

A new type of suture, called self-retaining suture (SRS), was developed for tissue approximation in plastic surgery and is now used for VUA. It is available

C. Tholomier (✉) • R. Valdivieso, M.D.
A.M. Alenizi, M.D.
Department of Surgery, Section of Urology, Centre Hospitalier de l'Université de Montréal, Montréal, QC, Canada
e-mail: come.tholomier@gmail.com

K. Zorn, M.D.
Department of Urology–Director of Robotic Surgery, University of Montreal, Montreal, Canada

J.W. Davis (ed.), *Robot-Assisted Radical Prostatectomy*, DOI 10.1007/978-3-319-32641-2_13

as a unidirectional barbed suture (V-Loc, Covidien, Mansfield, MA) or bidirectional (Quill, Angiotech, Vancouver, BC) to secure tension-free tissue approximation [14, 15]. The FDA approved it for soft-tissue closure in March 2009. The benefits of the V-Loc or the Quill sutures are similar: they allow for "stronger, more water-tight closures"; "fewer gaps and consistent tension and hold around closure"; "reduced tissue recoil during suturing"; and the "elimination of knot tying" [16, 17].

The V-Loc Suture in RARP

The main advantage of the self-retaining suture (SRS) V-Loc is the fact that both posterior reconstruction and VUA can be performed with the same inter-locked double arm suture, without the help of an assistant and without the need for knot tying. This significantly reduces operative time even for expert surgeons [18], thus reducing the global cost of the procedure. In a European setting, Massoud et al. determined that the cost reduction amounted to 199 euros [19].

The V-Loc suture achieves a tensile strength of 80 % after 7 days and it is fully absorbed by 180 days. The distance between the barbs is 0.025 inch (i.e., 40 barbs per inch). These unidirectional barbs prohibit suture slippage and distribute the tissue forces at several points so that tearing and ischemic changes are avoided if precise bites are taken.

Several randomized control trials have demonstrated that catheterization time, length of stay, and the incidence of urine leakage were lower in the V-Loc group [20, 21]. Moreover, return of urinary continence and complication rates were similar. This newer technique provides a safe, efficient, and cost-effective posterior reconstruction and VUA alternative during RARP.

The Vesicourethral Anastomosis: Surgical Technique

I. Hemostasis Control

Prior to engaging in the delicate VUA process, venous bleeding control should be managed as significant oozing can hamper visualization of key anatomic structures. In this effect, bleeding can be controlled by an increase in intra-abdominal pressure to 20 mmHg [8], usage of spot coagulation, hemostatic suture placement or clipping. In difficult cases where continued oozing is encountered, use of Surgicele and fibrin-based hemostats can be applied.

II. Bladder Neck Assessment

Larger prostates, the presence of a median lobe and a difficult bladder neck dissection could lead to a size discrepancy between the bladder neck and the urethral stump. To help with reducing the diameter of the bladder neck opening in these patients, an anterior "tennis racket" running suture can be used. Alternatively, lateral closure at the 3 and 9 o'clock positions can also be carried out with an absorbable suture.

Another detail to facilitate VUA is the release of the lateral bladder attachments to reduce any tension and minimize tearing of the bladder neck [22]. Care must always be made in such cases to properly identify the ureteral orifices to avoid possible injuries or obstruction.

III. Anterior Suspension to the Pubic Bone

Another technique used is the anterior suspension of the bladder neck to the pubic bone (Figs. 13.1 and 13.2). The surgeon places two pubourethral suspension stitches after dorsal vein complex (DVC) ligation, thus before starting VUA. The stitch is also passed through the DVC and the pubic bone to ensure additional support [23]. It has been shown that this technique promotes rapid recovery of urinary continence after RARP [7]. Conflicting results have been reported in the literature. They are summarized in Table 13.1. To the best of our knowledge, no studies have looked at the relation between VUA leakage and anterior suspension.

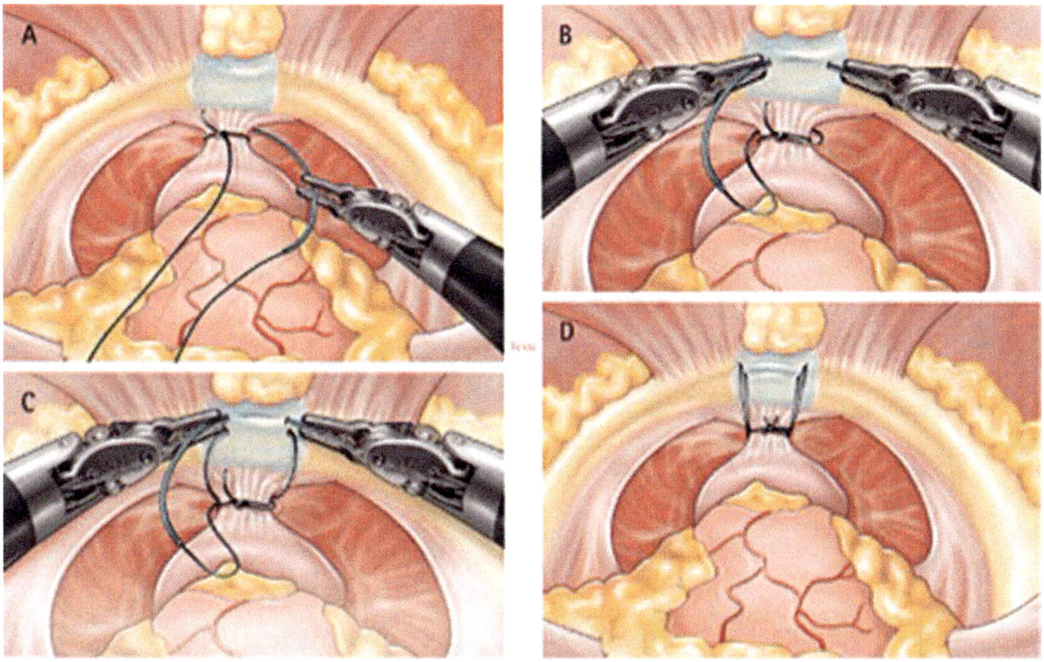

Fig. 13.1 *Anterior retropubic suspension.* (**a**) After ligation of the dorsal venous complex (DVC), the same suture is used to begin the anterior suspension. The needle is first passed between the DVC and the urethra. (**b**) The suture is passed at the posterior part of the pubic bone in the periosteum, holding the needle with the left needle driver at an angle of 90°, passing from left to right. (**c**) The suture is passed again between the DVC and the urethra from right to left and through the pubic bone. (**d**) View of the completed anterior suspension. (Reprinted with permission from John Wiley and Sons, license No. 3585701148571)

IV. Urethral Length Preservation

Maximizing urethral length has been correlated with better and earlier recovery of urinary continence especially for laparoscopic radical prostatectomy, where impressive results of 33 % vs. 15 % within 4 weeks ($p<0.05$) and a final continence rate of 89 % vs. 76 % ($p<0.05$) with no negative effects on positive surgical margin rates have been demonstrated [27, 28]. There is however a lack of studies concerning RARP.

The membranous urethral length is optimized at the step of the final division of the DVC and the urethra. Surgeon inspection of the prostatic apex should be performed along with careful assessment of initial transection. Similarly, once the anterior wall of the urethra is opened and the Foley catheter tip withdrawn, careful cutting of the posterior wall should be performed. Using this retro-apical approach (starting the transection at the posterior wall and at the apex of the urethra), combined with a synchronous (anterior and posterior) urethral transection, result in improved visualization, thus facilitating membranous urethral length preservation [29].

Furthermore, upon placement of the initial stitches for the posterior rhabdosphincter reconstruction, the traction of the distal periurethral tissues helps pull out of the pelvic musculature both the urethral stump and its mucosa—again favoring an excellent watertight, mucosa-to-mucosa, tension-free closure.

V. Posterior Rhabdosphincter Reconstruction

Rocco et al. developed in 2001 the posterior rhabdosphincter reconstruction (PRR) technique [11] and ultimately published the supportive data demonstrating its clinical benefits. Among the

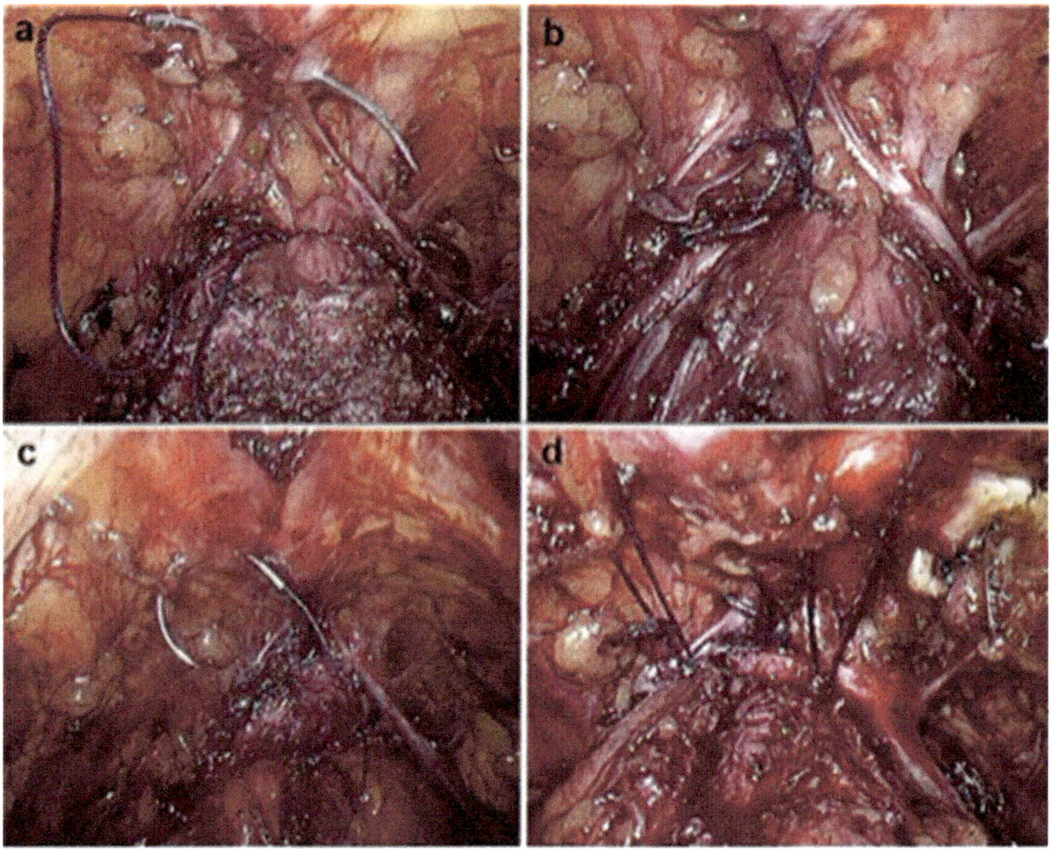

Fig. 13.2 *Anterior retropubic suspension with real images*

161 patients with clinically confined disease that underwent PRR, who were compared to a historical control group of 50 men, the former technique demonstrated excellent postoperative continence rates—72 % at day 3 after catheter removal following open radical prostatectomy [30]. While its impact on early continence is still debatable, the secondary endpoint of reduced VUA leakage is noteworthy [31].

The original posterior reconstruction of the rhabdosphincter consists of two steps where a 12-cm double-armed 2/0 quill suture on a RBI needle is used [32]. The first step is the apposition of the rhabdosphincter to the remaining Denonvilliers' fascia. The second step is the fixation of the Denonvilliers' fascia median raphe complex to the posterior bladder neck (Fig. 13.3). This helps preserving the urethra in its anatomic and functional position inside the pelvic floor.

A variety of modifications have been suggested since the initial technique from Rocco et al. was described. All of them aim at reinforcing the posterior musculofascial supporting plate even more. It has also been postulated that the combination of anterior and posterior reconstruction could lead to earlier continence recovery [33].

Gautam et al. and Coelho et al. reported various PRR techniques, showing their impact on continence recovery (Table 13.2). Conflicting results have been reported. To date, only one study (Menon et al.) was randomized, while all the others were control case studies. The former did not show any statistically significant difference, but includes less than 60 patients in each group. Most of the other studies do not have enough subjects, while the two biggest studies (Tewari et al. and Coelho et al.) show significant

Table 13.1 Contemporary RARP series with anterior suspension looking at postoperative continence rates

Series	Subjects (n)	Controls (n)			Continence	Comments
Noguchi et al. (2004)—CCS [24]	55	30			4w: 75 % vs. 13 % 12w: 89 % vs. 67 %	Statistically significant difference showing an advantage in immediate recovery of urinary continence
Hamada et al. (2014)—CCS [25]	30—AS + PR		30—AS + PR + UP	30—MULP alone	4w: 10 % vs. 50 % vs. 70 % 12w: 23 % vs. 90 % vs. 97 % 24w: 53 % vs. 100 % vs. 100 % ($p<0.0001$)	Significant difference when maximizing urethral length, more so than anterior suspension
Stolzenburg et al. (2011)—RCT [26]	90	90			2d: 10 % vs. 8 % 12w: 63 % vs. 63 %	No significant difference with bladder neck suspension. Better results when a nerve-sparing surgery was performed
Hurtes et al. (2012)—RCT [23]	39—AS + PR	33			15d: 5.9 % vs. 3.6 % 4w: 27 % vs. 7.1 % 12w: 45 % vs. 15 % 24w: 65 % vs. 58 %	Statistically significant difference at 1 and 3 months

AS anterior suspension, *d* day/days, *MULP* maximal urethral length preservation, *PR* posterior reconstruction, *w* week/weeks

difference especially in the first 4 weeks, meaning an earlier return to continence in the posterior reconstruction groups.

Only a few studies have compared vesicourethral anastomotic leaks with and without posterior reconstruction; and even fewer have enough patients to show statistical difference (Table 13.3). However, both studies from Coelho et al. and Menon et al. do show significant difference in favor of the posterior reconstruction technique.

We have previously described our surgical method to perform the PRR using the V-Loc180 suture [18, 40]. The first bite is taken from the 5 o'clock retrotrigonal area followed by the periurethral rectourethralis muscle at the same 5 o'clock position. The suture is then pulled through until the interlocked loops are stopped by the tissue, just like a knot. A second bite is taken from the midline retrotrigonal area behind the bladder, followed by a 6 o'clock bite of the periurethral tissue. A final 7 o'clock suture is performed on the bladder-side retrotrigonal tissue again while ensuring not to include any mucosa.

The left arm of the suture is then lifted cephalad and anteriorly with the left needle driver, while the open right needle driver stays on the bladder tissue to avoid tissue tears. The bladder can now be brought adjacent to the urethral stump via short and repetitive pulls.

VI. VUA

Once the posterior reconstruction is complete, the same left arm of the interlocked suture begins the VUA starting with a 6 o'clock, out-side-in, transmural bite of the bladder, followed by an inside-out bite of the posterior urethra. If backwalling of the mucosa is suspected, the assistant may pass the tip of the urethral catheter for orientation. The outside-in bites along the bladder and the inside-out urethral bites are continued from 6

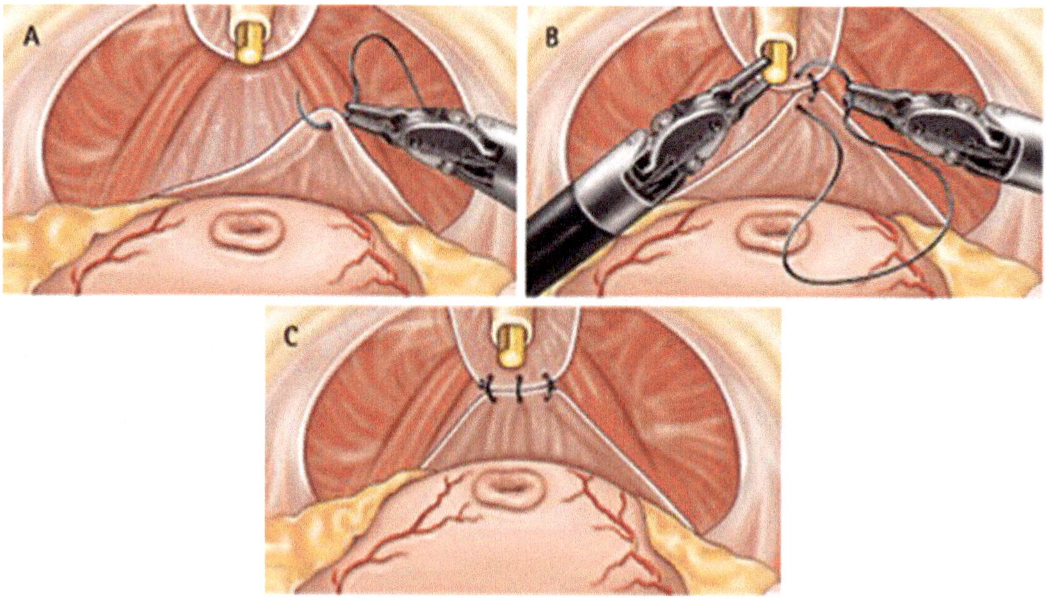

Fig. 13.3 *Posterior reconstruction of the rhabdomyosphincter.* (**a**) After removing the prostate specimen, the stitch is first passed through the Denonvilliers' fascia at the posterior face of the bladder. (**b**) The suture is passed through the musculofascial tissue beneath the urethra. Then it is passed two more times through the Denonvilliers' fascia and rhabdosphincter. (**c**) View of the completed posterior reconstruction, ready to begin vesicoureteral anastomosis. (Reprinted with permission from John Wiley and Sons, license No. 3585701148571)

to 10 o'clock. The right needle driver is used to avoid urethral tearing by straddling the suture.

If one were to complete the left side of the VUA now, it will obscure the posterior anastomosis. Therefore, we now use the right arm of the V-Loc suture to complete a synchronous anastomosis from an outside-in 5 o'clock bladder bite to a 5 o'clock inside-out urethral throw. It is important to make sure to avoid the neurovascular bundles and the rhabdosphincter muscle, which occurs most often when taking aggressive bites.

Repetitious bites are performed for the entire right side (5 to 12 o'clock) with final pass, each time independently, assuring adequate tension and thus getting rid of the need for the bedside assistant to follow tension. Now that the right anastomosis is completed, the arm is brought through the anterior urethral side and cut with a 2–3 cm stump. The left side is then completed from the 10 to 12 o'clock location again finishing on the anterior urethra. If bladder neck-urethral stump discrepancy does exist, surgeon may need to space bites on the bladder neck side in order to parachute the anastomosis. Fig.13.4 shows the tightening of the VLOC without the need to use knots or clips.

Before cutting the left arm, we instill 300 mL of normal saline in the bladder to verify watertight anastomosis (Fig. 13.5). If leakage was seen, further cinching of the suture or placement of additional V-Loc bites would be required. Now that the anastomosis is completed, the left arm of the V-Loc is used for retropubic suspension taking two passages into the posterior part of pubic symphysis, and then cutting it with a 2–3 cm stump. The two cut-ends are left untied allowing for a completely, knot-free reconstruction. In the event of a large bladder neck, where the last 2 cm of the V-Loc suture is required (which do not contain barbs), Lapra-Ty clips would help secure tension. In the case of a leak, bleeding, or lymph node dissection, a Jackson Pratt type abdominal drain is left inside the pelvic cavity.

Table 13.2 Contemporary RARP series of at least 50 patients who underwent rhabdosphincter reconstruction looking at postoperative continence

Series	Subjects (n)	Controls (n)	Reconstruction technique	Continence definition		Comment
				Strict 0 pad/day	0–1 Pad/day	
Kalisvaart et al. (2009)—CCS (level of evidence: III) [34]	50	50	Posterior reconstruction + anterior reconstruction	12w: 42 % vs. 21 %	NA	Statistically significant difference
Joshi et al. (2010)—CCS (III) [35]	53	54	Posterior reconstruction	12w: 25 % vs. 31 % 24w: 27 % vs. 49 %—defined as any involuntary urine loss	NA	No statistically significant difference
Woo et al. (2009)—CCS (III) [36]	69	63	Posterior only, 1-layer	No significant difference	90 vs. 150 ($p=0.01$)—using occasional (nondaily) security/safety pad	No significant difference between groups when strict definition of continence (0 pad/day) was applied
Tewari et al. (2008)—CCS (III) [37]	182 (Posterior + anterior) 304 (Anterior)	214	Total reconstruction and anterior only	NA	1w: 38 % vs. 27 % vs. 13 % 4–6w: 83 % vs. 59 % vs. 35 % 12w: 91 % vs. 77 % vs. 50 % 24w: 97 % vs. 86 % vs. 62 %	Statistically significant difference between controls and either form of reconstruction
Coelho et al. (2011)—CCS (III) [31]	437	330	Posterior reconstruction only, 2-layer	1w: 29 % vs. 23 % 4w: 52 % vs. 43 % 12w: 91 % vs. 92 % 24w: 97 % vs. 96 %	NA	Statistically significant difference between controls and subjects at 1 and 4 weeks. No difference for 12 and 24 weeks
Menon et al. (2008)—RCT (I) [38]	59	57	Total reconstruction, 1-layer	1d: 15 % vs. 7 % 2d: 14 % vs. 14 % 7d: 20 % vs. 16 % 30d: 42 % vs. 47 % ($p>0.1$)	1d: 34 % vs. 26 % 2d: 46 % vs. 49 % 7d: 54 % vs. 51 % 30d: 80 % vs. 74 % ($p>0.1$)	No statistically significant difference with both definition of continence

Adapted from Gautam et al. and Coelho et al. [31, 33]
CCS case control study, *d* day/days, *NA* not available, *RCT* randomized control trail, *w* week/weeks
Anterior reconstruction: the suture used to ligate the dorsal vein complex is passed through the periosteum of the symphysis pubis and ligated to the latter with a sliding knot technique [39]
Total reconstruction: combination of anterior and posterior reconstruction

Table 13.3 Contemporary RARP series with rhabdosphincter reconstruction looking at postoperative anastomotic leakage

Series	Subjects (n)	Controls (n)	Reconstruction technique	VUA leakage	Comments
Woo et al. (2009)—CCS (III) [36]	69	63	Posterior only, 1-layer	NA	No clinical urinary anastomotic leakage postoperatively in either group
Coelho et al. (2011)—CCS (III) [31]	437	330	Posterior reconstruction only, 2-layer	0.4 % vs. 2.1 % (p=0.036)	Statically significant difference in favor of the posterior reconstruction group
Zorn et al. (2011)—RCT (IIb) [21]	33	33	Posterior reconstruction	NA	No clinical urinary anastomotic leakage postoperatively in either group
Menon et al. (2008)—RCT (I) [38]	59	57	Total reconstruction, 1-layer	3.4 % vs. 8.7 % (p<0.05)	Statically significant difference in favor of the posterior reconstruction. However, clinical management was the same in each group (only patient in each cohort having to retain a catheter for more than the stipulated 1-week period)

CCS case control study, *d* day/days, *NA* not available, *RCT* randomized control trail, *w* week/weeks
Anterior reconstruction: the suture used to ligate the dorsal vein complex is passed through the periosteum of the symphysis pubis and ligated to the latter with a sliding knot technique [39]
Total reconstruction: combination of anterior and posterior reconstruction

Post-operative Considerations and Special Cases

I. Dealing with Post-operative Bladder Pain

The use of a prophylactic rectal suppository made of Belladonna (which contains the muscarinic receptor antagonists atropine and scopolamine) in conjunction to opium at the immediate conclusion of the surgery has been shown to significantly decrease postoperative pain, only for the first two postoperative hours, and also decrease 24-h morphine consumption [41]. Moreover, Lukasewycz et al. also demonstrated that this prophylactic rectal suppository helps reducing the irritative voiding symptoms, which represents most of the pain the patient voices.

II. Catheter Removal: Urinary Retention and VUA Leakage

Although uncommon, acute urinary retention after urethral catheter removal following RARP is an important reported complication [42]. To date, there is no general consensus on proper timing of catheter removal. Some high volume centers reported a retention rate of <1 % when the catheter was left for 5–7 days post RARP [31, 43]. On the other hand, early catheter removal after open or laparoscopic RP has been shown to increase the risk of urinary retention [44, 45]. Furthermore, in order to reduce the chance of urinary retention and any subsequent patient discomfort related to re-catheterization, some authors prefer to do cystography 3–7 days postoperatively [39, 42, 46]. In our experience, we test the anastomosis, intra-operatively, with 300

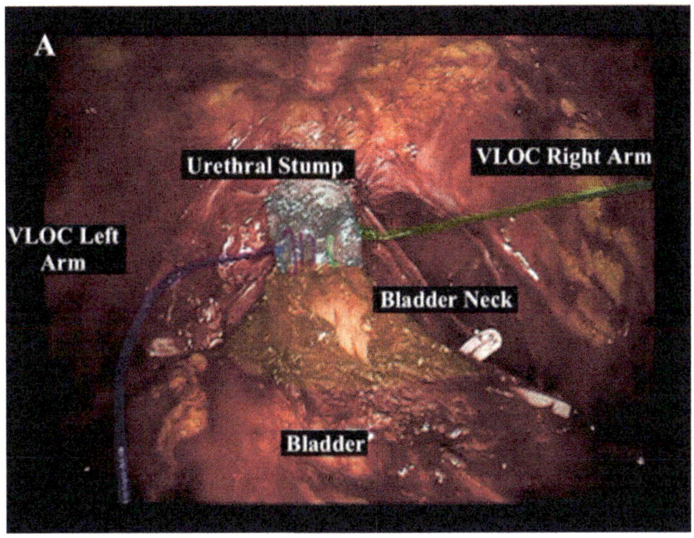

Fig. 13.4 *Tightening of the VLOC suture without using any knots or clips*

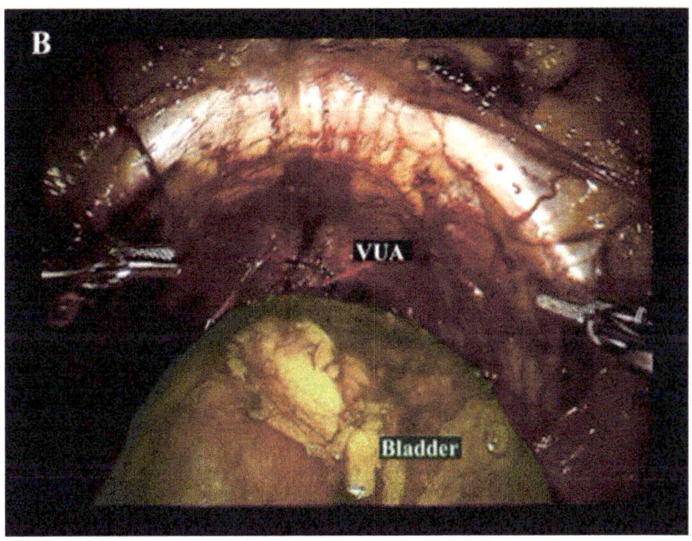

Fig. 13.5 *Verification of water-tightness*. 300 mL of saline instilled in the bladder to check for watertight anastomosis

mL of normal saline to verify water-tightness. If leakage is detected, urethral catheter is left in place for 7–10 days. However, if there is no evidence of leakage, urethral catheter is removed after 4 days.

VUA leakage is also a major cause of longer recovery time following radical prostatectomy (longer hospital stay, catheter duration, and days with an urinary drain). Management includes placing a catheter on mild traction, continuous antibiotics and taking the drain off suction with caution [47].

In a recently published article, we presented the results of 722 patients, who underwent RARP for localized prostate cancer [48]. We reported 0 bladder neck contractures, 3 vesicourethral anastomosis leakage (0.4 %) and 4 urinary retention needing Foley catheter replacement (0.6 %), demonstrating the excellent outcome of our vesicourethral anastomosis.

III. Bladder Neck Contracture

Bladder neck contractures can occur when the anastomosis narrows due to scarring and fibrosis. The actual mechanism is however poorly understood. The risk factors are likely to be excessive luminal narrowing at the site of the reconstruction, local tissue ischemia, failed mucosal apposition, and urinary leakage. A slow urinary stream should raise clinical suspicion. This can progressively result in acute urinary retention or overflow incontinence that may lead to kidney damage if not discovered early.

Bladder neck contracture rates after open radical retropubic prostatectomy are 5–32 % [49, 50], while they are only 0–3 % after laparoscopic radical retropubic prostatectomy [51, 52]. A study including 650 patients showed a rate of 1.1 % for robot-assisted radical prostatectomy. The diagnosis was made between 3 months and a year. Some possible causes of such a low rate certainly reside in the advantages of the da-Vinci console: better visualization, improved instrument maneuverability and decreased blood loss [5].

IV. Management of the Obese Patient

Obese patients also pose additional difficulties. In order to maximize the vision of the operative field, the Trendelenburg position can be increased, which results in a downward shift of the abdominal contents. To prevent clashing of the robotic arms and of the instruments, port placements should be optimized. Other important steps in order to improve the VUA in these cases would be to use the air seal trocar technology and/or bariatric trocars, to alter the trocar placement (more laterally), to use barbed sutures and to perform a modified posterior reconstruction [10]. All this is done in order to increase intra-pelvic working space and thus improve visualization.

Conclusion

The vesicourethral anastomosis is an important aspect of RARP, complicated to perform well since it is done towards the end of the operation, and which can lead to several important complications, namely bladder neck contracture and VUA leakage. The introduction of robotic surgery led to better outcomes specifically for the VUA due to the improved reconstructive capabilities. The Van Velthoven stitch is currently considered the standard of care for this procedure. However, the use of self-retaining barbed sutures, specifically V-Loc, looks promising as it helps to perform quicker and more reliable tissue tension for VUA, but also to improve patients' recovery.

Several techniques are now commonly used in order to maximize the anastomosis quality: tension-free, water-tightness, well-vascularized mucosa, and sparing of the neurovascular bundles. While incorporation of the posterior rhabdosphincter reconstruction technique may help promote earlier continence, the data favors its use to reduce VUA leakage.

References

1. Hu JC, Gu X, Lipsitz SR, Barry MJ, D'Amico AV, Weinberg AC, et al. Comparative effectiveness of minimally invasive vs open radical prostatectomy. JAMA. 2009;302(14):1557–64.
2. Berryhill Jr R, Jhaveri J, Yadav R, Leung R, Rao S, El-Hakim A, et al. Robotic prostatectomy: a review of outcomes compared with laparoscopic and open approaches. Urology. 2008;72(1):15–23.
3. Van Velthoven RF, Ahlering TE, Peltier A, Skarecky DW, Clayman RV. Technique for laparoscopic running urethrovesical anastomosis:the single knot method. Urology. 2003;61(4):699–702.
4. Krane LS, Bhandari M, Peabody JO, Menon M. Impact of percutaneous suprapubic tube drainage on patient discomfort after radical prostatectomy. Eur Urol. 2009;56(2):325–30.
5. Msezane LP, Reynolds WS, Gofrit ON, Shalhav AL, Zagaja GP, Zorn KC. Bladder neck contracture after robot-assisted laparoscopic radical prostatectomy: evaluation of incidence and risk factors and impact on urinary function. J Endourol. 2008;22(1):97–104.
6. Schlomm T, Heinzer H, Steuber T, Salomon G, Engel O, Michl U, et al. Full functional-length urethral sphincter preservation during radical prostatectomy. Eur Urol. 2011;60(2):320–9.
7. Patel VR, Coelho RF, Palmer KJ, Rocco B. Periurethral suspension stitch during robot-assisted laparoscopic radical prostatectomy: description of the technique and continence outcomes. Eur Urol. 2009;56(3):472–8.
8. Stolzenburg JU, Do M, Kallidonis P, Ghulam N, Hellawell G, Haefner T, et al. Hemostasis during

nerve-sparing endoscopic extraperitoneal radical prostatectomy. J Endourol. 2010;24(4):505–9.
9. Freire MP, Weinberg AC, Lei Y, Soukup JR, Lipsitz SR, Prasad SM, et al. Anatomic bladder neck preservation during robotic-assisted laparoscopic radical prostatectomy: description of technique and outcomes. Eur Urol. 2009;56(6):972–80.
10. Samavedi S, Abdul-Muhsin H, Pigilam S, Sivaraman A, Patel VR. Handling difficult anastomosis. Tips and tricks in obese patients and narrow pelvis. Indian J Urol. 2014;30(4):418–22.
11. Rocco F, Gadda F, Acquati P, Carmignani L, Favini P, Dell'Orto P, et al. Personal research: reconstruction of the urethral striated sphincter. Arch Ital Urol Androl. 2001;73(3):127–37.
12. Avant OL, Jones JA, Beck H, Hunt C, Straub M. New method to improve treatment outcomes for radical prostatectomy. Urology. 2000;56(4):658–62.
13. Zorn KC. Robotic radical prostatectomy: assurance of water-tight vesicourethral anastomotic closure with the Lapra-Ty clip. J Endourol. 2008;22(5):863–5.
14. Murtha AP, Kaplan AL, Paglia MJ, Mills BB, Feldstein ML, Ruff GL. Evaluation of a novel technique for wound closure using a barbed suture. Plast Reconstr Surg. 2006;117(6):1769–80.
15. Rosen AD. Use of absorbable running barbed suture and progressive tension technique in abdominoplasty: a novel approach. Plast Reconstr Surg. 2010;125(3):1024–7.
16. Greenberg JA, Einarsson JI. The use of bidirectional barbed suture in laparoscopic myomectomy and total laparoscopic hysterectomy. J Minim Invasive Gynecol. 2008;15(5):621–3.
17. Moran ME, Marsh C, Perrotti M. Bidirectional-barbed sutured knotless running anastomosis v classic Van Velthoven suturing in a model system. J Endourol. 2007;21(10):1175–8.
18. Zorn KC, Widmer H, Lattouf JB, Liberman D, Bhojani N, Trinh QD, et al. Novel method of knotless vesicourethral anastomosis during robot-assisted radical prostatectomy: feasibility study and early outcomes in 30 patients using the interlocked barbed unidirectional V-LOC180 suture. Can Urol Assoc J. 2011;5(3):188–94.
19. Massoud W, Thanigasalam R, El Hajj A, Girard F, Theveniaud PE, Chatellier G, et al. Does the use of a barbed polyglyconate absorbable suture have an impact on urethral anastomosis time, urethral stenosis rates, and cost effectiveness during robot-assisted radical prostatectomy? Urology. 2013;82(1):90–4.
20. Arslan M, Tuncel A, Aslan Y, Kozacioglu Z, Gunlusoy B, Atan A. Comparison of the urethrovesical anastomoses with polyglecaprone (Monocryl(R)) and bidirectional barbed (V-Loc 180(R)) running sutures in laparoscopic radical prostatectomy. Arch Ital Urol Androl. 2014;86(2):90–4.
21. Zorn KC, Trinh QD, Jeldres C, Schmitges J, Widmer H, Lattouf JB, et al. Prospective randomized trial of barbed polyglyconate suture to facilitate vesico-urethral anastomosis during robot-assisted radical prostatectomy: time reduction and cost benefit. BJU Int. 2012;109(10):1526–32.
22. Huang AC, Kowalczyk KJ, Hevelone ND, Lipsitz SR, Yu HY, Plaster BA, et al. The impact of prostate size, median lobe, and prior benign prostatic hyperplasia intervention on robot-assisted laparoscopic prostatectomy: technique and outcomes. Eur Urol. 2011;59(4):595–603.
23. Hurtes X, Roupret M, Vaessen C, Pereira H, Faivre d'Arcier B, Cormier L, et al. Anterior suspension combined with posterior reconstruction during robot-assisted laparoscopic prostatectomy improves early return of urinary continence: a prospective randomized multicentre trial. BJU Int. 2012;110(6):875–83.
24. Noguchi M, Noda S, Nakashima O, Matsuoka K, Kojiro M. Suspension technique improves rapid recovery of urinary continence following radical retropubic prostatectomy. Kurume Med J. 2004; 51(3-4):245–51.
25. Hamada A, Razdan S, Etafy MH, Fagin R, Razdan S. Early return of continence in patients undergoing robot-assisted laparoscopic prostatectomy using modified maximal urethral length preservation technique. J Endourol. 2014;28(8):930–8.
26. Stolzenburg JU, Nicolaus M, Kallidonis P, Do M, Dietel A, Hafner T, et al. Influence of bladder neck suspension stitches on early continence after radical prostatectomy: a prospective randomized study of 180 patients. Asian J Androl. 2011;13(6):806–11.
27. Mizutani Y, Uehara H, Fujisue Y, Takagi S, Nishida T, Inamoto T, et al. Urinary continence following laparoscopic radical prostatectomy: association with postoperative membranous urethral length measured using real-time intraoperative transrectal ultrasonography. Oncol Lett. 2012;3(1):181–4.
28. van Randenborgh H, Paul R, Kubler H, Breul J, Hartung R. Improved urinary continence after radical retropubic prostatectomy with preparation of a long, partially intraprostatic portion of the membraneous urethra: an analysis of 1013 consecutive cases. Prostate Cancer Prostatic Dis. 2004;7(3):253–7.
29. Tewari AK, Srivastava A, Mudaliar K, Tan GY, Grover S, El Douaihy Y, et al. Anatomical retro-apical technique of synchronous (posterior and anterior) urethral transection: a novel approach for ameliorating apical margin positivity during robotic radical prostatectomy. BJU Int. 2010;106(9):1364–73.
30. Rocco F, Carmignani L, Acquati P, Gadda F, Dell'Orto P, Rocco B, et al. Restoration of posterior aspect of rhabdosphincter shortens continence time after radical retropubic prostatectomy. J Urol. 2006;175(6):2201–6.
31. Coelho RF, Chauhan S, Orvieto MA, Sivaraman A, Palmer KJ, Coughlin G, et al. Influence of modified posterior reconstruction of the rhabdosphincter on early recovery of continence and anastomotic leakage rates after robot-assisted radical prostatectomy. Eur Urol. 2011;59(1):72–80.

32. Valero R, Schatloff O, Chauhan S, HwiiKo Y, Sivaraman A, Coelho RF, et al. Bidirectional barbed suture for bladder neck reconstruction, posterior reconstruction and vesicourethral anastomosis during robot assisted radical prostatectomy. Actas Urol Esp. 2012;36(2):69–74.
33. Gautam G, Rocco B, Patel VR, Zorn KC. Posterior rhabdosphincter reconstruction during robot-assisted radical prostatectomy: critical analysis of techniques and outcomes. Urology. 2010;76(3):734–41.
34. Kalisvaart JF, Osann KE, Finley DS, Ornstein DK. Posterior reconstruction and anterior suspension with single anastomotic suture in robot-assisted laparoscopic radical prostatectomy: a simple method to improve early return of continence. J Robot Surg. 2009;3(3):149–53.
35. Joshi N, de Blok W, van Muilekom E, van der Poel H. Impact of posterior musculofascial reconstruction on early continence after robot-assisted laparoscopic radical prostatectomy: results of a prospective parallel group trial. Eur Urol. 2010;58(1):84–9.
36. Woo JR, Shikanov S, Zorn KC, Shalhav AL, Zagaja GP. Impact of posterior rhabdosphincter reconstruction during robot-assisted radical prostatectomy: retrospective analysis of time to continence. J Endourol. 2009;23(12):1995–9.
37. Tewari A, Jhaveri J, Rao S, Yadav R, Bartsch G, Te A, et al. Total reconstruction of the vesico-urethral junction. BJU Int. 2008;101(7):871–7.
38. Menon M, Muhletaler F, Campos M, Peabody JO. Assessment of early continence after reconstruction of the periprostatic tissues in patients undergoing computer assisted (robotic) prostatectomy: results of a 2 group parallel randomized controlled trial. J Urol. 2008;180(3):1018–23.
39. Atug F, Kural AR, Tufek I, Srivastav S, Akpinar H. Anterior and posterior reconstruction technique and its impact on early return of continence after robot-assisted radical prostatectomy. J Endourol. 2012;26(4):381–6.
40. Valdivieso RF, Hueber PA, Zorn KC. Robot assisted radical prostatectomy: how I do it. Part II: surgical technique. Can J Urol. 2013;20(6):7073–8.
41. Lukasewycz S, Holman M, Kozlowski P, Porter CR, Odom E, Bernards C, et al. Does a perioperative belladonna and opium suppository improve postoperative pain following robotic assisted laparoscopic radical prostatectomy? Results of a single institution randomized study. Can J Urol. 2010;17(5): 5377–82.
42. Khemees TA, Novak R, Abaza R. Risk and prevention of acute urinary retention after robotic prostatectomy. J Urol. 2013;189(4):1432–6.
43. Agarwal PK, Sammon J, Bhandari A, Dabaja A, Diaz M, Dusik-Fenton S, et al. Safety profile of robot-assisted radical prostatectomy: a standardized report of complications in 3317 patients. Eur Urol. 2011;59(5):684–98.
44. Harpster LE, Brien J. Initial results using a running vesicourethral anastomosis following open radical retropubic prostatectomy. J Urol. 2007;177(1):118–22. discussion 22.
45. Nadu A, Salomon L, Hoznek A, Olsson LE, Saint F, de La Taille A, et al. Early removal of the catheter after laparoscopic radical prostatectomy. J Urol. 2001;166(5):1662–4.
46. Jeong IG, You D, Yoon JH, Hong S, Lim JH, Hong JH, et al. Impact of tamsulosin on urinary retention following early catheter removal after robot-assisted laparoscopic radical prostatectomy: a prospective randomized controlled trial. Int J Urol. 2014;21(2): 164–8.
47. Sukkarieh T, Harmon J, Penna F, Parra R. Incidence and management of anastomotic leakage following laparoscopic prostatectomy with implementation of a new anastomotic technique incorporating posterior bladder neck tailoring. J Robot Surg. 2007;1(3): 213–5.
48. Tholomier C, Bienz M, Hueber PA, Trinh QD, Hakim AE, Alhathal N, et al. Oncological and functional outcomes of 722 robot-assisted radical prostatectomy (RARP) cases: the largest Canadian 5-year experience. Can Urol Assoc J. 2014;8(5–6):195–201.
49. Kostakopoulos A, Argiropoulos V, Protogerou V, Tekerlekis P, Melekos M. Vesicourethral anastomotic strictures after radical retropubic prostatectomy: the experience of a single institution. Urol Int. 2004; 72(1):17–20.
50. Surya BV, Provet J, Johanson KE, Brown J. Anastomotic strictures following radical prostatectomy: risk factors and management. J Urol. 1990; 143(4):755–8.
51. Gonzalgo ML, Pavlovich CP, Trock BJ, Link RE, Sullivan W, Su LM. Classification and trends of perioperative morbidities following laparoscopic radical prostatectomy. J Urol. 2005;174(1):135–9. discussion 9.
52. Rassweiler J, Sentker L, Seemann O, Hatzinger M, Rumpelt HJ. Laparoscopic radical prostatectomy with the Heilbronn technique: an analysis of the first 180 cases. J Urol. 2001;166(6):2101–8.

Pelvic Lymph Node Dissection: Open Benchmarks with Lymphoscintigraphy

14

Daniel P. Nguyen, Philipp M. Huber, Tobias A. Metzger, Pascal Zehnder, and George N. Thalmann

Introduction

Radical prostatectomy (RP) is the gold standard for the surgical treatment of clinically localized prostate cancer [1, 2]. Since Hugh Hampton Young's first description of the intervention via the perineum in 1905 [3], RP has seen substantial changes, integrating increase in anatomical knowledge and improvements in surgical techniques to evolve into a safe, nerve-sparing procedure [4]. In addition, the popularization of retropubic RP by Walsh et al. in the 1980s gave a valuable opportunity for pelvic lymph node dissection (PLND) [5]. Yet, despite a significant amount of research dedicated to the subject, general consensus on the need for and the extent of PLND in conjunction with RP has not been reached. In fact, due to the stage migration of prostate cancer and probably to the introduction of minimally invasive techniques, a continuous decline in PLND rates has been observed [6]. The complexity of the debate is underscored by the fact that prostate cancer is a heterogeneous disease that encompasses a broad spectrum of biological behavior, from indolent to lethal. Thus, controversy surrounds not only PLND but also prostate cancer screening [7] and the necessity for radical therapy [8]. In this chapter, we will present open benchmarks for PLND in prostate cancer and explain why, in our opinion, an extended template is warranted when the indication for PLND is given.

D.P. Nguyen • P.M. Huber • T.A. Metzger
P. Zehnder • G.N. Thalmann, M.D. (✉)
Department of Urology, University Hospital of Bern, University of Bern, Anna-Seiler-Haus, Inselspital, Bern 3010, Switzerland
e-mail: Urology.berne@insel.ch

PLND as a Staging Procedure

Precise tumor staging identifies the extent and location of the malignancy, helps define malignant potential, and forms the basis for optimal therapeutic management. In continued efforts to assist clinicians with evidence-based and individualized decision-making, various tools predicting the probability of lymph node metastases according to serum prostate-specific antigen (PSA) levels, clinical stage, and preoperative biopsies have been developed [9–13]. Based on these prediction models, one may define patients in whom PLND should be performed, respectively in whom PLND may be omitted. The most recent nomogram was developed by Briganti et al. It constitutes the first algorithm based on a cohort of patients who underwent a more extended PLND, including only patients who had ten or more nodes removed. Unfortunately, its reliability is impacted by the fact that the majority of patients evaluated qualified as low risk, with approximately two-thirds having biopsy

J.W. Davis (ed.), *Robot-Assisted Radical Prostatectomy*, DOI 10.1007/978-3-319-32641-2_14

Gleason score 6 or less, while percentage of lymph node invasion was 8.3–11 % [11–13]. Therefore, prediction models do have inherent problems. They depend on the developmental cohort and thus reflect the experience of one or a few institutions. Given the variability in patient selection, staging procedure, surgeon experience, extent of PLND, and histopathologic tumor characteristics, these prediction models may lack generalizability. Nomograms can only attempt to predict the probability of finding positive nodes in an individual patient based on collected information about other patients. Furthermore, prediction models estimate the likelihood of nodal metastases but are unable to provide equally vital information about the number or location of these positive nodes. They also rely on Gleason score, which shows discrepancy between preoperative biopsy and pathologic specimen in more than 30 % of all cases [14, 15].

Radiological staging evaluation of prostate cancer includes computed tomography (CT) and magnetic resonance imaging (MRI). Despite steady advances, these imaging modalities still lack diagnostic accuracy in the staging of pelvic lymph nodes, with reported sensitivity for the detection of lymph node metastasis in the range of about 40 % for both tests [16]. In recent years, new concepts that include sentinel lymph node identification [17–22], diffusion-weighted MRI [23], and conventional or diffusion-weighted MR lymphangiography [24–26] have shown potential to detect diseased nodes. The role of sentinel lymph node techniques in defining lymphatic drainage of the prostate will be discussed below. As a staging procedure, the technique has a few setbacks. The prostate has many primary lymphatic landing sites in the pelvis [17, 18, 20–22]. Yet, only lymph nodes in proximity to the collimator are detected, and, consequently, those found outside the area explored may be missed. Furthermore, the technique is time-consuming, expensive, and dependent on the skills of the nuclear medicine specialist [19]. Finally, approximately 30 % of metastatic nodes are not sentinel nodes because tumor cells may obstruct lymphatics and compromise uptake of the nanocolloid [27]. Thus, for the time being, histopathologic examination of a meticulously performed PLND remains the most accurate and cost-effective staging procedure. The number of positive nodes, metastatic volume, and the presence of nodal extracapsular extension can be obtained [28], detailed information that is helpful for patient counseling about the risk of progression and stratifying men who may benefit from adjuvant therapy.

PLND Templates

Over the years, several PLND templates have been described. The minimal variant consists of removal of nodes in the obturator fossa or dorsal and along the external iliac vein only (Fig. 14.1). The limited variant (also termed standard) includes lymph nodes in the obturator fossa and dorsal and along the external iliac vein. Extended PLND, which additionally removes lymph nodes along the internal iliac vessels both medially and laterally and, in some cases, along the common iliac vessels, is the only variant that considers findings from anatomical and lymphoscintigraphic studies.

Anatomical Studies

Nearly 90 years ago, Cunéo and Marcille wrote that lymphatics from the prostate drain to lymph nodes located along the external iliac vein, in the obturator fossa, and along the internal iliac artery. Interestingly, they described that the medial chain of the common iliac lymph nodes ("groupe du promontoire") also receives direct afferents from the prostate [29]. Later on, Gil-Vernet described that lymphatics of the prostate gland drain into the periprostatic subcapsular network, from which three main ductal systems originate. These ducts run to the external iliac chain, the internal iliac chain, and to the presacral chain [30]. Weingärtner et al. underlined in an autopsy study that the number of nodes in the pelvis shows great interindividual variability, ranging from 8 to 56. The authors declared that 20 removed lymph nodes in the pelvis can be considered a representative dissection [31].

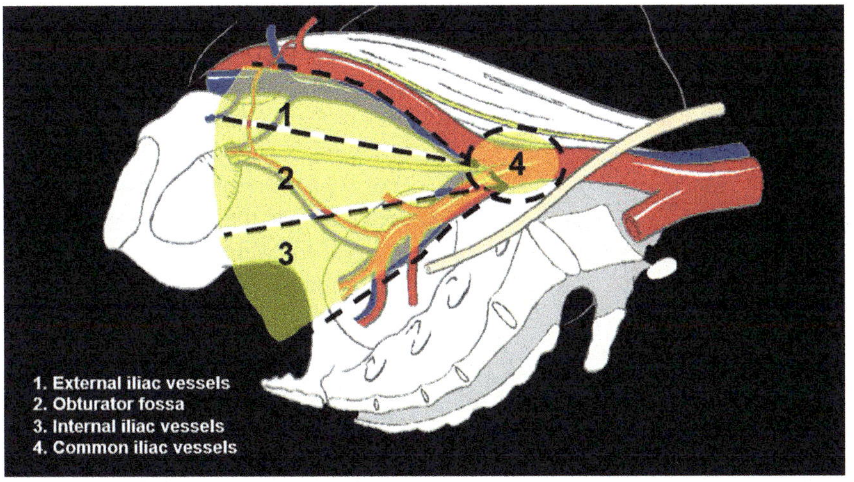

Fig. 14.1 PLND templates in prostate cancer. The minimal template includes lymph nodes in the obturator fossa or dorsal and along the external iliac vein. The limited ("standard") template includes lymph nodes in the obturator fossa and dorsal and along the external iliac vein. The extended template includes the internal iliac region additionally, and, in some institutions such as ours, lymph nodes along the common iliac vessels up to the ureter crossing

Lymphoscintigraphic Studies

Lymphoscintigraphy is based on the sentinel lymph node concept and aims to depict the first lymphatic landing site of the primary tumor. Recent mapping studies based on this technique have extended the knowledge acquired by anatomical studies with regard to lymphatic drainage of the prostate. Wawroschek et al. were the first to combine preoperative planar films with intraoperative gamma probe identification of sentinel lymph nodes after intraprostatic injection of ^{99m}Technetium in patients undergoing RP [17, 18]. A median of seven sentinel lymph nodes were detected per patient. Most men had sentinel nodes along the internal iliac artery alone (24 %) or in combination with other locations (32 %), which included the areas along the external iliac vein, the obturator fossa, and the presacral region. In 1055 men, 207 lymph node metastases were found, 205 of which were sentinel nodes. A limited PLND would have detected only 37 % of these metastases [18].

On the basis of this pioneering work, we used fusion imaging of three-dimensional single-photon emission computed tomography (SPECT) with CT/MRI after intraprostatic injection of ^{99m}Technetium [20]. SPECT/CT/MRI improves spatial resolution and orientation and allows for a more precise localization of ^{99m}Technetium-containing lymph nodes. This technique identified 317 sentinel lymph nodes in 34 patients with a median of ten per patient [3–19]. Locations of these primary landing sites of lymphatic drainage were external iliac/obturator fossa in 38 %, internal iliac in 25 %, presacral/pararectal in 8 %, common iliac in 16 %, paraaortic/caval in 12 %, and inguinal in 1 % (Fig. 14.2). Thus, the study revealed a more complex lymphatic drainage than was previously appreciated. Only little more than one-third of all sentinel lymph nodes would have been included within a limited template. In addition, only 63 % of the lymphatic landing sites were located inside the boundaries of an extended PLND limited to the iliac vessels distal to the bifurcation of the common iliac artery. By extending the dissection along common iliac vessels at least up to the ureter crossing, approximately 75 % of all nodes potentially harboring metastases would have been removed. Based on these findings, we argue that the extended PLND template should extend to the crossing of the ureter cranially (Fig. 14.1). In addition, the study emphasized that along the internal iliac artery

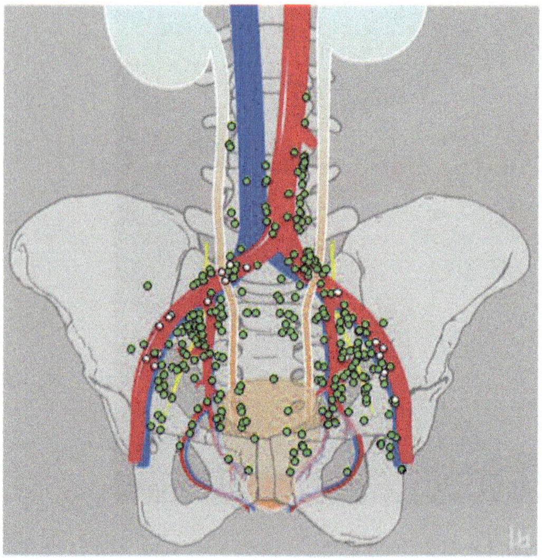

Fig. 14.2 Primary landing sites of the prostate [20]. Lymph nodes depict three-dimensional reconstruction of SPECT/CT/MRI data sets confirmed by intraoperative detection with a gamma probe. Green coded lymph nodes were visualized on direct view. White coded lymph nodes were located behind the represented vascular structures

and vein, sentinel lymph nodes are found both laterally and medially (presacral/pararectal region) to the vessels (Fig. 14.2).

Our results were reproduced in recent studies, using similar technique [21, 22]. Joniau et al., for instance, scintigraphically detected 470 sentinel lymph nodes in 74 patients, for a median number of six sentinel nodes per patient. A limited template would have removed lymph node metastases in only ten of 34 (29 %) patients. With an extended PLND including the external and internal iliac plus obturator regions, metastatic sites would have been resected in 26 of 34 patients (76 %). However, when including the common iliac region and the presacral chain, this number increased to 33 of 34 patients (97 %). The most common site for lymph node metastasis was the internal iliac region, alone or in combination with other sites (59 %) [22].

In summary, results from lymphoscintigraphic studies indicate that lymphatic drainage of the prostate shows large variability, with primary landing sites that include external iliac, obturator, internal iliac, common iliac, and presacral regions. Thus, lymph node metastases do not follow a predefined pathway of metastatic spread. It becomes evident that limited PLND misses a substantial number of primary landing sites of the prostate. Accordingly, recommended limits of extended PLND at our institution are (Fig. 14.1): the mid common region where the ureter crosses the iliac vessels cranially, the circumflex iliac vein and femoral canal distally, the upper limit of the external iliac vein laterally, the bladder medially, and the floor of the obturator fossa and the internal iliac vessels dorsally. Importantly, skeletonization of the tissue medial and lateral to the internal iliac vessels (presacral/pararectal region) should be done. It has to be noted that, even with the extended variant, approximately 25 % of the primary lymphatic landing sites lie outside the template and can be found up to the origin of the inferior mesenteric artery, as shown in our (20; Fig. 14.2) and Joniau et al. studies [22]. Nevertheless, when defining the extent of PLND, there must be a balance between potential benefits of removing all primary landing sites and risks of increased morbidity, compromised functional outcomes, longer surgery, and associated costs.

Outcomes After Extended PLND

Total Lymph Node Counts

With extended PLND, the median number of lymph nodes removed at RP is 21 (range 6–50) at our institution [32, 33]. This number is consistent with the above mentioned anatomical study from Weingärtner et al., who suggested that at least 20 lymph nodes removed enables adequate locoregional staging [31]. Heidenreich et al., comparing a historical cohort that underwent limited PLND with a more recent cohort that underwent extended PLND comprising the external iliac, internal iliac, obturator and common iliac as well as the presacral nodes, reported median number of removed lymph nodes of 11 [6–19] and 28 [21–46], respectively ($p<0.01$) [34]. In a study of patients who received laparoscopic RP, the mean number of lymph nodes removed was six for limited PLND and 18 for extended PLND ($p=0.002$)

[15]. Other recent analyses are in agreement with these numbers [11, 13]. Taken together, these studies demonstrate that extended PLND removes a median of 18–28 lymph nodes, whereas in limited PLND, only 6–11 lymph nodes are resected. Yet, although the number of total nodes removed gives an insight into the extent of PLND performed, the minimum number of lymph nodes for optimal staging remains unknown because of interindividual variability in lymph node counts [31]. Therefore, it is primarily the surgeon's dedication to clear a certain template (extended PLND) that is important.

Positive Lymph Node Counts and Location of Node Disease

Analyzing cohorts of patients operated on by different surgeons, investigators from both the United States and Europe demonstrated that removal of a greater number of lymph nodes at RP and PLND is associated with a linear increase in the probability of detecting lymph node invasion [35, 36]. These results corroborated those from the Surveillance Epidemiology and End Results (SEER) database [37]. Altogether, these data indirectly implied that, in general, an extended PLND template detects a higher percentage of lymph node invasion than a limited template. Indeed, while the proportion of patients with positive lymph nodes ranges from 7 to 12 % with limited PLND, it increases up to 23–26 % with extended PLND [32–34, 38]. Heidenreich et al. found twice as many positive nodes using the extended vs. the limited template (26 % vs. 12 %; $p<0.03$) [34]. Importantly, 42 % of all lymph node metastases were found outside the regions of limited PLND. Confirming these findings, by extending the boundary of PLND to include the internal iliac region, Wawroschek et al. detected an additional 35 % of patients with lymph node metastases [39]. In multivariable analysis, Touijer et al. reported a more than eightfold higher risk of positive nodes for extended vs. limited PLND [40]. In our own series, 58 % of all positive nodes were found along the internal iliac vessels. Furthermore, 20 % of patients had this as their sole site of node disease [32], which is consistent with Heidenreich et al. analysis [34], and, more recently, Joniau et al. mapping study [22]. Collectively, these studies indicate that PLND based on a limited template misses 40–60 % of all metastatic lymph nodes, under staging patients and leaving them with tumor disease.

Many have argued that the value of an extended template has yet to be proven in a prospective, randomized fashion. Clark et al. attempted to fill this void and conducted a study comparing limited and extended PLND in 123 patients. Percentages of lymph node invasion were not significantly different between the two groups; however, patients undergoing extended PLND had higher rates of complications. Although addressing an important issue, the study was underpowered to allow for a conclusion of noninferiority. In addition, it included patients the majority of whom were at low risk for lymph node metastases, even in those treated with extended PLND. The trial was further limited by the fact that in patients in the extended PLND group, dissection was performed on one side only independently of tumor location. Finally, the number of lymph nodes removed and pathological assessment were not described [41].

Overall, current evidence from our institution and others support the resection of lymph nodes located along the internal iliac vessels whenever PLND is indicated, as up to two-thirds of all positive lymph nodes are found in this area, and in one-fifth of all node-positive cases it is the sole site of disease.

Oncologic Outcomes

PLND May Offer a Chance for Cure in Patients with Minimal Lymph Node Disease

Despite the fact that RP and PLND provide excellent cancer control, at least 30 % of all patients will experience biochemical recurrence [42, 43], and a significant proportion of these men will ultimately die from disease progression [43–45]. In particular, evidence of lymph node invasion at RP has been associated with poor prognosis [46].

Nevertheless, there is accumulating evidence that a subset of node-positive patients have excellent outcomes, even without immediate hormonal therapy. In our cohort of 122 lymph node-positive patients with median follow-up of 5.6 years, cancer-specific survival probability was 85 % at 5 years and 60 % at 10 years. For patients with one, two, and three or more positive nodes, cancer-specific survival at 10 years was 72.1, 79.1, and 33.4 %, respectively. In multivariable analysis, the number of positive lymph nodes was identified as the most significant predictor of cancer-related death [47]. A recent update with a median follow-up of 15.6 years confirmed that a subset of patients with minimal node disease remain disease free [48]. These results would not seem possible if metastatic lymph nodes had been left in. Our results are in line with those from other institutions [49–51]. For instance, Touijer et al., evaluating 369 patients with lymph node invasion at RP who did not receive adjuvant therapy, documented that a considerable subset of these men (28 %) remain disease free at 10 years. The presence of three or more positive nodes conferred a significantly higher risk of biochemical recurrence [51]. Lymph node density, which is the ratio of number of positive nodes to total number of nodes removed, has also been used to demonstrate differences in survival outcomes among patients with lymph node metastases. Daneshmand et al. reported that patients with a density of 20 % or greater were at higher risk of clinical recurrence than those with a density of less than 20 % [49]. These data essentially agreed with those from Palapattu et al. who chose a 15 % cut-off point in the Johns Hopkins series [52].

Taken together, a subset of patients with node-positive disease have a good chance of asymptomatic long-term survival in the presence of minimal lymph node disease (two or less positive nodes, low metastatic volume). To what extent this prognosis is the result of a positive impact of PLND is still to be determined. PLND may also be beneficial in the context of adjuvant hormonal therapy. In the Mayo Clinic series, in which more than 90 % of node-positive patients received adjuvant hormonal therapy, 10-year event-free survival for patients with lymph node metastases was 80 % for systemic progression and 86 % for cancer death. Patients with one positive lymph node were at threefold higher risk for systemic progression and fourfold higher risk for prostate cancer-related death than node-negative patients. However, patients with two or more positive lymph nodes were twice more likely to experience systemic progression and prostate cancer-related death than those with one positive node [53].

Extended PLND May Offer Survival Benefit in Pathologically Node-Negative Patients

Some data suggest that the extent of PLND is associated with improved survival in pN0 patients. Bader et al. found increasing rates of PSA progression after removal of more than 14, 10-14, 5-9, and 0-4 lymph nodes in patients with pT1 and pT2 N0 prostate cancer [54]. Masterson et al. reported a significant correlation between number of nodes removed and freedom from biochemical recurrence for node-negative patients (hazard ratio 0.91; $p=0.01$) [35]. Performing a case-control study of node-negative patients, Heidenreich et al. found biochemical recurrence rates of 23 and 8 % in patients who underwent limited and extended PLND, respectively [55]. Joslyn and Konety analyzed the SEER database and reported that, among node-negative patients, a more extensive PLND (i.e., ten or more lymph nodes) confers a 15 % lower risk of cancer-specific death at 10 years compared to patients who did not undergo PLND [37].

These results lead to the assumption that extended PLND removes microscopic metastases that are not detected by routine pathologic processing, thereby providing survival benefit in a subset of patients. This hypothesis is supported by studies evaluating markers of micrometastasis by real-time RT-PCR and immunohistochemistry in pathologically node-negative patients. These assays detected occult metastasis in up to 30 % of all patients [56, 57]. Collectively, the available evidence suggests that not only the detection of positive nodes but also the removal of as many nodes as possible should be the main objective for PLND to improve outcome.

PLND in Low-Risk Prostate Cancer

Many surgeons consider PLND unnecessary in men with low-risk prostate cancer (serum PSA less than 10 ng/ml, pathologic Gleason score 6), which generally harbors lesser risk of nodal involvement [11]. Nevertheless, in our series, 11 % of patients with serum PSA less than 10 ng/ml had lymph nodes metastases. A 25 % incidence of lymph node metastases was seen in patients with pathologic Gleason score 7 or greater, while the risk of node disease was 3 % in patients with Gleason score 6 or less [58]. Weckermann et al. reported a slightly higher (7.4 %) percentage of lymph node invasion among patients with PSA 10 ng/ml or less and biopsy Gleason score 6 or less who underwent radio-guided resection of sentinel lymph nodes. Interestingly, 54 % of positive nodes were detected outside the limited PLND template [59]. Heidenreich et al. found a 6 % incidence of lymph node invasion in a similar population [60]. In North American series of patients with low-risk prostate cancer, the percentage of lymph node invasion was as low as 0.5 % [61, 62]. However, these studies are biased by the inclusion of patients treated with limited PLND, which may miss some positive nodes. Since the anatomical distribution of lymph node metastases is not different between patients with low-, intermediate-, and high-risk prostate cancer [32, 58, 59], the use of a limited template when performing PLND in the low-risk group is unjustified.

Altogether, the risk of lymph node invasion in low-risk patients ranges from 2 to 8 %. While many authors have come to the conclusion that PLND should not be performed in this group of patients, it should be pointed out that this population is probably at very low risk of dying from prostate cancer, even if left untreated, and the indication for RP should be questioned rather than that for PLND [8]. Finally, as mentioned previously, pathologic Gleason score is underestimated in the preoperative biopsies in approximately 30 % of all cases, especially in low-grade disease [14, 15], making the decision to perform PLND or not in this group difficult.

Complications of PLND

The most common complication associated with PLND is lymphocele formation. Lymphoceles can cause pain, fever, lymphedema, ileus, venous thrombosis, pulmonary embolism, and voiding dysfunction through extrinsic compression of the bladder. Injuries to the obturator nerve, ureter, and blood vessels may also occur during PLND. Reported complication rates after extended PLND range from 2 to 20 % [15, 32, 34, 58, 63]. Briganti reported that overall complication rates were higher in patients treated with extended PLND in comparison with limited PLND (19.8 % vs. 8.2 %; $p<0.001$) [63]. When specific complications were assessed, only the rate of lymphocele was significantly higher in patients treated with extended PLND (10.3 % vs. 4.6 %; $p=0.01$). Conversely, Heidenreich et al. showed no significant difference in numbers of intra- and perioperative complications and lymphocele formation between patients who underwent extended and limited PLND (8.7 % vs. 9 %). In our institution, secondary drainage of a lymphocele occurs in 2–3 % of all cases [32, 33, 47]. Finally, extended PLND has not been shown to influence functional outcomes after nerve-sparing RP [64, 65].

Morbidity of PLND can be minimized by the following measures: (1) with ligation, instead of clipping of lymphatics from the lower extremities, (2) saving all lymphatics lateral to the external iliac artery, (3) placement of two drains, one on each side of the pelvis, which are removed gradually every two days from the third postoperative day until the total amount drained is less than 50 ml/24 h, (4) injection of low molecular heparin into the upper arm instead of the thigh to avoid a local heparin effect. If a lymphocele occurs despite these precautions, ultrasound-guided placement of a cystostomy or nephrostomy tube into the lymphocele with continuous drainage will solve the problem. More invasive procedures are not necessary.

Final Words

Based on the findings reviewed above, when the indication for RP is given, whether open, laparoscopic, or robot-assisted, an extended PLND should be performed. Extended PLND increases the yield of both total lymph nodes and lymph node metastases independent of risk classification of prostate cancer. Importantly, two-thirds of all lymph node metastases are found laterally and medially to the internal iliac vessels [22, 32]. This finding is consistent with the description of primary landing sites of the prostate [18, 20]. Incorporating the available evidence to date, guidelines from the European Association of Urology and the National Comprehensive Cancer Network currently recommend extended PLND whenever indicated [1, 66]. In our opinion, the boundaries for an extended PLND should include: the mid-common region where the ureter crosses the common iliac vessels cranially, the circumflex iliac vein and femoral canal distally, the upper limit of the external iliac vein laterally, the bladder medially, and the floor of the obturator fossa and the internal iliac vessels dorsally. With adequate training and increasing experience, operative time is only marginally increased compared to limited PLND. Complications can be minimized by meticulous surgical technique, including ligation of the lymphatics coming from the legs and placement of bilateral wound drains.

Editor's Comments—Nguyen et al.

As detailed in the chapter to follow, the robotic technique to extended template lymph node dissection is part surgeon understanding of what nodes to obtain and part surgical skills. After years of developing the extended template technique with the robot from 2007 to 2012, I had sufficient data to show that the nodes and nodal yields increased [67]; however there was no way to know for sure that my technique was the same as developed by Studer and colleagues in Berne. Ultimately I had to travel there in person and observe cases and give some talks. What I learned was that the anatomy has to be moved around to find the nodes, and that the lymphoscintigraphy really identifies a wide, variable template of nodes. Attached are images from the visit showing how tedious learning process is—Figs. 14.3, 14.4, 14.5, 14.6, 14.7, and 14.8. For the rest of us, the knowledge gained can translate into an efficient extended template. In my hands I can do this in 30–45 min although early on this took around 90 min.

Fig. 14.3 Through an open approach the lymphoscintigraphy is performed. The Geiger counter is quite large and not feasible for laparoscopic access

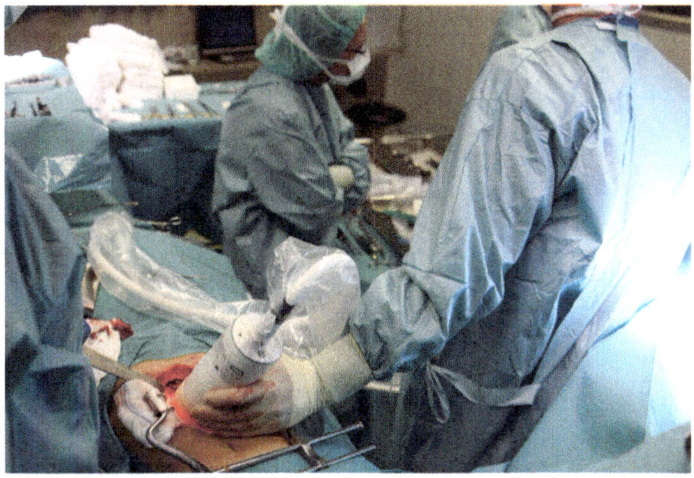

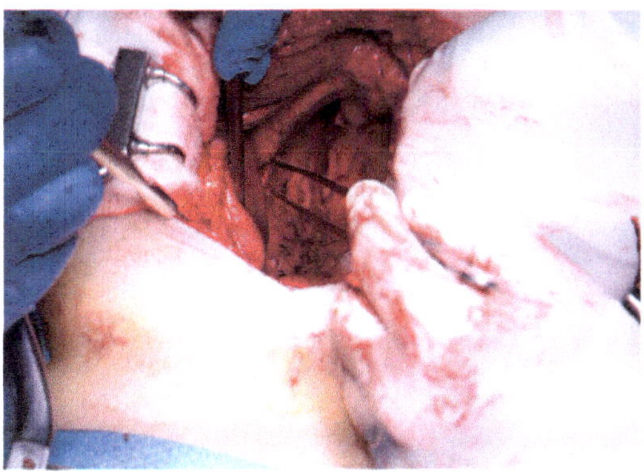

Fig. 14.4 The template is exposed with their open approach and extraperitoneal

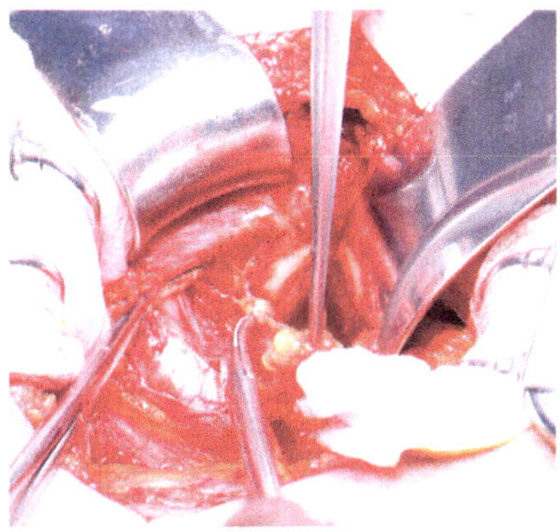

Fig. 14.5 The template is dissected along the left external iliac artery

Fig. 14.6 A laptop software package shows the imaging progress—nodes with signaling are still present

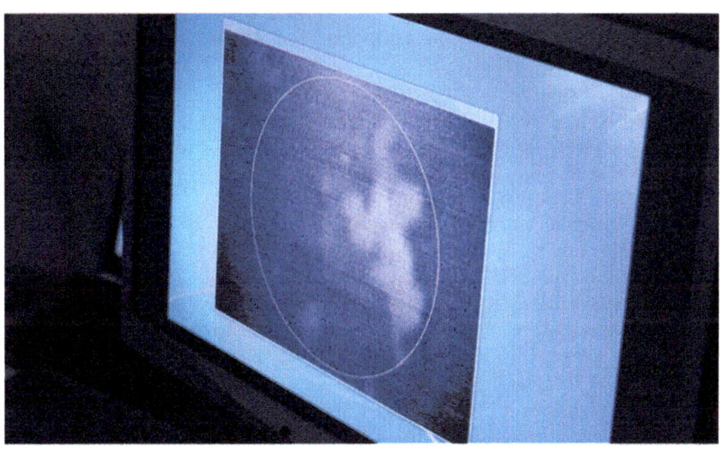

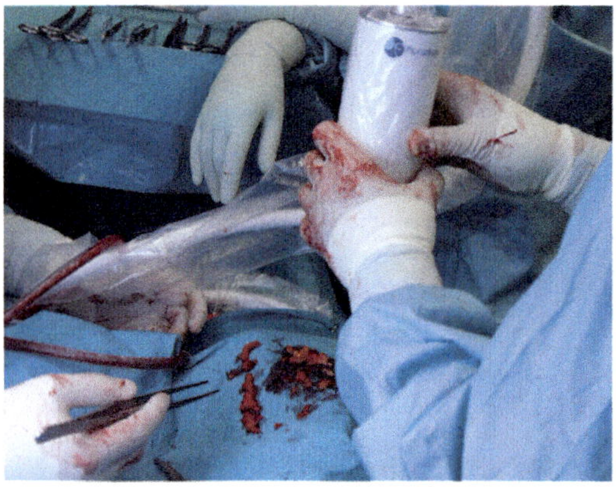

Fig. 14.7 The lymph nodes removed are re-examined on the back table for signaling

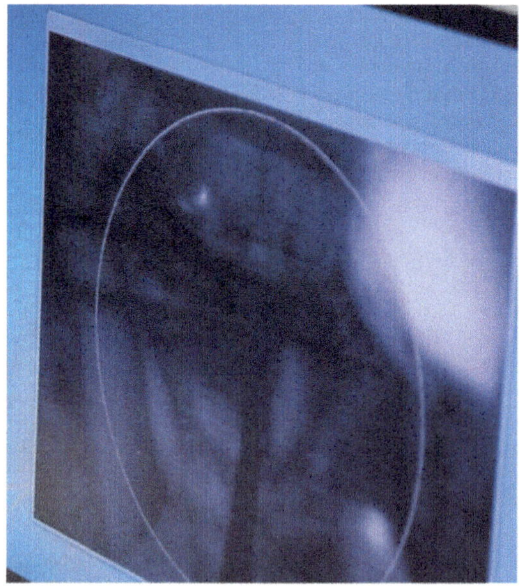

Fig. 14.8 The field is re-examined for remaining signaling such as in the *upper left corner*, and the images rechecked until all tissue with signaling are removed

References

1. Heidenreich A, Bastian PJ, Bellmunt J, et al. EAU guidelines on prostate cancer. Part 1: screening, diagnosis and local treatment with curative intent-update 2013. Eur Urol. 2014;65:124–37.
2. Bill-Axelson A, Holmberg L, Ruutu M, et al. Radical prostatectomy versus watchful waiting in early prostate cancer. New Engl J Med. 2011;364:1708–17.
3. Young HH. The early diagnosis and radical cure of carcinoma of the prostate: being a study of 40 cases and presentation of a radical operation which was carried out in four cases. Bull Johns Hopkins Hosp. 1905;16:315–21.
4. Kessler TM, Burkhard FC, Studer UE. Nerve-sparing open radical retropubic prostatectomy. Eur Urol. 2007;51:90–7.
5. Walsh PC. Anatomic radical retropubic prostatectomy. In: Walsh PC, Retik AB, Vaughan Jr ED, Wein AJ, editors. Campbell's urology, vol. III. 7th ed. Philadelphia: WB Saunders; 1997. p. 2565–88. Chapter 86.
6. Feifer AH, Elkin EB, Lowrance WT, et al. Temporal trends and predictors of pelvic lymph node dissection in open or minimally invasive radical prostatectomy. Cancer. 2011;117:3933–42.
7. Carlsson S, Vickers AJ, Roobol M, et al. Prostate cancer screening: facts, statistics, and interpretation in response to the US Preventive Services Task Force Review. J Clin Oncol. 2012;30:2581–4.
8. Vickers AJ, Eastham JA, Scardino PT. Radical prostatectomy versus observation for prostate cancer. N Engl J Med. 2012;367:1467–8.
9. Cagiannos I, Karakiewicz P, Eastham JA, et al. A preoperative nomogram identifying decreased risk of positive pelvic lymph nodes in patients with prostate cancer. J Urol. 2003;170:1798–803.
10. Makarov DV, Trock BJ, Humphreys EB, et al. Updated nomogram to predict pathologic stage of prostate cancer given prostate-specific antigen level, clinical stage, and biopsy Gleason score (Partin tables) based on cases from 2000 to 2005. Urology. 2007;69:1095–101.
11. Briganti A, Chun FK, Salonia A, et al. Validation of a nomogram predicting the probability of lymph node invasion among patients undergoing radical prostatectomy and an extended pelvic lymphadenectomy. Eur Urol. 2006;49:1019–26.
12. Briganti A, Karakiewicz PI, Chun FK, et al. Percentage of positive biopsy cores can improve the ability to predict lymph node invasion in patients undergoing radical prostatectomy and extended pelvic lymph node dissection. Eur Urol. 2007;51:1573–81.
13. Briganti A, Larcher A, Abdollah F, et al. Updated nomogram predicting lymph node invasion in patients with prostate cancer undergoing extended pelvic lymph node dissection: the essential importance of percentage of positive cores. Eur Urol. 2012;61:480–7.
14. Moussa AS, Kattan MW, Berglund R, Yu C, Fareed K, Jones JS. A nomogram for predicting upgrading in patients with low- and intermediate-grade prostate cancer in the era of extended prostate sampling. BJU Int. 2010;105:352–8.
15. Eden CG, Arora A, Rouse P. Extended vs standard pelvic lymphadenectomy during laparoscopic radical

prostatectomy for intermediate- and high-risk prostate cancer. BJU Int. 2010;106:537–42.
16. Hövels AM, Heesakkers RA, Adang EM, et al. The diagnostic accuracy of CT and MRI in the staging of pelvic lymph nodes in patients with prostate cancer: a meta-analysis. Clin Radiol. 2008;63:387–95.
17. Wawroschek F, Vogt H, Wengenmair H, et al. Prostate lymphoscintigraphy and radio-guided surgery for sentinel lymph node identification in prostate cancer: technique and results of the first 350 cases. Urol Int. 2003;70:303–10.
18. Weckermann D, Dorn R, Trefz M, Wagner T, Wawroschek F, Harzmann R. Sentinel lymph node dissection for prostate cancer: experience with more than 1,000 patients. J Urol. 2007;177:916–20.
19. Warncke SH, Mattei A, Fuechsel FG, Z'Brun S, Krause T, Studer UE. Detection rate and operating time required for gamma probe-guided sentinel lymph node resection after injection of Technetium-99 m nanocolloid into the prostate with and without preoperative imaging. Eur Urol. 2007;52:126–32.
20. Mattei A, Fuechsel FG, Bhatta Dhar N, et al. The template of the primary lymphatic landing sites of the prostate should be revisited: results of a multimodality mapping study. Eur Urol. 2008;53:118–25.
21. Ganswindt U, Schilling D, Müller AC, Bares R, Bartenstein P, Belka C. Distribution of prostate sentinel nodes: a SPECT-derived anatomic atlas. Int J Radiat Oncol Biol Phys. 2011;79:1364–72.
22. Joniau S, Van Den Bergh L, Lerut E, et al. Mapping of pelvic lymph node metastases in prostate cancer. Eur Urol. 2013;63:450–8.
23. Thoeny HC, Froehlich JM, Triantafyllou M, et al. Metastases in normal-sized pelvic lymph nodes: detection with diffusion-weighted MR imaging. Radiology. 2014;273:125–35.
24. Heesakkers RA, Hövels AM, Jager GJ, et al. MRI with a lymph-node-specific contrast agent as an alternative to CT scan and lymph-node dissection in patients with prostate cancer: a prospective multicohort study. Lancet Oncol. 2008;9:850–6.
25. Birkhäuser FD, Studer UE, Froehlich JM, et al. Combined ultrasmall superparamagnetic particles of iron oxide-enhanced and diffusion-weighted magnetic resonance imaging facilitates detection of metastases in normal-sized pelvic lymph nodes of patients with bladder and prostate cancer. Eur Urol. 2013;64:953–60.
26. Triantafyllou M, Studer UE, Birkhäuser FD, et al. Ultrasmall superparamagnetic particles of iron oxide allow for the detection of metastases in normal sized pelvic lymph nodes of patients with bladder and/or prostate cancer. Eur J Cancer. 2013;49:616–24.
27. Weckermann D, Dorn R, Holl G, Wagner T, Harzmann R. Limitations of radioguided surgery in high-risk prostate cancer. Eur Urol. 2007;51:1549–58.
28. Fleischmann A, Schobinger S, Schumacher M, Thalmann GN, Studer UE. Survival in surgically treated, nodal positive prostate cancer patients is predicted by histopathological characteristics of the primary tumor and its lymph node metastases. Prostate. 2009;69:352–62.
29. Cunéo B, Marcille M. Topographie des ganglions iliopelviens. Bull Mem Soc Anat Paris 1901;653–663
30. Gil-Vernet JM. Prostate cancer: anatomical and surgical considerations. Br J Urol. 1996;78:161–8.
31. Weingärtner K, Ramaswamy A, Bittinger A, Gerharz EW, Vöge D, Riedmiller H. Anatomical basis for pelvic lymphadenectomy in prostate caner: results of an autopsy study and implications for the clinic. J Urol. 1996;156:1969–71.
32. Bader P, Burkhard FC, Markwalder R, Studer UE. Is a limited lymph node dissection an adequate staging procedure for prostate cancer? J Urol. 2002;168:514–8.
33. Bader P, Burkhard FC, Markwalder R, Studer UE. Disease progression and survival of patients with positive lymph nodes after radical prostatectomy. Is there a chance of cure? J Urol. 2003;169:849–54.
34. Heidenreich A, Varga Z, Von Knobloch R. Extended pelvic lymphadenectomy in patients undergoing radical prostatectomy: high incidence of lymph node metastasis. J Urol. 2002;167:1681–6.
35. Masterson TA, Bianco FJ, Vickers AJ, et al. The association between total and positive lymph node counts, and disease progression in clinically localized prostate cancer. J Urol. 2006;175:1320–4.
36. Briganti A, Chun FK, Salonia A, et al. Validation of a nomogram predicting the probability of lymph node invasion based on the extent of pelvic lymphadenectomy in patients with clinically localized prostate cancer. BJU Int. 2006;98:788–93.
37. Joslyn SA, Konety BR. Impact of extent of lymphadenectomy on survival after radical prostatectomy for prostate cancer. Urology. 2006;68:121–5.
38. Stone NN, Stock RG, Unger P. Laparoscopic pelvic lymph node dissection for prostate cancer: comparison of the extended and modified techniques. J Urol. 1997;158:1891–4.
39. Wawroschek F, Wagner T, Hamm M, et al. The influence of serial sections, immunohistochemistry, and extension of pelvic lymph node dissection on the lymph node status in clinically localized prostate cancer. Eur Urol. 2003;43:132–7.
40. Touijer KA, Rabbani F, Otero JR, et al. Standard versus limited pelvic lymph node dissection for prostate cancer in patients with a predicted probability of nodal metastasis greater than 1 %. J Urol. 2007;178:120–4.
41. Clark T, Parekh DJ, Cookson MS, et al. Randomized prospective evaluation of extended versus limited lymph node dissection in patients with clinically localized prostate cancer. J Urol. 2003;169:145–7.
42. Bianco FJ, Scardino PT, Eastham JA. Radical prostatectomy: long-term cancer control and recovery of sexual and urinary function ("trifecta"). Urology. 2005;66(5 Suppl):83–94.
43. Ward JF, Blute ML, Slezak J, Bergstralh EJ, Zincke H. The long-term clinical impact of biochemical recurrence of prostate cancer 5 or more years after radical prostatectomy. J Urol. 2003;170:1872–6.

44. Freedland SJ, Humphreys EB, Mangold LA, et al. Risk of prostate cancer-specific mortality following biochemical recurrence after radical prostatectomy. JAMA. 2005;294:433–9.
45. Stephenson AJ, Kattan MW, Eastham JA, et al. Prostate cancer-specific mortality after radical prostatectomy for patients treated in the prostate-specific antigen era. J Clin Oncol. 2009;27:4300–5.
46. Eggener SE, Scardino PT, Walsh PC, et al. Predicting 15-year prostate cancer specific mortality after radical prostatectomy. J Urol. 2011;185:869–75.
47. Schumacher MC, Burkhard FC, Thalmann GN, Fleischmann A, Studer UE. Good outcome for patients with few lymph node metastases after radical retropubic prostatectomy. Eur Urol. 2008; 54:344–52.
48. Seiler R, Studer UE, Tschan K, et al. Removal of limited nodal disease in patients undergoing radical prostatectomy: long-term results confirm a chance for cure. J Urol. 2014;191:1280–5.
49. Daneshmand S, Quek ML, Stein JP, et al. Prognosis of patients with lymph node positive prostate cancer following radical prostatectomy: long-term results. J Urol. 2004;172:2252–5.
50. Briganti A, Karnes JR, Da Pozzo LF, et al. Two positive nodes represent a significant cut-off value for cancer specific survival in patients with node positive prostate cancer. A new proposal based on a two-institution experience on 703 consecutive N+ patients treated with radical prostatectomy. Eur Urol. 2009;55:261–70.
51. Touijer KA, Mazzola CR, Sjoberg DD, et al. Long-term outcomes of patients with lymph node metastasis treated with radical prostatectomy without adjuvant androgen-deprivation therapy. Eur Urol. 2014;65:20–5.
52. Palapattu GS, Allaf ME, Trock BJ, et al. Prostate specific antigen progression in men with lymph node metastases following radical prostatectomy: results of long-term followup. J Urol. 2004;172:1860–4.
53. Boorjian SA, Thompson RH, Siddiqui S, et al. Long-term outcome after radical prostatectomy for patients with lymph node positive prostate cancer in the prostate specific antigen era. J Urol. 2007;178:864–70.
54. Bader P, Spahn M, Huber R, Echtle D, Frohneberg D. Limited dissection in prostate cancer may miss lymph node metastases and determines outcome of apparently pN0 prostate cancer. Eur Urol Suppl. 2004;3:16. abstract 55.
55. Heidenreich A, Ohlmann CH, Polyakov S. Anatomical extent of pelvic lymphadenectomy in patients undergoing radical prostatectomy. Eur Urol. 2007;52:29–37.
56. Pagliarulo V, Hawes D, Brands FH, et al. Detection of occult lymph node metastases in locally advanced node-negative prostate cancer. J Clin Oncol. 2006;24:2735–42.
57. Miyake H, Hara I, Kurahashi T, Inoue T, Eto H, Fujisawa M. Quantitative detection of micrometastases in pelvic lymph nodes in patients with clinically localized prostate cancer by real-time reverse transcriptase-PCR. Clin Cancer Res. 2007;13:1192–7.
58. Schumacher MC, Burkhard FC, Thalmann GN, Fleischmann A, Studer UE. Is pelvic lymph node dissection necessary in patients with a serum PSA < 10 ng/ml undergoing radical prostatectomy for prostate cancer? Eur Urol. 2006;50:272–9.
59. Weckermann D, Goppelt M, Dorn R, Wawroschek F, Harzmann R. Incidence of positive pelvic lymph nodes in patients with prostate cancer, a prostate-specific antigen (PSA) level of ≤10 ng/mL and biopsy Gleason score of ≤6, and their influence on PSA progression-free survival after radical prostatectomy. BJU Int. 2006;97:1173–8.
60. Heidenreich A, Pfister D, Thüer D, Brehmer B. Percentage of positive biopsies predicts lymph node involvement in men with low-risk prostate cancer undergoing radical prostatectomy and extended pelvic lymphadenectomy. BJU Int. 2011;107:220–5.
61. Makarov DV, Humphreys EB, Mangold LA, et al. Pathological outcomes and biochemical progression in men with T1c prostate cancer undergoing radical prostatectomy with prostate specific antigen 2.6 to 4.0 vs 4.1 to 6.0 ng/ml. J Urol. 2006;176:554–8.
62. Berglund RK, Sadetsky N, DuChane J, Carroll PR, Klein EA. Limited pelvic lymph node dissection at the time of radical prostatectomy does not affect 5-year failure rates for low, intermediate and high risk prostate cancer: results from CaPSURE. J Urol. 2007;177:526–9.
63. Briganti A, Chun FK, Salonia A, et al. Complications and other surgical outcomes associated with extended pelvic lymphadenectomy in men with localized prostate cancer. Eur Urol. 2006;50:1006–13.
64. Burkhard FC, Kessler TM, Fleischmann A, Thalmann GN, Schumacher M, Studer UE. Nerve sparing open radical retropubic prostatectomy-does it have an impact on urinary continence? J Urol. 2006;176:189–95.
65. Gandaglia G, Suardi N, Gallina A, et al. Extended pelvic lymph node dissection does not affect erectile function recovery in patients treated with bilateral nerve-sparing radical prostatectomy. J Sex Med. 2012;9:2187–94.
66. NCCN Clinical Practice Guidelines in Oncology (NCCN Guidelines®) Prostate Cancer v2.2014.

Pelvic Lymph Node Dissection: Robotic Surgery Efficiency and Space-Creation Techniques to Achieve an Extended Template

15

John W. Davis

Introduction

Prior to robotic platforms, the laparoscopic approach to pelvic lymph node dissection (L-PLND) was one of the first minimally invasive options in urology in the 1990s [1–3]. The rationale was to sample the obturator node spaces to determine if pN1 disease could be determined to help decide on hormonal therapy versus local therapy. The median nodal yield of 6.5 in the Shackley series [1] was similar to open results when such a standard template was the goal. Of interest, this early series heavily relied on experienced laparoscopic general surgeons in the UK, as experience among urologic surgeons was only developing. Herrell et al. compared the emerging L-PLND and compared it to open and mini-laparotomy. The yields were equivalent at 8–9 range [4]. Many years later, it is eye opening that these procedures took a median 2.8 h of procedure time. The tools were minimal including monopolar cautery and early model clip appliers. Absent were Ligasure's and intracorporeal sewing techniques to handle vascular issues. Early robotic systems such as the Zeus from Computer Motion made the operation slightly easier, but the understanding of anatomic goals was the same—sample the obturator space. In Fig. 15.1, you can see a screenshot from an old video made with Zeus and Socrates systems in which telementoring during robotic-PLND was demonstrated. As the figure shows, the basic goal was to incise the peritoneum, identify the external iliac vein and obturator nerve, and avoid injury to the nerve and vessels.

J.W. Davis, M.D. (✉)
Department of Urology, Uro-surgical Prostate Cancer Program, The University of Texas M.D. Anderson Cancer Center, Houston, TX, USA
e-mail: jdhdavis@aol.com

The Template Changes to Extended

As described earlier in the chapter from Nguyen et al. experience with extended templates changed our understanding of the landing zones of lymph nodes from the prostate. As illustrated in Fig. 15.2a, b, the standard template only captured the small area under the external iliac vein and over the obturator nerve, leaving significant tissue behind. Figure 15.1 from the Nguyen chapter can be compared side by side with Fig. 15.2a in this chapter. As they concluded:

> *In our opinion, the boundaries for an extended PLND should include: the mid-common region where the ureter crosses the iliac vessels cranially, the circumflex iliac vein and femoral canal distally, the upper limit of the external iliac vein laterally, the bladder medially and the floor of the obturator fossa and the internal iliac vessels dorsally.*

J.W. Davis (ed.), *Robot-Assisted Radical Prostatectomy*, DOI 10.1007/978-3-319-32641-2_15

For robotic surgeons, the question becomes how to expose similar anatomy, and to deliver the nodes safely and efficiently. The exposure starts very differently in that the approach is mostly transperitoneal, and therefore the bladder and extraperitoneal spaces have to be exposed. Figure 15.3a–d shows the typical initial exposure shots transperitoneally. For E-PLND, the urachus and space of Retzius can be divided and exposed. The sigmoid colon is best mobilized out of the way to expose the higher aspects of the template.

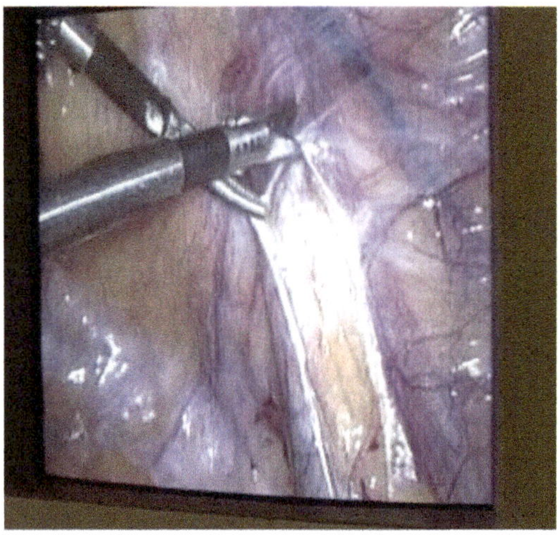

Fig. 15.1 Early robotic PLND with the Zeus system (Computer Motion) showing a basic attempt to clear obturator space nodes. Photo courtesy Mike Fabrizio and Ingolf Tuerk

However, the bowel and bladder can still be in the way of finding the hypogastric artery and lower aspects of the template.

There are two methods we have utilized for exposure. Early, we utilized Vicryl sutures as "marionette" strings to pull the bladder laterally and expose the template [5] (Fig. 15.4).

An alternate method is to use the third arm for exposure. The lateral aspect of the urachus/median umbilical ligament is grasped and pushed contralaterally and upwards. The dissecting instruments work underneath this arm. This refers to a left-sided two-arm setup with right-side assistant. For the right side, the third arm pulls contralateral to the left. As dissection progresses, generally this arm can be tightened to improve exposure. Specific to the right side, on some occasions, the bowel is in the way and sometimes not. If it is in the way, then go back to the suture retraction trick—tie a Vicryl to the right urachus/median umbilical ligament and pull it out of the third arm port and clamp on tension. Then the third arm can directly retract bowel downwards and expose the hypogastric spaces.

Once the spaces are figured out, then the surgeon can think of three different areas of dissection: (1) templates included in the easy/standard obturator space, (2) the extended template that will come out en bloc, and (3) the hard-to-get spaces that need separate attention. Figure 15.5 shows a completed dissection including such

a b

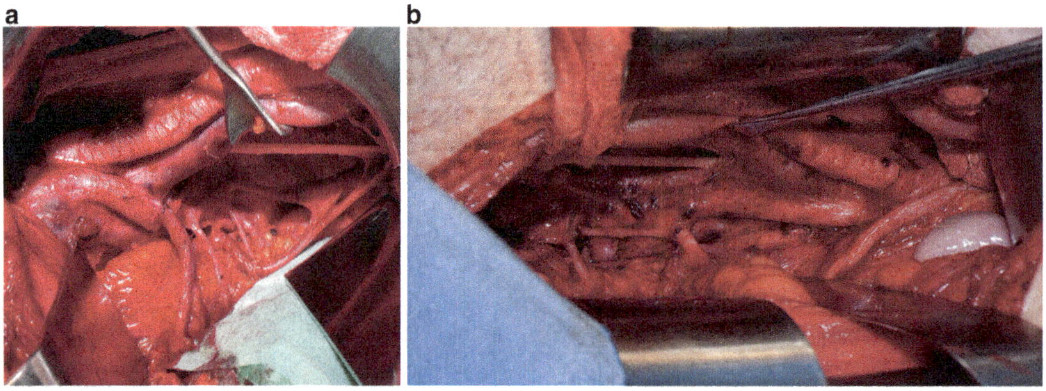

Fig. 15.2 (**a**) *Above*: Completed open extended pelvic lymph node dissection (*left side*), courtesy of Urs Studer. (**b**) *Below*: Completed open extended pelvic lymph node dissection by Paul Lange after case observations with Professor Studer, courtesy of Paul Lange

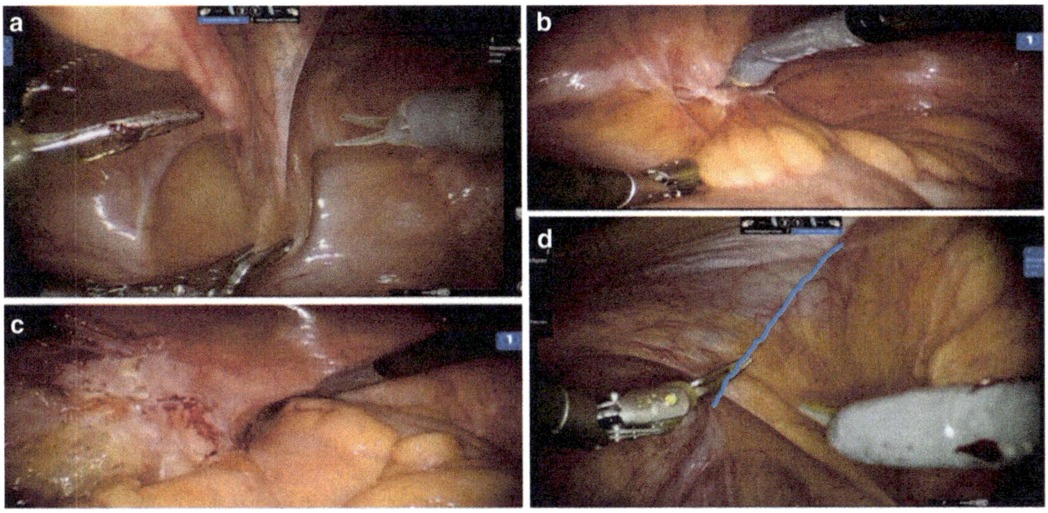

Fig. 15.3 (**a–d**) The initial setup requires entering the space of retzius (**a**), and moving the sigmoid colon out of the way with lateral dissection (**b**). Gravity then allows the sigmoid to fall cephalad (**c**). Alternatively, you can simply dissect down the medial umbilical ligament and go straight into the pelvic node space leaving the urachus up (**d**: *blue line* is the dissection plane)

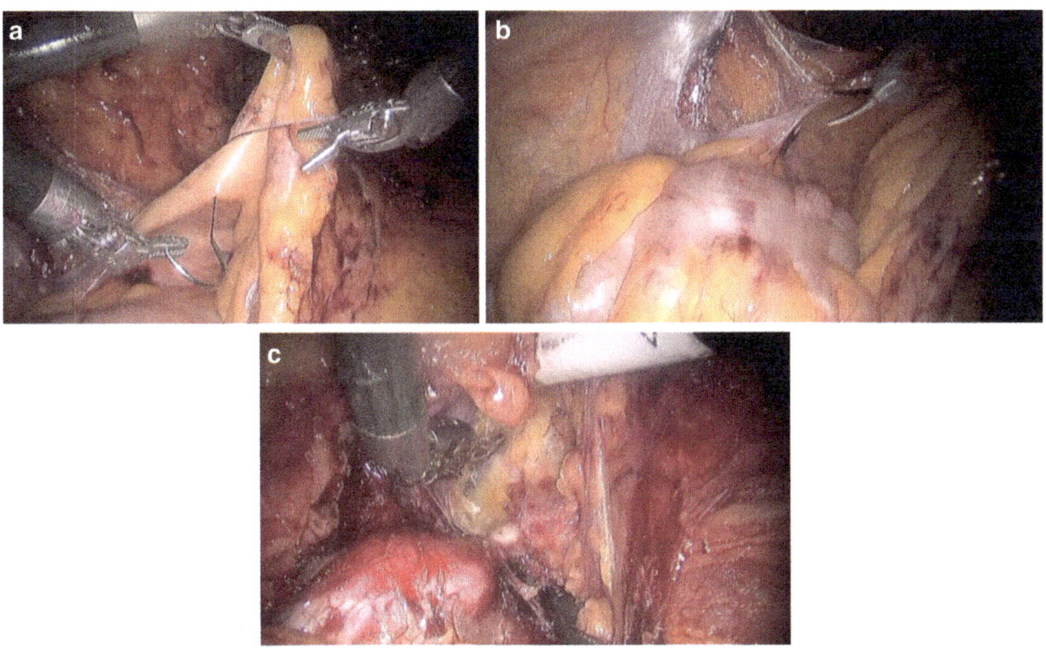

Fig. 15.4 (**a–c**) (**a**) The marionette Vicryl string is sewn around the left side of the urachus and exteriorized through the assistant port and pulled on tension. (**b**) The peritoneum and sigmoid colon are mobilized, and (**c**) the suction pulls the ureter medial as dissection carries from the hypogastric distally to the obliterated branch

areas designated in the cartoon inlays. From the numbering scheme listed, we would argue that region 2 is the standard obturator template. Region 1 is external iliac medial to the artery—this is fairly easy to get to. Region 3 represents the lymph nodes in the triangular space behind

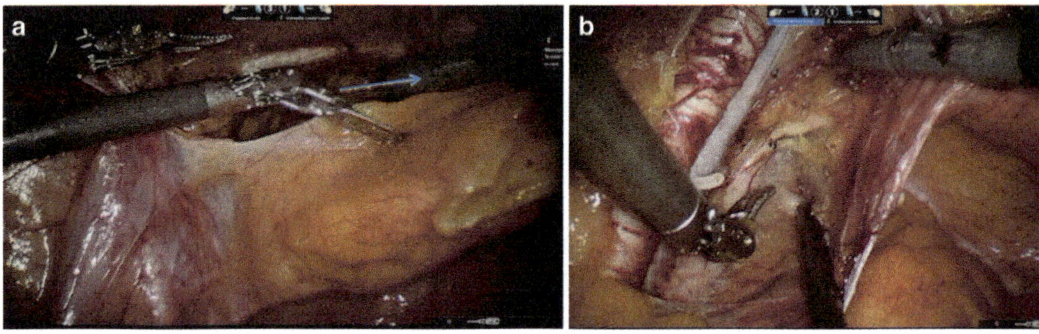

Fig. 15.5 (**a**, **b**) The third arm grasper can push the bladder contralaterally and anterior in the direction of the *blue arrow* (**a**). The camera and first and second arms can work under the third arm (**b**). With the sigmoid out of the way, vas divided, and ureter retracted ventrally by the suction, the dissection can proceed to identify the external iliac artery/hypogastric artery division, the obliterated artery, and the external iliac vein. Note that the tension provided by the third arm pulls the obliterated artery sideways and outwards such that the medial hypogastric space can be oriented and dissected

the junction of the external lilac artery and vein. This triangle can be separated and the nodes mobilized—they will connect with region 2 behind the vein. The red line would indicate the proximal extent of a typical standard template while region 3 would indicate the proximal extent for an extended template. Region 4 represents the sub-obturator spaces. These can be split and rolled along with region 2. However, the region is distinct in that there are many different vessels in the area that will need attention with clips or bipolar current. The distal extent connects with a fatty layer overlying the endopelvic fascia. This represents a difficult aspect of communicating technique with medical illustration versus still or video images from actual cases. If you refer back to the illustration from Nguyen in the previous chapter, there is the vague ending point at the far left side of the diagram where the zones fan out in the distal pelvis. How do you know when you are done? Comparing our operative photo from a left dissection to the right-sided illustration, we would suggest that region 1 on the illustration corresponds to our region 1–3. Region 2 is sub-obturator and refers to our region 4. Region 3 is hypogastric and refers to our region 5. The point of our splitting up region 5 is that these nodes are in and around several branches of the hypogastric artery and often have to be plucked out in smaller packets to make it clear on the level of Fig. 15.2a image from Professor Studer (Fig. 15.6).

More Attention to the Hard-to-Reach Areas

As we described in the chapter on "making spaces," there are certain parts of an EPLND that need specific dissection steps that are different from standard templates. In order to find the triangular space, the dissection must split the external iliac artery and vein near the take-off of the hypogastric artery. This is distinct from a radical dissection template where the dissection goes full lateral to the artery. In this case, you can just dissect lateral to the external iliac artery and then move down the space of the psoas muscle and find the obturator nerve again. For prostate, the goal is to preserve lateral external iliac artery lymphatics—they are of low yield and will help reduce lymphedema complications. As Fig. 15.7 shows, the triangle is opened and the proximal lymphatics clipped, taking care to identify and protect the obturator nerve. This packet of lymphatics will then connect with the obturator space and can be flipped back into the obturator space and the combined bloc extracted.

The sub-obturator and hypogastrics spaces will inevitably hide additional low areas of nodes that often are anchored by surrounding vascular branches. As Fig. 15.8 shows, additional nodes can be plucked from these spaces under the obturator nerve.

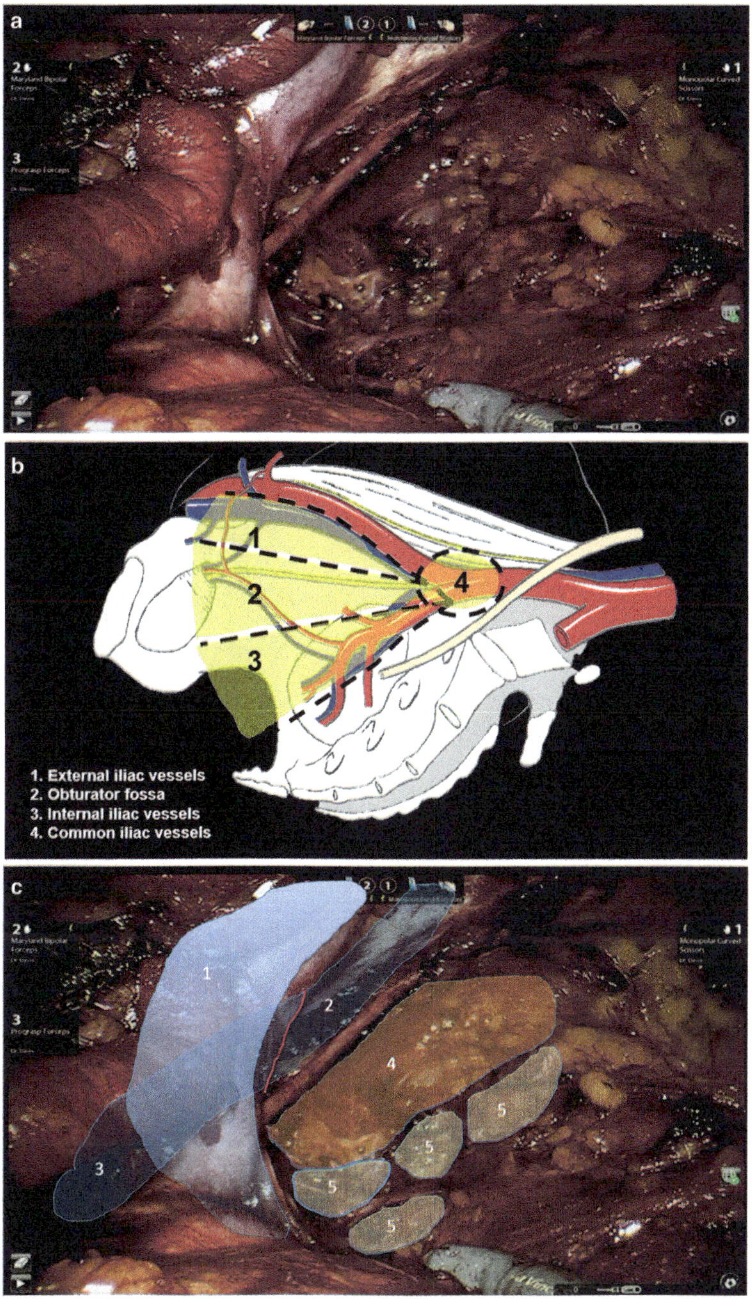

Fig. 15.6 (**a**–**c**) A completed left-side template is shown (**a**) with the similar diagram from Nguyen's chapter (**b**). For the same operative image (**c**), we have drawn specific zones of dissection and descriptions: (1) a typical external iliac artery/vein dissection (leaving lateral artery alone), (2) a typical obturator space with the *red line* showing a typical stopping point proximal, (3) additional nodes behind the triangular space, (4) sub-obturator space that can go en bloc with the obturator in a split and roll method, and (5) the remaining hypogastric artery planes that need additional "pluck" dissection to clear

Extending the Extended Template

The lymphoscintigraphy studies such as Joniau et al. [6] show that a handful of nodes can exist even outside of the above-described reasonable EPLND template. These additional areas can be along the common iliac artery near the ureter crossing, as well as the pre-sacral space. In some patients on clinical trials with locally advanced/regional cN1 disease, we have performed full cystectomy templates with much higher zones of dissection (Fig. 15.9).

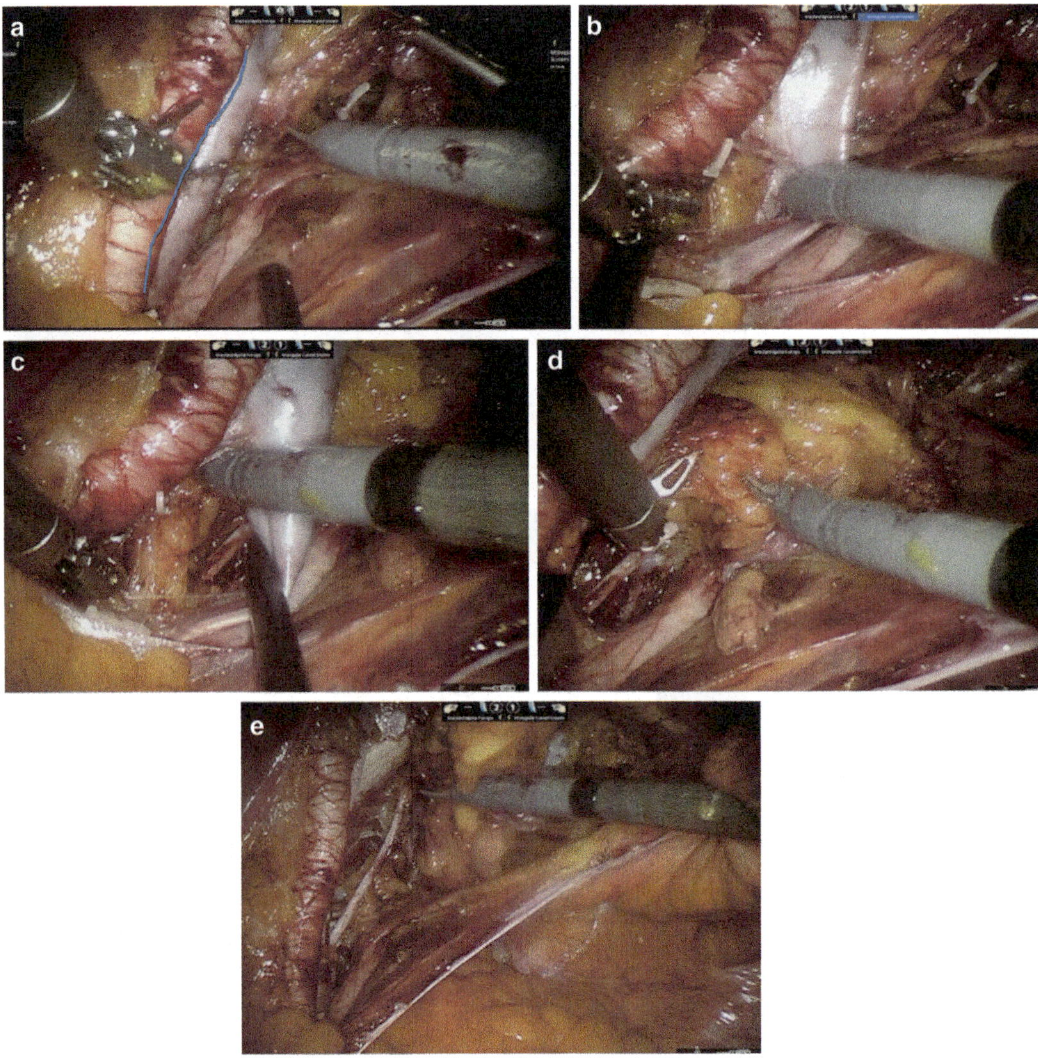

Fig. 15.7 (**a**–**e**) To clear the triangular space, the plane is cut between the external iliac artery and vein (**a**—*blue line*). The artery and vein can be separated gently near the hypogastric artery (**b**). The obturator nerve can be seen again in the triangle and the proximal lymphatics clipped and cut here (**c**). The triangular lymphatics can be rolled forward into the obturator space to remove with the obturator nodes (**d**). The finished appearance with the nodes ready to place in an extraction bag (**e**)

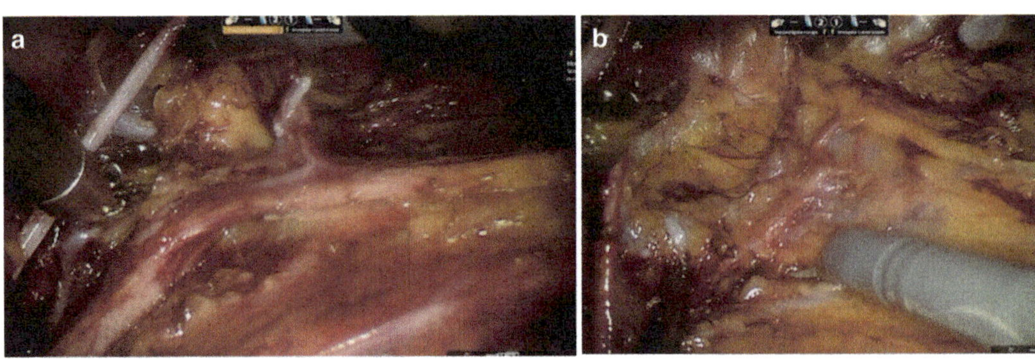

Fig. 15.8 (**a**, **b**) At the end of the dissection, the hypogastric is re-inspected and additional nodes plucked in and round the minor branches

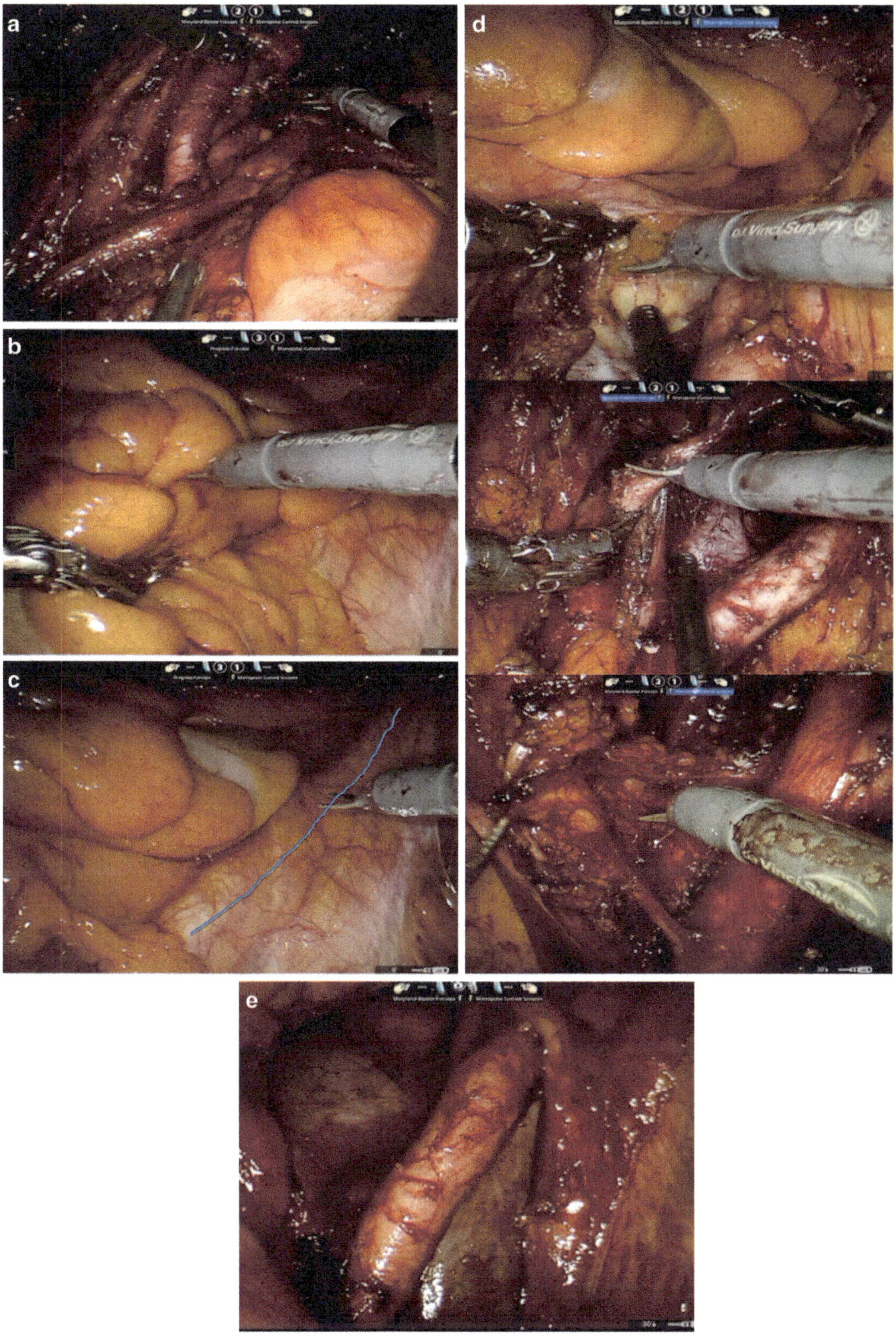

Fig. 15.9 (**a**–**e**) A left-sided dissection is shown with the ureter mobilized and the left common iliac nodes retrieved (**a**). On the right side, the sigmoid colon can be raised up with the third arm (**b**), and the peritoneum incised per the *blue line* (**c**). The pre-sacral space can be accessed and cleared. The suction here is touching the sacrum just past the crossing left common iliac vein. Additional pre-sacral space is seen in (**d**) between the common iliac arteries. Dissection further up the aorta demonstrates access to the internal iliac artery (**e**)

References

1. Shackley DC, Irving SO, Brough WA, et al. Staging laparoscopic pelvic lymphadenectomy in prostate cancer. BJU Int. 1999;83:260–4.
2. Gershman A, Daykhovsky L, Chandra M, et al. Laparoscopic pelvic lymphadenectomy. J Laparoendoscopic Surg. 1990;1:63–8.
3. Schuessler WW, Pharand D, Vancaillie TG. Laparoscopic standard lymph node dissection for cancer of the prostate. Is it accurate? J Urol. 1993;150:898–901.
4. Herrell SD, Trachtenberg J, Theodorescu D. Staging pelvic lymphadenectomy for localized carcinoma of the prostate: a comparison of 3 surgical techniques. J Urol. 1997;157:1337–9.
5. Davis JW, Shah JB, Achim M. Robot-assisted extended pelvic lymphadenectomy at the time of radical prostatectomy—a video based illustration of technique, results, and unmet patient selection needs. BJU Int. 2011;108(6 Pt 2):993–8.
6. Joniau S, Van den Bergh L, Lerut E, et al. Mapping of pelvic lymph node metastases in prostate cancer. Eur Urol. 2013;63:450–8.

16 Innovation and Orientation Challenges: Posterior "Retzius-Sparing" Technique

Patrick H. Tuliao and Koon Ho Rha

Introduction

Several authors in this book discuss strategies to improve urinary continence—at the urethral dissection, reconstruction layers, and even nerve sparing. In this chapter, the group from Yonsei presents a technique of robot-assisted radical prostatectomy that is completely through the pouch of Douglas. The initial approach is identical to the posterior approach to the seminal vesicles. However the dissection then continues and landing on key anatomy shifts to an upside-down look. The chapter presents the relevant outcomes and rationale for pursuing this technique as another way to improve urinary control recovery.

During its infancy, the robotic platform with its three-dimensional view, tremor filtration, endo-wrist action, and scaling of motion held promise to have a significant impact during radical prostatectomy [1]. However, the clinical significance of this was initially unclear. Several years after its introduction, there are now available data that demonstrate the advantages of robot-assisted radical prostatectomy (RARP) compared to the other techniques in terms of surgical outcome [2–5]. Such evidence was not available early on because, like all surgical procedures, RARP entails a learning curve.

For the purpose of discussion, conventional approach (C-RARP) was used to describe the RARP technique wherein a great majority of the dissection and prostatectomy are carried out approaching the prostate anteriorly. This technique was developed based on the principles of the open retropubic radical prostatectomy technique as described by Walsh and the laparoscopic radical prostatectomy technique as popularized by Montsouris [6].

RARP however is far from a static technique and continues to evolve as more surgeons utilize it. When performing the C-RARP approach, the urinary bladder and its supporting structures are taken down to facilitate the prostatectomy phase. Consequently, there is a need for some form of reconstruction [7, 8], sling [9] or suspension [10] procedure in an attempt to re-approximate anatomic status quo.

In contrast, the posterior or Retzius-sparing (RS-RARP) approach was recently developed to avoid tearing down supporting structures to the bladder and urethra, thus precluding the need to do additional reconstructive procedures.

P.H. Tuliao • K.H. Rha, M.D., Ph.D., F.A.C.S. (✉)
Department of Urology, Urological Science Institute, Yonsei University College of Medicine, 50 Yonsei-ro, Seodaemun-gu, Seoul 120-752, South Korea
e-mail: khrha@yuhs.ac

J.W. Davis (ed.), *Robot-Assisted Radical Prostatectomy*, DOI 10.1007/978-3-319-32641-2_16

Retzius-Sparing Radical Prostatectomy

In their article describing the results of the first 200 cases of RS-RARP, Galfano described their technique in detail. Ports were placed as illustrated in Fig. 16.1. The whole prostatectomy and urethrovesical anastomosis was performed through a 5–7 cm incision in the parietal peritoneum in the anterior aspect of the pouch of Douglas [11]. After seminal vesicle and vas deferens dissection and incision, the posterolateral surface of the prostate was dissected from the Denonvilliers' fascia. The bladder was then separated from the prostate's base and then the anterior prostate is freed from the dorsal venous plexus. The apex was identified and the urethra was incised to complete the prostatectomy. The urethrovesical anastomosis was then accomplished via a modified van Velthoven technique beginning in the 12 O' clock position. None of these steps required taking down the bladder, ligating the dorsal vein complex, or the deliberate opening of the endopelvic fascia. A 30° lens which was pointing upwards was recommended except during the vas deferens and seminal vesicle dissection.

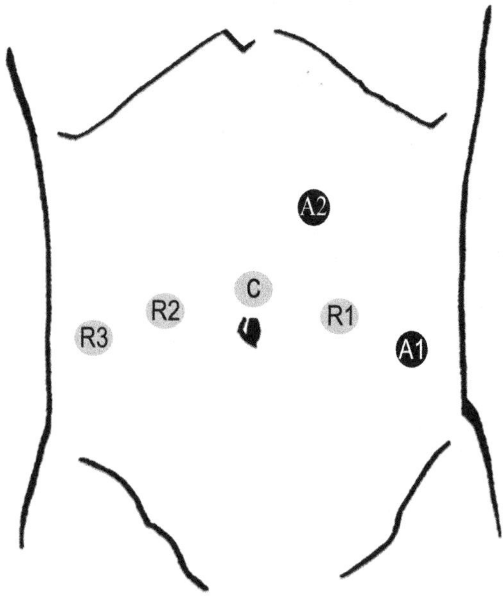

Fig. 16.1 Port placement for Retzius-sparing robot-assisted radical prostatectomy. *C* camera port, *A1* and *A2* assistant ports, *R1*, *R2*, and *R3* robotic arms

For their first 200 cases using the RS-RARP technique, the aforementioned authors reported overall positive margin rates of 15 and 45 % in pathologic stage T2 and T3 tumors, respectively. Continence recovery 7 days after catheter removal was 75 % using a no-pad definition and 91 % using a one-safety liner definition. Overall continence after 1 year was 96 %. Erectile function after 1 year was at 76 %. With regard to the learning curve of RS-RARP, this study showed improvement in terms of positive surgical margin rates when comparing the initial 100 to the latter 100 cases. Urinary continence and erectile function were not significantly different for these two groups.

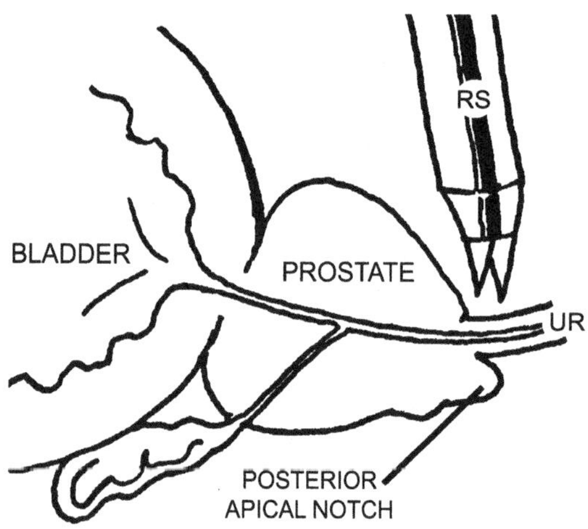

Fig. 16.2 The posterior apical notch may be incised during urethral incision. UR urethra, RS robotic scissors

So far, the only institution outside of Europe that has reported using RS-RARP is in the Yonsei University College of Medicine in Seoul, Korea [12]. In their report of a single surgeon's experience on his first 50 patients, Lim et al. described their technique to be similar to the steps described by Galfano et al. with a few modifications (Fig. 16.2). Bladder neck dissection was carried out by removing the perivesical fat until the detrusor muscles are visualized while retracting the prostate downwards. Closure of the peritoneal incision after the urethrovesical anastomosis was routinely done. And during pelvic lymph node dissection, instead of prolonging the original incision, separate longitudinal incisions were made from the base towards the apex of the triangle formed by the medial umbilical ligament, vas deferens, and the abdominal wall (base).

In the same study, compared to the conventional anterior approach of RARP, RS-RARP was found to have similar intraoperative blood loss, complication rates, and positive margin rates. When using a definition of no pads, continence recovery was found to be significantly better 1 month after the surgery for RS-RARP. Unfortunately, erectile function was not reported in the study.

In both publications about RS-RARP, there was no need for reconstruction or suspension techniques. This lack of need for additional steps also leads to a shortening of the operative time which consequently decreases anesthesia-related complications and may help decrease operating room costs. Furthermore, the advantage of RS-RARP appears to be its excellent urinary continence outcome.

RS-RARP offers several advantages. It allows a 360° access to the prostate which enables the surgeon to perform intra-fascial nerve-sparing prostatectomy. It also makes prostatectomy possible without necessarily violating the endopelvic fascia and the veil of Aphrodite or transecting the puboprostatic ligaments and dorsal veins which preserves as much periprostatic tissue and supporting structures as possible [11, 12].

Challenges and Techniques

With any surgical procedure, there remain challenges to overcome. For RARP, one such challenge is apical dissection. Proper dissection of the apex decreases the risk of developing positive surgical margins, lessens injury to the neurovascular bundle, and helps preserve urethral length. With C-RARP, the prostatic apex is quite arguably the most common sites of positive surgical margins. This can be partially explained anatomically by the lack of a distinct capsule in the anterior prostatic surface [13]. Also, the apex is in the deepest part of the pelvic cavity and is in very close proximity to the deep venous complex and the urethral sphincter. When approached from the anterior, the posterior prostatic apex is more difficult to visualize. Adding to the difficulty is the great variability in apical anatomy. In some cases, there is a portion of the posterior apex that protrudes posterior to the urethra. The surgeon can easily cut into this posterior apical notch (Fig. 16.3) and, when it harbors malignancy, develop positive margins.

Several techniques to facilitate apical dissection without sacrificing functional recovery have been described. When approaching from the anterior, ligation of the deep venous complex and removal of the prostatic anterior fat pad have been demonstrated early on by Ahlering et al. to decrease positive margin rates by improving apical visualization and dissection [14]. Somewhat related to this, cold incision of the deep venous complex prior to its suture ligation was associated with lower apical margins compared to when suturing was done before ligation [15]. Lastly, lateral dissection of the apex, by transferring the camera to a lateral port, has been shown to decrease dorso-apical margins [16]. The anatomical retro-apical technique was described by Tewari et al. in 2010 [17]. This technique involved approaching the prostate from the posterior surface while using an upward-pointing 30° lens. Posterior apical dissection is carried out after separation of the prostate from the rectal wall. According to the article, margin positive rates were lower in the 209 cases of retro-apical dissection compared to cases of the traditional anterior dissection. This was despite a higher incidence of more advanced cancer in the former group. This technique was externally validated on Asian men with prostate cancer by Ou et al. [18]. They noted however that the dissection was more difficult in larger prostates and men with smaller pelvis or higher body mass indexes.

Although still theoretical because it currently lacks literature support, RS-RARP potentially may facilitate apical dissection by providing better visualization of the posterolateral aspects of the apex. This should enable the surgeon to easily identify and avoid cutting into a posterior apical notch whenever it is present.

For RS-RARP, apical positive margins do not appear to be as much of a problem as was anteriorly located margins. In their article comparing C-RARP and RS-RARP, Lim et al. [12] noted a significantly higher incidence of positive margins in RS-RARP (8 %) vs. a propensity-matched group of C-RARP cases (0 %). However, when they compared the anterior margins of the first 25 cases with the latter 25 cases of RS-RARP, there was a decrease in the incidence of the anterior positive margins. As mentioned earlier, a deficiency of the capsule in the anterior prostate may have contributed to this occurrence. The improvement in outcomes can be explained by familiarity with the procedure and evolution of

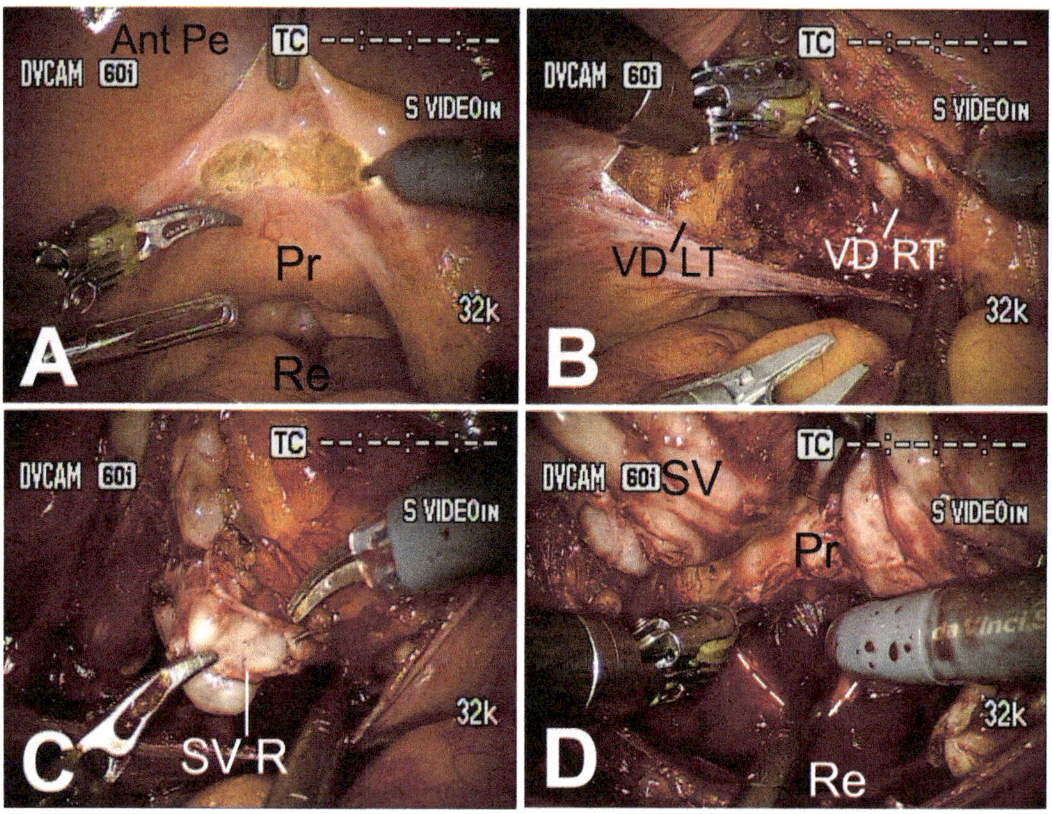

Fig. 16.3 Key steps in Retzius-sparing robot-assisted radical prostatectomy. (**a**) Making a 5–7 cm incision on the parietal peritoneum. (**b**) Identification and ligation of the vas deferens. (**c**) Dissection of the seminal vesicle. (**d**) Separation of the posterior prostate from the Denonvilliers' fascia (outlined in *white broken lines*). (**e**) Dissection of the posterolateral prostate (outlined in *white broken lines*), with preservation of the neurovascular bundle whenever oncologically safe. (**f**) Identification and incision of the prostatovesical junction. (**g**) Dissection of the anterior surface of the prostate with the bladder neck outlined in white broken lines. (**h**) Isolation and transection of the urethra (outlined in *white broken lines*). *Pr* prostate, *Re* rectum, *Ant Pe* anterior peritoneum, *VD LT* left vas deferens, *VD RT* right vas deferens, *SV R* right seminal vesicle, *NVB* neurovascular bundle, *BN* bladder neck, *DVC* dorsal vein complex, *Ur* urethra

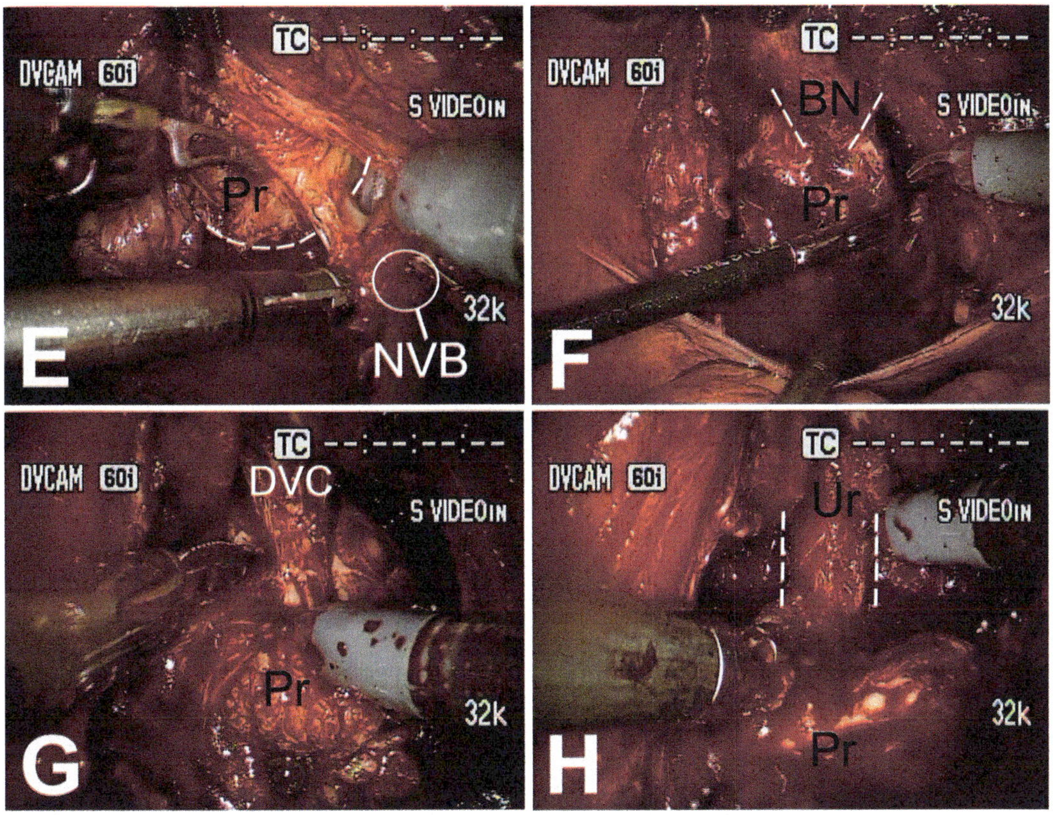

Fig. 16.3 (continued)

the technique. Speaking from experience, the anterior positive margins may be avoided during RS-RARP if the following steps are followed. After separation of the prostate from the bladder neck, anterior dissection is started by identifying the layer of fat anterior to the prostate. Once the fatty plane is identified, it is developed laterally and then the dissection is carried towards the apex. Making incisions directed at an acute angle away from the prostate rather than directly parallel to the prostate prevents cutting into the prostatic capsule.

Another challenge in RS-RARP is the urethrovesical anastomosis. Because RS-RARP is carried out completely from the posterior of the bladder and prostate, the posterior bladder limits movements in the area approaching the anterior abdominal wall. Consequently, the urethrovesical anastomosis is accomplished with the robotic camera pointing upwards as opposed to pointing downwards when performing C-RARP. Although it is still possible to complete the anastomosis using a zero degree lens, it is more economical to use an upward-pointing 30° lens [11]. In addition, although not exclusive to RS-RARP, using barbed sutures for the anastomosis has been shown to increase operative efficiency. In their randomized trial comparing the use of barbed vs. monofilament suture for the anastomosis, Zorn et al. noted a significant reduction in mean anastomosis time as well as in posterior reconstruction time when using the barbed vs. the monofilament suture (11.3 vs. 17.2 min, $p<0.01$) [19]. The advantage of using a barbed suture is that there is less chance of slippage and therefore lesser need to readjust suture tension. The capacity of the barbed suture for self-retention also decreases the need for help from the bedside assistant and knotting of the ends after anastomosis may be omitted. Using barbed sutures shortens the anastomosis time, which translates into shorter operative time, and less operating room expenses.

The Learning Curve of RS-RARP

In its simplest definition, the learning curve is the rate at which someone learns something new or the course of progress made in learning something new. When learning a new surgical procedure, performance and outcomes tend to improve with increasing experience. Graphically speaking, plotting surgical performance or outcomes against the level of experience produces a learning curve. Assessment of the surgical learning curve cannot be made by examining a procedure in its entirety, but is generally made using measurements of the (1) surgical process and (2) patient outcomes. For RARP, the intraoperative time, amount of blood loss, and surgical margins are commonly used variables to evaluate the former while length of hospital stay, rate of complications, continence rate, and potency rates are usually used for the latter.

The learning curve for C-RARP has been considerably analyzed over the years. In fact, in terms of oncologic and functional outcomes, it can be argued that the learning curve for C-RARP has already been overcome [20–22]. In contrast, there is paucity of data regarding RS-RARP. The most plausible explanation for this is the relative novelty of the technique, limiting its acceptability and general utility. If we follow the definition of a learning curve as previously stated, it is still too early to make any conclusions with regard to RS-RARP. However, basing it on the experience of Galfano et al. with their first 200 RS-RARP cases, it can be cautiously stated that results will significantly improve after the first 100 cases have been performed [11]. This is of course not to say that the results of the initial 100 cases were unacceptable based on present standards. At best, more studies are required before the learning curve of RS-RARP can be ascertained.

References

1. Pasticier G, Rietbergen JB, Guillonneau B, Fromont G, Menon M, Vallancien G. Robotically assisted laparoscopic radical prostatectomy: feasibility study in men. Eur Urol. 2001;40(1):70–4.
2. Asimakopoulos AD, Pereira Fraga CT, Annino F, Pasqualetti P, Calado AA, Mugnier C. Randomized comparison between laparoscopic and robot-assisted nerve-sparing radical prostatectomy. J Sex Med. 2011;8(5):1503–12.
3. Porpiglia F, Morra I, Lucci Chiarissi M, Manfredi M, Mele F, Grande S, Ragni F, Poggio M, Fiori C. Randomised controlled trial comparing laparoscopic and robot-assisted radical prostatectomy. Eur Urol. 2013;63(4):606–14.
4. Willis DL, Gonzalgo ML, Brotzman M, Feng Z, Trock B, Su LM. Comparison of outcomes between pure laparoscopic vs robot-assisted laparoscopic radical prostatectomy: a study of comparative effectiveness based upon validated quality of life outcomes. BJU Int. 2012;109(6):898–905.
5. Di Pierro GB, Baumeister P, Stucki P, Beatrice J, Danuser H, Mattei A. A prospective trial comparing consecutive series of open retropubic and robot-assisted laparoscopic radical prostatectomy in a centre with a limited caseload. Eur Urol. 2011;59(1):1–6.
6. Tewari A, Peabody J, Sarle R, Balakrishnan G, Hemal A, Shrivastava A, Menon M. Technique of da Vinci robot-assisted anatomic radical prostatectomy. Urology. 2002;60(4):569–72.
7. Rocco F, Carmignani L, Acquati P, et al. Restoration of posterior aspect of rhabdosphincter shortens continence time after radical retropubic prostatectomy. J Urol. 2006;175:2201–6.
8. Gondo T, Yoshioka K, Hashimoto T, et al. The powerful impact of double-layered posterior rhabdosphincter reconstruction on early recovery of urinary continence after robot-assisted radical prostatectomy. J Endourol. 2012;26(9):1159–64.
9. Takenaka A, Tewari AK, Leung RA, Bigelow K, El-Tabey N, Murakami G, Fujisawa M. Preservation of the puboprostatic collar and puboperineoplasty for early recovery of urinary continence after robotic prostatectomy: anatomic basis and preliminary outcomes. Eur Urol. 2007;51(2):433–40.
10. Hurtes X, Rouprêt M, Vaessen C, Pereira H, Faivre d'Arcier B, Cormier L, Bruyère F. Anterior suspension combined with posterior reconstruction during robot-assisted laparoscopic prostatectomy improves early return of urinary continence: a prospective randomized multicentre trial. BJU Int. 2012;110(6):875–83.
11. Galfano A, Di Trapani D, Sozzi F, Strada E, Petralia G, Bramerio M, Ascione A, Gambacorta M, Bocciardi AM. Beyond the learning curve of the Retzius-sparing approach for robot-assisted laparoscopic radical prostatectomy: oncologic and functional results of the first 200 patients with ≥1 year of follow-up. Eur Urol. 2013;64(6):974–80.

12. Lim SK, Kim KH, Shin TY, Han WK, Chung BH, Hong SJ, Choi YD, Rha KH. Retzius-sparing robot-assisted laparoscopic radical prostatectomy: combining the best of retropubic and perineal approaches. BJU Int. 2014;114(2):236–44.
13. Walz J, Burnett AL, Costello AJ, et al. A critical analysis of the current knowledge of surgical anatomy related to optimization of cancer control and preservation of continence and erection in candidates for radical prostatectomy. Eur Urol. 2010;57:179–92.
14. Ahlering TE, Eichel L, Edwards RA, Lee DI, Skarecky DW. Robotic radical prostatectomy: a technique to reduce pT2 positive margins. Urology. 2004;64(6):1224–8.
15. Lei Y, Alemozaffar M, Williams SB, Hevelone N, Lipsitz SR, Plaster BA, Amarasekera CA, Ulmer WD, Huang AC, Kowalczyk KJ, Hu JC. Athermal division and selective suture ligation of the dorsal vein complex during robot-assisted laparoscopic radical prostatectomy: description of technique and outcomes. Eur Urol. 2011;59(2):235–43.
16. Sasaki H, Miki J, Kimura T, Sanuki K, Miki K, Takahashi H, Egawa S. Lateral view dissection of the prostato-urethral junction to reduce positive apical margin in laparoscopic radical prostatectomy. Int J Urol. 2009;16(8):664–9.
17. Tewari AK, Srivastava A, Mudaliar K, et al. Anatomical retroapical technique of synchronous (posterior and anterior) urethral transection: a novel approach for ameliorating apical margin positivity during robotic radical prostatectomy. BJU Int. 2010;106:1364–73.
18. Ou YC, Hung SW, Wang J, Yang CK, Cheng CL, Tewari AK. Retro-apical transection of the urethra during robot-assisted laparoscopic radical prostatectomy in an Asian population. BJU Int. 2012;110 (2 Pt 2):E57–63.
19. Zorn KC, Trinh QD, Jeldres C, et al. Prospective randomized trial of barbed polyglyconate suture to facilitate vesicourethral anastomosis during robot-assisted radical prostatectomy: time reduction and cost benefit. BJU Int. 2012;109:1526–32.
20. Ficarra V, Novara G, Rosen RC, Artibani W, Carroll PR, Costello A, Menon M, Montorsi F, Patel VR, Stolzenburg JU, Van der Poel H, Wilson TG, Zattoni F, Mottrie A. Systematic review and meta-analysis of studies reporting urinary continence recovery after robot-assisted radical prostatectomy. Eur Urol. 2012;62(3):405–17.
21. Ficarra V, Novara G, Artibani W, Cestari A, Galfano A, Graefen M, Guazzoni G, Guillonneau B, Menon M, Montorsi F, Patel V, Rassweiler J, Van Poppel H. Retropubic, laparoscopic, and robot-assisted radical prostatectomy: a systematic review and cumulative analysis of comparative studies. Eur Urol. 2009;55(5):1037–63.
22. Ficarra V, Novara G, Ahlering TE, Costello A, Eastham JA, Graefen M, Guazzoni G, Menon M, Mottrie A, Patel VR, Van der Poel H, Rosen RC, Tewari AK, Wilson TG, Zattoni F, Montorsi F. Systematic review and meta-analysis of studies reporting potency rates after robot-assisted radical prostatectomy. Eur Urol. 2012;62(3):418–30.

Bibliography

Breyer BN, Davis CB, Cowan JE, Kane CJ, Carroll PR. Incidence of bladder neck contracture after robot-assisted laparoscopic and open radical prostatectomy. BJU Int. 2010;106(11):1734–8.

Carter SC, Konijeti R, Hu J. Selective suture ligation of the dorsal vein complex during robot-assisted laparoscopic radical prostatectomy. J Endourol. 2012;26(12):1576–7.

Eastham JA, Kattan MW, Riedel E, Begg CB, Wheeler TM, Gerigk C, Gonen M, Reuter V, Scardino PT. Variations among individual surgeons in the rate of positive surgical margins in radical prostatectomy specimens. J Urol. 2003;170:2292–5.

Kojima Y, Takahashi N, Haga N, Nomiya M, Yanagida T, Ishibashi K, Aikawa K, Lee DI. Urinary incontinence after robot-assisted radical prostatectomy: pathophysiology and intraoperative techniques to improve surgical outcome. Int J Urol. 2013;20(11):1052–63.

Koutlidis N, Mourey E, Champigneulle J, Mangin P, Cormier L. Robot-assisted or pure laparoscopic nerve-sparing radical prostatectomy: what is the optimal procedure for the surgical margins? A single center experience. Int J Urol. 2012;19(12):1076–81.

Leroy TJ, Thiel DD, Duchene DA, Parker AS, Igel TC, Wehle MJ, Goetzl M, Thrasher JB. Safety and peri-operative outcomes during learning curve of robot-assisted laparoscopic prostatectomy: a multi-institutional study of fellowship-trained robotic surgeons versus experienced open radical prostatectomy surgeons incorporating robot-assisted laparoscopic prostatectomy. J Endourol. 2010;24(10):1665–9.

Menon M, Tewari A, Peabody J, VIP Team. Vattikuti Institute prostatectomy: technique. J Urol. 2003; 169(6):2289–92.

Patel VR, Schatloff O, Chauhan S, Sivaraman A, Valero R, Coelho RF, Rocco B, Palmer KJ, Kameh D. The role of the prostatic vasculature as a landmark for nerve sparing during robot-assisted radical prostatectomy. Eur Urol. 2012;61(3):571–6.

Patel VR, Tully AS, Holmes R, Lindsey J. Robotic radical prostatectomy in the community setting - the learning curve and beyond: initial 200 cases. J Urol. 2005;174:269–72.

Rocco B, Cozzi G, Spinelli MG, Coelho RF, Patel VR, Tewari A, Wiklund P, Graefen M, Mottrie A, Gaboardi F, Gill IS, Montorsi F, Artibani W, Rocco F. Posterior musculofascial reconstruction after radical prostatectomy: a systematic review of the literature. Eur Urol. 2012;62(5):779–90.

Sammon J, Perry A, Beaule L, Kinkead T, Clark D, Hansen M. Robot-assisted radical prostatectomy: learning rate analysis as an objective measure of the acquisition of surgical skill. BJU Int. 2010;106:855–60.

Tewari AK, Patel ND, Leung RA, et al. Visual cues as a surrogate for tactile feedback during robotic-assisted laparoscopic prostatectomy: posterolateral margin rates in 1340 consecutive patients. BJU Int. 2010;106:528–36.

Getting Out: Closure, Prevention, and Management of Hernias

17

Maxim J. McKibben, Michael E. Woods, and Raj S. Pruthi

Epidemiology of Closure Complications

After several decades of experiences with laparoscopic surgery, data regarding incidence of TSH is robust. A recent large systematic review across laparoscopic surgery found a 0–5.2 % incidence of TSH for an overall incidence of 0.5 % [2]. In laparoscopic GI surgery, a meta-analysis demonstrated an overall incidence of 0.74 % with 23.9-month follow-up. The lowest rate of TSH was in bariatric surgery (0.57 %), and the highest was laparoscopic colorectal surgery, with a 1.47 % incidence [3]. In robotic gynecologic surgery, the incidence of port-site hernia was 0.6 % in a recent 500-patient series [4].

Data for TSH after minimally invasive radical prostatectomy are fewer, but a reasonable body of literature exists. Several large single-surgeon series demonstrate a relatively wide range of TSH, from 0.4 to 5.3 %, though these are largely observational series with heterogeneous closure techniques, follow-up protocols, and definitions [5–8]. A recent study examining SEER-Medicare data compared rates of incisional hernia repair claims after open and minimally invasive radical prostatectomy (MIRP). Among 3199 MIRP and 6795 open prostatectomies, the frequency of incisional hernia repair was 5.3 % in the MIRP group and 1.9 % in the open group, and a significant difference remained after controlling for multiple covariates including surgeon experience [9]. Though the rate of TSH following RARP is relatively low, incident cases usually result in a second surgery, and because TSH may represent a technical oversight, some attention is owed to closure technique.

Pathogenesis of Trocar-Site Hernia

Trocar Size

Many theories regarding the etiology of trocar-site hernia have been posited, but few have been definitely demonstrated in well-designed studies. Large trocar size is an obvious etiologic factor, as larger facial defects should be more prone to herniation. Indeed, large studies regarding TSH suggest that nearly all hernias occur in ports ≥10 mm (96 %), though there are rare 5 mm hernias reported (4 % of all TSH) [2]. Most surgeons now utilize bladeless radially expanding trocars, which when compared to cutting trocars produce significantly small fascial defects, and likely decrease the risk of hernia [11].

M.J. McKibben, M.D. • M.E. Woods, M.D., F.A.C.S.
R.S. Pruthi, M.D., F.A.C.S.
Department of Urology, University of North Carolina at Chapel Hill, 170 Manning Drive, 2115 Physicians Office Building, CB#7235, Chapel Hill, NC 27599-7235, USA

J.W. Davis (ed.), *Robot-Assisted Radical Prostatectomy*, DOI 10.1007/978-3-319-32641-2_17

Table 17.1 Trocar-site hernia rates in robot-assisted radical prostatectomy

Author	Patient no.	Follow-up	Cases (% of incidence)	Port size, fascial closure, etc.
Carlsson [9]	3199 (SEER claims data)	3.1 Years	168 (5.3 %)	"Minimally invasive prostatectomy"; some laparoscopic prostatectomy included
Liss [10]	735 Vertical 235 Transverse	38.7 Months	40/735 (5.4 %) 1/265 (0.4 %)	–
Kang [8]	498	18 Months	2 (0.4 %)	12 mm, only 12 mm ports closed
Fuller [7]	250	35 Months	12 (4.8 %)	12 mm closed. 10/12 hernias at midline extraction site. Two hernias were from 8 mm ports
Chiong [6]	441	13 Months	4 (0.9 %)	All hernias were 12 mm bladeless without fascial closure

Closure of Trocar-Site Fascia

In RARP, essentially all experts recommend closure of the 12 mm midline trocar-site fascia, but there is no consensus regarding closure of non-midline or smaller ports, as there is a very small risk of hernia from ports less than 10 mm. A systematic review of studies of TSH showed an increased rate of incisional hernia in series where trocar-site fascia is not closed (1.5 %) versus closed (0.6 %) [2].

Incision Orientation

Orientation of the trocar incisions (vertical versus transverse) appears to play a role in the rate of incisional hernia. A Cochrane review of abdominal surgery found a significantly decreased rate of hernia when transverse rather than vertical incisions were used [12]. Two large single-surgeon series of RARP found similar results; when a vertical camera port/specimen extraction incision was used, the rate of hernia was 5.3–5.4 %, which decreased dramatically to 0.4–0.6 % with a transverse incision [5, 10]. This difference is thought to be due to the difference in directional forces on the fascia when abdominal strain is applied.

Host Factors

Patient factors associated with poor wound healing such as obesity, poor nutrition, diabetes, and COPD have traditionally been thought to increase the risk of TSH, but this has not been borne out in well-designed studies [2, 13, 14]. The morbidly obese are at higher risk for preperitoneal hernias because of higher intra-abdominal pressure, but this may be due to the tendency to improperly close facial defects in very obese patients [15]. Umbilical wound infection after laparoscopy has been shown to be a predisposing etiologic factor for development of TSH [16].

Closure Techniques and Technology

Techniques for fascial closure are many. Some utilize devices such as the Carter-Thomason ClosureSure™ (CooperSurgical, Trumbull, CT), or the Endo Close™ (Covidien, Mansfield, MA) which may be helpful in obese patients when significant adiposity makes it difficult to locate fascia for closure. These devices also allow for full-thickness closure of peritoneum, muscle, and anterior fascia, which is probably preferable to anterior fascial closure, as partial abdominal wall or subfascial herniation can still occur with anterior fascial closure [17]. Bioabsorbable mesh plugs have demonstrated promise, but studies are small with short follow-up [18]. No large, randomized studies regarding the various closure methods have yet demonstrated superiority or inferiority of a given technology with regard to hernia rates, as the baseline rate is low. Suture material used for fascial closure is based on physician preference. High-strength, slowly absorbing sutures such as polydioxanone (PDS™, Ethicon, USA) or polyglactin (Vicryl™, Ethicon, USA) are the most commonly used. Similarly, interrupted or running suture technique is a matter of surgeon preference, as neither is demonstrably better [7, 19].

Presentation, Diagnosis, and Management

TSH can be divided into acute versus late onset. In acute-onset TSH, there is dehiscence of the anterior and posterior fascial planes, along with peritoneum (Fig. 17.1a). There may be gross breakdown of the wound with drainage, and patients may present with signs or symptoms of small bowel obstruction. These are uniformly managed with surgical repair. In late-onset hernia (Fig. 17.1b), there is also dehiscence of the anterior and posterior fascial planes, but in contrast to the peritoneal defect seen in acute onset, the hernia contents are usually contained by peritoneum [20]. A special category of hernia (Fig. 17.1c) that is relatively uncommon is protrusion of abdominal contents through all fascial layers and the skin as well.

Acute-onset TSH patients usually present in the first days to weeks after surgery, and late-onset patients present several months to as many as 10 years after surgery [14, 22]. Common late presentations include presence of a bulge with exertion or Valsalva, or constant painful bulge if omentum or bowel is incarcerated, which is less common. Diagnosis is often made clinically with physical exam, and computed tomography is used to confirm diagnosis [20]. MRI may be useful in cases where the hernia is very small in size and CT findings are not definitive [3].

With concern for bowel obstruction or incarceration, immediate surgical repair is warranted. Larger defects that allow for entry and exit of bowel with minimal risk of incarceration, and in these patients, delayed intervention may be feasible, but is usually required at some point, unless the patient is a poor surgical candidate. Repair can be laparoscopic or open, and often liberation of the herniated abdominal contents and isolation and repair of the fascial defect is sufficient for repair, but occasionally bowel resection and more advanced fascial repair techniques (i.e., mesh) is required Fig. 17.2.

The Authors' Preferences

The authors utilize bladeless, radially expanding trocars, and perform fascial closure of the 12 mm camera/extraction port, but no fascial closure of the remaining ports (8 and 5 mm). We generally do not use any of the previously mentioned closure devices, but rather perform direct fascial closure with polydioxanone (PDS™, Ethicon, USA), or polyglactin (Vicryl™, Ethicon, USA).

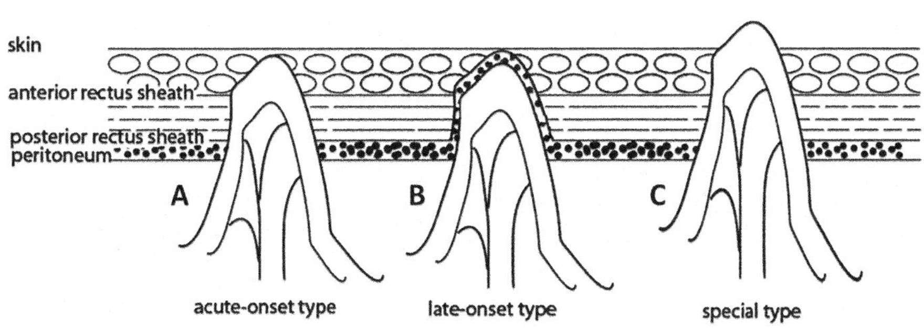

Fig. 17.1 Tonouchi [20] trocar-site hernia classification (*adapted from Lee 2014* [21] *with permission from author*)

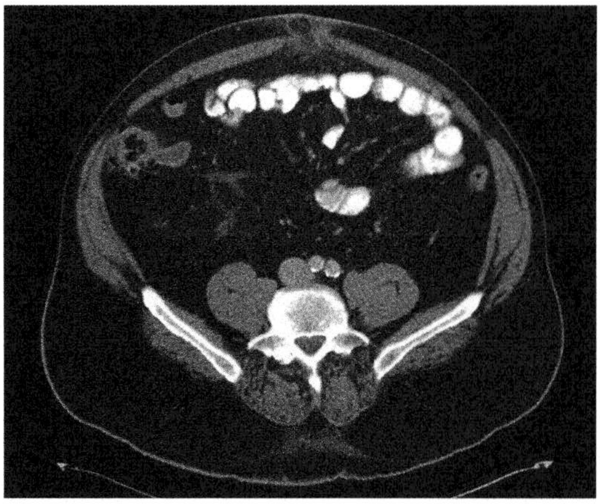

Fig. 17.2 Midline trocar-site hernia with incarcerated and necrotic omentum. Patient taken for emergent mesh repair 1.5 years after robot-assisted radical prostatectomy

Recommendations for Prevention of TSH

1. Transverse midline camera/extraction-site incision, rather than vertical.
2. Use of bladeless, radially expanding trocars rather than cutting trocars.
3. Closure of midline camera port.
4. Closure of all port sites ≥10 mm.
5. Closure of any port site that is stretched or manipulated significantly.
6. Full-thickness fascial closure, including peritoneum if possible.

Conclusion

TSH is an underdiagnosed and underappreciated complication of RARP, occurring in up to 5 % of patients. This avoidable complication often leads to a second surgery for correction, with possible bowel resection and other attendant surgical risks. Though factors affecting wound healing such as diabetes mellitus, poor nutrition, COPD, and obesity may contribute to hernia formation, this has not been definitively demonstrated in large studies. The use of bladeless radially expanding trocars, transverse camera port/specimen extraction incision, and closure of all ports ≥10 mm will likely minimize this complication in patients undergoing RARP, further reducing the morbidity of radical prostatectomy.

References

1. Sood A, Jeong W, Peabody JO, Hemal AK, Menon M. Robot-assisted radical prostatectomy: inching toward gold standard. Urol Clin North Am. 2014;41(4):473–84.
2. Helgstrand F, Rosenberg J, Bisgaard T. Trocar site hernia after laparoscopic surgery: a qualitative systematic review. Hernia. 2011;15(2):113–21.
3. Owens M, Barry M, Janjua A, Winter D. A systematic review of laparoscopic port site hernias in gastrointestinal surgery. Surgeon. 2011;9(4):218–24.
4. Clark LH, Soliman PT, Odetto D, et al. Incidence of trocar site herniation following robotic gynecologic surgery. Gynecol Oncol. 2013;131(2):400–3.
5. Beck S, Skarecky D, Osann K, Juarez R, Ahlering TE. Transverse versus vertical camera port incision in robotic radical prostatectomy: effect on incisional hernias and cosmesis. Urology. 2011;78(3):586–90.
6. Chiong E, Hegarty PK, Davis JW, Kamat AM, Pisters LL, Matin SF. Port-site hernias occurring after the use of bladeless radially expanding trocars. Urology. 2010;75(3):574–80.
7. Fuller A, Fernandez A, Pautler SE. Incisional hernia after robot-assisted radical prostatectomy—predisposing factors in a prospective cohort of 250 cases. J Endourol. 2011;25(6):1021–4.
8. Kang DI, Woo SH, Lee DH, Kim IY. Incidence of port-site hernias after robot-assisted radical prostatectomy with the fascial closure of only the midline 12-mm port site. J Endourol. 2012;26(7):848–51.
9. Carlsson SV, Ehdaie B, Atoria CL, Elkin EB, Eastham JA. Risk of incisional hernia after minimally invasive and open radical prostatectomy. J Urol. 2013;190(5):1757–62.
10. Liss MA, Skarecky D, Morales B, Osann K, Eichel L, Ahlering TE. Preventing perioperative complications of robotic-assisted radical prostatectomy. Urology. 2013;81(2):319–23.
11. Tarnay CM, Glass KB, Munro MG. Incision characteristics associated with six laparoscopic Trocar-Cannula systems: a randomized, observer-blinded comparison. Obstetr Gynecol. 1999;94(1):89–93.
12. Brown SR, Goodfellow P. Transverse verses midline incisions for abdominal surgery. Cochrane Database Syst Rev. 2005;4.
13. Ramachandran CS. Umbilical hernial defects encountered before and after abdominal laparoscopic procedures. Int Surg. 1998;83(2):171–3.
14. Nassar A, Ashkar K, Rashed A, Abdulmoneum M. Laparoscopic cholecystectomy and the umbilicus. Br J Surg. 1997;84(5):630–3.

15. Cottam DR, Gorecki PJ, Curvelo M, Weltman D, Angus LG, Shaftan G. Preperitoneal herniation into a laparoscopic port site without a fascial defect. Obesity Surg. 2002;12(1):121–3.
16. Mayol J, Garcia-Aguilar J, Ortiz-Oshiro E, Jose A, Fernandez-Represa JA. Risks of the minimal access approach for laparoscopic surgery: multivariate analysis of morbidity related to umbilical trocar insertion. World J Surg. 1997;21(5):529–33.
17. Bemelman WA. Prevention and treatment of postoperative complications after laparoscopic colorectal resections. Cuesta MA, Bonjer HJ (Eds.). Treatment of Postoperative Complications After Digestive Surgery. Springer 2014. Pg 247–258.
18. Moreno-Sanz C, Picazo-Yeste JS, Manzanera-Diaz M, Herrero-Bogajo ML, Cortina-Oliva J, Tadeo-Ruiz G. Prevention of trocar site hernias: description of the safe port plug technique and preliminary results. Surg Innov. 2008;15(2):100–4.
19. Hodgson NC, Malthaner RA, Ostbye T. The search for an ideal method of abdominal fascial closure: a meta-analysis. Ann Surg. 2000;231(3):436–42.
20. Tonouchi H, Ohmori Y, Kobayashi M, Kusunoki M. Trocar site hernia. Arch Surg. 2004;139(11): 1248–56.
21. Lee J, Zheng XJ, Ng CY. Trocar site hernias from using bladeless trocars: should fascial closure be performed? J Surg Case Rep. 2014;2014(5):rju044.
22. Bowrey D, Blom D, Crookes P, et al. Risk factors and the prevalence of trocar site herniation after laparoscopic fundoplication. Surg Endosc. 2001;15(7):663–6.

18 Robot-Assisted Laparoscopic Radical Prostatectomy – Extraperitoneal and Transperitoneal Technique

Vineet Agrawal and Jean Joseph

Introduction

Radical prostatectomy (RP) remains the gold standard in the surgical management for patients with clinically localized prostate cancer (PC) [1]. RP can be performed by open retropubic (ORP), perineal, laparoscopic (LRP), or robot-assisted laparoscopic approaches. Many parts of the world, esp. the USA and Europe, have witnessed a dramatic increase in number of robot-assisted radical prostatectomy (RARP) in the last decade [2]. The proven benefits of minimally invasive surgery coupled with a steep learning curve associated with LRP have played a part in wide dissemination of RARP. Critics however argue that aggressive patient-directed marketing and hospital competition have had a large role in this extraordinary expansion of RARP. They also point to lack of good-quality evidence demonstrating superiority of RARP over ORP/LRP and the issue of increased cost [3].

V. Agrawal, M.D., FRCSEd (Uro)., FEBU
Department of Urology, The Guthrie Clinic, Sayre, PA, USA
e-mail: agrawal_vineet@guthrie.org

J. Joseph, M.D., M.B.A. (✉)
Departments of Urology and Oncology, Center for Robotic Surgery and Innovation, University of Rochester Medical Center, Rochester, NY, USA
e-mail: Jean_Joseph@urmc.rochester.edu

This chapter summarizes historical perspective, surgical preparation, procedural step- by-step, peri- and postoperative management, outcomes, and the future of RARP.

Historical Perspective

The first case report of RARP was published in 2001, 9 years following initial description of LRP [4, 5]. Evolution of RARP was driven by the need to mitigate challenges inherent in performing standard LRP and its steep learning curve. Operating in the deep confines of the pelvis during a LRP requires advanced laparoscopic skills, especially in reconstructive steps of the procedure. This had prevented wide dissemination of LRP. The da Vinci® Surgical system (Intuitive Surgical, Sunnyvale, CA, USA), approved in 1999 and first used for cardiac surgery heralded a new era in minimally invasive surgery. When applied to prostatectomy, the 10- to 12-fold magnified 3-D vision, ergonomic superiority, wristed tremor-free instruments with 7° of freedom, and motion scaling provide greater dexterity and precision in performing the procedure, particularly the vesicourethral anastomosis (VUA).

Since the initial description of RARP, several early adopters of this technology spearheaded by the Vattikuti Institute in Detroit, Michigan, USA, have driven surgical advances and refinement in

J.W. Davis (ed.), *Robot-Assisted Radical Prostatectomy*, DOI 10.1007/978-3-319-32641-2_18

the technique of RARP [6, 7]. The technique has now been standardized with over 80 % of RP in the USA routinely performed using the roboti-assisted technology [8].

RARP was the first robot-assisted surgical procedure to achieve widespread use. It has helped paved the way for robotic utilization in other procedures across not only urology but also many other surgical disciplines [9].

Indications/Contraindications and Patient Selection

Patients diagnosed with organ-confined PC who opt for radical prostatectomy are candidates for RARP. Standard indications and contraindications found in open and laparoscopic surgery also apply to RARP. Challenging scenarios such as patients with large prostateor large median lobe, high body mass index, prior prostate or abdominal surgery, and pelvic radiation are best dealt with once the learning curve of performing RARP has been overcome.

Preoperative Preparation

The preoperative and preanesthesia screening to determine suitability for undergoing RARP is identical to that performed before open surgery.

Perioperative Preparation

We perform an antibiotic bowel preparation with Neomycin (1 g tid) and Metronidazole (500 mgs tid) administered the day before the procedure. 5000 units of low-molecular-weight heparin are injected subcutaneously prior to arrival in the operating room. A single dose of intravenous Cephalosporin antibiotic is administered at the time of induction of anesthesia. Intravenous (IV) fluids are run slowly to keep the total infused volume less than 1.5–2 l until the VUA is complete to avoid flooding the surgical field.

Operative Procedure

The following section outlines our technique of RARP. We have recently switched to using the four arm da Vinci Xi surgical system.

Patient Positioning and Setup

Position-related injuries can be a source of morbidity and must be avoided. Patients are placed supine over a beanbag on a split leg operating table. Following induction of general endotracheal anesthesia and insertion of IV lines and oro-gastric tube, the patient is secured to the table with activation of the vacuum beanbag. This is to prevent sliding down when placed in the Trendelenburg position. Arms are adducted in egg crate protective foams to prevent brachial plexus injury. The legs are abducted on a spreader bar to allow the patient cart to be positioned, and access to the perineum if needed. Leg abduction should be kept to a minimum to avoid hip dislocation. Stockings and sequential compression devices are placed on the legs for deep vein thrombosis prophylaxis. All pressure points are well padded to avoid pressure sores. A rectal examination is performed for intraoperative clinical staging. Abdomen is shaved and prepped from the level of the nipples to the upper thigh followed by draping of the operative field.

A 16F Foley catheter with 10 cc of water in the balloon is inserted in the sterile field. The patient is then placed in Trendelenburg position.

Extraperitoneal Access and Trocar Placement

Our favored approach is an open Hasson "cut-down" technique. The approach is obtained consistently in a controlled manner with clear visualization of anatomical landmarks.

The instruments required to create the potential extraperitoneal space include an OMS-XB2 (Oval) Extraview™ balloon dilator trocar (Autosuture, Norwalk, CT) or a spacemaker™ trocar, a 0° laparoscope, 2 "S"-shaped retractors, and a 15 cm long smooth trocar (12 mm 512 XD, Ethicon Endo-Surgery, Cincinnati, OH). We prefer to use a separate scope for this step. The robotic camera and scope system are difficult to maneuver due to their weight.

After a 3 cm left peri-umbilical skin, subcutaneous tissue is bluntly spread to expose the anterior rectus sheath over which a 1 cm incision is made. A 0 vicryl purse string suture is placed on the anterior sheath and the underlying rectus muscle is gently retracted laterally to reveal the posterior rectus sheath. A balloon trocar with a 10 mm 0° camera is inserted in the space of Retzius, staying above the posterior rectus sheath. The balloon is inflated and creation of the extraperitoneal space is visualized. Placement of a fist over the left side of the lower abdomen as the balloon inflates ensures uniform extraperitoneal space creation on either side of midline. Important landmarks are inferior epigastric arteries, external iliac vessels, and pubic symphysis. Once the space is adequately created, the balloon trocar with the camera is withdrawn. A 10/12 15 cm smooth trocar with a beveled tip is inserted into the extraperitoneal space created followed by connecting the gas tubing to keep the space insufflated with CO_2 up to a pressure of 15 mmHg. This trocar is smooth and a key to our approach. All subsequent trocar insertions are under vision. To facilitate this the beveled edge of the camera trocar is used to sweep the peritoneum cephalad off the transversalis fascia, further enlarging the extraperitoneal space. Care is taken to avoid an inadvertent peritoneal opening. The first trocar to be inserted is a 12 mm assistant trocar (150 mm Excel 512 XD), which we prefer to place on the right side, as our bedside assistant is left handed. Next, a hypodermic needle is inserted at the site of the right 8 mm robotic trocar insertion to identify and avoid injury to the inferior epigastric vessels. The trocar is inserted 8–10 mm caudad to the camera trocar on a line joining the umbilicus to the anterior superior iliac spine (ASIS). This is repeated on the left side to insert the left 8 mm robotic trocar. Another 8 mm robotic trocar is inserted 5 mm cephalad to the left ASIS for the fourth arm. Finally, a 5 mm trocar is inserted 5 mm about 6 cm lateral to the camera trocar on the right side. A Xeroform gauze is tightly wrapped around the camera trocar to prevent gas leakage. The previously placed purse string suture is tightened to narrow the opening around the trocar.

After docking of patient cart to the trocars, a 0° da Vinci camera is inserted. Initial instruments used are Maryland bipolar and Prograsp forceps in left and fourth robotic arm, respectively, while scissors are inserted in right robotic arm with the assistant using 12 mm assistant trocar for clipping and 5 mm trocar for suction/irrigation.

Transperitoneal Access, Creation of Pneumoperitoneum, Trocar Placement, Bladder Dissection, and Exposure of Space of Retzius

Holding up the skin on either side of umbilicus ensures that the visceral peritoneum is lifted away from intra-abdominal contents. A towel clip placed in the umbilicus can be used to lift in very obese patients. A Veress needle is inserted perpendicularly in the umbilicus with its proper placement confirmed by two clicks of the needle. Gas tubing is connected to the needle to create pneumoperitoneum with CO_2 up to a pressure of 15 mmHg. We insert a 10/12 mm camera trocar with visual obturator using a 10 mm 0° camera through an incision just left to umbilicus. All subsequent trocars are inserted under vision. A hypodermic needle is inserted at the site of the 8 mm robotic trocar insertion to identify and avoid injury to the inferior epigastric vessels. The trocar is inserted 8–10 mm caudad to the camera trocar on either side of the umbilicus on a line joining it to the ASIS. Another 8 mm robotic trocar is inserted 5 mm cephalad to the left ASIS for the fourth arm. With our bedside assistant being left handed, we prefer to place a 12 mm assistant trocar about 5 mm cephalad to the right ASIS. Finally, a 5 mm trocar is inserted 5 mm cephalad to the camera trocar on the right side. The Trendelenburg position is adjusted as necessary to keep the bowels sufficiently out of the operative field.

After docking of patient cart and fixing the robotic arms to the trocars, a 0° da Vinci camera is inserted.

The bladder is dropped down by dissecting the urachus off the anterior abdominal wall, following the dissection lateral to both medial umbilical ligaments in a caudad direction in an inverted "U" fashion. The lower limits of the dissection are the vasa on either side. Following an avascular plane between the bladder and abdominal wall allows the bladder to drop posteriorly and helps expose the space of Retzius. Fat overlying the puboprostatic ligaments, dorsal vein complex (DVC), and the anterior aspect of the prostate is removed. The superficial branch of the DVC is coagulated using bipolar cautery and divided.

Subsequent steps of RARP that are common to both the trans- and extraperitoneal access techniques are described below. While some surgeons routinely perform early posterior approach to dissection of the seminal vesicles, we prefer the anterior approach whereby the seminal vesicle dissection is performed after the bladder neck dissection.

Endopelvic Fascia Dissection

Opening the space of Retzius exposes the endopelvic fascia. A sharp cut is made in the endopelvic fascia just lateral to the prostate with the cut extended in the direction of the apex. A combination of sharp and blunt dissection is used to separate Levator ani muscle on the pelvic floor off the lateral prostate fascia. This dissection is carried out caudad until the "notch" between the urethra and dorsal venous complex (DVC) is sufficiently exposed. We prefer to take down the puboprostatic ligaments.

Dorsal Vessel Complex Ligation

We use a barbed 2/0V-Lok™ suture on an SH needle to secure the DVC in a figure of eight fashion. The needle is inserted in the plane between the urethra and DVC in a right-to-left direction. We perform anterior suspension of this suture to the pubic symphysis.

Bladder Neck Transection

The plane between prostate and bladder is identified and a combination of "burn-and-push" technique is employed. This plane is developed laterally on either side and carried to the midline. The anterior bladder neck is incised in the midline at which point the Foley catheter can be observed. After transection of the posterior bladder neck, the anterior layer of Denonvilliers' fascia is exposed and incised, allowing identification of the vas deferens and the seminal vesicles.

Vas Deferens and Seminal Vesicle Dissection

The vas is divided between Hem-o-lok clips. Next, the seminal vesicle is skeletonized, avoiding thermal injury to the laterally placed neurovascular bundle (NVB). Prograsp forceps and the assistant retractor are used to provide anterior and cranial traction of the left and right seminal vesicle, respectively, to facilitate the next step.

Incision of Denonvilliers' Fascia

The posterior layer of Denonvilliers' fascia is incised in the midline close to the prostate. A plane between the prostate anteriorly and the rectum posteriorly is developed with the dissection carried distally in the direction of the apex. The plane of dissection leaves the most posterior layer of Denonvilliers' fascia on the rectum.

Securing the Prostatic Pedicle

The prostatic pedicles are controlled using Hem-o-lok clips. We tend to avoid any thermal energy to avoid inadvertent damage to the NVB.

Neurovascular Bundle Sparing

Scissors are used to incise the lateral prostatic fascia along the prostate and the NVB is gently dissected off of the prostatic capsule. This dissection is carried toward the apex. A combination of antegrade and retrograde dissection is performed.

Apical Dissection

The previously secured DVC is incised. Further dissection leads to the plane between prostatic apex and urethra. Once the anterior urethra wall is exposed, it is sharply cut. The urethra is transected a few millimeters distal to the prostatic apex. Care is taken to avoid injury to the anterolaterally coursing NVB near the prostatic apex. Division of posterior urethral wall and the rectourethralis muscle frees the specimen. The specimen is examined for adequacy of resection margins.

Posterior Reconstruction

Two separate 3/0 9-in. V-Lok™ sutures are used to perform the posterior reconstruction incorporating posterior rhabdosphincter, Denonvilliers' fascia, and the longitudinal fibers posterior to the bladder that were previously covering the seminal vesicles. The sutures are cinched to approximate the bladder neck to urethra. The sutures are suspended to Cooper's ligament after VUA has been completed. This is a technical modification we have been using with the aim of improving early return of urinary continence by providing a sling-like effect.

Vesicourethral Anastomosis

We use two separate 2/0 9-in. Vicryl suture on an RB-1 needle to perform a running anastomosis. The initial throw is placed in an inside-out fashion in the urethra at the 5 O' clock position and then through the bladder in an outside-in fashion. The suture is then run in a clockwise direction to 11 O' clock ensuring good mucosa-to-mucosa apposition, cinching as we go along. This completes the posterior layer. For the anterior layer, a second suture is run in an anticlockwise direction from 4 to 10 O' clock position. The two sutures are tied separately providing two distinct suture lines avoiding reliance on a single knot. A 20F 2-way Foley catheter is inserted with 30 cc of water in the balloon. Filling the bladder with about 180 cc of saline and observing for leak verifies the integrity of the anastomosis.

The robot is undocked after removal of instruments.

Drain Placement

A 19F Blake drain is inserted and exits via the left-sided fourth arm trocar. The drain is positioned over the pelvis ensuring that it does not lie over the anastomosis that can result in falsely high output due to suction. 3/0 silk suture is used to anchor the drain to the skin.

Specimen Extraction and Wound Closure

The entrapment bag string is transferred from the assistant's 12 mm port to the robotic 12 mm camera port. The umbilical incision is extended and the specimen is extracted. We close the fascia with 3–4 interrupted 0-polyglactin sutures. Care is taken to ensure that bowel is not caught in the suture line. Gaps between sutures are eliminated so that there is no possibility of herniation of the bowel. The Trendelenburg positioning is reversed at this point.

All the ports are removed under vision. The 12 mm right-sided assistant trocar incision is closed by placement of deep 0 polyglactin (Vicryl) suture in a figure of eight fashion to prevent hernia formation. We do not routinely close the 8 mm robotic trocar incisions. All skin incisions are closed with 4/0 Monocryl sutures. Steristrips and dressings are applied over the incision and local anesthetic is infiltrated at each trocar site prior to the reversal of anesthesia.

Postoperative Care

On reversal from anesthesia, patient is transferred to PACU and to the 23-h stay unit a few hours later. Clear liquid diet is administered initially and the diet is advanced as tolerated. Patients ambulate the same day. They receive thromboembolic prophylaxis with subcutaneous low-molecular-weight heparin as well as intermittent pneumatic compression device for the duration of their hospitalization. 15 cc of water is removed from the balloon the morning after the procedure. The drain is removed when the output is <75 cc in an 8-h shift. Most patients are discharged within 24 h of their surgery. Foley catheter is removed in 7–10 days.

Pros and Cons of Extraperitoneal and Transperitoneal Technique

The advantages of the transperitoneal technique include familiarity with the anatomy and the instruments and adequate space for dissection. Dropping the bladder down helps with releasing tension at the time of VUA. The disadvantages include potential for peritoneal urine leak due to communication of the VUA site with the peritoneal cavity. There is a slight increased risk of bowel injury, ileus, and adhesions.

The advantages of the extraperitoneal technique include need for less steep Trendelenburg position (10–15 compared to 15–25°), feasibility of the procedure in patients with extensive prior abdominal procedures, and a slightly lesser risk of ileus. The disadvantages include lack of adequate space for dissection and suturing [10].

Outcomes

Several retrospective studies have shown that RARP is associated with lower blood loss, transfusion rates, and a shorter length of stay compared to ORP. A systematic review in 2012 which retrieved 110 eligible studies on RARP outcomes showed that the mean operative time was 152 min, blood loss 166 ml, transfusion rate 2 %, mean catheterization time 6.3 days, and length of hospital stay 1.9 days [11]. The mean complication rate was 9 %, with most of the complications of the low grade. Lymphocele/lymphorrhea (3.1 %), urine leak (1.8 %), and reoperation (1.6 %) were the most prevalent complications.

Functional outcomes of RARP were the subject of a systematic review in 2012 [12]. The 12-month urinary incontinence rates ranged from 4 to 31 % with a mean value of 16 % using a no-pad definition. This review concluded that age, body mass index, comorbidity index, lower urinary tract symptoms, and prostate volume were preoperative predictors of urinary incontinence after RARP. As for potency after RARP, another systematic review from the same year concluded that potency after RARP is influenced by several factors [13]. Twelve- and twenty-four-month potency rates ranged from 54–90 % to 63–94 %, respectively.

Early measures of oncological success such as positive surgical margin rates (PSM) indicate excellent outcomes in experienced hands. Mean PSM rates were 15 % for all comers and 9 % in pathologically localized (pT2) PC [14]. Studies assessing the long-term oncologic outcomes of RARP with regard to biochemical recurrence, metastases-free, and cancer-specific mortality-free survival are still lacking as RARP has been a rather recent introduction but a recent study looking at 10-year outcome data was published [15]. One hundred and ten patients who underwent RARP 10 years ago were followed for a mean period of 121 months. Biochemical recurrence-free survival, metastasis-free survival, and cancer-specific survival rates at 10 years were 73.1 %, 97.5 %, and 98.8 %, respectively.

Techniques to Improve Outcomes

RARP has continued to evolve rapidly over time with various studies published describing technical modifications that aim to improve outcomes. Most of the effort has been focused on quality-of-life issues such as early return and overall continence or potency. Other modifications focus on oncological outcomes and patient comfort.

Techniques employed in an attempt to improve early return and overall continence include anterior anastomotic urethral suspension [16], bladder neck preservation [17], intussusception or tubularization [18], sparing of puboprostatic ligament or pubovesical complex [19], sling construction [20], intraoperative cooling [21], posterior reconstruction [22], and additional modifications to the posterior reconstruction (anterior, posterior, or total reconstruction) [23].

Refinements in NVB preservation include development and preservation of the lateral prostatic fascia ("veil of Aphrodite") [24], intraoperative cooling [25], and athermal or tension-free dissection [26].

Suprapubic instead of urethral drainage of bladder has been attempted with the aim of reducing patient discomfort with similar outcomes in terms of continence and stricture rate [27].

Robot-Assisted Prostatectomy: Recent Advances and Future

It remains to be seen if the recent introduction of the latest model of the da Vinci surgical platform, the Xi model equipped with overhead arm architecture, thinner instruments with longer shafts, and integrated energy source will provide any additional benefits over the existing S and Si models during performance of an RARP [28]. Currently, it is felt that the ability of this model to access previously difficult-to-reach anatomical spaces may have more advantages for procedures in urology other than RARP such as nephroureterectomy, and non-urological procedures. In addition, the landscape of RARP and indeed other robot-assisted laparoscopic procedures is in a state of constant evolution with several robotic platforms (SOFIE, Amadeus, Raven) and instruments anticipated to be introduced in the future [29]. Some of these newer platforms are portable and can be attached to the operating table.

In the future, some or all of these following modalities may be routinely used to enhance the outcomes of an RARP. The ProPep nerve monitoring system is designed to improve the performance of nerve sparing during an RARP. Robotically manipulated transrectal ultrasound (ViKY System; EndoControl Medical, Grenoble, France) monitors the prostate and periprostatic anatomy providing the console surgeon with real-time anatomic information during an RARP [30].

Recently, a feasibility study of successfully performing a nerve-sparing perineal robot-assisted radical prostatectomy was performed in three cadaver models [31]. A single port was used for the procedure and total operative time was 89 min. Clinical studies comparing this novel technique with the standard RARP techniques are awaited.

Single-site RARP in 20 patients has been reported although wide dissemination of this technique has not occurred due to the technical difficulties [32]. Further refinements in the specific instruments (VeSPA) used to perform single-site robot-assisted surgery may change this.

Conclusions

Systematic reviews and meta-analyses have shown that RARP is associated with functional and oncological outcomes no inferior to open and laparoscopic radical prostatectomy. For the foreseeable future, an increasing number of prostatectomies will continue to be performed robotically, as surgeons seek to deliver an effective procedure with limited invasiveness. Continued heated debate among the urological community will call for further cost–benefit analysis.

References

1. Bill-Axelson A, Holmberg L, Garmo H, et al. Radical prostatectomy or watchful waiting in early prostate cancer. N Engl J Med. 2014;370(10):932–42.
2. Barbash GI, Friedman B, Glied SA, et al. Factors associated with adoption of robotic surgical technology in US hospitals and relationship to radical prostatectomy procedure volume. Ann Surg. 2014; 259(1):1–6.
3. Laviana AA, Williams SB, King ED et al, Robot assisted radical prostatectomy: the new standard? Minerva Urol Nefrol. 2015;67(1):47–53.
4. Binder J, Kramer W. Robotically-assisted laparoscopic radical prostatectomy. BJU Int. 2001;87: 408–10.
5. Schuessler WW, Kavoussi LR, Clayman RV, et al. Laparoscopic radical prostatectomy: initial case report. J Urol. 1992;147:246A. Abstract no. 130.

6. Menon M, Shrivastava A, Tewari A, et al. Laparoscopic and robot assisted radical prostatectomy: establishment of a structured program and preliminary analysis of outcomes. J Urol. 2002;168(3):945–9.
7. Menon M, Tewari A, Baize B, et al. Prospective comparison of radical retropubic prostatectomy and robot-assisted anatomic prostatectomy: the Vattikuti Urology Institute experience. Urology. 2002;60(5):864–8.
8. Chang SL, Kibel AS, Brooks JD, et al. The impact of robotic surgery on the surgical management of prostate cancer in the USA. BJU Int. 2015;115(6):929–36
9. Ng AT, Tam PC. Current status of robot-assisted surgery. Hong Kong Med J. 2014;20(3):241–50.
10. Lee JY, Diaz RR, Cho KS, et al. Meta-analysis of transperitoneal versus extraperitoneal robot-assisted radical prostatectomy for prostate cancer. J Laparoendosc Adv Surg Tech A. 2013;23(11):919–25.
11. Novara G, Ficarra V, Rosen RC, et al. Systematic review and meta-analysis of perioperative outcomes and complications after robot-assisted radical prostatectomy. Eur Urol. 2012;62(3):431–52.
12. Ficarra V, Novara G, Rosen RC, et al. Systematic review and meta-analysis of studies reporting urinary continence recovery after robot-assisted radical prostatectomy. Eur Urol. 2012;62(3):405–17.
13. Ficarra V, Novara G, Ahlering TE, et al. Systematic review and meta-analysis of studies reporting potency rates after robot-assisted radical prostatectomy. Eur Urol. 2012;62(3):418–30.
14. Novara G, Ficarra V, Mocellin S, et al. Systematic review and meta-analysis of studies reporting oncologic outcome after robot-assisted radical prostatectomy. Eur Urol. 2012;62(3):382–404.
15. Diaz M, Peabody JO, Kapoor V, et al. Oncologic outcomes at 10 years following robotic radical prostatectomy. Eur Urol. 2015;67(6):1168–76.
16. Patel VR, Coelho RF, Palmer KJ, et al. Periurethral suspension stitch during robot-assisted laparoscopic radical prostatectomy: description of the technique and continence outcomes. Eur Urol. 2009;56(3):472–8.
17. Freire MP, Weinberg AC, Lei Y, et al. Anatomic bladder neck preservation during robotic-assisted laparoscopic radical prostatectomy: description of technique and outcomes. Eur Urol. 2009;56(6):972–80.
18. Yanagida T, Koguchi T, Hata J, et al. Current techniques to improve outcomes for early return of urinary continence following robot-assisted radical prostatectomy. Fukushima J Med Sci. 2014;60(1):1–13.
19. Asimakopoulos AD, Annino F, D'Orazio A, et al. Complete periprostatic anatomy preservation during robot-assisted 1 laparoscopic radical prostatectomy (RALP): the new pubovesical complex-sparing technique. Eur Urol. 2010;58(3):407–17.
20. Kojima Y, Takahashi N, Haga N, et al. Urinary incontinence after robot-assisted radical prostatectomy: pathophysiology and intraoperative techniques to improve surgical outcome. Int J Urol. 2013;20(11):1052–63.
21. Finley DS, Osann K, Chang A, et al. Hypothermic robotic radical prostatectomy: impact on continence. J Endourol. 2009;23(9):1443–50.
22. Gautam G, Rocco B, Patel VR, et al. Posterior rhabdosphincter reconstruction during robot-assisted radical prostatectomy: critical analysis of techniques and outcomes. Urology. 2010;76(3):734–41.
23. Hurtes X, Rouprêt M, Vaessen C, et al. Anterior suspension combined with posterior reconstruction during robot-assisted laparoscopic prostatectomy improves early return of urinary continence: a prospective randomized multicentre trial. BJU Int. 2012;110(6):875–83.
24. Savera AT, Kaul S, Badani K, et al. Robotic radical prostatectomy with the "Veil of Aphrodite" technique: histologic evidence of enhanced nerve sparing. Eur Urol. 2006;49(6):1065–73.
25. Finley DS, Osann K, Skarecky D, et al. Hypothermic nerve-sparing radical prostatectomy: rationale, feasibility, and effect on early continence. Urology. 2009;73(4):691–6.
26. Ahlering TE, Eichel L, Skarecky D. Evaluation of long-term thermal injury using cautery during nerve sparing robotic prostatectomy. Urology. 2008;72(6):1371–4.
27. Sammon JD, Trinh QD, Sukumar S, et al. Long-term follow-up of patients undergoing percutaneous suprapubic tube drainage after robot-assisted radical prostatectomy (RARP). BJU Int. 2012;110(4):580–5.
28. Wilson TG. Advancement of technology and its impact on urologists: release of the da Vinci Xi, a new surgical robot. Eur Urol. 2014;66(5):793-4
29. Cathelineau X, Sanchez-Salas R, Sivaraman A. What is next in robotic urology? Curr Urol Rep. 2014;15(12):460.
30. Hung AJ, Abreu AL, Shoji S, et al. Robotic transrectal ultrasonography during robot-assisted radical prostatectomy. Eur Urol. 2012;62(2):341–8.
31. Laydner H, Akca O, Autorino R, et al. Perineal robot-assisted laparoscopic radical prostatectomy (P-RALP): feasibility study in the cadaver model. J Endourol. 2014;28(12):1479-86
32. Kumar P, Kommu SS, Challacombe BJ, et al. Laparoendoscopic single-site surgery (LESS) prostatectomy—robotic and conventional approach. Minerva Urol Nefrol. 2010;62(4):425–30.

Part II

Peri-operative Care and Safety

Perioperative Medical Evaluation of the Patient Undergoing RARP

19

Sunil Kumar Sahai

Introduction

Since the introduction of robotic-assisted robotic prostatectomy (RARP) in the care of the prostate cancer patient, it has become the surgical treatment of choice [1]. While the various intraoperative and postoperative concerns for RARP have been extensively reported in the literature [2, 3], little attention has been paid to the role of the evaluation of medical issues in the perioperative period. In this chapter, I seek to point out perioperative medical concerns that the surgical team will need to take into consideration prior to a patient undergoing RARP. One of the great advantages in treating men with prostate cancer is that there is no rush to action. Unlike some other cancers, where doubling time of the tumor is measured in days or weeks, a more measured approach can be taken; especially when faced with the medically complex patient. In order to determine the medical complexity of the cancer patient, a thorough history and physical are needed [4]. In our practice, most cancer patients presenting for perioperative evaluation have sufficient documentation of prior surgical procedures; however, complete documentation of the presence and severity of comorbidities and prior chemotherapy or radiation treatment regimens is frequently absent. A careful history and physical examination accompanied by evidence-based targeted testing before surgery are needed to reduce the likelihood of adverse perioperative outcomes [5, 6]. Potential triggers for initiating a perioperative medical evaluation are presented in Table 19.1. The medical evaluation should ideally be done by a primary care physician familiar with the patient, or if not available a consultant physician familiar with the perioperative implications of a patient undergoing a robotic prostatectomy. In general, the issues with RARP tend to be the same issues that occur other surgeries that utilize Trendelenburg positioning and pneumoperitoneum, and guideline statements such as those by the European Association for Endoscopic Surgery should be consulted [7].

Medical History

In our perioperative medicine clinic, we approach every patient as a brand new patient to the institution, despite the fact that they may have been seen by numerous care teams in the past. By starting out with a blank slate, we are frequently able to uncover medical comorbidities previously not documented, or forgotten by the patient [8]. The approach to the medical his-

S.K. Sahai, M.D., F.A.A.P., F.A.C.P. (✉)
Department of General Internal Medicine, The Internal Medicine Perioperative Assessment Center, The University of Texas MD Anderson Cancer Center, 1515 Holcombe Blvd, Houston, TX 77030, USA
e-mail: ssahai@mdanderson.org

J.W. Davis (ed.), *Robot-Assisted Radical Prostatectomy*, DOI 10.1007/978-3-319-32641-2_19

Table 19.1 Potential triggers for perioperative medical consultation

Cardiac/vascular • Coronary artery disease • Congestive heart failure • Arrhythmias • Peripheral vascular disease • CVA/TIA • Intravascular stents	Gastrointestinal disease • History of Crohn's disease or ulcerative colitis • On immunosuppressants/biologicals
Pulmonary • COPD • Asthma • Smoker: active or >20 pack year • Suspected sleep apnea	Rheumatologic disease • Rheumatoid arthritis/lupus • On immunosuppressants/biologicals
Hypertension • History of hypertension • Systolic blood pressure >180 mmHg • Diastolic blood pressure >110 mmHg	Hepatic • Hepatitis/ascites • History of coagulopathy • Abnormal liver function tests
Other endocrine • Uncontrolled thyroid disease • Adrenal insufficiency	Renal • Dialysis • Creatinine >2.0
Anticoagulation issues • Recent vascular stents • Atrial fibrillation • DVT/PE	Hematologic • Coagulopathy • Thrombophilia • Transfusion reactions
Diabetes • NIDDM/IDDM • Elevated fasting glucose • Insulin pumps	HIV/AIDS • Or other immunosuppression
Obesity	Alcohol/drug abuse • With suspected metabolic derangements

tory is systematic and template driven, ensuring a high degree of conformity between providers. Medical comorbid conditions involving the cardiovascular, cerebrovascular, pulmonary, and renal systems are extensively documented. Additionally, cardiovascular interventions such as surgery, artificial valves, and placement of stents and pacemakers are documented and double-checked against source documentation. A current medication list is generated and double-checked against the actual bottles and actual patient compliance. Patients on anticoagulants and antiplatelet medications are reviewed in terms of indication, dosage, and the need for bridging interventions for the perioperative period. Source documentation from outside physicians and hospitals is requested in an expedited manner, and in return, our assessments are shared with those physicians who may be treating the patient in the post-discharge setting.

Of particular importance is determining if the patient has had prior diagnosis of cancer, and the nature of any treatments provided. If the patient has received treatment known to cause toxicity to the cardiovascular, pulmonary, or renal systems, any potential long-term effects affecting the patient need to be documented.

Cardiac History

It is well known that more men die *with* prostate cancer, and then *from* prostate cancer [9]. For the majority of men with early-stage prostate cancer, death from heart disease is more common than death from prostate cancer [10]. As such, it behooves both the perioperative team and treating urologist to determine the greater long-term risk to the patient in terms of morbidity and mortality. Fortunately, prostate surgery in general carries a relatively low risk of perioperative cardiovascular complications [3, 11].

In a recent prospective review of complications from RARP, Agarwal et al. [12] showed that the presence of preexisting cardiac comorbidities was predictive of a greater likelihood of medical complications after multivariate analysis. Additionally, there are isolated case reports in the literature [13] and at our institution concerning increased perioperative cardiac complications in patients with cardiac stents undergoing RARP. As such, our practice has evolved to incorporate the following general guidelines.

1. A thorough cardiac history is documented, including dates, locations, and type of cardiac stents.
2. For any patient who is less than 1 year from stent placement, a cardiology consultation is requested to assess risk of perioperative cardiac issues, including risk from premature discontinuation of dual-antiplatelet agents.
3. Patients with stents less than 1 year old are discussed with the treating urologist to determine if surgery can be delayed or other therapies can be initiated in order to complete 1 year of dual antiplatelet therapy.
4. Those patients on dual-antiplatelet agents are told to withhold clopidogrel, ticagrelor, or prasugrel only 5 days before the procedure.
5. Patients with cardiac stents are told to switch to or remain on low-dose aspirin throughout the entire perioperative period, with resumption of a second agent within 48 h of surgery.
6. Patients with known history of cardiac intervention such as bypass or PTCA are told to remain on low-dose aspirin throughout the perioperative period.

While the use of aspirin during the perioperative period was initially controversial, the concern about perioperative cardiac in-stent thrombosis [14] and studies showing the relative safety of aspirin have seen its widespread adoption [15, 16]. Recent studies [17, 18] have led to conflicting conclusions about the efficacy of perioperative aspirin use; however, at our institution, we feel that with the prothrombotic nature of cancer patients, its use is justified [19].

In regard to congestive heart failure, it is essential to determine the etiology of the heart failure and ejection fraction prior to surgery. Patients may have received anthracycline-based chemotherapy for an unrelated cancer in the past, and may have unrecognized heart failure [20]. In a prospective observational study of 31 patients, Rosendal et al. showed that RARP resulted in 8 % decrease in cardiac output during capnoperitoneum and increased afterload by 17 % [21]. As such, in those patients with ischemic cardiomyopathy, coronary perfusion and oxygen supply to the heart may be compromised. In the fragile patient with heart failure and an ejection fraction less than 40 %, we recommend that a cardiology consultation be obtained for risk assessment and optimization of heart function. In these situations, the slow progression of prostate cancer allows time for thoughtful preoperative optimization of cardiac issues.

Cerebrovascular History

Of concern to some practitioners not familiar with RARP is the issue of cerebrovascular compromise in steep Trendelenburg position. Of particular concern is the combination of positioning and pneumoperitoneum leading to cerebral edema. For the elderly, there is a concern for vascular compromise and also postoperative mental status changes due to increased intracranial pressure. As such, a thorough neurological and mental status history is recommended to establish a baseline prior to surgery. The literature at this time is contradictory. Kalmar et al. monitored thirty-one patients and found no adverse changes in regional cerebral oxygenation and cerebral perfusion pressure [22]. However, Schram showed that cerebrovascular autoregulation deteriorates over time during steep Trendelenburg of 40–45 % [23]. In light of conflicting data and a limited literature, we recommend that the positioning be titrated to be as shallow as needed for the operation. Additionally, we recommend a slow transition to Trendelenburg of 15° at a time, allowing for the patient to reach a state of hemodynamic equilibrium before the next positioning change.

Ophthalmologic History

In a recent review of ocular complications of RARP by Kan et al. the most common issue encountered is corneal abrasions [24]. Corneal abrasions are thought to occur due to steep Trendelenburg positioning leading to conjunctival chemosis and subsequent corneal exposure due to incomplete closure of the eyelids. Depending on the study cited, the risk of corneal abrasions is between 0.2 and 3 % [25–27]. Fortunately, with education and proper precautions, the incidence of corneal abrasions can be reduced to 0 % [28].

A devastating complication of steep Trendelenburg is ischemic optic neuropathy which may lead to blindness [24]. Thorough discussion of this complication is beyond the scope of this chapter, and further details can be found in the review by Kan et al. [24]. In the Trendelenburg position, one concern is increased ocular pressure worsening glaucoma symptoms. In the review by Kan et al. the question remains open, however; the authors do suggest ophthalmology consultation for patients with open-angle glaucoma who may be at risk for a prolonged operation [24].

Pulmonary History

Steep Trendelenburg accompanied by pneumoperitoneum can reduce pulmonary compliance; as such, documentation of the presence of chronic obstructive pulmonary disease or pulmonary fibrosis may be adversely affected. Other airway complications include subcutaneous emphysema, stridor, and pulmonary and laryngeal edema [29, 30]. In practice however, it is not necessary to subject all patients with a history of COPD to further evaluation. Patients who have an adequate functional status and do not need supplemental oxygen on a daily basis will not benefit from further testing.

Diabetes

It is well known that diabetes in itself is a risk for postoperative complications from deranged glucose metabolism. In regard to referral for medical evaluation, patients with adequate glycemic control do not require further evaluation. For those with fluctuating blood sugars and poor control of their sugars, evaluation by an internist or endocrinologist may be helpful. Patients with type 1 diabetes or insulin pumps should have a perioperative management plan outlined prior to surgery. While the risk of postoperative complications increases in a linear fashion with hemoglobin A1c levels, surgical and oncologic urgency also plays a role in determining the best time to operate [31]. For the poorly controlled diabetic with a hemoglobin A1c above 9 %, it may be prudent to delay surgery until better glycemic control is reached.

Obesity

As the population of the world increases, the obesity epidemic will leave no country unscathed. As such, the careful evaluation of the obese man before surgery should focus on the metabolic syndrome and potentially undiagnosed comorbidities of diabetes, hypertension, and cardiac disease. Many morbidly obese men are simply unable to achieve an adequate level of exercise to quantify functional status before surgery. Additionally, there needs to be a high index of suspicion for undiagnosed sleep apnea in the morbidly obese population. Patients with morbid obesity tend to be challenges for surgical and anesthesia team members, and in general have a higher postoperative complication rate in regard to venous thromboembolism, surgical site infections, and postoperative cardiac complications [32]. While all these challenges are present in the obese patient undergoing RARP, it appears that RARP is just as efficacious as those undergoing laparoscopic radical prostatectomy (LRP) [26, 33–35].

Conclusion

In summary, while robotic-assisted robotic prostatectomy is associated with a lower perioperative morbidity than traditional open prostatectomy, it is still a major surgical procedure requiring careful medical evaluation of the patient. The presence of medical comorbidities may adversely impact surgical outcomes, and increase postoperative complications. Medical evaluation by a consultant physician well before surgery will allow time for perioperative optimization and adequate risk assessment of the patient.

References

1. Sood A, Jeong W, Peabody JO, Hemal AK, Menon M. Robot-assisted radical prostatectomy: inching toward gold standard. Urol Clin North Am. 2014;41(4):473–84.
2. Gainsburg DM. Anesthetic concerns for robotic-assisted laparoscopic radical prostatectomy. Minerva Anestesiol. 2012;78(5):596–604. Epub 2012/03/15. eng.
3. Novara G, Ficarra V, Rosen RC, Artibani W, Costello A, Eastham JA, et al. Systematic review and meta-analysis of perioperative outcomes and complications after robot-assisted radical prostatectomy. Eur Urol. 2012;62(3):431–52. Epub 2012/07/04. eng.
4. Sahai SK. Perioperative assessment of the cancer patient. Best Pract Res Clin Anaesthesiol. 2013;27(4):465–80. Epub 2013/11/26. eng.
5. Vazirani S, Lankarani-Fard A, Liang L-J, Stelzner M, Asch SM. Perioperative processes and outcomes after implementation of a hospitalist-run preoperative clinic. J Hosp Med. 2012;7(9):697–701.
6. Wijeysundera DN. Preoperative consultations by anesthesiologists. Curr Opin Anaesthesiol. 2011; 24(3):326–30.
7. Neudecker J, Sauerland S, Neugebauer E, Bergamaschi R, Bonjer HJ, Cuschieri A, et al. The European Association for Endoscopic Surgery clinical practice guideline on the pneumoperitoneum for laparoscopic surgery. Surg Endosc. 2002;16(7):1121–43.
8. Sahai SK. IMPAC+head & neck surgery: the metrics. [Lecture]. Unpublished Data. 2008
9. Satariano WA, Ragland KE, Eeden SKVD. Cause of death in men diagnosed with prostate carcinoma. Cancer. 1998;83(6):1180–8.
10. Ketchandji M, Kuo YF, Shahinian VB, Goodwin JS. Cause of death in older men after the diagnosis of prostate cancer. J Am Geriatr Soc. 2009;57(1):24–30. Pubmed Central PMCID: Pmc2956511, Epub 2008/12/05. eng.
11. Rabbani F, Yunis LH, Pinochet R, Nogueira L, Vora KC, Eastham JA, et al. Comprehensive standardized report of complications of retropubic and laparoscopic radical prostatectomy. Eur Urol. 2010;57(3):371–86. Epub 2009/12/01. eng.
12. Agarwal PK, Sammon J, Bhandari A, Dabaja A, Diaz M, Dusik-Fenton S, et al. Safety profile of robot-assisted radical prostatectomy: a standardized report of complications in 3317 patients. Eur Urol. 2011;59(5):684–98. Epub 2011/02/18. eng.
13. Thompson J. Myocardial infarction and subsequent death in a patient undergoing robotic prostatectomy. AANA J. 2009;77(5):365–71. Epub 2009/11/17. eng.
14. Llau JV, Lopez-Forte C, Sapena L, Ferrandis R. Perioperative management of antiplatelet agents in noncardiac surgery. Eur J Anaesthesiol. 2009;26(3): 181–7. Epub 2009/02/28. eng.
15. Nowfar S, Kopp R, Palazzi-Churas K, Derweesh IH, Kane CJ. Initial experience with aspirin use during robotic radical prostatectomy. J Laparoendosc Adv Surg Tech A. 2012;22(3):225–9. Epub 2012/03/08. eng.
16. Leyh-Bannurah SR, Hansen J, Isbarn H, Steuber T, Tennstedt P, Michl U, et al. Open and robot-assisted radical retropubic prostatectomy in men receiving ongoing low-dose aspirin medication: revisiting an old paradigm? BJU Int. 2014;114(3):396–403. Epub 2013/10/17. eng.
17. Rossini R, Musumeci G, Capodanno D, Lettieri C, Limbruno U, Tarantini G, et al. Perioperative management of oral antiplatelet therapy and clinical outcomes in coronary stent patients undergoing surgery. Results of a multicentre registry. Thromb Haemost. 2014;2:113(1). Epub 2014/10/03. Eng.
18. Devereaux PJ, Mrkobrada M, Sessler DI, Leslie K, Alonso-Coello P, Kurz A, et al. Aspirin in patients undergoing noncardiac surgery. N Engl J Med. 2014;370(16):1494–503. Epub 2014/04/01. eng.
19. Sherman KL, Obi SH, Aranha GV, Yao KA, Shoup MC. Heparin-coated stents do not protect cancer patients from cardiac complications after noncardiac surgery. Am Surg. 2009;75(1):61–5. Epub 2009/02/14. eng.
20. Bonita R, Pradhan R. Cardiovascular toxicities of cancer chemotherapy. Semin Oncol. 2013; 40(2):156–67.
21. Rosendal C, Markin S, Hien MD, Motsch J, Roggenbach J. Cardiac and hemodynamic consequences during capnoperitoneum and steep Trendelenburg positioning: lessons learned from robot-assisted laparoscopic prostatectomy. J Clin Anesth. 2014;26(5):383–9. Epub 2014/08/05. eng.
22. Kalmar AF, Foubert L, Hendrickx JF, Mottrie A, Absalom A, Mortier EP, et al. Influence of steep Trendelenburg position and CO(2) pneumoperitoneum on cardiovascular, cerebrovascular, and respiratory homeostasis during robotic prostatectomy. Br J Anaesth. 2010;104(4):433–9. Epub 2010/02/20. eng.
23. Schramm P, Treiber AH, Berres M, Pestel G, Engelhard K, Werner C, et al. Time course of cerebro-

vascular autoregulation during extreme Trendelenburg position for robotic-assisted prostatic surgery. Anaesthesia. 2014;69(1):58–63.
24. Kan KM et al. Ocular complications in robotic-assisted prostatectomy: a review of pathophysiology and prevention. Minerva Anestesiol. 2015;81(5): 557–66.
25. Danic M, Chow M, Alexander G, Bhandari A, Menon M, Brown M. Anesthesia considerations for robotic-assisted laparoscopic prostatectomy: a review of 1,500 cases. J Robotic Surg. 2007;1(2):119–23. English.
26. Kwon YS, Leapman M, McBride RB, Hobbs AR, Collingwood SA, Stensland KD, et al. Robotic-assisted laparoscopic prostatectomy in men with metabolic syndrome. Urol Oncol. 2014;32(1):40.e9–e16.
27. Nakamura L, Nunez R, Andrews P, Ferrigni R, Humphreys M, Swanson S, et al. Older age does not impact perioperative complications after robot-assisted radical prostatectomy. J Robotic Surg. 2011;5(3):201–8. English.
28. Banerjee KMD, Zdravka Zafirova MD, Avery Tung MD. Corneal abrasions during laparoscopic prostatectomy: mechanisms and prevention. Abstract presented at: American Society of Anesthesiologists Annual Meeting, October 19, 2008; Orlando, Florida. 2008
29. Kilic OF et al. Effects of steep Trendelenburg position for robotic-assisted prostatectomies on intraand extra-thoracic airways in patients with or without chronic obstructive pulmonary disease. Br J Anaesth. 2015; 114(1):70–6.
30. Hong JY, Oh YJ, Rha KH, Park WS, Kim YS, Kil HK. Pulmonary edema after da Vinci-assisted laparoscopic radical prostatectomy: a case report. J Clin Anesth. 2010;22(5):370–2. Epub 2010/07/24. eng.
31. Underwood P, Askari R, Hurwitz S, Chamarthi B, Garg R. Preoperative A1C and clinical outcomes in patients with diabetes undergoing major noncardiac surgical procedures. Diabetes Care. 2014;37(3):611–6.
32. King DR, Velmahos GC. Difficulties in managing the surgical patient who is morbidly obese. Crit Care Med. 2010;38(9 Suppl):S478–82. Epub 2010/08/28. eng.
33. Sundi D, Reese AC, Mettee LZ, Trock BJ, Pavlovich CP. Laparoscopic and robotic radical prostatectomy outcomes in obese and extremely obese men. Urology. 2013;82(3):600–5. Pubmed Central PMCID: Pmc3758791, Epub 2013/07/19.eng.
34. Bae JJ, Choi SH, Kwon TG, Kim TH. Advantages of robot-assisted laparoscopic radical prostatectomy in obese patients: comparison with the open procedure. Korean J Urol. 2012;53(8):536–40. Pubmed Central PMCID: Pmc3427837, Epub 2012/09/06. eng.
35. Moskovic DJ, Lavery HJ, Rehman J, Nabizada-Pace F, Brajtbord J, Samadi DB. High body mass index does not affect outcomes following robotic assisted laparoscopic prostatectomy. Can J Urol. 2010;17(4):5291–8. Epub 2010/08/26. eng.

Patient Positioning and Safety in Steep Trendelenburg

20

Cooper R. Benson and Jay B. Shah

Patient Positioning

Proper patient positioning is critical to the success of performing an RARP and it is the job of the entire operating room team to ensure that the positioning is safe for the patient. Since the transition from pure laparoscopic prostatectomy to RARP using the da Vinci system, there have been many modifications in the setup for the procedure including patient positioning and site of robotic patient cart docking. Binder and Kramer, in 2001, described their initial technique utilizing supine position with the legs on spreader bars to accommodate the patient cart between the legs [1]. In a variation designed to allow greater access to the perineum and rectum, the Vattikuti approach pioneered by Menon utilized the lithotomy position with the lower extremities placed in Allen Yellofin stirrups [2].

Lower Extremity Positioning

There are several options for positioning the lower extremities during RARP. They are largely based on surgeon preference and all are acceptable and safe. Low-lithotomy position is the most commonly described technique for positioning for RARP. In lithotomy the knees are flexed, the heels are seated correctly in the trough of the boot, and the knee is aligned with the opposite shoulder. The low-lithotomy position can be difficult to accomplish in patients with joint disease of the hip or knee and it carries a slightly increased risk of neuropraxia. However, the easy access to the perineum and rectum during the operation can greatly facilitate the application of perineal pressure to improve visualization of the urethral stump and it allows easier execution of rectal insufflation to check for rectal injury. A second technique is to keep the patient supine but instead of lithotomy utilize a split-leg table. The split-leg technique still allows the robot to be docked between the patient's legs but avoids the hip and knee limitations of the low-lithotomy position. As a third option, the patient may be kept completely supine on the table without spreading the legs. This option also avoids the hip and knee limitations of the lithotomy position but it must be used with a side-docking approach since the robot cannot be placed between the legs.

The split-leg and pure supine positions require less setup time at the beginning of the operation but do not allow the ready access to the perineum and rectum afforded by the lithotomy positioning. As such, surgeons who are earlier in their learning curve may prefer the low-lithotomy position: rectal insufflation can provide greater

C.R. Benson, M.D. (✉) • J.B. Shah
Department of Urology, MD Anderson Cancer Center, University of Texas-Houston Division of Urology, Houston, TX, USA
e-mail: cooper.r.benson@uth.tmc.edu; jbshah@mdanderson.org

J.W. Davis (ed.), *Robot-Assisted Radical Prostatectomy*, DOI 10.1007/978-3-319-32641-2_20

reassurance against inadvertent rectal injury (or early recognition of injury) and application of perineal pressure may allow easier suturing of the urethro-vesical anastomosis. At our institution, the surgeons are equally split between the low-lithotomy positioning and the supine side-dock positioning. Regardless of the positioning chosen for the lower extremities, compression stockings and mechanical sequential compression devices (SCDs) should be used for all patients to decrease the risk of deep venous thrombosis secondary to venous stasis. In addition, for the lithotomy positioning, there should be adequate padding around the calf to prevent compartment syndrome, rhabdomyolysis, and nerve injury [3–5].

Patient Immobilization

In order to accomplish robotic pelvic surgery, steep Trendelenburg is required, which uses gravity to move the intestines cephalad out of the surgical field. The table may be padded with gel pads or egg crates secured to the table, a beanbag, and/or utilize 3 M Reston Foam®, which prevents the patient from slipping more cephalad on the table while in Trendelenburg position. Some surgeons utilize shoulder pads to prevent slippage, but our preference is not to use these pads, due to their association with brachial plexus neuropraxia and injury [6]. If chest straps are used, care should be taken to ensure that the shoulders are in neutral position and that chest wall movement is not restricted. The arms are tucked to the side in a neutral position with palms facing medial and arms pronated using foam pads to support and protect the arms and the sheets to secure the arms during the case. Additionally, foam is typically placed around the hands and a rolled piece of foam in the hands for support. It is also important to ensure that tubing from intravenous lines and wiring from hemodynamic monitoring devices function properly and do not cause skin abrasions from inadvertent contact.

Once patient positioning, prepping, and draping have been completed and robotic ports have been placed, the patient cart of the da Vinci system is docked. The robot may be docked either between the legs (if patient is in lithotomy or split-leg position) or off to one side of the patient. The original description of the RARP technique uses docking between the legs. Uffort and Jensen described their experience utilizing side docking of the robot [7]. The benefits of side docking the robot include shorter setup and positioning time [7, 8]. Side docking the robot also obviates the need for lithotomy positioning and associated hazards, albeit it can also be used with lithotomy if needed or based on surgeon preference [8]. The new Xi da Vinci system has more flexibility in regard to docking the patient cart, and also allows easier transition between different anatomic quadrants of the abdomen for other procedures without re-docking. As experience grows with the Xi model in the coming years, we anticipate an increase in the percentage of surgeons employing the side-dock technique for RARP (Figs. 20.1, 20.2, 20.3, and 20.4).

Patient Safety

It is useful to have a robotics team, composed of circulating and scrub nurses who are trained and more experienced in robotic surgery, which makes the setup and the operation itself more efficient. It allows the nuances of positioning to be learned faster and it improves operating room time and efficiency. Additionally, utilizing checklists may help to reduce errors in positioning and also in re-evaluating positioning during the course of the operation. Song and colleagues introduced the use of a second time-out after 3 or

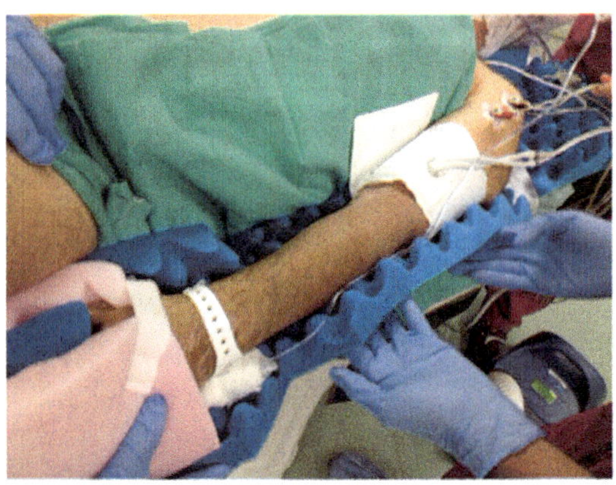

Fig. 20.1 Padding and positioning of upper extremity

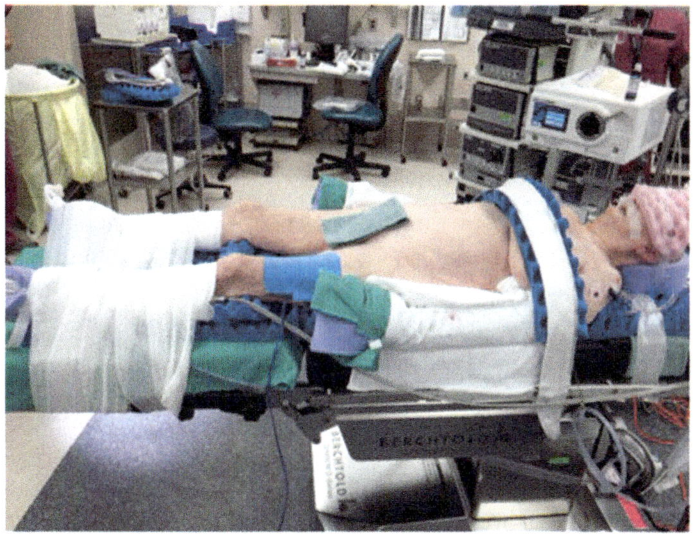

Fig. 20.2 Split-leg supine positioning in preparation for side-docking technique

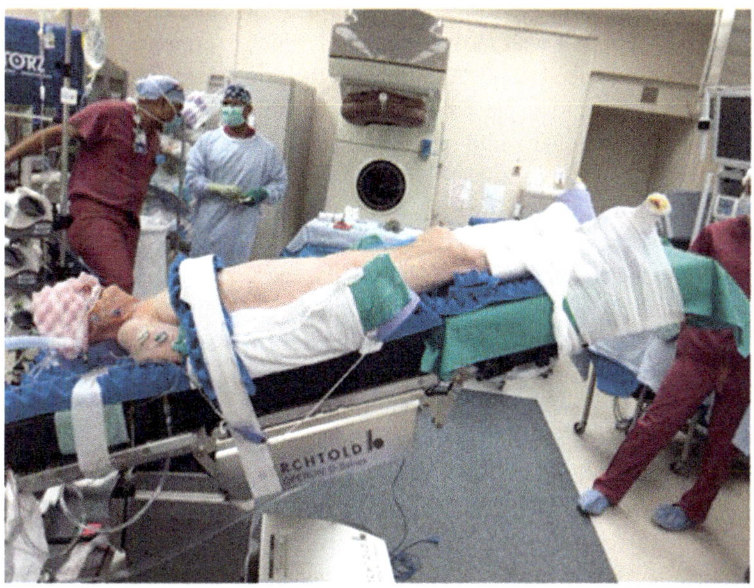

Fig. 20.3 Demonstrating testing steep Trendelenburg positioning for the case

4 h as a way to communicate with the entire operating room team in the middle of the case and a means to ensure patient safety for longer procedures [17]. In the second time-out the extremities are evaluated, positioning, padding, and straps are checked, ensuring that the SCDs are functioning and additionally evaluating the patient and the case overall, serving as a safety checkpoint.

The entire operating room team is responsible for maintaining patient safety during an RARP. Patient factors including body mass index (BMI), previous orthopedic surgery, and medical comorbidities require additional consideration. Certainly, the patient's body habitus and BMI impact the techniques in patient positioning and padding and typically require additional maneuvers to secure the patient safely. Obese patients present a challenge for RARP and require us to alter our approach to securing the patient in the steep Trendelenburg position. In addition to using 3 M Reston® foam to prevent cephalad migration while in Trendelenburg, we sometimes utilize a

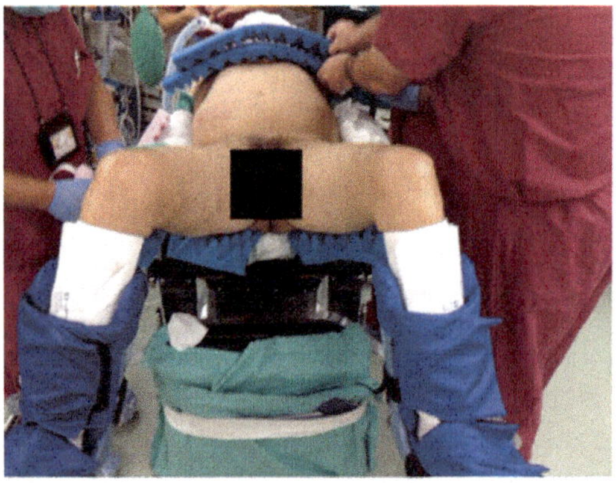

Fig. 20.4 Standard lithotomy positioning

soft strap placed over egg crate foam on the chest to better secure the patient. It is critical to make sure that a chest strap is not so tight as to cause shoulder injury, brachial plexus neuropraxia, or restriction of chest wall movement, all of which have been described [3, 4]. Additionally, the arm boards may need to be placed parallel to the table to provide additional width so that the arms can be positioned safely. Protective padding allows for even distribution of pressure across the body surface to prevent excessive compression and uneven pressure or stretching that could cause inadvertent skin, muscle, or nerve injury. For obese patients, we recommended testing steep Trendelenburg to ensure that the patient is well secured and protected and that there is no cephalad migration so that it can be adjusted before starting the procedure.

There are many physiologic changes that occur as a result of Trendelenburg positioning and CO_2 pneumoperitoneum. An exhaustive review of the physiologic consequences of pneumoperitoneum and positioning is beyond the scope of this text; however, there are several important considerations that must be kept in mind. Gravitational migration of the intestines and abdominal pannus toward the lungs limits the extent of diaphragmatic excursions during breathing. In addition, excessively tight strapping of the chest to prevent patient movement can restrict the movement of chest wall muscles. These both cause altered lung mechanics including decreased pulmonary compliance, decreased vital capacity, and decreased functional residual capacity, all of which lead to increased ventilation-perfusion mismatch and shunting. The majority of patients are able to handle this increased work of breathing without issues. However, in select situations involving patients with morbid obesity and/or severe pulmonary disease, the ventilatory restriction is to a degree that they cannot handle [9]. In these cases, compromise of lung function will be evident immediately after placing the patient in the steep Trendelenburg position. For these rare cases, the surgeon must decide to perform the RARP with minimal Trendelenburg, convert to open prostatectomy, or abort the procedure altogether. Steep Trendelenburg position also increases intracranial pressure (ICP) and may be associated with cerebral edema. However, several studies have shown that this is associated with neither compromised cerebral perfusion nor residual neurologic sequela [10–12]. Ischemic optic neuropathy has been described as a complication of prolonged Trendelenburg, but it is a rare event [16].

Position-related complications associated with skin, muscle, and nerve injury are also of concern. These types of complications are a function of improper positioning and padding but are also a function of prolonged operative time and surgeon experience [9]. Di Pierro and colleagues demonstrated that with increasing experience the number of positioning-related complications declined significantly [13]. During the procedure, it is important to monitor the integrity of the positioning, which can be done by anesthesia to monitor migration and also by the circulating nurses to ensure that the legs stay in good position in stirrups [3].

Upper and lower extremity musculoskeletal and nerve injuries are well-described complications associated with improper positioning. As mentioned previously, upper extremity brachial plexus injuries have been described especially with the use of a shoulder strap and may occur if the body slips cephalad while in steep Trendelenburg [3, 4]. Lower extremity injuries in patients that are in prolonged lithotomy include nerve and muscle injury and also potential for deep vein thrombosis [3–5, 13–15].

Lower extremity rhabdomyolysis and compartment syndrome have been described as a consequence of prolonged lithotomy (>4 h), malposition of the legs, and other patient factors such as BMI and history of vascular disease [3–5, 9, 14]. Pridgeon and colleagues described the UK experience in which there were nine cases (0.29 %) of lower extremity compartment syndrome in a series of 3110 RARPs [14]. This may be a function of compression of the popliteal artery while in stirrups and also decreased perfusion associated with the steep Trendelenburg positioning [9]. Nerve injuries may be a result of over-stretching with prolonged hip flexion, abduction or external rotation, as well as pressure point injury. During RARP, several different nerves are at risk, including the peroneal, femoral, sciatic, and obturator nerves [16]. Peroneal nerve injury may be related to direct pressure due to malposition of the legs in lithotomy; this presents as foot drop and/or a sensory deficit on the anterolateral lower leg and dorsal foot [16]. In their series of 179 RARP cases performed using the lithotomy position, Manny and colleagues reported lower extremity neuropathy in 1.68 % of their patients [15].

Given the risks associated with using the lithotomy position for prolonged periods of time or in patients with lower extremity joint disease, some investigators have explored the use of supine positioning [7]. Koc and colleagues described their experience with using a split-leg table, and they found a different pattern of nerve injuries associated with this position [6]. Overall 1.3 % of 377 patients experienced lower extremity neuropathy after RARP with split-leg table. Specifically, split-leg table puts the femoral nerve more at risk for injury, which manifests as hip flexion weakness or anterior thigh paresthesia.

Conclusions

Patient positioning and safety are of utmost importance for the entire operative team and are critical to the success of an RARP. It is important we pay close attention to positioning, pressure points, and securing of patients on the operating room table. Creating a specialized robotic surgery team, including circulating and scrub nurses, that have the training and experience to assist with proper positioning and setup for an RARP is advantageous. Developing a checklist and safety time-outs are useful to maintain proper positioning techniques and preserve patient safety throughout the duration of the operation. We have the responsibility to our patients to not only treat their disease but also to do no harm while doing so. Using the strategies and positioning techniques discussed in this chapter can allow an operative team to maintain patient safety while performing an RARP. In the following chapters, we will further discuss the steps and techniques for an RARP as we hope to provide a road map for a successful RARP.

Editor's Note

Empirically, I have observed that patients with a BMI of <40 tend to do well with steep Trendelenburg position, while caution for >40 in terms of risk of high ventilation pressures, acidosis, and more risk of moving on the table. Benson and Shah provide several tips and tricks for safe positioning. I would emphasize that for larger patients who occupy the width of the bed and have heavy arms, consider leaving the arm boards in place and parallel to the body, as there is too much pressure when wrapped in sheets and hanging off the table edges. My modification is to then run the chest strap inside the arms but out of the brachial plexus, and to be sure that the pelvis is right at the edge of the bed in lithotomy to provide a good anchor. The Reston foam is a promising alternative some of my colleagues use to provide stability that does not depend upon strap pressure points. For all cases, wrap IVs and monitoring lines with lots of gauze pads and keep pressure off the skin.

References

1. Binder J, Kramer W. Robotically-assisted laparoscopic radical prostatectomy. BJU Int. 2001;87:408–10.
2. Tewari A, Peabody J, Sarle R, Balakrishnan G, Hemal A, Shrivastava A, Menon M. Technique of da Vinci

robot-assisted anatomic radical prostatectomy. Urology. 2001;60:569–72.
3. Wolf Jr JS, Marcovich R, Gill IS, et al. Survery of neuromuscular injuries to the patient and surgeon during urologic laparoscopic surgery. Urology. 2000;55:831–6.
4. Mattei A, Di Pierro GB, Rafeld V, Konrad C, Beutler J, Danuser H. Positioning injury, rhabdomyolysis and serum creatinine kinase concentration course in patients undergoing robot-assisted radical prosatatectomy and extended pelvic lymph node dissection. J Endourol. 2013;27:45–51.
5. Koc G, Tazeh NN, Joudi FN, Winfield HN, Tracy CR, Brown JA. Lower extremity neuropathies after robot-assisted laparoscopic prostatectomy on a split-leg table. J Endourol. 2012;26:1026–9.
6. Chitlik A. Safe positioning for robotic-assisted laparoscopic prosatatectomy. AORN J. 2011;94:37–45.
7. Uffort EE, Jensen JJ. Side docking the robot for robotic laparoscopic radical prostatectomy. JSLS. 2011;15:200–2.
8. Chan ES, Yee C, Lo K, Chan C, Hou S, Ng C. Side-docking technique for robot-assisted urologic pelvic surgery. Urology. 2013;82:1300–3.
9. Collins S, Lehman DS, McDougall E et al: AUA BLUS Handbook of Laparoscopic and Robotic Fundamentals. American Urological Association Education and Research, Inc. Available at http://www.auanet.org/common/pdf/education/BLUS-Handbook.pdf.
10. Kalmar AF, Dewaele F, Foubert L, Hendrickx JF, Heeremans EH, Struys MMRF, Absalom A. Cerebral haemodynamic physiology during steep Trendelenburg position and CO_2 pneumoperitoneum. Br J Anaesth. 2012;108:478–84.
11. Closehn D, Treiber AH, Berres M, Sebastiani A, Werner C, Engelhard K, Schramm P. Robotic assisted prostatic surgery in the Trendelenburg position does not impair cerebral oxygenation measured using two different monitors. Eur J Anaesth. 2014;31:104–9.
12. Kim MS, Bai SJ, Lee JR, Choi YD, Kim YJ, Choi SH. Increase in intracranial pressure during carbon dioxide pneumoperitoneum with steep Trendelenburg positioning proven by ultrasonographic measurement of optic nerve sheath diameter. J Endourol. 2014;28:801–6.
13. Di Pierro GB, Wirth JG, Ferrari M, Danuser H, Mattei A. Impact of a single-surgeon learning curve on complications, positioning injuries and renal function in patients undergoing robot assisted radical prostatectomy and extended pelvic lymph node dissection. Urology. 2014;84:1106–11.
14. Pridgeon S, Bishop CV, Adshead J. Lower limb compartment syndrome as a complication of robot-assisted radical prostatectomy: the UK experience. BJU Int. 2013;112:485–8.
15. Manny TB, Gorbachinsky I, Hemal AK. Lower extremity neuropathy after robot assisted laparoscopic radical prostatectomy and radical cystectomy. Can J Urol. 2010;17:5390–3.
16. Cadeddu JA, Richstone L, Ogan K. (2015) Laparoscopy and robotics. American Urological Association Education and Research, Inc.: AUA University. Available at https://www.auanet.org/university/core_topic.cfm?coreid=129.
17. Song JB, Vemana G, Mobley JM, Bhayani SB. The second "time-out:" a surgical safety checklist for lengthy robtotic surgeries. Patient Saf Surg. 2013;7:19.

Safety Checklist for Training and Assessment in Robot-Assisted Prostate Surgery

21

Catherine Elizabeth Lovegrove, Prokar Dasgupta, and Kamran Ahmed

Introduction

Evidence has consistently demonstrated the manifold differences in the technical and non-technical skill requirements between robotic, laparoscopic and open surgeries. With increasing use of robot-assisted radical prostatectomy (RARP) in the operating room (OR) for treating prostate cancer, it is important that training and assessment be evaluated to ensure that they continue to equip surgeons with the skills required for safe, competent practice.

Surgical Safety

Medical error and compromised patient safety can be attributed to human factors often beyond the conscious control of individuals. Latent environmental factors impose external pressures on the healthcare system. Medical legislation, training and assessment incorporate evidence-based medicine into health services, externally influencing surgical practice. This is important in establishing minimum standards for doctors and surgeons and in identifying inadequate health-care services. These methods should be evaluated to encompass new surgical techniques and results of new research to ensure continued effectiveness and benefit to patient safety.

Adverse events in surgery arise from deficiencies in technical and non-technical skills that training and assessment are designed to rectify. To harness the full benefits of robotics, it is necessary that trainees develop skills specific to the technology. They must also improve their knowledge of generic and procedure-specific techniques such as RARP. Adjusting training and assessment to ensure these outcomes is one method of maintaining patient safety and ensuring competent use of innovative surgical methods.

Checklists

Checklists are used both to protect patient safety and measure surgical competence. Objective structured assessment of technical skills (OSATS) have been employed in training (in gynaecology and ophthalmology), in assessment and in measuring learning curves for procedures. OSATS comprises a global rating scale and a checklist. The former scores familiarity with generic surgical skills, such as tissue handling, and the latter examines a series of specific tasks. Global rating scales assess skills and knowledge and are subjectively scored by an examiner using

C.E. Lovegrove, B.Sc. (Hons) (✉)
P. Dasgupta, M.D., F.E.B.U., F.R.C.S. (Urol)
K. Ahmed, M.B.B.S., M.R.C.S., Ph.D.
MRC Centre for Transplantation, NIHR Biomedical Research Centre, Guy's Hospital, King's College London, 5th Floor Tower Wing, London SE1 9RT, UK
e-mail: catheronelovegrove1@gmail.com

J.W. Davis (ed.), *Robot-Assisted Radical Prostatectomy*, DOI 10.1007/978-3-319-32641-2_21

a Likert scale; this reduces value in objectively assessing competence. Conversely, checklists objectively record whether certain steps have been completed within a defined procedure.

Available Safety Checklists

To date, only non-specific measures have been designed to augment patient safety in the robotic operating theatre. All have been developed to address a certain aim. Consequently, the designs of individual checklists differ. These have been used around the world, in a variety of settings and in a range of surgical modalities (Table 21.1). Available checklists include:

1. World Health Organisation (WHO) Surgical Safety Checklist.
2. Song et al: "The second "time-out": a surgical safety checklist for lengthy robotic surgeries."
3. Ahmed et al: "Development and content validation of a surgical safety checklist for operating theatres that use robotic technology" [1].
4. Global Evaluation and Assessment of Robotic Skills (GEARS).
5. RARP Assessment Score.

World Health Organisation (WHO) Surgical Safety Checklist [2–4] (Fig. 21.1)

The WHO surgical checklist acknowledges that any operation entails avoidable error and is employed in a multitude of surgical settings. This checklist was based on the guidelines of the WHO for surgical patients and intended as a broad, universally applicable measure to increase patient safety and avoid adverse events associated with surgery. It is the only checklist that has objective evidence to demonstrate that mortality rate and operative outcomes improve with its use. Beginning before initiation and finishing after the completion of the technical procedure 19, issues are examined at various times within an operation. "Sign in" focuses on preparing the patient to ensure the correct individual, procedure, anaesthesia, oxygenation and evaluation of any difficulties that have been encountered or anticipated thus far. Prior to the first skin incision teamwork, preparation, reaffirmation of the patient, operation and any adverse events are conducted. Finally, before the patient leaves the OR the team confirm what procedure took place, conduct a surgical count and plan post-operative care based

Table 21.1 Status of current checklists

Checklist	Generic or robot specific	Validation	Effect on surgical process or patient health
World Health Organisation (WHO) Surgical Safety Checklist	Generic checklist for all surgical settings	Validated	Reduced mortality rate and avoidable error
Song et al: "The second "time-out": a surgical safety checklist for lengthy robotic surgeries"	Generic checklist for all surgical settings	Validated	Minimal intrusion on surgical process
Ahmed et al: "Development and content validation of a surgical safety checklist for operating theatres that use robotic technology"	Robot-specific checklist	Validated	Future plan to implement and further validate the checklist in the setting of urological robot-assisted surgery
Global Evaluation and Assessment of Robotic Skills (GEARS)	Robot-specific checklist	Validated	Monitor progression of surgical skills
RARP Assessment Score	Checklist specific to robot-assisted radical prostatectomy	Validated	Demonstrate learning curve for procedural steps No data on effects on surgery or patients to date

World Health Organization

SURGICAL SAFETY CHECKLIST (FIRST EDITION)

Before induction of anaesthesia ▸▸▸▸▸▸▸▸▸	Before skin incision ▸▸▸▸▸▸▸▸▸▸▸▸▸▸	Before patient leaves operating room
SIGN IN	**TIME OUT**	**SIGN OUT**
☐ PATIENT HAS CONFIRMED • IDENTITY • SITE • PROCEDURE • CONSENT	☐ CONFIRM ALL TEAM MEMBERS HAVE INTRODUCED THEMSELVES BY NAME AND ROLE	NURSE VERBALLY CONFIRMS WITH THE TEAM:
☐ SITE MARKED/NOT APPLICABLE	☐ SURGEON, ANAESTHESIA PROFESSIONAL AND NURSE VERBALLY CONFIRM • PATIENT • SITE • PROCEDURE	☐ THE NAME OF THE PROCEDURE RECORDED
☐ ANAESTHESIA SAFETY CHECK COMPLETED	ANTICIPATED CRITICAL EVENTS	☐ THAT INSTRUMENT, SPONGE AND NEEDLE COUNTS ARE CORRECT (OR NOT APPLICABLE)
☐ PULSE OXIMETER ON PATIENT AND FUNCTIONING	☐ SURGEON REVIEWS: WHAT ARE THE CRITICAL OR UNEXPECTED STEPS, OPERATIVE DURATION, ANTICIPATED BLOOD LOSS?	☐ HOW THE SPECIMEN IS LABELLED (INCLUDING PATIENT NAME)
DOES PATIENT HAVE A: KNOWN ALLERGY? ☐ NO ☐ YES	☐ ANAESTHESIA TEAM REVIEWS: ARE THERE ANY PATIENT-SPECIFIC CONCERNS?	☐ WHETHER THERE ARE ANY EQUIPMENT PROBLEMS TO BE ADDRESSED
DIFFICULT AIRWAY/ASPIRATION RISK? ☐ NO ☐ YES, AND EQUIPMENT/ASSISTANCE AVAILABLE	☐ NURSING TEAM REVIEWS: HAS STERILITY (INCLUDING INDICATOR RESULTS) BEEN CONFIRMED? ARE THERE EQUIPMENT ISSUES OR ANY CONCERNS?	☐ SURGEON, ANAESTHESIA PROFESSIONAL AND NURSE REVIEW THE KEY CONCERNS FOR RECOVERY AND MANAGEMENT OF THIS PATIENT
RISK OF >500ML BLOOD LOSS (7ML/KG IN CHILDREN)? ☐ NO ☐ YES, AND ADEQUATE INTRAVENOUS ACCESS AND FLUIDS PLANNED	HAS ANTIBIOTIC PROPHYLAXIS BEEN GIVEN WITHIN THE LAST 60 MINUTES? ☐ YES ☐ NOT APPLICABLE	
	IS ESSENTIAL IMAGING DISPLAYED? ☐ YES ☐ NOT APPLICABLE	

THIS CHECKLIST IS NOT INTENDED TO BE COMPREHENSIVE. ADDITIONS AND MODIFICATIONS TO FIT LOCAL PRACTICE ARE ENCOURAGED.

Fig. 21.1 WHO Surgical Safety Checklist [4]

on individual patient characteristics and the difficulties encountered within the operation.

Use of the WHO Surgical Safety Checklist was evaluated through 30-day patient follow up. Haynes et al. identified numerous benefits associated with the implementation of the checklist in eight hospitals and cities. These included:

- Reduction in all complications from 11 to 7 %; $P<0.001$.
- Reduction in in-hospital death rate from 1.5 to 0.8 %; $P=0.003$.
- Reduction in surgical site infection; $P<0.001$.
- Reduction in unplanned re-operation; $P=0.047$.

Positive changes were found to occur whether or not an observer was present, though significant change in death rate was found only to have occurred in lower-income centres.

The checklist is a generic measure for use in many fields of surgery, creating a defined point where the full surgical team takes the opportunity to clarify intentions, progress and forward planning from an operation. Whether the benefits are related to increased awareness of causes of error or improved situational awareness and team working is difficult to ascertain. Nevertheless, the benefits of the WHO Surgical Safety Checklist cannot be overlooked and have been appreciated all over the globe with centres from all continents and economic backgrounds employing this measure.

Song et al: "The Second "Time-Out": A Surgical Safety Checklist for Lengthy Robotic Surgeries" [5] (Fig. 21.2)

This study was conducted in acknowledgment of the fact that, despite many surgical benefits, unique aspects of robotic surgery predispose to patient-related complications. The most problematic issues from procedures were identified through a literature search that provided insight into complications and their associated causes.

General Patient Considerations	Surgeon Considerations	Anesthesia Considerations	Nursing Considerations
☐ Turn all room lights on	☐ Determine if the length of surgery is usual for the operation	☐ Check vital signs	☐ Check if surgical counts are intact
☐ Verify patients's head and eye placement and padding	☐ Evaluate progression of surgery	☐ Evaluate extent of blood loss	☐ Check equipment for proper function
☐ Verify patients's upper and lower extermity placement and padding	☐ Identify cause(s) of prolonged operative time	☐ Evaluate patient's urine output	☐ Check for placement and function of pneumatic compression devices
☐ Check for pooling of preparation solutions at buttocks and lower back	☐ Evaluate need for conversion to another approach	☐ Evaluate need for antibiotic redosing	☐ Update administration on room time and discuss need to provide additional robotic trained nurses
☐ Check extremities for mottle appearance	☐ Evaluate need for help from another surgeon	☐ Evaluate need to draw labs	
☐ Verify sufficient padding at pressure points	☐ Evaluate surgeon and surgical assistant fatigue		
☐ Verify tightnes of straps	☐ Evaluate surgeon and surgical assistant need for a break		

Fig. 21.2 Second time out [5]

The checklist comprised four key areas:

1. General patient considerations.
   Patient positioning is an important factor contributing to adverse, avoidable patient outcomes post-operatively. These include neuropathy or blindness from increased intra-ocular pressure from prolonged time spent in steep Trendelenburg positioning. Consequently, Song et al. advocate that all care providers review patient positioning and monitor for signs of any shift that may have occurred inadvertently from long operating times. Based on a review of the most commonly injured nerves they suggest protection of the ulnar nerve at the elbow, brachial plexus at the shoulder, common peroneal nerve at the head of the fibula, saphenous nerve at the medial condyle of the tibia and obturator and femoral nerves at the hip.
2. Surgical considerations.
   In order that surgeons do not lose track of time or become so absorbed in the procedure that they forget to maintain awareness of what is happening in the OR as a whole, Song et al. suggest taking the opportunity to reflect on the progress of the operation thus far. In so doing, problems and difficulties may be addressed to avoid long operating times, evaluate their progress and consult others for assistance where required. Furthermore, the second time out provides surgeons and theatre staff with opportunity to check on the physical and mental state of all involved in the operation to avoid complications associated with burn-out of professionals.
3. Anaesthesia considerations.
   Alongside the physical dangers of prolonged operating times, physiological dangers jeopardise patient wellbeing. In this stage of the checklist, the authors advocate monitoring of vital signs, fluid volumes, urine output and blood loss thus far. By monitoring physiological function at a set point in the operation, evaluation of the surgery is conducted, enabling changes to be made to protect patients from inadvertent harm. Such changes may include altering the surgical approach, modifying the pneumoperitoneum or administering additional prophylactic antibiotics.
4. Nursing considerations.
   The second time out provides a definite opportunity for nursing staff to reflect on patient position and equipment function. Technical

failures from faulty apparatus can prolong operative time and predispose to adverse patient outcomes such as thromboembolic events or inadvertent injury from failing to retrieve all instruments from the operative field. Longer surgeries have been associated with increased incidence of lapses such as those mentioned above, thus a second time out provides opportunity to avoid these mistakes.

Ahmed et al: "Development and Content Validation of a Surgical Safety Checklist for Operating Theatres That Use Robotic Technology" [1] (Fig. 21.3)

Similar to Song et al., Ahmed et al. recognised the need for a checklist specifically designed with robotic surgery in mind. They sought to develop a measure that also focused on patient safety, though adopted a different approach to identifying causes of error. Through systematic risk analysis a four-stage checklist was constructed with 22 items. In utilising in-depth, systematic analysis hazards pertinent to robotic surgery were identified and addressed in the study. By encompassing existing checklists within the robotic checklist, account was taken for risks that are common to open, laparoscopic and robotic settings, ensuring that no danger was overlooked. The stages encompassed successive parts of robotic surgery:

1. Anaesthetic room.
   Measures common to the WHO Surgical Safety Checklist are evaluated in addition to robot-specific considerations such as evaluating the function of important equipment to guard against technical failures.
2. Operating theatre—before the procedure.
   Similar to Song et al., Ahmed et al. realised the importance of patient positioning in robotic surgery that is associated with prolonged operating times. Hazards unique to robotic surgery, such as docking and positioning of the robot, was addressed in addition to promoting non-technical communication skills between the surgeon and assistant.
3. Operating theatre—after the procedure.
   Similar to items preceding the operation and the WHO Surgical Safety Checklist, robot de-docking and instrument removal were considered in this stage. Furthermore, evaluation of any technical faults from equipment was deemed important to guard against any future failures that may jeopardise patient or operative outcomes.
4. Handover to recovery.
   Using the structure of the WHO Surgical Safety Checklist, the checklist for robotic surgery deemed the handover of patient information essential in safeguarding their future care. Additionally, reflection, evaluation and discussion of complications encountered are undertaken as a measure to avoid future problems.

Global Evaluation and Assessment of Robotic Skills (GEARS) [6] (Fig. 21.4)

Developed in consultation with expert robotic surgeons, GEARS is a measure specific to robotic surgery used in assessing the technical ability of trainees. Surgeons considered the pertinent differences of robotic surgery over open and laparoscopic disciplines to construct a global rating scale specific to the unique attributes required when operating. Six domains are evaluated:

- Depth perception
- Bimanual dexterity
- Efficiency
- Force sensitivity
- Autonomy
- Robotic control

GEARS is designed for use in robotic surgery, though is not specific to one procedure. It was evaluated in surgeons of all experiences and in several operations over a 2-year period. It demonstrated higher scores in expert robotic surgeons over novices ($P=0.004$) and in attending surgeons over post-graduate trainee surgeons ($P<0.05$).

KING'S College LONDON

Surgical Safety Checklist for Robotic Suygery

ANAESTHETIC ROOM:	
1. RELEVANT HISTORY CHECKED? Such as pre-medications, fasting time, drug/alcohol history or any obstructive airway conditions.	
2. AIRWAY ASSESSED? Check for dentures/crowns/birdges/loose tooth and any other obstructions.	
3. EQUIPMENT CHECKED? Check anaesthetic / monitoring equipments for faults. Ensure all equipments are switched on.	
OPERATING THEATRE- BEFORE PROCEDURE:	
4. OPERATING TABLE CORRECTLY ADJUSTED?	
5. PATIENT CORRECLY POSITIONED/SECURED? Check that leg straps are not applied too tightly and that gel pads have been put in place.	
6. SURGICAL INSTRUMENTS COUNTED?	
7. EQUIPMENT CHECKED? Confirm preliminary checks for robot has been completed. Check all equipments for faults.	
8. CORRECT MARKING SITE AND INSERTION OF PORTS?	
9. ROBOT DOCKED AND CORRECTLY POSITIONED?	
10. PORTS PLACED ADEQUATELY TO AVOID ARM COLLISION?	
11 EFFECTIVE COMMUNICATION BETWEEN LEAD AND ASSISTING SURGEON?	
OPERATING THEATRE- AFTER PROCEDURE:	
12. ROBOT CORRECTLY DE-DOCKED?	
13. SPECIMEN RETRIEVAL BAGS/OTHER INSTRUMENTS REMOVED? Such as needles, swabs, vasular clip etc.	
14. SPECIMENS CORRECTLY LABELLED?	
15. SURGICAL INSTRUMENTS COUNTED?	
16. EQUIPMENT PROBLEMS REPORTED? Please make a formal report of any faults with the robot or any other euipment to be dealt with as soon as possible	
17. PATIENT'S CHART UPDATED?	
18. ANAESTHETIST PRESENT TO MONITOR RECOVERY?	
HANDOVER TO RECOVERY:	
19. ACCURATE HANDOVER OF DETAILS? Ensure that all patient and procedure details are passed on a accurately to the recovery team	
20. RECOVERY PLANS DISCUSSED? Ensure discussion of recovery plans between surgical and recovery teams	
21. COMPLICATIONS DISCUSSED?	

Debrief: Please note any comments or corcerns:

____

____

Fig. 21.3 Safety checklist for robot-assisted surgery [1]

GEARS bridges the gap between identifying requirements for robotic surgeons and evaluating their technical performance to promote good outcomes that maximise patient safety. It has been employed to monitor progression of skills with increasing experience to determine the learning curve associated with generic robotic skills within specified procedures.

Depth perception

1	2	3	4	5
Constantly overshoots target, wide swings, slow to correct		Some overshooting or missing of target, but quick to correct		Accurately directs instruments in the correct plane to target

Bimanual dexterity

1	2	3	4	5
Uses only one hand, ignores nondominant hand, poor coordination		Uses both hand, but does not potimize interaction between hands		Expertly uses both hands in a complementary way to provide best exposure

Efficiency

1	2	3	4	5
Inefficient efforts; many uncertain movements; constantly changing focus or persisting without progress		Slow, but planned movements are reasonably organized		Confident, efficient and safe conduct, maintains focus on task, fluid progression

Force sensitivity

1	2	3	4	5
Rough moves, tears tissue, injures nearby structures, poor control, frequent suture breakage		Handles tissues reasonably well, minor trauma to adjacent tissue, rare suture breakage		Applies appropriate tension, negligible injury to adjacent structures, no suture breakage

Autonomy

1	2	3	4	5
Unable to complete entire task, even with verbal guidance		Able to complete task safely with moderate guidance		Able to complete task independently without prompting

Robotic control

1	2	3	4	5
Consistently does not optimize view, hand position, or repeated collisions even with guidance		View is sometimes not optimal. Occasionally needs to relocate arms. Occasional collisions and obstruction of assistant.		Controls camera and hand position optimally and independently. Minimal collisions or obstruction of assistant

Fig. 21.4 GEARS [6]

RARP Assessment Score (Fig. 21.5)

Though relevant to robotic methods, the aforementioned checklists do not assess intra-operative ability for specific procedures. To address this paucity, the RARP Assessment Score was constructed using Healthcare Failure Mode and Effect Analysis, a specific, systematic method of risk analysis adapted for use in the healthcare setting. For the first time, this created a safety and assessment checklist for the assessment of technical skills of surgeons performing RARP.

Comprising five steps, HFMEA combines expert experience with brainstorming techniques to list failures and failure modes.

Step 1: Define the HFMEA Topic

A specific process, usually related to patient safety or adverse events, is chosen for analysis. In this case, RARP using a trans-abdominal approach was chosen as the operation for analysis.

Step 2: Assemble the Team

A Multi-Disciplinary Team (MDT) of experts brainstorm the topic. Thirteen surgeons were involved through specific suggestions or through observing them operating. Anaesthetists, anaesthetic assistants, scrub nurses and theatre staff were involved.

Name:......................
Date: ..../..../
D'Amico risk:............
cTNM Stage: T....N....M....
Patient's BMI: .....kg/m²
Prostate Volume.....cc

SCORING
1=Unacceptable
5= Excellent

STEP	DIFFICULTY	#	PROCESS	SUB-PROCESS DEFINITIONS	0	1	2	3	4	5
Preparation of operative field	I	1	Robot set-up & patient positioning	Lithotomy position, angulation in Trendelenberg position, legs spread on adhesive covering						
	I	2	Pneumoperitoneum & port placement	If Veress needle used: appropriate insufflation (12-15mmHg) & placement of first trocar						
				If Hasson technique is used: appropriate incision & placement of first trocar						
				Insert secondary ports under direct camera vision in correct position						
	II	3	Laparoscopic adhesiolysis *(if applicable)*	Lysis of abdominal adhesions						
	I	4	Initiation of console, ensuring robot is docked safely	Appropriate docking of the robot						
				Clean operative field by lysing pelvic adhesions up to sigmoid colon using 4th arm for mobilization & retraction						
Dissection of the bladder & prostate	II	5	Drop bladder from anterior wall	Correct opening of peritoneum						
				Good dissection in prevesical space of Retzius						
	II	6	Expose prostatic apex & endopelvic fascia *(varies)*	Remove fat over pubo-prostatic ligaments						
				Incise endopelvic fascia & mobilise prostate to reach membranous urethra						
				Incise puboprostatic ligaments (optional at this point)						
	II	7	Stitching & division of dorsal venous plexus *(varies)*	Suture Dorsal Venous Complex (if applicable)						
				Cut Dorsal Venous Plexus using cold instruments or stapler (if applicable)						
	II/III	8	Anterior bladder neck transection	Bladder traction by 4th arm/or traction by a stay suture on back of prostate						
				Dissect anterior bladder from prostate-vesical junction in correct plane, incise anterior bladder neck						
	III	9	Posterior bladder neck transection	Transect posterior bladder neck						
				Dissect & incise prostatovesical musculature						
	III	10	Seminal vesicle dissection	Identify seminal vesicles & vasa deferentia. Clip artery to vas deferentia						
				Dissect vasa deferentia & seminal vesicles						
	III	11	Posterior Dissection	Retract seminal vesicles anteriorly & cranially to expose Denonvilliers' fascia						
				Enter fascia in midline, mobilise prostate from rectum to develop rectal plane to reach apex						
	IV	12	Dissection of prostate pedicle & neurovascular bundle. Nerve preservation Y/N *(varies)*	Incise lateral prostatic fascia lateral to prostate & release neurovascular bundle from prostate capsule						
				Identify, clip & divide prostatic vascular pedicles						
				Use scissors & minimal traction to dissect neurovascular bundle						
				Dissection in right plane (intra-, inter-, extrafascial)						
				Avoid use of clips near apical stump						
	IV	13	Apical dissection of prostate *(varies)*	If not completed yet: incise puboprostatic ligaments & incise deep venous complex						
				Selective suturing of deep venous plexus (if applicable)						
				Examine apex of prostate to ensure that apical margins are avoided						
				Divide urethra						
Anastomosis & closure	III	14	Vesico-urethral anastomosis	Stabilisation of posterior sphincteric complex with a "Rocco" stitch (optional)						
				Modified Van Velthoven technique with a running suture (variable)						
				Anterior fixation & reconstruction (optional)						
	I	15	Inspection of abdomen	Haemostasis if necessary						
				Drain inserted & secured with suture (if applicable)						
				Hold specimen bag with grasper inserted through port (appropriate instructions/views for assistant)						
	I	16	Finalising	Remove instruments & ports from abdomen under direct vision & robot de-docked safely						
				Close skin layer						
	III	17	Lymph node dissection *(varies)*	Bilateral lymph node dissection						
				Extended or limited nodal dissection						

*Difficulty Definition
I (lowest level of difficulty); IV (highest level of difficulty)

Score	0	1	2	3	4	5
Definition	NA	Unacceptable	Poor	Acceptable	Good	Excellent

Fig. 21.5 RARP assessment score [12]

Step 3: Graphically Describe the Process (Mapping)

Create a map or diagram to break the process into processes and sub-processes.

Patients' journeys from anaesthetic room to theatre and recovery ward were observed. Discussion with surgeons and combinations of anaesthetists, anaesthetic assistants, scrub nurses and theatre staff explored how RARP steps differ with patients, hospitals and surgeons. The map was continually revised and recommendations of the Pasadena Consensus Panel were reviewed and incorporated [7]. It identified ten main steps with 30 sub-steps to be evaluated by HFMEA. This was internationally circulated to surgeons for content validation.

Step 4: Conduct a Hazard Analysis

"Failure modes" and "failure mode effects" are considered, allocated probability and severity hazard scores and assessed for "single point weaknesses," "detectability" and "existing control measures," constructing an HFMEA hazard analysis table.

Hazard analysis was conducted in an international, multi-institutional teleconference with experts. Severity and probability scores allocated according to predefined definitions producing a hazard score for each failure mode [8].

Three phases of RARP were identified by HFMEA (Fig. 21.6):

1. Preparation of the operative field.
2. Dissection of the bladder and prostate.
3. Anastomosis and closure.

Step 5: Actions and Outcome Measures

Interventions are designed to address the failure modes and effects requiring further action. Single point weaknesses and failure modes and effects with a hazard score equal to or greater than 8 were included as "key steps" in the initial design. "Detectable" steps and those with existing control measures were excluded. After content validation with ERUS members, the RARP Checklist was formed and a defined rating scale added to enable use as an assessment and safety tool.

Once developed, the RARP Assessment Score was validated according to a range of parameters:

Content Validation

Content validation was undertaken at various stages with the MDT according to parameters outlined by Van der Vleuten et al. [9].

Distribution of the HFMEA process map, hazard analysis table, initial checklist and final

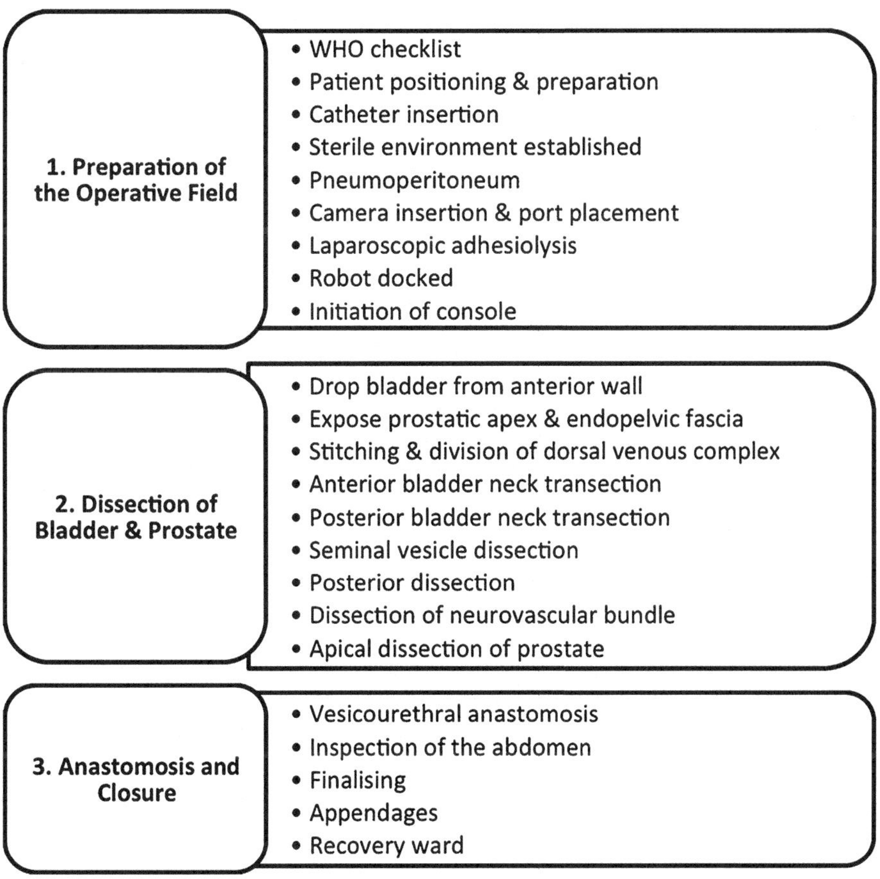

Fig. 21.6 Phases of RARP after hazard analysis

RARP Checklist to an international team of experts resulted in content validity.

Construct Validity

To determine if the checklist could differentiate between levels of experience, two videos of RARP were distributed to three experts. One showed an expert surgeon and one represented a less experienced surgeon. Each rater scored the videos individually and results were compared.

Inter-Rater Reliability

The expert and novice videos were used to examine concordance between raters' scores and consider to what extent agreement occurred due to chance.

Feasibility, Acceptability and Educational Impact

A questionnaire addressing feasibility, acceptability and educational impact was distributed to mentors and fellows. This included questions regarding their views on the importance of the checklist, its ease of use and its application to training.

This found the RARP Assessment Score to be relevant and acceptable.

Cost Effectiveness

Cost effectiveness was appraised by considering the financial cost involved in using and developing the checklist as an assessment tool. Costs encountered were negligible. During implementation, some trainees and mentors chose to print the checklist, accounting for a small cost. Others avoided this by filling in electronic forms.

Discussion

Checklist assessments are used both to protect patient safety and to measure surgical competence. Global rating scales assess skills and knowledge and are subjectively scored by an examiner using a Likert scale; this reduces value in objectively assessing competence. Conversely, checklists objectively record whether certain steps have been completed within a defined procedure.

As discussed, the unique characteristics of surgical modalities recommend the use of specific training and assessment tools. Current surgical assessment largely concentrates on the traditional operating environment and laparoscopy. This leaves patients vulnerable to the effects of error in the context of RARP. Studies demonstrate that new surgical modalities require different skills, which are not addressed in the WHO Surgical Safety Checklist.

The European Robotic Urology Section's (ERUS) Robotic Curriculum Pilot Study II evaluated technical skills through a global rating scale (GEARS) and non-technical skills through a similar rating system; Non-Technical Skills for Surgeons (NOTSS) [10]. Though relevant to robotic methods, these did not assess competence for specific procedures. Specific control measures to protect patient safety in the robotic setting and individual procedures can reduce the likelihood and severity of hazards occurring. In addition to the subjectivity of the global rating scale, the generic nature of existing assessments indicate the need for more specific, objective tools, such as checklists, to be developed to measure surgical competence in robotic techniques.

Assessments of varying designs have been developed to measure the different traits of competence [9]. To be effective in encouraging proficiency and identifying practice that does not reach an acceptable standard, each must be carefully constructed and evaluated according to a range of parameters (Table 21.2). Without considering these factors, the usefulness of an assessment is reduced.

Any training tool or assessment must be developed to address a specific aspect of competence (measurement-driven instruction). Ensuring "content validity" and "face validity" allow the aim to be effectively addressed in the design phase, so the tool is fit-for-purpose. Literature review, expert opinion or focus groups, quantitative surveys and qualitative interviews can be used. A controlled pilot study is necessary during

Table 21.2 Parameters for validation

Parameter	Definition	Outcome measure
Face validity	Extent to which the examination resembles the situation in the real world	Workplace vs. laboratory, human vs. animal vs. synthetic tissue
Content validity	Extent to which the intended content domain is being measured by the assessment exercise	Task components of the assessment procedure
Construct validity	Extent to which a test is able to differentiate between a good and bad performer	Significance of difference between ≥2 groups (e.g. experienced vs. inexperienced)
Concurrent validity	Extent to which the results of the test correlate with gold-standard tests known to measure the same domain	Correlation analysis with other assessment methods
Predictive validity	Extent to which this assessment will predict future performance	Follow-up assessments, proficiency gain curves
Inter-rater reliability	Extent of agreement between ≥2 assessors/observers	Correlation between 2 blind/non-blind assessors
Inter-item reliability	Extent to which different components of a test correlate (internal consistency)	Correlation of test items
Inter-test reliability	Ability of a test to generate similar results when applied at 2 time points	Correlations between test and retest
Acceptability	Extent to which assessment procedure is accepted by subjects in assessment	Survey results
Educational impact	Extent to which test results and feedback contribute to improve the learning strategy on behalf of the trainer and the trainee	Survey results, proficiency gain curves
Cost effectiveness	Technical and non-technical requirements for implementation of test into clinical practice	Costs generated by one test (US $)

validation to confirm inter-rater reliability using two blinded assessors. To examine test-retest reliability, the pilot study should be repeated with the same subjects and assessors at a different time. Inter-item reliability may be verified by comparing results of different tests. Construct validity is determined by examining individuals of differing expertise. Finally, concurrent validity may be assessed if a gold-standard method exists.

Prior to implementation, feasibility, acceptability, educational impact and cost effectiveness must be evaluated. Feasibility and acceptability can be appraised through surveys and interviews. Delivering constructive feedback and re-examining subsequent tests addresses educational impact while cost analysis depends on the geographical location and assessment environment [11].

To date, the WHO Surgical Safety Checklist has been validated through its implementation, demonstrating positive effects on mortality, adverse events and operative outcomes [2]. The study by Song et al. undertook content validation in the design phase by encompassing results of an extensive literature search and implementation demonstrated feasibility, though a short follow-up period limited the validation of all parameters [5]. Ahmed et al. undertook extensive content validation, using HFMEA to identify the hazards associated with robotic technology in surgery. The checklist is yet to be implemented in a large-scale setting, thus other parameters of reliability and validity were not assessed. GEARS was validated in terms of usefulness, reliability and construct validity, demonstrating positive results in all fields. Results indicate great promise for implementation and adaptation of the assessment tool to evaluate specific procedures, enhancing the protection of patient safety [6]. Finally, the RARP Assessment Score was also validated extensively with positive outcomes when implemented in a pilot study of 17 surgical fellows. More wide-scale distribution is necessary to fully ascertain the benefits of this assessment checklist despite good initial results.

At present, developed checklists indicate promising results; however, more substantial evidence is required on a larger scale to truly ascertain the relative benefits and drawbacks of each tool. At the highest level of evidence lie randomised controlled trials, surrounded by a myriad of ethical questions when designing studies. The logistics and ethics of randomising surgeons and patients to examine the value to individual checklists could be problematic, though use of simulation technology and team-based scenarios may alleviate such pressures. In time, this is likely the route required to further augment surgical training, assessment and provide the greatest level of protection to patients while exploiting the benefits of individual surgical modalities.

Conclusions

A multi-institutional, international study employed a methodical approach to designing the RARP Checklist using HFMEA to augment patient safety. Systematic development involved experts from centres in the USA, Belgium and Italy. Extensive content validation formed a 17-stage checklist to assess technical competence in important sub-steps of RARP where poor technique most jeopardises patient safety. This can guard against adverse events when used as a safety and assessment tool to ensure that surgeons do not undertake steps prematurely. The RARP Checklist promotes the technical skills required for the procedure, helping trainees to harness these skills in a safe manner enabling urologists to exploit the benefits of robotic surgery.

References

1. Ahmed K, Khan N, Khan MS, Dasgupta P. Development and content validation of a surgical safety checklist for operating theatres that use robotic technology. BJU Int. 2013;111(7):1161–74.
2. Haynes AB, Weiser TG, Berry WR, Lipsitz SR, Breizat AH, Dellinger EP, et al. A surgical safety checklist to reduce morbidity and mortality in a global population. N Engl J Med. 2009;360(5):491–9.
3. Patel J, Ahmed K, Guru KA, Khan F, Marsh H, Shamim Khan M, et al. An overview of the use and implementation of checklists in surgical specialities—a systematic review. Int J Surg. 2014;12(12):1317–23.
4. WHO International. WHO surgical safety checklist and implementation manual: World Health Organisation; (cited 2014 12.12.2014). http://www.who.int/patientsafety/safesurgery/ss_checklist/en/.
5. Song JB, Vemana G, Mobley JM, Bhayani SB. The second "time-out": a surgical safety checklist for lengthy robotic surgeries. Patient Saf Surg. 2013;7(1):19.
6. Goh AC, Goldfarb DW, Sander JC, Miles BJ, Dunkin BJ. Global evaluative assessment of robotic skills: validation of a clinical assessment tool to measure robotic surgical skills. J Urol. 2012;187(1):247–52.
7. Montorsi F, Wilson TG, Rosen RC, Ahlering TE, Artibani W, Carroll PR, et al. Best practices in robot-assisted radical prostatectomy: recommendations of the Pasadena Consensus Panel. Eur Urol. 2012;62(3):368–81.
8. DeRosier J, Stalhandske E, Bagian JP, Nudell T. Using health care failure mode and effect analysis: the VA National Center for Patient Safety's prospective risk analysis system. Jt Comm J Qual Improv. 2002;28(5):248–67. 09.
9. Vleuten CPM. The assessment of professional competence: developments, research and practical implications. Adv Health Sci Educ. 1996;1(1):41–67.
10. ERUS. ERUS Pilot Study for European Robotic Curriculum 2013 (cited 2014 06.02.14). http://www.uroweb.org/fileadmin/sections/ERUS/fellowship/docs/Curriculum.pdf.
11. Ahmed K, Miskovic D, Darzi A, Athanasiou T, Hanna GB. Observational tools for assessment of procedural skills: a systematic review. Am J Surg. 2011;202(4):469–80. e6.
12. Lovegrove C, Novara G, Mottrie A, Guru KA, Brown M, Challacombe B, et al. Structured and Modular Training Pathway for Robot-assisted Radical Prostatectomy (RARP): Validation of the RARP Assessment Score and Learning Curve Assessment. European Urology. 2016;69(3):526–35.

22 Immediate Postoperative Care Following Robot-Assisted Radical Prostatectomy

Janet E. Baack Kukreja, Claudia Berrondo, and Jean Joseph

Introduction

Robot-assisted radical prostatectomy (RARP) provides patients the unique opportunity to undergo a major oncologic operation with a relatively quick recovery. Many patients return to work and/or normal life activities a few days after their surgery and catheter removal. Over the last 30 years there have been many programs designed to improve patient recovery from intra-abdominal and pelvic operations [1]. These programs are often collectively called Fast-Track or Enhanced Recovery After Surgery (ERAS). ERAS pathways are designed for early discharge and promotion of patient recovery [1]. One of the main goals of ERAS is reduction in postoperative ileus with early feeding, early ambulation, and avoidance of narcotic pain medications [1].

ERAS principles are important in preventing ileus, which is still the leading cause of RARP delay in discharge past POD 1, which occurs in about 2% of patients [2]. Robotic surgery often allows for a quick recovery and discharge POD 1 [3]. However, as many as 10–15% of patients may require a longer hospital stay of 2 days or more after RARP [4]. Thus, it is essential that perioperative care pathways are considered in the quest of improving recovery post-RARP [3]. RARP in combination with ERAS allows for optimal patient recovery. The RARP postoperative care starts in the office once a patient has decided on surgery as the treatment modality. The nature, risks, and benefits of surgery must be thoroughly explained while the discussing all the management options, as per the informed consent process. Patient education of the preoperative, operative, and postoperative phases of care are addressed, reducing postoperative stress and anxiety about the surgical option [5, 6]. Proper education in the office setting helps clarify patient and family expectations. Patients must be informed of the criteria for discharge, and the steps necessary to reach them. Attentive perioperative care is essential to early discharge and complication prevention [7]. When patients are instructed on all the necessary steps to qualify for discharge on POD1, they report high level of satisfaction with their hospitalization and discharge process post-RARP on POD 1 [8, 9].

J.E. Baack Kukreja, M.D. (✉) • C. Berrondo, M.D.
Department of Urology, University of Rochester Medical Center, Rochester, NY, USA
e-mail: Janet_Kukreja@urmc.rochester.edu; Claudia_Berrondo@urmc.rochester.edu

J. Joseph, M.D., M.B.A.
Departments of Urology and Oncology, Center for Robotic Surgery and Innovation, University of Rochester Medical Center, Rochester, NY, USA
e-mail: Jean_Joseph@urmc.rochester.edu

J.W. Davis (ed.), *Robot-Assisted Radical Prostatectomy*, DOI 10.1007/978-3-319-32641-2_22

Setting Up a Robotic-Assisted Radical Prostatectomy Recovery Pathway

It is essential for the care team to be involved with the entire spectrum of care in the RARP recovery pathway. Without a team approach to RARP recovery, it is difficult to consistently discharge patients on POD 1. The preparation starts prior to admission to the hospital. Patient education of the preprocedure preparation, surgery, and postoperative RARP plans and schedules are essential for understanding the recovery pathway [10]. When the patient is aware of expectations postoperatively, his anxiety level is lowered, allowing better pain management, and facilitates cooperation with the care team, making all aspects of the recovery easier [6]. Patient-centered care is best achieved by educating the patient, his partner or family in the planning, delivery of his care, and all aspects of the recovery process planning. This eases anxiety for all parties and improves postoperative care plan adherence [9, 11].

Involving the anesthesia team is important in reaching the intraoperative goals of ERAS programs. Anesthesia providers are instrumental in maintaining normothermia, avoidance of fluid overload, intraoperative, and immediate postoperative pain control [11, 12]. Maintenance of normothermia reduces postoperative surgical infections [13]. Avoidance of fluid overload reduces postoperative ileus [11]. Excessive intraoperative fluid administration can lengthen the procedure, particularly the vesicourethral anastomosis stage, when the surgical team has to spend additional time to evacuate the resultant high urine output from the operative field. Additionally, prevention of postoperative nausea and vomiting begins in the operating room, which is essential to staying on an RARP recovery pathway [13].

Nursing in all phases of care must be involved in the ERAS plans for RARP patients [14]. Nursing awareness of the ERAS pathway for RARP is essential to encouraging patient participation in their recovery [14]. Immediately upon admission to the short stay, observation unit or urology floor, it is essential the nurses get the patient involved in their own care [14]. Importantly, postoperative nursing helps provide orientation to the pain medications available, educate patients on symptoms. Patients have to be oriented to the unit layout and instructed on expected milestone related to ambulation around the unit as they recover. Catheter care teaching includes explaining to the patient where to place the catheter when ambulating, versus when seating or supine.

Postoperative care providers (e.g., residents, physician assistant, nurse practitioner, inpatient medicine, or hospitalists) must also be familiar with the ERAS RARP pathway. Knowledge of the ERAS pathway for RARP patients is essential in keeping patients on the pathway [14]. Order sets either preprinted for paper orders or standard RARP computer order sets should be available to providers to help with standardization of patient care (see Table 22.2 for an example order set) [15]. Standardization of the pathway will lead to a system that works together in all phases of care, allows for patients to participate in their care, and has early discharge and early return to normal life [15].

Early Feeding

Early feeding is defined by resumption of oral intake within the first few hours after surgery [1]. It is almost never necessary to utilize a nasogastric tube after RARP [2]. Even in the setting of an extensive lysis of adhesions, patients can be streamlined to early feeding [2]. Clear liquids can be safely offered immediately after the operation. If a clear liquid diet is tolerated, patients are automatically advanced to regular diet the following morning. Our practice is to have the patient order breakfast the evening of surgery. We routinely administer scheduled doses of metoclopramide postoperatively which serves as a prokinetic and an antiemetic [16]. Erythromycin has also been used as a prokinetic at some centers [17]. Routine proton pump inhibitors or H2 blockers may be administered based on the patient's risk for peptic ulcer disease, and at the discretion of the surgeon. These decrease postoperative peptic and duodenal stress ulcers associated with ketorolac; however, they also increase the risk of *Clostridium difficile* [18, 19].

After tolerating breakfast the first day after surgery, patients are considered suitable for discharge. There is no requirement of flatus or bowel movements prior to discharge. All patients are discharged with a stool softener, such as docusate, to avoid straining for bowel movements over the next month.

Early Ambulation

Engaging the patients in early ambulation is critical to an early discharge. It has been our nurses' initiative to ambulate patients overnight and encourage routine activity. This leads to mobilization within hours of the patients leaving the OR [14]. Early ambulation gives the patient confidence in a POD 1 discharge and additionally reduces postoperative ileus [1, 11].

Postoperative Pain Control

Postoperative pain control begins in the operating room with local anesthesia infiltration in the incisions and administration of a belladonna and opium suppository prior to the start of the RARP [20, 21]. There are a few ways to address postoperative pain control with both scheduled medications and as needed medications. It is safe and effective to administer ketorolac, scheduled or as needed with acetaminophen, or in combination with narcotic tablets [22, 23].

Alternatively, narcotics can be avoided all together. Scheduled acetaminophen and ketorolac are very effective in reducing narcotic needs [24]. The addition of tramadol as needed for breakthrough pain helps avoid the narcotic side effects. Avoidance of narcotics helps with prevention of postoperative ileus. Additional medications that can be included in the postoperative pain regimen to avoid narcotics include scheduled celecoxib and pregabalin [24]. Antimuscarinics and antispasmodics (e.g., oxybutynin and hyoscyamine) should be offered as needed for postoperative bladder spasms. [23] Lidocaine jelly 2% can often be helpful for catheter related discomfort at the urethral meatus [23]. Patients are educated by nursing on what bladder spasms are and when they would want to ask for these medications to manage such symptoms. If the patient begins to show early signs of ileus, methylnaltrexone 12 mg subcutaneously has been reported as promising in some studies at reversing the narcotic related side effects [25, 26].

An additional method of pain control is a transverse abdominal plan (TAP) block. This can be performed by the surgical or anesthesia team [27]. However, these are unlikely to be necessary in RARP patients. Consideration could be given to TAP blocks for postoperative pain control in patients with chronic narcotic use.

Discharge with acetaminophen/oxycodone or acetaminophen/hydrocodone combination tablets, oxybutynin as needed for bladder spasms, and over the counter ibuprofen as needed is our current routine home pain regimen.

Cardiopulmonary Care

If a beta-blocker has been started or was a routine medication for the patient preoperatively, this should be continued postoperatively. There is no benefit reported in the literature for those patients not previously administered a beta-blocker to start this in the postoperative period [28].

Incentive spirometers should be provided to patients because these are low cost; however, early ambulation usually provides sufficient postoperative pulmonary exercise [29].

Antibiotic Prophylaxis in Radical Prostatectomy

Antibiotic prophylaxis at the time of prostatectomy has been shown to decrease the rate of urinary tract infections and surgical site infections postoperatively [30, 31]. The American Urologic Association (AUA) recommends antibiotic prophylaxis at the time of surgery for all patients undergoing surgery with entry into the genitourinary tract [30]. The duration of antibiotic prophylaxis should be limited to 24 h based on the results of a randomized clinical trial, which demonstrates that 1 day of perioperative antibiotic prophylaxis was equivalent to 4 day duration [30, 32]. The antibiotics of choice are a first or second generation Cephalosporins, Aminoglycosides, Aztreonam with Metronidazole or Clindamycin. Alternative antibiotics include Ampicillin/Sulbactam or Fluoroquinolones [30].

Venous Thromboembolism Prophylaxis

Venous thromboembolism (VTE) prophylaxis is essential in preventing postoperative thromboembolic complications. Despite major reductions in VTE, after surgery for urologic malignancy due to the systematic application of preventative recommendations, the occurrence of such events remains high [33]. Extended pelvic lymph node dissections may contribute to increased rates of VTE [34]. The increase in relative risk for VTE following a pelvic lymph node dissection is between 31.6 (95 % CI 12.4–80.6) and 69.6 (95 % CI 35.3–137.4) for the first 14 days after prostatectomy with 73 % of the VTE events diagnosed within that same time frame [35, 36]. Contemporary reports VTE rates within 30 days following radical prostatectomy range from 1 to 11 % [35–40]. Given the increased risk, it is standard to provide patients with VTE prophylaxis. In our experience, intermittent pneumatic compression device application with low molecular weight heparin (LMWH) (e.g., Enoxaparin 40 mg or Dalteparin 5000 units) is safe and effective at reducing postoperative VTE in RARP patients.

In patients not following the care pathway (e.g., prolonged hospitalization with ileus, readmission), extended duration prophylactic anticoagulation for 28 days with LMWH is helpful in preventing VTE [41, 42]. Additionally patients at very high risk of developing a VTE (e.g., factor V Liden deficiency, history of VTE) consideration should be given for discharge with 28 days of prophylactic anticoagulation using low molecular weight heparin [43].

Presentation with a postoperative VTE should prompt a scan of the pelvis to investigate if a lymphocele is compressing a pelvic vein as a cause of VTE development.

Pelvic Drain Removal

Some urologists may not leave pelvic drains, but the majority of surgeons leave a drain after prostatectomy [44]. If the surgeon has left a pelvic drain, it is important for the provider team to have a plan for removal. Prior to drain removal, patient participation in ambulation is needed to ensure the output remains below the surgeons' threshold for removal. Surgeons must set a cutoff value for drain removal prior to discharge, for both extraperitoneal and intraperitoneal RARP. Most drains can be removed prior to discharge. It is our practice to remove intraperitoneal RARP drains if the output is less than 100 ml for the last 8 h, and for extraperitoneal less than 75 ml over the same time period, regardless of lymph node dissection status.

Discharge Postoperative Day 1

With appropriate patient selection and patient preparation, discharging the same day is feasible [27, 45]. However, in general, discharge the morning after is more often expected postoperatively.

Expectations must be set preoperatively for anticipated discharge on POD 1 [5]. A reason to keep the RARP patient overnight is because these patients are often hypovolemic after fluid restriction for surgery preparation and the intraoperative fluid restriction, thus commonly requiring at least a mild resuscitation [12]. Even though a short overnight stay is usually indicated, it is uncommon for the patients after RARP to have any electrolyte or hematological abnormalities, thus avoidance of postoperative labs is usually appropriate [29]. Even though postoperative labs are often unnecessary, if there is a large blood loss during surgery, high drain outputs or clinical indication specific to a patient, labs may be indicated [29].

Once the patient has tolerated a regular breakfast, ambulated sufficiently, pain is controlled with all oral medication, had catheter teaching, and usually after pelvic drain removal, the patient is ready for discharge. The RARP patient is often discharged less than 24 h after entrance into the operating room. Discharge is held for abdominal distention and pain that cannot be managed with oral medications; however, this is rare. No signs of bowel function are necessary to discharge the patient, unless they are not tolerating clear or regular diet.

Catheter Removal

Cystogram

Catheter removal at postoperative day 7–10 allows for a low chance of urinary retention and a high chance of complete healing of the urethrovesical anastomosis [29]. It is unnecessary to obtain a cystogram prior to catheter removal [46].

Antibiotics

One of the key questions associated with catheter removal is when and for how long antibiotics are needed. Although there is no evidence that the time of catheter removal is a high risk window for the development of a symptomatic UTI, there is a belief that manipulation of the catheter in the presence of bacteriuria during the removal process may predispose to the subsequent development of UTI. For this reason, many providers administer antibiotic prophylaxis around the time of catheter removal [47]. However, this practice is controversial. Although the use of prophylactic antibiotics may reduce the number of symptomatic urinary tract infections, it is unclear whether the benefits outweigh the risks of developing *Clostridium difficile* infection or selection for antibiotic-resistant bacteria [48–51].

Current national society guidelines also differ on recommendations for antibiotic prophylaxis at the time of urinary catheter removal. The position of the Infectious Diseases Society of America is that prophylactic antimicrobials should not be administered routinely to patients at the time of catheter removal [50]. The AUA recommends consideration of antibiotic prophylaxis for catheter removal after urinary tract surgery when the catheter is in place for greater than 48–72 h in high risk patients. The AUA defines high risk individuals as patients with advanced age, anatomic abnormalities of the urinary tract, poor nutrition, smoking, chronic steroid use, immunodeficiency, prolonged hospitalization, distant coexistent infection, all of which are commonly present in patients undergoing radical prostatectomy. With the growing prevalence of resistant bacteria and *Clostridium difficile* infections, administration of prophylactic antibiotics at the time of catheter removal after prostatectomy should only be considered in high risk patients or in patients where urinary tract infection would be especially harmful. For patients in whom providers decide to use prophylactic antibiotics, the AUA recommends 24 h or less of antibiotic coverage. The preferred choice is a Fluoroquinolone or Trimethoprim–Sulfamethoxazole. Alternative antibiotics include Aminoglycosides and/or Ampicillin, first or second generation Cephalosporins or Amoxicillin/Clavulanate [2]. Randomized clinical trials are necessary to determine the utility of antibiotic prophylaxis for catheter removal after radical prostatectomy as well as the appropriate type and duration of therapy. Until high quality evidence exists, antibiotic prophylaxis for catheter removal should be considered in high risk patients according to the AUA recommendations.

Conclusions

Proper patient and family education of the perioperative care plan is key to a rapid recovery. Most patients undergoing RARP are candidates for discharge on POD 1. Earlier discharge or discharge immediately post-op is possible. In our experience, we have discharged a number of patients the afternoon or evening of the day of surgery. Our patients are routinely discharged less than 24 h from the time of arrival to the hospital. Hospital length of stay is often used as a surrogate marker of recovery. The goal, however, should not be on timing of discharge, but rather a rapid and successful recovery, and avoidance of readmission. Every patient presents unique sets of physiological or social issues that can impact all aspects of the recovery, in addition to factors under the control of the surgical team. While patient care is individualized, care pathways are helpful in eliminating wasteful variations in practice patterns, and set standards to continue to improve from Table 22.1.

Table 22.1 Review of a pathway

Phase of care	Intervention
Preoperative	Patient education Preoperative subcutaneous heparin prophylaxis
Intraoperative	Belladonna and opium suppository Avoidance of fluid overload Maintenance of normothermia Intermittent pneumatic compression (IPC) stockings
Postoperative care day of surgery	Clear liquid diet Ambulation within first few hours after leaving the operating room Metoclopramide 5 mg IV every 6 h Ketorolac 15 mg IV every 6 h As needed acetaminophen with oxycodone or hydrocodone every 4 h IV morphine or hydromorphone for break through pain control Oxybutynin 5 mg as needed for bladder spasms Enoxaparin 40 mg every 24 h IPC stockings Restarting home medications IV fluid resuscitation as needed for hemodynamics and urine output Starting Foley catheter teaching
Postoperative day 1	Regular diet at 5:00 a.m. Discontinue IV fluids Last dose of antibiotic All medications by mouth Continue ambulation Complete Foley catheter teaching Pelvic drain removal Discharge after breakfast
Postoperative day 7–10	Foley catheter removal in the office

Table 22.2 Post-Operative Order Set Example

Diet	
Diet clear liquid	Diet effective now, starting today
Diet regular	Diet effective 0500, starting tomorrow
Nursing	
Notify provider	Starting today notify provider: Systolic blood pressure: <100 and > 160, Diastolic blood pressure: < 40 and > 100, Heart rete: < 60 and > 100, Respirations: < 10 and > 30, Temperature: > 38.5, Urine output <120ml for 4 hours
Vital signs	Every 4 hours
Intake and output	Every 8 hours
Jackson Pratt drain to bulb suction	Measure and record every 8 hours
Catheter care	Every 8 hours, catheter in cath-secure
Ambulate patient	3 times daily, start today
Foley leg bag teaching	One time, foley leg bag teaching

Table 22.2 (continued)

Medications	
Sodium chloride IV OR Lactated ringers IV	150 ml/hr, intravenous
Cefoxitin IV OR Clindamycin 600mg IV + gentamicin 80mg IV	1 g, every 8 hours, for 3 doses OR Every 8 hours, for 3 doses
Metoclopramide IV	5mg, every 6 hours
Acetaminophen 1000mg	1 tablet, oral, every 8 hours
Tramadol 50mg	1 tablet, oral, every 4 hours prn, mild pain
	2 tablet, oral, every 4 hours prn, moderate pain
Ketorolac IV	15 mg, every 6 hours (limit 5 days)
Oxycodone 5mg	1 tablet, oral, every 4 hours prn, mild pain
	2 tablet, oral, every 4 hours prn, moderate pain
Hydrocodone 5mg	1 tablet, oral, every 4 hours prn, mild pain
	2 tablet, oral, every 4 hours prn, moderate pain
Hydromorphone IV	0.5 mg, every 2 hours prn, breakthrough pain
Docusate sodium 100 mg	Oral, 2 times daily
Oxybutynin	5 mg, oral, every 8 hours prn, bladder spasms
Ondansetron IV	4 mg, every 4 hours prn, nausea
Promethazine IV	12.5 mg, every 6 hours prn, nausea
Pantoprazole	40 mg, oral, every morning, starting today
Home Medication Reconciliation	
Venous Thromboembolism Prophylaxis (Choose one of the following + IPCs)	
If patients classified as moderate, high and very high risk: enoxaparin	40 mg, subcutaneous, every 24 hours
Patients ≥120kg: enoxaparin	40 mg, subcutaneous, every 12 hours
All patients with creatinine clearance <30ml/min: enoxaparin	30 mg, subcutaneous, every 24 hours
Intermittent pneumatic compression (IPC)	With assessment every 8 hours Instructions: while in bed

References

1. Fearon KCH. Overview: key elements and the impact of enhanced recovery care. In: Francis N, Kennedy RH, Ljungqvist O, Mythen MG, editors. Manual of fast track surgery recovery for colorectal surgery. New York, NY: Springer; 2012.
2. Pierorazio PM, Mullins JK, Ross AE, Hyams ES, et al. Trends in immediate perioperative morbidity and delay in discharge after open and minimally invasive radical prostatectomy (RP): a 20-year institutional experience. BJU Int. 2013;112:45–53.
3. Nelson B, Kaufman M, Broughton G, Cookson MS, Change SS, Herrell SD, Baumgartner RG, Smith JA. Comparison of length of hospital stay between radical retropubic prostatectomy and robot assisted laparoscopic prostatectomy. J Urol. 2007;177:929–31.
4. Trinh QD, Sammon J, Sun M, et al. Perioperative outcomes of robot-assisted radical prostatectomy compared with open radical prostatectomy: results from the nationwide inpatient sample. Eur Urol. 2012; 61(4):679–85.
5. Jenkins JT, Burch JL. Preoperative optimisation and conditioning of expectations. In: Francis N, Kennedy RH, Ljungqvist O, Mythen MG, editors. Manual of fast track surgery recovery for colorectal surgery. New York, NY: Springer; 2012.
6. Starnes SN, Sims TW. Robotic prostatectomy surgery. Urol Nurs. 2006;26(2):138–40.
7. Parrado CL, Gregorio SA, Martin-Martinez Q, Martin-Vega A, Caballero JG, Pena Barthel JJ. Impact of a clinical pathway in patient care following surgery on laparoscopic radical prostatectomy. Qual Manag Health Care. 2008;17(3):234–41.
8. Kirsh ED, Worwag EM, Sinner M, et al. Using outcomes data and patient satisfaction surveys to develop policies regarding minimum length of hospitalization after radical prostatectomy. Urology. 2000;56:101–6.
9. Magheli A, Nina K, Lein M, Hinz S, Kempkensteffen C, Gralla O. Impact of fast-track postoperative care on intestinal function, pain and length of hospital stay after laparoscopic radical prostatectomy. J Endourol. 2011;25(7):1143–7.
10. Inman DM, Jacobson TM, Maxson PM, Wang H, Lohse CM. Effects of urinary catheter education for

patients undergoing prostatectomy. Urol Nurs. 2013; 33(6):289–98.
11. Kehlet H, Wilmore DW. Evidence-based surgical care and the evolution of fast-track surgery. Ann Surg. 2008;248:189–98.
12. Awad H, Walker CM, Shaikh M, Dimitrova GT, Abazza R, O'Hara J. Anesthetic considerations for robotic prostatectomy: a review of the literature. J Clin Anesth. 2012;24:494–504.
13. Mythen MG, Michael S. Anesthetic contributions in enhanced recovery. In: Francis N, Kennedy RH, Ljungqvist O, Mythen MG, editors. Manual of fast track surgery recovery for colorectal surgery. New York, NY: Springer; 2012.
14. Starnes DN, Sims TW. Care of the patient undergoing robotic-assisted prostatectomy. Urol Nurs. 2006;26(2): 129–36.
15. Carter F, Kennedy RH. Setting up and enhanced recovery programme. In: Francis N, Kennedy RH, Ljungqvist O, Mythen MG, editors. Manual of fast track surgery recovery for colorectal surgery. New York, NY: Springer; 2012.
16. Habib AS, Gan TJ. CON: postoperative nausea and vomiting database research: limitations and opportunities. Anesth Analg. 2010;110(2):412–4.
17. Gralla O, Haas F, Knol D, et al. Fast-track surgery in laparoscopic radical prostatectomy: basic principles. World J Urol. 2007;25:185–91.
18. Mazaris EM, Varkarakis I, Chrisofos M, et al. Use of nonsteroidal anti-inflammatory drugs after radical retropubic prostatectomy: a prospective, randomized trial. Urology. 2008;72(6):1293–7.
19. Janarthanan S, Ditah I, Phil M, Adler DG, Ehrinpreis MN. *Clostridium difficile*-associated diarrhea and proton pump inhibitor therapy: a meta-analysis. Am J Gastroenterol. 2012;107:1001–10.
20. Fawcett WJ. Pain control after surgery. In: Francis N, Kennedy RH, Ljungqvist O, Mythen MG, editors. Manual of fast track surgery recovery for colorectal surgery. New York, NY: Springer; 2012.
21. Lukasewycz S, Holman M, Kozlowski P, et al. Does a perioperative belladonna and opium suppository improve postoperative pain following robotic assisted laparoscopic radical prostatectomy? Results of a single institution randomized study. Can J Urol. 2010; 17(5):5377–82.
22. Webster TM, Herrell SD, Chang SS, Cookson MS, Baumgartner RG, Anderson LW, Smith JA. Robotic assisted laparoscopic radical prostatectomy versus retropubic radical prostatectomy: a prospective assessment of postoperative pain. J Urol. 2005;174(3):912–4.
23. Woldu SL, Weinberg AC, Bergman A, Shapiro EY, Korets R, Motamedinia P, Badani KK. Pain and analgesic use after robot-assisted radical prostatectomy. J Endourol. 2014;28(5):544–8.
24. Trabulsia EJ, Patela J, Viscusib ER, Gomellaa LG, Lallasa LD. Preemptive multimodal pain regimen reduces opioid analgesia for patients undergoing robotic-assisted laparoscopic radical prostatectomy. Urology. 2010;76(5):1122–4.
25. Yu CS, Chun HK, Stambler N, Carpenito J, Schulman S, Tzanis E, et al. Safety and efficacy of methylnaltrexone in shortening the duration of postoperative ileus following segmental colectomy: results of two randomized, placebo-controlled phase 3 trials. Dis Colon Rectum. 2011;54:570–8.
26. Anissian L, Schwartz HW, Vincent K, Vincent HK, Carpenito J, Stambler N, et al. Subcutaneous methylnaltrexone for treatment of acute opioid-induced constipation: phase 2 study in rehabilitation after orthopedic surgery. J Hosp Med. 2012;7:67–72.
27. Dudderidge TJ, Doyle P, Mayer EK, et al. Evolution of care pathway for radical laparoscopic prostatectomy. J Endourol. 2012;26:660–5.
28. Fleisher LA, Fleischmann KE, Auerbach AD et al. ASS/AHA guideline on perioperative cardiovasuclar evaluation and management of patients undergoing noncardiac surgery. J Am College Cardiol. In Press. Accessed 6 Sept 2014. http://content.onlinejacc.org/article.aspx?articleid=1893784.
29. Kaufman MR, Baumgartner RG, Anderson LW, Simth JA, Chang AA, Herrell SD, Cookson MS. The evidence-based pathway for peri-operative management of open and robotically assisted laparoscopic prostatectomy. BJU Int. 2007;99(5):1103–8.
30. Wolf JS, Bennett CJ, Dmochowski RR, Hollenbeck BK, Pearle MS, Schaeffer AJ. Best practice policy statement on urologic surgery antimicrobial prophylaxis. J Urol. 2008;179(4):1379–90.
31. Grabe M. Controversies in antibiotic prophylaxis in urology. Int J Antimicrob Agents. 2004;23 Suppl 1:S17–23.
32. Terai A, Ichioka K, Kohei N, Ueda N, Utsunomiya N, Inoue K. Antibiotic prophylaxis in radical prostatectomy: 1-day versus 4-day treatments. Int J Urol. 2006;13:1488–93.
33. Rice KR, Brassell SA, McLeod DG. Venous thromboembolism in urologic surgery: prophylaxis, diagnosis, and treatment. Rev Urol. 2010;12(2–3): e111–24.
34. Eifler JB, Levinson AW, Hyndman ME, Trock BJ, Pavlovich CP. Pelvic lymph node dissection is associated with symptomatic venous thromboembolism risk during laparoscopic radical prostatectomy. J Urol. 2011;185(5):1661–5.
35. Augustin H, Hammerer P, Graefen M, et al. Intraoperative and perioperative morbidity of contemporary radical retropubic prostatectomy in a consecutive series of 1243 patients: results of a single center between 1999 and 2002. Eur Urol. 2003; 43:113.
36. Heinzer H, Hammerer P, Graefen M, et al. Thromboembolic complications rate after radical retropubic prostatectomy. Impact of routine ultrasonography for the detection of pelvic lymphoceles and hematomas. Eur Urol. 1998;33:86.
37. Clément C, Rossi P, Aissi K, Barthelemy P, Guibert N, Auquier P, et al. Incidence, risk profile and morphological pattern of lower extremity venous thromboembolism after urological cancer surgery. J Urol. 2011;186(6):2293–7.
38. Hammond J, Kozma C, Hart JC, Nigam S, Daskiran M, Paris A, et al. Rates of venous thromboembolism

among patients with major surgery for cancer. Ann Surg Oncol. 2011;18(12):3240–7.
39. Joudi FN, Allareddy V, Kane CJ, et al. Analysis of complications following partial and radical nephrectomy for renal cancer in a population based sample. J Urol. 2007;177:1709.
40. Andriole GL, Smith DS, Rao G, et al. Early complications of contemporary anatomical radical retropubic prostatectomy. J Urol. 1994;152(5 Pt 2):1858–60.
41. Van Hemelrijck M, Garmo H, Holmberg L, Bill-Axelson A, Carlsson S, Akre O, et al. Thromboembolic events following surgery for prostate cancer. Eur Urol. 2013;63(2):354–63.
42. Kibel AS, Creager MA, Goldhaber SZ, Richie JP, Loughlin KR. Late venous thromboembolic disease after radical prostatectomy: effect of risk factors, warfarin and early discharge. J Urol. 1997;158:2211–5.
43. Rasmussen MS, Jørgensen LN, Wille-Jørgensen P. Prolonged thromboprophylaxis with low molecular weight heparin for abdominal or pelvic surgery. Cochrane Database Syst Rev. 2009;1:CD004318.
44. Sharma S, Kim HL, Mohleremail JL. Routine pelvic drainage not required after open or robotic radical prostatectomy. Urology. 2007;69(2):330–3.
45. Martinemail AD, Nunez RN, Andrews JR, Martin GL, Andrews PE, Castle EP. Outpatient prostatectomy: too much too soon or just what the patient ordered? Urology. 2010;75(2):421–4.
46. Guru KA, Seereiter PJ, Sfakianos JP, Huston AD, Mohler JL. Is a cystogram necessary after robot-assisted radical prostatectomy? Urol Oncol. 2007;25:465–7.
47. Wazait HD, van der Meullen J, Patel HR, et al. Antibiotics on urethral catheter withdrawal: a hit and miss affair. J Hosp Infect. 2004;58:297–302.
48. Banks JA, McGuire BB, Loeb S, Shrestha S, Helfand BT, Catalona WJ. Bacteriuria and antibiotic resistance in catheter urine specimens following radical prostatectomy. Urol Oncol. 2013;31:1049–53.
49. Marschall J, Carpenter CR, Fowler S, Trautner BW, Program CDCPE. Antibiotic prophylaxis for urinary tract infections after removal of urinary catheter: meta-analysis. BMJ. 2013;346:f3147.
50. Hooton TM, Bradley SF, Cardenas DD, et al. Diagnosis, prevention, and treatment of catheter-associated urinary tract infection in adults: 1009 International Clinical Practive Guidelines from the Infectious Disease Society of America. Clin Infect Dis. 2010;50:625–63.
51. Lusardi G, Lipp A, Shaw C. Antibiotic prophylaxis for short-term catheter bladder drainage in adults. Cochrane Database Syst Rev. 2013;7:CD005428.

Part III

Outcomes

23 Penile Rehabilitation: Recovering Erectile Function Following Prostate Cancer Treatment

Jonathan Clavell-Hernandez and Run Wang

Introduction

The American Cancer Society estimated that about 233,000 new cases of prostate cancer would be diagnosed in the year 2014 [1]. Given the improvement in detection and treatment modalities, prostate cancer patients are diagnosed at an earlier stage that can be both cured and controlled. Radical prostatectomy and radiation therapy are highly effective in improving cancer survival. However, despite the improved treatment efficacy, secondary effects such as erectile dysfunction (ED) still remain as a major concern for both physicians and patients. Alemozaffar et al. [2] attempted to predict erectile function after prostate cancer patients undergoing radical prostatectomy (RP), external radiotherapy (RT) and brachytherapy. Pretreatment sexual health related quality of life score, age, serum prostate-specific antigen level, race/ethnicity, body mass index, and intended treatment details were associated with functional erections 2 years after treatment. They found that 48 % of patients ($n=1027$) with functional erections prior to treatment reported erectile dysfunction 2 years after treatment. In the prostatectomy cohort, 60 % of patients with prior functional erections reported ED, along with 42 and 37 % of the external radiotherapy and brachytherapy cohorts, respectively. The Prostate Cancer Outcomes study revealed 60 % of men experienced self-reported erectile dysfunction 18 months after radical prostatectomy, and only 28 % of men reported erections firm enough for intercourse at a 5-year follow-up [3]. This pernicious effect on sexual function has wider effects on men's quality of life and general well-being. Even more, many urologists believe more patients would accept surgical treatment if it were not for the possibility of developing post-operative ED [4].

Previous reviews have reported that ED after radical prostatectomy may take up to 4 years to recover, with as many as 20–80 % of these patients never returning to normal erectile function [5]. Penile rehabilitation consists of understanding the mechanisms that cause erectile dysfunction and utilizing pharmacologic agents, devices or interventions to promote male sexual function before and after any insult to the penile erectile physiologic axis [6]. For the past decade many researchers have pursued to define effective treatment modalities to improve ED after prostate cancer treatment. Despite the understanding of the mechanisms and well-established rationale for post-prostate treatment penile rehabilitation, there is still no consensus regarding effective rehabilitation programs. This

J. Clavell-Hernandez • R. Wang (✉)
Division of Urology, Department of Surgery, University of Texas Medical School at Houston and MD Anderson Cancer Center, 6431 Fannin, Suite 6.018, Houston, TX 77030, USA
e-mail: run.wang@uth.tmc.edu

J.W. Davis (ed.), *Robot-Assisted Radical Prostatectomy*, DOI 10.1007/978-3-319-32641-2_23

chapterreviews a contemporary series of trials and studies pertaining to penile rehabilitation after prostate cancer treatment.

Pathophysiology of Post-prostatectomy ED

The pathophysiology of ED after prostate cancer treatment has been found to be multifactorial. There is evidence that changes of neuropraxia, ischemic and hypoxic insults, fibrotic remodeling, and apoptosis contribute to erectile dysfunction even after meticulous dissection in attempt to preserve the neurovascular bundle during prostatectomy [7, 8]. Neuropraxia ensues due to mechanical stretching of cavernous nerves during prostate retraction, thermal injury to nerve tissue from electrocautery use, inflammation from surgical trauma, and nerve ischemia secondary to damage to blood supply during surgery. Studies have shown that even in the most cautious dissection during nerve-sparing prostatectomy, a certain degree of neuropraxia occurs. These nerves tend to recover slowly and may take up to 3 years to recover their baseline status [9].

The persistent lack of erections after neuropraxia can itself set up a cascade of harmful processes to erectile function. Wang summarized the mechanism of how chronic impotence promotes poor oxygenation of the corporeal bodies, which consequently leads to cavernosal fibrosis and transformation of the trabecular smooth muscle through collagen, which itself leads to the loss of the veno-occlusive mechanism required to maintain erections. Furthermore, ligation of accessory internal pudendal arteries during prostatectomy decreases arterial inflow. The combination of nerve damage with decreased arterial inflow may exacerbate hypoxia and ultimately result in apoptosis (Fig. 23.1) [8, 10].

Radiotherapy also causes ED by damaging the neurovascular bundle, penile vasculature, and cavernosal tissue, although the impact to these components is different. Stember et al. [11] reported that there are three mechanisms of injury contributing to the development of ED after radiation therapy. The first mechanism is vasculogenic. Radiation precipitates fibrosis and ischemia by damaging endothelial cells in penile arteries and sinusoids of the corpora cavernosum in a dose- and time-dependent manner. Secondly, neurovascular injury occurs but to a much lesser extent. Zelefsky and Eid [12] classified neurogenic injury in 3 % of post-RT patients in a penile Duplex Doppler-based study. The third major effect is the dose-dependent ultrastructural changes that generate corporal fibrosis, venous leakage and therefore, inability to maintain erections. In many occasions radiation is accompanied by androgen deprivation therapy (ADT) which by itself has been found to decrease erectile function, ejaculation and libido [13].

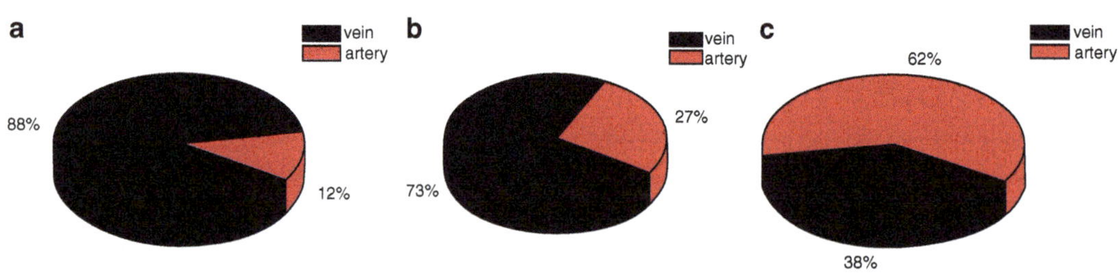

Fig. 23.1 (**a**–**c**) The blood composition in the corpus cavernosum by the following formula: $A\% = [\text{Measured SO2} - V(\text{SO2})] / [A(\text{SO2}) - V(\text{SO2})]$; $V\% = 1 - A\%$. (**a**) Flaccid group: arterial blood accounts for 12 %, and venous blood accounts for 88 % in the corpus cavernosum. (**b**) In the Traction group: arterial blood accounts for 27 %, and venous blood accounts for 73 % in the corpus cavernosum. (**c**) VED therapy group: arterial blood accounts for 62 %, and venous blood accounts for 38 % in the corpus cavernosum. Lin HC et al. *Asian J Androl. 2013* (15):387–390

After understanding the mechanisms that promote ED after prostate cancer treatment, multiple studies have been focused on evaluating ways to increase oxygenation of the cavernosal bodies, decrease tissue fibrosis and apoptosis, and consequentially improve erectile function. The role of penile rehabilitation is to maintain tissue oxygenation and prevent tissue fibrosis until the cavernosal nerves recover from neuropraxia with the return of spontaneous nocturnal tumescence.

Phosphodiesterase 5 Inhibitors

Since entering the market in 1998, phosphodiesterase-5 inhibitors (PDE5i) revolutionized the treatment of ED. Its relatively safe profile and ease of use have made them popular among patients and physicians. PDE5is decrease the breakdown of cyclic guanosine monophosphate (cGMP) that increases the efflux of intracellular calcium ions and result in smooth muscle relaxation and erection. This mechanism is potentiated by nitric oxide production stimulated by cavernous nerves [14, 15]. Clinical trials using PDE5is presented in this review are summarized in Table 23.1.

A number of studies have investigated the role of PDE5is in post-prostate cancer treatment patients, and many of these reported higher International Index of Erectile Function (IIEF) scores (Fig. 23.2) and spontaneous erection rates [16–19]. Padma-Nathan et al. [19] performed the first multicenter, double-blind, randomized, placebo-controlled trial to our knowledge evaluating the effects of nightly sildenafil on erectile function after bilateral nerve-sparing RP. They randomized 125 patients into three parallel fixed-dose treatment groups: placebo and 50 mg or 100 mg sildenafil. Trial enrollment ended prematurely because of a 'lack of treatment effect', but 82 men completed the trial and 76 completed the post-washout evaluation period. After an 8-week washout period, only one of 25 patients (4 %) in the placebo arm was potent, vs. 14 of 51 patients (27 %) in the sildenafil 50 and 100 mg groups combined. The significant difference of $p = 0.016$ suggested that nightly sildenafil has a benefit for penile rehabilitation after prostatectomy. Critics of this study state that the placebo rate was lower than that specified by the investigators [20]. Also, treatment administration began 1 month after surgery and there was a significant patient dropout rate, which may call into question the statistical power of the study.

Montorsi et al. [21] published the REINVENT penile rehabilitation after prostatectomy trial in 2008. REINVENT was a 628-patient, multicenter, double-blind placebo-controlled trial in which patients with a baseline IIEF score of >26 were randomized into taking nightly vardenafil, on-demand vardenafil, or placebo for 9 months. Primary outcome was percentage of patients achieving an Erectile Function domain of the IIEF (IIEF-EF) score >21. After the 9-month treatment period, on-demand vardenafil was associated with more patients scoring ≥22 compared to placebo. However, results from this trial did not support nightly vardenafil over on-demand dosing, and as a matter of fact found no improvement in IIEF score after washout for either protocol compared with placebo. Limitations to this study are that dropout rates ranged between 31 and 35 % in the study arms and there was no defined limit in drug usage in the on-demand arm, therefore creating doubt that the two study arms truly represented different dosage patterns. The authors concluded that their data argue against the use of nightly PDE5i in the treatment of post-prostatectomy ED.

Pavlovich et al. [22] found similar results when they randomized 100 preoperatively potent men who had undergone nerve-sparing RP to receive either nightly sildenafil and on-demand placebo (nightly sildenafil group), or on-demand sildenafil and nightly placebo (on-demand sildenafil group; with a maximum on-demand dose of 6 tablets/month) starting the day after surgery for 12 months. All men had previously completed a pre-surgery IIEF-EF survey and had a score of ≥26 before undergoing nerve-sparing RP. Surgeons prospectively recorded the quality of neurovascular bundle (NVB) preservation and this was quantified using a nerve sparing score (NSS) of one to four, with higher scores representing better preservation. The double-blind

Table 23.1 Penile rehabilitation after prostate cancer treatment: summary of clinical trials using oral PDE5is

Author	Year	*N*	Follow-up	Study design	Prostate CA treatment modality	ED treatment (treatment period)	Significant findings
Padma-Nathan	2008	125	44 Weeks	Prospective, double blind, randomized, placebo-controlled	RP	Nightly sildenafil vs. placebo (36 weeks)	Sildenafil had higher IIEF score and increased nocturnal rigidity
Pavlovich	2013	100	13 Months	Prospective, double-blind, randomized	RP	Daily sildenafil with on demand placebo vs. daily placebo with on demand sildenafil (12 months)	No difference in IIEF scores between treatments
Montorsi	2008	628	13.5 Months	Prospective, double-blind, randomized, placebo-controlled	RP	Nightly vardenafil vs. on-demand vs. placebo (9 months)	On-demand group had significantly more patients with IIEF >22 After a washout period, there was no difference in EF between groups
Montorsi	2013	423	13.5 Months	Prospective double-blind, randomized, placebo-controlled	RP	Tadalafil nightly vs. on-demand vs. placebo (9 months)	– Daily Tadalafil had significantly higher IIEF at 9 months treatment period – After washout, no difference in EF between groups – Tadalafil daily: protection from penile length loss
Mulhall	2013	298	12 Weeks	Prospective, double-blind, randomized, placebo-controlled	RP	Avanafil on-demand 100 mg vs. 200 mg vs. placebo (12 weeks)	On-demand Avanafil 100 mg or 200 mg improved drug-assisted EF – Washout period not assessed
Ilic	2012	27	2 Years	Prospective double-blind, randomized, placebo controlled	RT	Prophylactic daily sildenafil vs. placebo (6 months)	Daily sildenafil did not result in improved EF at 2 years
Zelefsky	2014	279	2 Years	Prospective double-blind, randomized, placebo controlled	RT	Daily sildenafil vs. placebo (6 months)	Daily sildenafil = improved overall EF
Pisansky	2014	242	1 Year	Prospective double-blind, randomized, placebo controlled	RT	Daily Tadalafil vs. placebo (24 weeks)	Daily tadalafil did not result in improved EF

PDE5i phosphodiesterase-5 inhibitors, *RP* radical prostatectomy, *RT* radiotherapy, *IIEF* international index of erectile function, *EF* erectile function

Questions	Response options
Q1. How often were you able to get an erection during sexual activity? **Q2.** When you had erections with sexual stimulation, how often where your erections hard enough for penetration?	0 = No sexual activity 1 = Almost never/never 2 = A few times (much less than half the time) 3 = Sometimes (about half the time) 4 = Most times (much more than half the time) 5 = Almost always/always
Q3. When you attempted sexual intercourse, how often were you able to penetrate (enter) your partner? **Q4.** During sexual intercourse, how often were you able to maintain your erection after you had penetrated (entered) your partner?	0 = Did not attempt intercourse 1 = Almost never/never 2 = A few times (much less than half the time) 3 = Sometimes (about half the time) 4 = Most times (much more than half the time) 5 = Almost always/always
Q5. During sexual intercourse, how difficult was it to maintain your erection to completion of intercourse?	0 = Did not attempt intercourse 1 = Extremely difficult 2 = Very difficult 3 = Difficult 4 = Slightly difficult 5 = Not difficult
Q6. How many times have you attempted sexual intercourse?	0 = No attempts 1 = One to two attempts 2 = Three to four attempts 3 = Five to six attempts 4 = Seven to 10 attempts 5 = More than 11 attempts
Q7. When you attempted sexual intercourse, how often was it satisfactory to you?	0 = Did not attempt intercourse 1 = Almost never/never 2 = A few times (much less than half the time) 3 = Sometimes (about half the time) 4 = Most times (much more than half the time) 5 = Almost always/always
Q8. How much have you enjoyed sexual intercourse?	0 = No intercourse 1 = No enjoyment 2 = Not very enjoyable 3 = Fairly enjoyable 4 = Highly enjoyable 5 = Very highly enjoyable
Q9. When you had sexual stimulation or intercourse, how often did you ejaculate? **Q10.** When you had sexual stimulation or intercourse, how often did you have the feeling of orgasm or climax?	0 = No sexual stimulation/intercourse 1 = Almost never/never 2 = A few times (much less than half the time) 3 = Sometimes (about half the time) 4 = Most times (much more than half the time) 5 = Almost always/always
Q11. How often have you felt sexual desire?	1 = Almost never 2 = A few times (much less than half the time) 3 = Sometimes (about half the time) 4 = Most times (much more than half the time) 5 = Almost always/always
Q12. How would you have rate your level of sexual desire?	1 = Very low/none at all 2 = Low 3 = Moderate 4 = High 5 = Very high
Q13. How satisfied have you been with your overall sex life? **Q14.** How satisfied have you been withyour sexual relationship with your partner?	1 = Very dissatisfied 2 = Moderately dissatisfied 3 = About equally satisfied and dissatisfied 4 = Moderately satisfied 5 = Very satisfied
Q15. How do you rate your confidence that you could get and keep an erection?	1 = Very low 2 = Low 3 = Moderate 4 = High 5 = Very high

SCORING

Domain	*Erectile function*	*Intercourse satisfaction*	*Orgasmic function*	*Sexual desire*	*Overall satisfaction*
Questions:	1.____	6.____	9.____	11.____	13.____
	2.____	7.____	10.____	12.____	14.____
	3.____	8.____			
	4.____				
	5.____				
	15.____				
Total score	____ (1-30)	____ (0-15)	____ (0-10)	____ (2-10)	____ (2-10)

Fig. 23.2 The International Index of Erectile Function is a validated tool for detecting erectile dysfunction. It addresses the relevant domains of male sexual function and has been linguistically validated in ten languages. All questions in the above questionnaire are preceded by the phrase "Over the past 4 weeks…." Source: http://www.aafp.org/afp/2000/0101/p95.html. Reprinted [56]

study period included quality-of-life assessments at 1, 3, 6, 9, and 12 months after RP, and at 13 months after a washout period. Compliance in returning questionnaires ranged from 60 to 96 % per time-point, but was balanced between groups. After adjusting for potential confounding factors, no significant differences were found in erectile function between treatments (nightly vs. on-demand sildenafil) at any single time-point after RP. The summary NSS was the only factor that was consistently found to have a significant association with EF outcomes in all longitudinal multivariable models. A 1-unit increase in NSS was associated with an absolute increase in IIEF-EF score of 1.65 ($p=0.005$). This study had factors that weakened its findings. First, fearing that patients would not want to be randomized to a placebo-only group, a pure placebo arm was not part of the trial. Ninety percent of subjects were Caucasian, which may not necessarily be generalizable to all populations. Moreover, the study period in the trial was only 13 months, which is short of the 18–24 months duration recommended by some authors.

In a recent study, Mulhall et al. [23] found that 3 months of treatment with the newly approved PDE5i avanafil taken on-demand significantly improved drug-assisted erectile function after prostatectomy. They randomized 298 patients with post-RP ED of 6 months or more to on-demand 100 or 200 mg avanafil or placebo for 12 weeks. At the end of treatment 100 mg (31 %) and 200 mg (41 %) avanafil groups responded that treatment improved their erections when compared to placebo (10.7 %). Treatment efficacy was also statistically significant when stratifications by age, ED baseline severity, and type of RP were performed. Dropout rates ranged from 8 to 24 % between groups, with the largest amount in the placebo group in which 14 of 24 patients discontinued from the study withdrew their consent. This fact raises the possibility that these patients perceived lack of treatment efficacy. Sustained effect on unassisted EF and long-term response to treatment were not assessed in this study.

The REACTT conducted by Montorsi et al. [24] trial attempted to compare the efficacy of tadalafil daily and on demand vs. placebo in improving unassisted erectile function and reducing loss of penile length following nerve-sparing RP. Four hundred twenty-three patients were randomized into 9 months of treatment with tadalafil 5 mg once daily, tadalafil 20 mg on demand, or placebo followed by a 6-week washout period and 3 months open-label tadalafil once daily (all patients). Drop out rates were 14–18 % between groups. They found that after 9 months of treatment there was a significant difference in reaching the target IIEF-EF $\geq$22 in the tadalafil once daily group compared to placebo. Nonetheless, after the drug free washout period, there was no significant difference in EF between groups with 20.9, 16.9 and 19.1 % of patients reaching target IIEF-EF in the tadalafil once daily, on demand and placebo groups, respectively. After the open-label tadalafil once daily period IIEF-EF scores increased in all treatment groups. Regarding penile length, there was significantly less shrinkage of penile length observed in the daily tadalafil group (2.2 mm) compared to other groups (7.9 mm on demand, 6.3 mm placebo) at 9 months of treatment. This data suggests that PDE5is may play a role in the preservation of cavernosal integrity by protecting against structural changes after post-prostatectomy neuropraxia [24–27].

As stated earlier, the etiology of post-RT erectile dysfunction appears to be more related to vascular (endothelial) dysfunction rather than neural injury. There are studies in which patients treated with sildenafil or tadalafil had improved flow-mediated dilation and some authors suggest these medications have a protective effect in the vascular endothelium [28, 29]. Ilic et al. [30] examined whether early prophylactic sildenafil is effective in reducing long-term ED in prostate cancer patients treated with radiation. A total of 27 men were randomized at a 1:1 ratio to receive either sildenafil citrate 50 mg or placebo every night starting 1 month after completion of radiotherapy for a total of 6 months. The primary outcome of this trial was erectile function measured at 2 years post treatment using IIEF-5 score. The trial was closed after 32 months due to a poor accrual of patients. There was no significant difference in treatment compliance between groups with 95.1 and 96 % compliance of men in sildenafil and placebo groups, respectively. They found a significant difference in IIEF-5 scores by week four of the study and at 6 months ($p=0.02$ and $p=0.02$, respectively). However, there was no difference in erectile function between groups at 2 years after treatment ($p=0.48$), therefore suggesting that regular use of sildenafil after RT for prostate cancer does not improve long-term EF. This study was grossly underpowered by its small study cohort size and early study termination.

A larger study conducted by Zelefsky et al. [31] investigated if adjuvant daily sildenafil preserved EF during and after radiotherapy. They randomized 279 patients who were to undergo radiation therapy with or without neo-adjuvant ADT into taking prophylactic daily sildenafil 50 mg vs. placebo. Treatment was initiated 3 days pretreatment and continued daily for 6 months and outcomes were analyzed for 24 months after RT. As expected, ADT patients tended to experience worse erectile function outcomes than non-ADT patients. Among patients not receiving ADT (90 %) there was a significant difference in EF and IIEF scores during RT and 24 months between groups. At 24 months, 81.6 % of the sildenafil group and 56 % of placebo patients reported functional erections. There were no differences in EF outcomes among external beam radiation therapy compared with brachytherapy or a combined-modality treatment. The greatest improvement in IIEF scores and overall EF was at 6 and 12 months after treatment, suggesting that a longer course of PDE5i may be required to provide even better functional outcomes.

More recently, Pisansky et al. [32] conducted the first multicenter, stratified, placebo-controlled, double-blinded, parallel-group study to our knowledge to evaluate tadalafil for ED prevention in men treated with radiotherapy for prostate cancer. Two hundred forty-two men with localized prostate adenocarcinoma and intact erectile function scheduled to receive radiotherapy were randomized 1:1 into receiving 5 mg of tadalafil daily vs. placebo. Baseline as well as radiotherapy characteristics were balanced well, with no significant differences between groups. Treatment was started within 7 days after initiation of external radiotherapy or the date of brachytherapy and was to continue for 24 consecutive weeks. Participants reported IIEF scores before radiotherapy and up to 1 year after treatment. Intensity modulation was used in 98 % of patient treated with external radiotherapy with a median dose of 78.0Gy. Eighty five percent of patients undergoing brachytherapy received iodine 125, and palladium 103 was used for the remainder. At weeks 28 and 30, they found no statistically significant difference between patients receiving tadalafil (79 %) and those receiving placebo (74 %). Moreover, tadalafil did not result in a statistically significant difference in improved sexual function at 1 year when compared to placebo. They concluded that daily use of tadalafil did not result in improved erectile function when compared to placebo. However, testing for other tadalafil dosing schedules, larger study cohorts and longer follow-ups could yield different results.

The question still remains on whether the use of PDE5is as a penile rehabilitation regimen would improve spontaneous EF in patients after prostate cancer treatment. We found only one meta-analysis and systematic review on the use of oral PDE5is for treating ED after nerve-sparing RP. Wang et al. [33] screened 77 studies of which eight randomized controlled trials met inclusion criteria for their review. Some of these studies were analyzed in our review [19, 23, 24]. They attempted to systematically assess the efficacy and safety of oral PDE5is for post-bilateral nerve sparing RP ED. Erectile function was measured using the IIEF scores, Sexual Encounter Profile question 2 (SEP-2, "Were you able to insert your penis into your partner's vagina?" [yes/no]), Sexual Encounter Profile question 3 (SEP-3, "Did your erection last long enough for you to have successful intercourse?" [yes/no]) and the Global Assessment Question (GAQ, "Has the treatment you have been taking during this study improved your erection?" [yes/no]). The meta-analysis showed that treatment with PDE5is resulted in clinically favorable outcomes in term of IIEF scores, SEP-2, SEP-3 and GAQ success rate when compared to placebo. They also found a trend, but no statistical significance, that responsiveness to PDE5is was associated with longer treatment duration, higher dosage, on-demand dosing, use of sildenafil and preoperative mild ED. Although this data provides compelling evidence for the use of PDE5is as a primary treatment for post-RP ED, there remains an opportunity for the development of appropriately designed RTCs with sufficiently long-term follow-up to address PDE5i use, dosage, and duration of treatment in penile rehabilitation.

Vacuum Erection Devices

As mentioned earlier, patients have been found to suffer from penile shrinkage after radical prostatectomy. Fraiman et al. [34] demonstrated that there was a decrease in penile dimensions after RP. The flaccid and erect measurements of length and circumference decreased almost 10 %, mostly between the first 4 and 8 months after nerve-sparing RP. The vacuum erection device (VED) has gained popularity among patients and physicians due to its low complication rates, few side effects, and cost-effectiveness when compared to other penile rehabilitation modalities. VED causes erections by creating negative pressure around the penis and drawing both venous and arterial blood into the corpus cavernosum sinusoids.

Although previous studies suggested that VED could preserve penile length and aid in the return of spontaneous erections, there was no basic scientific evidence demonstrating that VED therapy improved penile length after RP. Lin et al. designed a study to explore the mechanism of VED in penile rehabilitation by analyzing cavernous oxygen saturation (SO2) in rats after bilateral cavernous nerve crush (BCNC), therefore mimicking ED after RP. They randomized 30 adult male rats into three groups: sham surgery with no cavernous crush, surgery with BCNC and no therapy, and surgery with BCNC and VED therapy. Penile length and penile blood gas were analyzed in all three groups. They found that VED therapy was effective in preventing penile shortening and penile circumference reduction. Moreover, VED therapy preserved erectile function by increasing oxygen saturation level in penile cavernous tissue and therefore, alleviating tissue hypoxia. This helps inhibit apoptosis and prevent cavernous tissue fibrosis [35].

Welliver et al. [36] confirmed these findings by showing that the use of VED significantly increased both glanular and corporal oximetry, hence improving penile overall oxygen saturation. The VED device contains a constriction ring used at the base of the penis that aids in maintaining erections for intercourse. However, it also decreases oxygen saturation after 30 min of use. Therefore, the use of the constriction band is not recommended in penile rehabilitation [37, 38].

There are few clinical trials that evaluate the effect of VED after prostate cancer treatment. Köhler et al. [39] randomized 28 men with baseline IIEF scores of >11, to start daily VED use 1 month after nerve-sparing RP or start VED on-demand prior to intercourse 6 months after surgery. They found that men who had completed early VED use had significantly greater IIEF scores and stretched penile length (2 cm) compared to the on-demand group. However, at last follow-up (mean 9.5 months, 6–12 months) there was no significant difference in outcomes, and none of the patients reported unassisted EF sufficient for intercourse. This in turn suggests the need for longer rehabilitation periods and the importance of neural pathway regeneration for successful penile rehabilitation.

A prospective clinical trial by Raina et al. [40] of 109 patients randomized into using daily VED vs. no treatment found that at the end of 9 months, 80 % of those using VED had erections sufficient for intercourse and were less likely to report penile shrinkage (85 % vs. 23 %, respectively). Another prospective study by Raina and colleagues evaluated the long-term effects in EF after RP with the early use of VED and other non-oral ED treatments. One hundred forty-one patients who had undergone nerve-sparing RP were motivated to participate in early penile rehabilitation. At 1- and 5-year follow-up, 80 and 62 % of men, respectively, were sexually active. After 5 years 71 % of sexually active men had natural erections sufficient for penetration without assistance. Most patients used either VED alone or in combination with another ED treatment modality. Unfortunately, this study has major limitations, as there was no control group, and protocol details or nerve-sparing status were not revealed. However, it does recognize VED as a valuable and effective treatment in penile rehabilitation [41].

A retrospective study by Basal et al. reviewed 203 patients who underwent bilateral nerve-sparing RP and utilized PDE5is, VED, the combination of PDE5i and VED or no treatment for penile rehabilitation. They attempted to study the erectile function recovery period (EFRP) in patients with mild, moderate or no preoperative ED. Patients with mild ED yielded the shortest EFRP with a mean recovery period of 8.73 ± 5.67 months after surgery. Only PDE5is and combination PDE5is and VED groups had a beneficial effect on EFRP [42]. We believe VED has an important role in penile rehabilitation. Unlike other therapies, VED can ensure multiple erections on a daily basis early in the penile rehabilitation period and thus prevent early penile hypoxia which may lead to fibrosis and consequently a decrease in stretch penile length and long-term ED. Its mechanism causing erections works independently of the neural pathway and thus overcomes problems generated by neuropraxia. Most importantly, VED can be used safely with other treatment modalities to achieve better EF results. A summary of clinical trials that assess VED and other non-oral modalities are presented in Table 23.2.

Intraurethral Therapy

Intraurethral alprostadil (IUA) is a urethral suppository that delivers prostaglandin E1 (PGE1). PGE1 acts locally by increasing levels of cyclic adenosine 3′,5′-cyclic monophosphate (cAMP) within erectile tissue. IUA acts indirectly in the erectile tissue through the urethra [15, 43]. This urethral suppository bypasses the neural pathway in the corpora cavernosum and generally does not cause systemic side effects. The most common side-effect is urethral burning and penile pain.

McCullough et al. [43] reported the first randomized, prospective trial to study the effect of nightly Medicated Urethral System for Erection (MUSE, Vivus Inc. Mountain View, CA, USA) (Fig. 23.3). A total of 212 men were randomized into taking IUA or sildenafil nightly. IUA was titrated from 125 to 250 μg after 1 month of treatment for better toleration. Dropout rates were 19 % for the sildenafil group and 30 % for IUA group. Most dropouts occurred with the increase in IUA dosage secondary to pain. Compliance rates were 98 and 79 % for sildenafil and IUA groups, respectively. IIEF scores increased in the IUA and SC groups from a mean of 9.9 and 10.4 at 1-month to 15.28 and 17.65 at study end, respectively. At 9 months, there were no statistically significant differences in the IIEF-EF score and successful intercourse rates. The only statistically significant difference between groups in erections, assessed by the global assessment question (GAQ, “Has the treatment you have been taking during this study improved your erection?” [yes/no]), occurred at 6 months in favor of IUA (76 % vs. 60 %). It is possible this benefit occurred in the period of neuropraxia when PDE5i are not expected to be effective.

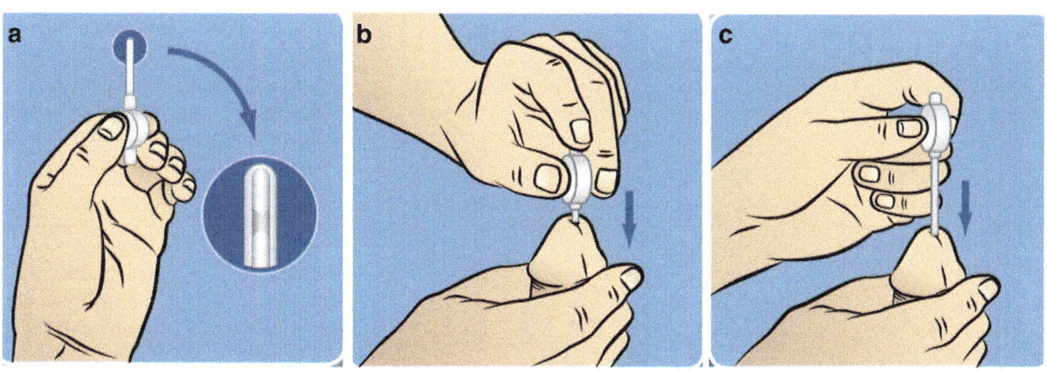

Fig. 23.3 Medicated urethral system for erection (MUSE, Vivus Inc. Mountain View, CA, USA). (**a**) Device used for insertion of the intraurethral suppository. The *curved arrow* shows the medicated pellet. (**b**) While keeping the penis stretched, insert the device up to the collar of the applicator and then push the button on the applicator. Source: www.muserx.com

Table 23.2 Penile rehabilitation after prostate cancer treatment: summary of clinical trials using non-oral modalities

Author	Year	*N*	Follow-up	Study design	Prostate CA treatment modality	ED treatment (treatment period)	Significant findings
Köhler	2007	28	6–12 Months	Prospective, randomized	RP	Daily VED vs. no treatment (6 months)	At 6 months, early VED had better IIEF and penile length. No difference at last follow-up between groups
Raina	2010	141	5 Years	Prospective, no control	RP	VED and other non-oral therapies (9 months)	Most men who tried non-oral agents, with or without VED, remained sexually active after 5 years
McCullough	2010	212	9 Months	Prospective, randomized	RP	IUA vs. sildenafil (9 months)	No difference in IIEF and intercourse success between treatments
Montorsi	1997	30	12 Weeks	Prospective randomized	RP	ICI versus no treatment (12 weeks)	ICI has higher rate of spontaneous erections compared with controls
Mulhall	2005	132	18 Months	Prospective, no control	RP	Sildenafil ± ICI (12 months)	Treatment group had more spontaneous erections and higher IIEF compared with controls Men on rehabilitation are more likely to respond to treatment
Mulhall	2009	84	2 Years	Retrospective, no control	RP	Sildenafil ± ICI Early (2 months) vs. Delayed (7 months)	Early better delayed group in unassisted erections
Fode	2014	68	18 Months	Retrospective	RP	PVS w PDE5i vs. No PVS w PDE5i (6 weeks)	No significant difference, though trend of better IIEF score in patients using PVS

RP radical prostatectomy, *VED* vacuum erection devices, *IUA* intraurethral alprostadil, *ICI* intracavernosal injection therapy, *PVS* penile vibratory stimulation, *IIEF* international index of erectile function score

Normal therapeutic doses of IUA range between 500 and 1000 μg. Nonetheless, we found no clinical trials that assess these doses in patients undergoing prostate cancer treatment. Although IUA can improve erections in patients with ED, its use after prostate cancer treatment is limited in the medical community. This is most likely secondary to cost and the lack of quality randomized controlled trials to prove its overall effectiveness in patients undergoing prostate cancer treatment.

Intracavernosal Injection

Intracavernosal injection (ICI) consists of PGE1 alprostadil alone or in combination with papaverine and phentolamine. Phentolamine is an α-blocker that causes smooth muscle relaxation and papaverine is a nonspecific phosphodiesterase inhibitor that increases both cAMP and cGMP in the cavernous tissue. These agents in combination act as vasoactive agents that aid in increasing blood flow to the corpus cavernosum, hence causing erections and penile engorgement.

The first treatment studied as a penile rehabilitation strategy was ICI by Montorsi et al. [44] in 1997. Thirty patients who underwent bilateral nerve-sparing RP were randomized to either receive alprostadil injections three times per week for 12 weeks vs. no treatment. After 6 months, 67 % of men in the treatment group vs. 20 % in the control group achieved spontaneous erections sufficient for penetration. The researchers concluded that the injections of alprostadil decreased the hypoxia-induced tissue damage. Reported complications were minor and the therapy proved to be well tolerated.

Mulhall et al. [45] published the only long-term follow-up prospective study that assessed ICI in penile rehabilitation. Men with preoperative erections who underwent RP were treated with early sildenafil and those who did not respond were switched to ICI three times per week. A total of 58 patients received penile rehabilitation treatment vs. 74 who were allowed to have treatment on-demand off-protocol. Patients who were not compliant with therapy for at least 12 months were excluded from the study group. IIEF scores were assessed for 18 months. At 18 months after prostatectomy, 52 % of the rehabilitation group vs. 19 % of the control group reported unassisted spontaneous erections. Ninety-five percent of patients responded to ICI and 64 % to sildenafil in the study group, vs. 76 and 24 % in the control group, respectively. Limitations of this study include lack of randomization and intention-to-treat, and selection bias.

In a similar study in 2009, Mulhall et al. [46] attempted to define if EF outcomes were better with early institution of penile rehabilitation. Forty-eight patients in the early group and 36 patients in the delayed group were instructed to obtain three erections per week using sildenafil initially, and if unsuccessful, then intracavernous injections. Penile rehabilitation started at a mean time of 2 months and 7 months after RP in the early and delayed groups, respectively. At 2 years after surgery, 48 % of the early group and 30 % of the delayed group had unassisted erections hard enough for penetration. There was also a statistical significant difference in those achieving an IIEF-EF score >25 between groups. Even though this is a retrospective study and selection bias could have altered results, this study unveils evidence that timing of penile rehabilitation is of paramount importance.

ICI has been proven effective for treatment of ED after prostate cancer treatment. However, we are still in need of clinical trials with long-term follow-up that assess its role in penile rehabilitation.

Penile Vibratory Stimulation

The use of penile vibratory stimulation (PVS) was first described by Sobrero et al. in 1965 [47]. Advancements in technology and technique led to the development of devices that stimulate penile erection in men with ED and ejaculation in men with spinal cord injury. PVS works through the stimulation of branches of the pudendal nerves along the penile shaft. The stimulation causes a reflex parasympathetic erection through the activation of nerve terminal endings that release nitric oxide and inhibit

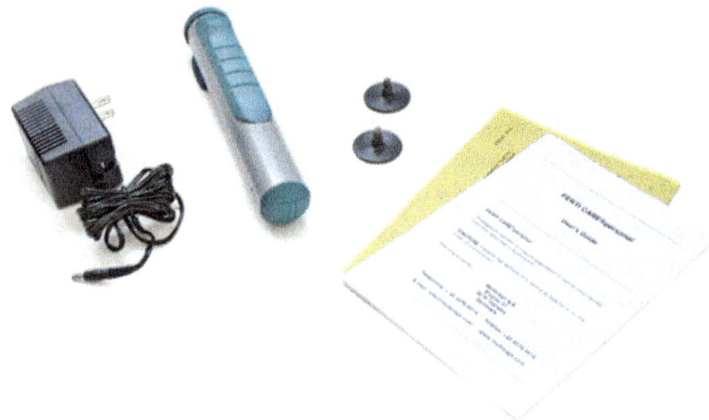

Fig. 23.4 The Ferticare vibrator®: was used at an amplitude of 2 mm and a vibration frequency of 100 Hz. It was applied to the frenulum once daily, with a sequence consisting of 10 s of stimulation followed by a 10 s rest and repeated for a total of 10 times. Source: http://medicalvibrator.com

sympathetic fibers. The resultant effect is the liberation of cGMP and cAMP. Both of these cause cavernosal smooth muscle dilation and penile engorgement [48].

Fode and colleagues presented the first prospective randomized study aimed to examine the effect of PVS on penile rehabilitation in patients undergoing nerve-sparing RP. Sixty-eight patients were randomized into using PVS with oral PDE5is vs. oral PDE5is without the use of PVS. The Ferticare vibrator® (Fig. 23.4) was used at an amplitude of 2 mm and a vibration frequency of 100 Hz. It was applied to the frenulum once daily, with a sequence consisting of 10 s of stimulation followed by a 10 s rest and repeated for a total of 10 times. Patients in the study group were instructed in stimulating the frenulum once daily for at least 1 week before surgery and after catheter removal for a period of 6 weeks. IIEF scores were evaluated at 3, 6, and 12 months after surgery. Results showed that IIEF scores were higher in the PVS group at all times, though no difference reached significance. At 12 months after surgery 53 % had reached an IIEF score of at least 18, compared to 32 % of patients in the control group ($p=0.07$) [49]. Patient compliance and PDE5i type, frequency, or dosages were not presented in this study. Furthermore, stopping PVS use after 6 weeks raises the question if a longer treatment period would have yielded different outcomes. Although this study had significant limitations, it showed that PVS is both acceptable and tolerable for patients. Most importantly, it also pioneers the use of PVS as an agent in erection rehabilitation after nerve-sparing RP.

Low-Intensity Extracorporeal Shockwave Therapy

The use of low-intensity extracorporeal shockwave (LI-ESW) attempts to alter the underlying pathophysiology of the erectile mechanism. Shockwaves (SWs) applied to targeted tissue cause mechanical stress and micro-trauma that catalyze a set of biological reactions that result in neovascularization of the tissue [50]. Even though this mechanism is not completely understood, recent animal studies revealed that corpora harvested from rats treated with LI-ESWT result in increased smooth muscle and endothelial content, along with upregulation of vascular endothelial growth factor (VEGF), neuronal NO synthase and von Willebrand factor [51].

Human clinical studies have seen a high tolerability and an increase of IIEF-EF scores in patients and high with mild and severe ED treated with this noninvasive modality [52, 53]. These led Vardi and colleagues to develop the first randomized, double-blind, sham controlled clinical trial to evaluate the use of LI-ESWT in ED [54]. The sham treatment in this study consisted of an identical probe that looked, sounded and felt the same but did not produce any SWs to the targeted tissue. IIEF-EF scores and penile hemodynamics were assessed at 3 and 6 months in 67 randomized participants with ED who could previously achieve erections with PDE5is. A 4-week PDE5i washout period was performed prior to the initiation of a 9-week treatment period, consisting of 2 sessions per week for 3 weeks that were repeated after a 3-week no-treatment interval. Results showed that the overall satisfaction, ability to penetrate, and mean IIEF-EF scores of patients in the treatment group were significantly higher than those in the control group. Penile hemodynamics also revealed a significantly improved resting and maximal post-ischemic penile blood flow in LI-ESWT participants. Although the study cohort was relatively small and prostate cancer treatment patients were excluded, this study demonstrated that this modality might serve as an adjunct to penile rehabilitation in the near future.

Currently there are no clinical trials that assess LI-ESWT in patients undergoing prostate cancer treatment. Although there are more questions than answers regarding the mechanism and therapeutic use of LI-ESWT for improvement of EF, this modality could 1 day take part in post-prostatectomy penile rehabilitation programs.

Conclusion

The majority of studies available assess the use of PDE5i in penile rehabilitation, most likely because they are well known and widely available. PDE5s are well tolerated and have been proven to improve early assisted sexual function when compared to placebo. Nonetheless, the use of PDE5is has not been proven to significantly improve in unassisted erections in the long-term when compared to placebo. Many clinical trials studying other treatment modalities presented in this chapter lacked placebo control. However, due to the nature of these modalities such as PVS, ICI, and VEDs it is difficult to create a believable hoax modality to eliminate the placebo effect.

Currently there is no standard treatment algorithm or clinical guideline for EF recovery after prostate cancer treatment. Limited robust studies exist for post-RP patients and even less for post-RT. A survey demonstrated that these factors have not hindered AUA urologists from including penile rehabilitation programs in their practices [55]. Although today's treatment options are limited, advancements in research and technology will ultimately create and refine management options for penile rehabilitation. Recent therapeutic advances such as PVS, LI-ESWT, impulse magnetic field therapy, nanotechnology, and endovascular treatment may open new ways that can revolutionize treatment of ED [48]. Recent trials have shown that most therapies are well-tolerated and aid in some degree on EF recovery. However, we currently do not have tangible evidence to recommend an irrefutable penile rehabilitation algorithm. We are confident that advancements in research and technology will ultimately create and refine management options for penile rehabilitation. Penile rehabilitation pioneers and researchers all over the world may gather this information to launch clinical trials that 1 day will delineate an algorithm for ED after radical prostatectomy.

Author Contributions JCH and RW contributed to the concept and design of the study and drafted, revised, and approved the manuscript. JCH contributed to the acquisition and analysis of data.

References

1. What are the key statistics about prostate cancer? Am Cancer Soc http://www.cancer.org/cancer/prostate-cancer/detailedguide/prostate-cancer-key-statistics. Accessed 8 Apr 2014.
2. Alemozaffar M, Regan MM, Cooperberg MR, Wei JT, Michalski JM, et al. Prediction of erectile function following treatment for prostate cancer. JAMA. 2011;306:1205–14.
3. Penson DF, McLerran D, Feng Z, Li L, Albertsen PC, Gilliland FD, et al. 5-year urinary and sexual outcomes after radical prostatectomy: results from the Prostate Cancer Outcomes Study. J Urol. 2008;179(5 Suppl):S40–4.
4. Sanda MG, Dun RL, Michalski J, Sandler HM, Northouse L, et al. Quality of life and satisfaction with outcome among prostate-cancer survivors. N Engl J Med. 2008;358:1250–61.
5. Zippe CD, Pahlajani G. Penile rehabilitation following radical prostatectomy: role of early intervention and chronic therapy. Urol Clin North Am. 2007;34:601–18. viii.

6. Hakky TS, Baumgarten AS, Parker J, Zheng Y, Kongnyuy M, et al. Penile rehabilitation: the evolutionary concept in the management of erectile dysfunction. Curr Urol Rep. 2014;15:393.
7. Mccullough AR. Rehabilitation of erectile function following radical prostatectomy. Asian J Androl. 2008;10:61–74.
8. Wang R. Penile Rehabilitation after radical prostatectomy: where do we stand and where are we going? J Sex Med. 2007;4:1085–97.
9. Walsh PC, Marschke P, Ricker D, Burnett AL. Patient reported urinary continence and sexual function after anatomic radical prostatectomy. Urology. 2000;55:58–61.
10. Mulhall JP, Slovick R, Hotaling J, Aviv N, Valenzuela R, et al. Erectile dysfunction after radical prostatectomy: hemodynamic profiles and their correlation with the recovery of erectile function. J Urol. 2002;167:1371–5.
11. Stember DS, Mulhall JP. The concept of erectile function preservation (penile rehabilitation) in the patient after brachytherapy for prostate cancer. J Brachyther. 2012;11:87–96.
12. Zelefsky MJ, Eid JF. Elucidating the etiology of erectile dysfunction after definitive therapy for prostate cancer. Int J Radiat Oncol Biol Phys. 1998;40:129–33.
13. Sharifi N, Gulley JL, Dahut WL. Androgen deprivation therapy for prostate cancer. JAMA. 2005;294:238–44.
14. Gontero P, Kirby R. Proerectile pharmacological prophylaxis following nerve-sparing radical prostatectomy. Prostate Cancer Prostatic Dis. 2004;7(3):223–6.
15. Alba F, Wang R. Current status of penile rehabilitation after radical prostatectomy. Urology. 2010;16:93–101.
16. Mccullough AR, Levine LA, Padma-Nathan H. Return of nocturnal erections and erectile function after bilateral nerve-sparing radical prostatectomy in men treated nightly with sildenafil citrate: subanalysis of a longitudinal randomized double-blind placebo-controlled trial. J Sex Med. 2008;5:476–84.
17. Bannowsky A, Schulze C, Vander-Horst C, Hautmann S, Jünemann KP. Recovery of erectile function after nerve-sparing radical prostatectomy: improvement with nightly low-dose sildenafil. BJU Int. 2008;101:1279–83.
18. Pace G, Del Rosso A, Vicentini C. Penile rehabilitation therapy following radical prostatectomy. Disabil Rehabil. 2010;32:1204–8.
19. Padma-Nathan H, McCullough AR, Levine LA, Lipshultz LI, Siegel R, et al. Randomized, double-blind, placebo-controlled study of postoperative nightly sildenafil citrate for the prevention of erectile dysfunction after bilateral nerve-sparing radical prostatectomy. Int J Impot Res. 2008;20:479–86.
20. Lim KB, Deyoung L, Brock G. Chronic PDE5 inhibitor altered cavernosal protein expression-use in identifying protein biomarker for erectile recovery post trauma. J Sex Med. 2006;3 suppl 5:383.
21. Montorsi F, Brock G, Lee J, Shapiro J, Van Poppel H, et al. Effect of nightly versus on-demand vardenafil on recovery of erectile function in men following bilateral nerve-sparing radical prostatectomy. Eur Urol. 2008;54:924–31.
22. Pavlovich CP, Levinson AW, Su LM, Mettee LZ, Feng Z, et al. Nightly vs on-demand sildenafil for penile rehabilitation after minimally invasive nerve-sparing radical prostatectomy: results of a randomized double-blind trial with placebo. BJU Int. 2013;112:844–51.
23. Mulhall JP, Burnett AL, Wang R, McVary KT, Moul JW, et al. A phase 3, placebo controlled study of the safety and efficacy of avanafil for the treatment of erectile dysfunction after nerve sparing radical prostatectomy. J Urol. 2013;189:2229–36.
24. Montorsi F, Brock G, Stolzenburg JU, Mulhall JP, Moncada I, et al. Effects of tadalafil treatment on erectile function recovery following bilateral nerve-sparing radical prostatectomy: a randomized placebo-controlled study (REACTT). Eur Urol. 2014;65:587–96.
25. Berookhim BM, Nelson CJ, Kunzel B, Mulhall JP, Narus JB. Prospective analysis of penile length changes after radical prostatectomy. BJU Int. 2013. doi:10.1111/bju.12443.
26. Nelson CJ, Scardino PT, Eastham JA, Mulhall JP. Back to baseline: erectile function recovery after radical prostatectomy from the patients' perspective. J Sex Med. 2013;10:1636–43.
27. Mostafa ME, Senbel AM, Mostafa T. Effect of chronic low-dose tadalafil on penile cavernous tissues in diabetic rats. Urology. 2013;81:1253–60.
28. Desouza C, Parulkar A, Lumpkin D, Akers D, Fonseca VA. Acute and prolonged effects of sildenafil on brachial artery flow-mediated dilation in type 2 diabetes. Diabetes Care. 2002;25:1336–9.
29. Rosano GM, Aversa A, Vitale C, Fabbri A, Fini M, et al. Chronic treatment with tadalafil improves endothelial function in men with increased cardiovascular risk. Eur Urol. 2005;47:214–20.
30. Ilic D, Hindson B, Duchesne G, Millar JL. A randomized, double-blind, placebo-controlled trial of nightly sildenafil citrate to preserve erectile function after radiation treatment for prostate cancer. J Med Imaging Radiat Oncol. 2012;57:81–8.
31. Zelefsky MJ, Shasha D, Branco RD, Kollmeier M, Baser RE, et al. Prophylactic sildenafil citrate for improvement of erectile function in men treated by radiotherapy for prostate cancer. J Urol. 2014. doi:10.1016/j.juro.2014.02.097.
32. Pisansky TM, Pugh SL, Greenberg RE, Pervez N, Reed DR, et al. Tadalafil for prevention of erectile dysfunction after radiotherapy for prostate cancer the radiation therapy oncology group [0831] randomized clinical trial. JAMA. 2014;311(13):1300–7.
33. Wang X, Wang X, Liu T, He Q, Wang Y, et al. Systematic review and meta-analysis of the use of phosphodiesterase type 5 inhibitors for treatment of erectile dysfunction following bilateral nerve-sparing radical prostatectomy. PLoS One. 2014;9(30):e91327. doi:10.1371/journal.pone.0091327.
34. Fraiman MC, Lepor H, McCullough AR. Changes in penile morphometrics in men with erectile dysfunction after nerve-sparing radical retropubic prostatectomy. Mol Urol. 1999;3:109–15.

35. Lin HC, Yang WL, Zhang JL, Dai YT, Wang R. Penile rehabilitation with a vacuum erectile device in an animal model is related to an antihypoxic mechanism: blood gas evidence. Asian J Androl. 2013;15:387–90.
36. Welliver Jr RC, Mechlin C, Goodwin B, Alukal JP, et al. A pilot study to determine penile oxygen saturation before and after vacuum therapy in patients with erectile dysfunction after radical prostatectomy. J Sex Med. 2014;11(4):1071–7.
37. Monga M, Utz W, Reddy P, Kohler T, Hendlin K, et al. Early use of the vacuum constriction device following radical retropubic prostatectomy: a randomized clinical trial. South Central Section of the AUA 85th annual meeting 2006; abstract book, p. 98 (Abstract 50).
38. Bosshardt RJ, Farwerk R, Sikora R, Sohn M, Jakse G. Objective measurement of the effectiveness, therapeutic success and dynamic mechanisms of the vacuum device. Br J Urol. 1995;75:786–91.
39. Kohler TS, Pedro R, Hendlin K, Utz W, Ugarte R, et al. A pilot study on the early use of the vacuum erection device after radical retropubic prostatectomy. BJU Int. 2007;100(4):858–62.
40. Raina R, Agarwal A, Ausmundson S, Lakin M, Nandipati KC, et al. Early use of vacuum constriction device following radical prostatectomy facilitates early sexual activity and potentially earlier return of erectile function. Int J Impot Res. 2006;18:77–81.
41. Raina R, Pahlajani G, Agarwal A, Jones S, Zippe C. Long-term potency after early use of a vacuum erection device following radical prostatectomy. BJU Int. 2010;106:1719–22.
42. Basal S, Wambi C, Acikel C, Gupta M, Badani K. Optimal strategy for penile rehabilitation after robot-assisted radical prostatectomy based on preoperative erectile function. BJU Int. 2013;111(4):658–65.
43. McCullough AR, Hellstrom WG, Wang R, Lepor H, Wagner K, et al. Recovery of erectile function after nerve sparing radical prostatectomy and penile rehabilitation with nightly intraurethral alprostadil versus sildenafil citrate. J Urol. 2010;183:2451–6.
44. Montorsi F, Guazzoni G, Strambi LF, Da Pozzo LF, Nava L, et al. Recovery of spontaneous erectile function after nerve-sparing radical retropubic prostatectomy with and without early intracavernous injections of alprostadil: results of a prospective, randomized trial. J Urol. 1997;158(4):1408–10.
45. Mulhall J, Land S, Parker M, Waters WB, Flanigan RC. The use of an erectogenic pharmacotherapy regimen following radical prostatectomy improves recovery of spontaneous erectile function. J Sex Med. 2005;2(4):532–40.
46. Mulhall JP, Parker M, Waters BW, Flanigan R. The timing of penile rehabilitation after bilateral nerve-sparing radical prostatectomy affects the recovery of erectile function. BJU Int. 2009;105:37–41.
47. Sobrero AJ, Stearns HE, Blair JH. Technic for the induction of ejaculation in humans. Fertile Steril. 1965;16:765–7.
48. Stein MJ, Lin H, Wang R. New advances in erectile technology. Ther Adv Urol. 2014;6(1):15–24.
49. Fode M, Borre M, Ohl D, Lichtbach J, Sønksen J. Penile vibratory stimulation in the recovery of urinary continence and erectile function after nerve-sparing radical prostatectomy: a randomized, controlled trial. BJU Int. 2014. doi:10.1111/bju.12501.
50. Gruenwald I, Appel B, Kitrey N, Vardi Y. Shockwave treatment of erectile dysfunction. Ther Adv Urol. 2013;5(2):95–9.
51. Liu J, Zhou F, Li GY, Wang L, Li HX, et al. Evaluation of the effect of different doses of low energy shock wave therapy on the erectile function of streptozotocin (STZ)-induced diabetic rats. Int J Mol Sci. 2013;14:10661–73.
52. Vardi Y, Appel B, Jacob G, Massarwi O, Gruenwald I. Can low-intensity extracorporeal shockwave therapy improve erectile function? A 6-month follow-up pilot study in patients with organic erectile dysfunction. Eur Urol. 2010;58:243–8.
53. Gruenwald I, Appel B, Vardi Y. Low-intensity extracorporeal shock wave therapy—a novel effective treatment for erectile dysfunction in severe ED patients who respond poorly to PDE5 inhibitor therapy. J Sex Med. 2012;9:259–64.
54. Vardi Y, Appel B, Kilchevsky A, Gruenwald I. Does low intensity extracorporeal shock wave therapy have a physiological effect on erectile function? Short-term results of a randomized, double-blind, sham controlled study. J Urol. 2012;187:1769–75.
55. Tal R, Teloken P, Mulhall JP. Erectile function rehabilitation after radical prostatectomy: practice patterns among AUA members. J Sex Med. 2011;8:2370–6.
56. Rosen RC, Riley A, Wagner G, Osterlow IH, Kirkpatrick J, Mishra A. The international index of erectile dysfunction (IIEF): a multidimensional scale for assessment of erectile dysfunction. Urology. 1997;49:822–30.

Structured Reporting of RARP Complications: Are We Making Measurable Progress?

24

John Michael DiBianco, Arvin K. George, and Piyush K. Agarwal

Introduction

Recently, the urologic profession has followed the lead of the general surgeons in defining and quantifying complications with each surgical procedure. At the beginning of the nineteenth century, E. A. Codman introduced the concept of a "end results system" to track hospital outcomes and since then, this has been a central measure in our health care system [1]. Today, the Centers for Medicare & Medicaid Services (CMS) and the Affordable Care Act have further expanded the use of outcomes data through incentive-based reimbursement schemes in an attempt to improve surgical outcomes [2, 3]. Outcomes have previously guided change in surgical techniques. For example, the transition to laparoscopy from open surgical procedures largely followed observations that patients treated with laparoscopic surgery experienced less postoperative pain, improved cosmesis, fewer infections and blood transfusions, and shorter hospital stays [4]. The advent of RAS provided multiple mechanical and ergonomic advantages over standard laparoscopic procedures [5]. The first robot-assisted laparoscopic surgery in humans was performed in 1997 [5]. Since the first robot-assisted radical prostatectomy (RARP) reported in 2000, there has been a prompt increase in utilization, with an almost fourfold surge in robot-assisted prostatectomies between 2005 and 2008 alone, reaching an incidence of 60,000 procedures annually in the United States in 2008 [1, 6–8]. The initial diffusion of robot-assisted surgery has garnered controversy, especially with respect to the appropriate utilization of the technique, procedural costs, reimbursement issues, and complications [5, 7].

Similar to other new surgical procedures, RAS has an initial *learning curve* for most surgical teams. As more procedures are performed over time, operative times decrease, and fewer complications result [9, 10]. Since the first RARP in the year 2000, surgical outcomes and complication rates have seemingly improved; although this conclusion largely results from high-volume single center series [11, 12]. However, initial reports, prior to the publication by Agarwal et al. did not report outcomes from RARP in a standardized fashion [12, 13]. This lack of standardization in reporting early and delayed postoperative complications made it difficult to interpret the safety and efficacy profiles of RARP case series, thereby making it challenging to directly compare outcomes with open radical prostatectomy series. However, many open surgical series also failed to

J.M. DiBianco, M.D. • A.K. George, M.D.
P.K. Agarwal, M.D. (✉)
Urologic Oncology Branch, Center for Cancer Research, National Institutes of Health, National Cancer Institute, Building 10, Hatfield Clinical Research Center, Room 2W-3952 10 Center Drive MSC 1210, Bethesda, MD 20892-1210, USA
e-mail: john.dibianco@yahoo.com; Arvin.george@nih.gov; piyush.agarwal@nih.gov

J.W. Davis (ed.), *Robot-Assisted Radical Prostatectomy*, DOI 10.1007/978-3-319-32641-2_24

categorize complications in a standardized fashion. In the 1990s, numerous attempts in the general surgery literature suggested methods of standardized reporting of surgical adverse events, but generally, these failed to gain wide acceptance [14–17].

Today, several systems of reporting complications currently exist, including the: Clavien–Dindo classification of surgical complications, Memorial Sloan-Kettering Center Classification modification (MSKCC), Accordion, National Surgical Quality Improvement Program (NSQIP), and National Cancer Institute Common Toxicity Criteria (NCT-CTC) [2, 18–22]. In 1992, Clavien introduced *T92*, a grading system that assessed the severity of complications based on the intervention required to alleviate them [23]. In 2002, Martin et al. modified T92 slightly producing a similar classification referred to as the Memorial Sloan-Kettering Cancer Center severity grading system [24]. In 2004, Dindo et al. proposed a modification to T92, increasing the levels of severity available for classification of a complication and specifically identifying if the complication required general anesthesia or admission to intensive care to resolve it, or if it caused organ failure [25].

The Clavien–Dindo classification system offers many advantages over the nonspecific and inconsistent ranking of surgical outcomes data that existed previously. The Clavien–Dindo system avoided previous terms such as minor, moderate, and major, which often were not explicitly defined or uniformly applied to adverse postoperative events [18, 22, 23]. The Clavien–Dindo system ranks the severity of postoperative adverse events according to the therapy or intervention needed to remedy the complication. In its current iteration, it consists of a five-tiered list of complication severity based on the type of therapy needed to treat the complications [18]. By using the medical record to identify the intervention needed to remedy the complication, the opportunity to overlook or downgrade complications is minimized [18]. The system has been widely used in surgery and urology reports and has been evaluated for interobserver variation in categorizing complications across seven centers with an 89 % agreement in identifying and ranking complications [18].

Complications Associated with RARP

Currently, minimally invasive radical prostatectomy has a lower risk profile than the corresponding open surgical procedures [10]. Previous studies have demonstrated significant improvement in the rates of overall complications as surgeons overcome their individual learning curves [9, 10, 26]. In bariatric surgery, procedure volume correlated with surgical skill, reduced complications, reoperations, readmissions, and emergency room (ER) visits. However, years in bariatric surgical practice, formal fellowship training, and practice in a teaching or nonteaching setting did not correlate with reduced complications, reoperations, readmissions, or ER visits [27]. It is noteworthy that an assessment of surgical skill, obtained from review of a representative video-taped procedure by peer surgeons and blinded to the identity of the operators, correlated closely with surgical skill as assessed by complication rates [27]. How best to expedite the learning curve for RARP remains elusive.

Preoperative

Medical/Anesthesia Related

As with all medical and surgical approaches and procedures, proper patient selection is perhaps the most critical initial step. General anesthesia is required for RARP, contributing a relatively well-defined set of anesthetic-associated complications whose frequency and severity are related to the baseline demographics and comorbidities of the patient [28]. It is recognized that even in the hands of an experienced robotic surgeon, certain patient characteristics will dictate increased surgical risks. In patients undergoing RARP, a BMI>30, prostate gland >70 g or a gland having a large median lobe, previous prostate or other pelvic surgery, and a history of radiation, are associated with higher risks of surgical complications [29]. Armed with this information, urologists and patients can make more educated decisions when weighing the risks and benefits of selected surgery. Present trends indicate that we may be placing more patients on active surveillance than in previous years [30]. In a large experience, Agarwal et al. reported a correlation of medical and surgical complications of patients undergoing RARP to the patient's baseline characteristics, including the independent prediction of increased medical adverse events in patients with cardiopulmonary comorbidities and increased PSA levels [12]. Additionally, presence of gastric reflux and increasing age or Gleason score were independently associated with surgical complications [12].

Cardiorespiratory

RARP requires CO_2 pneumoperitoneum which may result in hypercarbia, oliguria, subcutaneous emphysema, and organ hypoperfusion [28]. A CO_2 pressure of 15 mmHg is commonly used, although 20 mmHg has been shown to be safe, in urologic laparoscopic surgeries [28, 31]. Some surgeons alter the intraoperative CO_2 insufflation pressure, depending on their experience and the course of the surgery, as higher pressures may allow for a modest tamponade-like effect on bleeding from venous sinuses, the source of most intraoperative blood loss [32–34]. Rates of cardiac and respiratory complications associated with radical prostatectomy are reported to range between 0.9–4.3 % and 1.2–6.7 % respectively [10].

Thromboembolic

The majority of patients undergoing radical prostatectomy are considered to be at high risk for venous thrombosis and embolization by the ACCP guidelines [35–37]. Thromboembolic events are potentially lethal medical complications of virtually all types of major surgery and are recognized to be increased in patients with cancer, including prostate cancer (PCa) [38]. As reported by Kim et al. thromboembolic events are increased with longer operative times, which are more frequently associated with more extensive and complicated surgeries [39]. Historically, with ORP, pulmonary embolism (PE) was the most common cause of death, which has now diminished due to thromboprophylaxis such as routine perioperative anticoagulation, early ambulation, compression stockings [36, 37].

The increased use of laparoscopic techniques, compared to open procedures, has reduced thromboembolic complications. Patients undergoing open retropubic prostatectomy (ORP) have a significantly higher risk of thromboembolic events compared to those treated with RARP; in one recent report, thromboembolic risk was increased almost fourfold with the ORP vs. RARP (RR 3.8, 99 % CI 1.42–9.99) [40]. Thromboembolic events and current rates of PE for patients undergoing RARP overall is ~0.2 % [37]. This statistic is informed by the specific mix of patient demographics and comorbidities, which correlate with the incidence of venous thromboembolism (VTE). Specifically, for patients treated with RARP, an increased frequency of VTE is seen in association with: increasing age (>60 years), history of thrombosis, procoagulant states, pT4 disease, Gleason score of $\geq$8, obesity, personal and family history of PE, venous disease (superficial or deep venous thrombosis), and surgery-related parameters, such as, an RARP lasting more than 60 min, complicated by extensive tissue injury or infection, or combined with lymph node dissection [29, 40]. In a large experience, RARP with lymph node dissection placed patients at an especially high risk. Studying 3544 patients undergoing both open and RARP, the investigators observed almost an eightfold increase in deep venous thrombosis (RR 7.80, 95 % CI 3.51–17.32) and a sixfold increase in pulmonary embolism (RR 6.29, 95 % CI 2.11–18.73) associated with radical prostatectomy that included lymph node dissection [40]. Increased risks associated with lymph node dissection also included wound, respiratory, cardiovascular and neuromuscular events and more than doubled readmission rates (14.6 % vs. 6.3 %) [40].

Position Related

When a patient is placed in a steep Trendelenburg position for RARP and the patient's arms are tucked, access to the patient's airway and intravenous sites may be limited, thereby compromising the ease of maintaining fluid, medication, and oxygen administration, and ventilation [28]. Trendelenburg position and maintenance of pneumoperitoneum can increase intracranial and intrathoracic pressure and can cause subcutaneous head and neck swelling, decrease pulmonary compliance, and increase risk of pulmonary edema [41]. These complications, fortunately, are rarely associated with long-term morbidity [41]. While exceedingly sporadic in occurrence, and predominantly associated with spinal surgery, blindness postoperatively with RARP has an incidence of 0.02–0.10 % [42, 43]. It is a devastating event if irreversible and is more likely to occur in long procedures (≥8 h) where the patient remains in steep Trendelenburg [42, 43]. This phenomenon is not completely understood; it may be related to increased intraocular pressures leading to retinal ischemia [42].

Placing the patient in a steep Trendelenburg with adduction of the arms has been associated with other complications including: compressive neuropathies or myopathies (rhabdomyolysis), musculoskeletal pain, edema, and neuropraxia. Neuropathy, resulting from an underlying nerve injury, may occur from positioning, usually the result of excessive external pressure (ischemia) and/or neural stretching [28]. The risk for such injuries increases with stirrups (lithotomy position) and the duration of surgery. Neuropathies attributed to RARP positioning have been reported to include involvement of the brachial, ulnar, femoral, and peroneal nerves. Most neuropathic complications resulting from patient positioning can be avoided by special attention to alleviating the pressure of operative equipment against the patient, intermittent repositioning if feasible, and shorter durations of surgery. Importantly, most neuropathies improve or resolve with time. Analyzing data from 61,656 patients who underwent minimally invasive RP in the National Inpatient Sample database, Wen et al. found that positioning-related complications occurred at a rate of 0.4 % with ophthalmic complications being predominant. These investigators reported that standard laparoscopic procedures were highly associated with the occurrence of positioning injuries (odds ratio [OR] = 2.88, $P<0.01$), whereas RARP procedures (OR = 0.93, $P>0.4$) were not, and that positioning injuries increased inpatient costs and extended LOS by almost 400 and 300 %, respectively [44].

Operative

Device/Robot Related

Robot malfunction or failure may occur occasionally during surgery [45]. In a survey of 176 surgeons performing RARP, 100 reported having had at least one irrecoverable, intraoperative, robot malfunction; approximately 46 % (80/176) were preoperative and were resolved by rescheduling the intended procedure (58 %) or converting to another type of procedure (19 % were converted to ORP and 15 % to standard laparoscopic prostatectomy) [45]. In only 5 % of cases was another robotic surgical system available for the intended procedure [45]. By far, more problematic from a patient safety standpoint, are malfunctions of the robot *during* active surgery. With respect to intraoperative robot malfunctions, 36 % (63/176) occurred before starting the vesicourethral anastomosis and the remaining 18 % (32/176) occurred before completion of the anastomosis [45–47]. The majority of intraoperative robot malfunctions resulted in conversion to open radical retropubic or standard laparoscopic prostatectomy [45]. Chen et al. reporting on a series of 400 urologic cases, found 14 cases of robot malfunction: four were critical and required conversion to standard laparoscopy and one was noncritical and the procedure was rescheduled [47]. These investigators and others have identified the da Vinci surgical system as highly reliable, with rare critical and irrecoverable malfunctions, ranging from 0.2 to 2.6 %; with even lower rates (0.4 %) being reported from large multi-institutional studies [10, 45–49]. Since 1993, the U.S. Food and Drug Administration has maintained the Manufacturer And User Facility Device Experience (MAUDE) database which has focused on adverse events associated with robotic surgery, primarily using the Zeus and Da Vinci robotic systems. Note: most information and procedures now relate, almost exclusively, to the Da Vinci system, since, in 2003, manufacturers of the Zeus and Da

Vinci systems merged to produce and promote only the Da Vinci Surgical System (Intuitive Surgical, Sunnydale, CA) [19, 46, 48]. In a report assessing device malfunctions (product use errors and product quality problems) that resulted in patient injury between the years 2000 and 2007, Andonian et al., found a total failure rate of 0.38 %, representing 189 malfunction events [19]. Of the total malfunction events, 4.8 % (9/189) were associated with some degree of patient injury [19]. Notably, between 2003 and 2007, there was a decline in device robot malfunctions that required conversions to open surgical procedures from 94 to 16 % [19]. It should be noted that the MAUDE database, while large, has been criticized for its accuracy. It is an open, voluntary forum that allows patients and healthcare personnel, to post and write about their experiences. There is no requirement to report and no accuracy assurance; hence, it is suspected to be incomplete and perhaps biased.

Nonprostate Tissue Injury

Injury to the structures and tissues within the operative field may inadvertently occur during RARP. In the era of laparoscopic surgery, bowel, rectal, vascular (especially the aorta, iliac, and gonadal vessels), nervous, and/or genitourinary system injury can occur when trocars or other instruments are placed through the abdominal wall and into the peritoneal cavity. Although uncommon, each of these potential injuries, are complications that have been reported during RARP, and are accepted to be more common in prolonged or more extensive procedures, such as those requiring lymph node dissection. The obturator nerve, for example, a potential target of injury with lymph node dissection, requires special attention during RARP to minimize harm. Precise rates of nonprostate tissue injury are not well defined as current classification schemes do not specifically catalog these problems. In studies reporting uncommon nonprostate tissue injuries, the Martin–Donat criteria has been used to facilitate the comprehensive and accurate reporting of urologic complications and the Clavien–Dindo classification has been used to define severity [50].

The average rate of vascular complications, usually perforation or incision, resulting from RARP is approximately 2.7 % and is recognized to generally decline with increased surgeon/surgical team experience and increased case volumes [9]. Bowel and rectal injury during RARP have been reported at rates ranging from 0.7 to 2.4 % and are not different in frequency from those reported prior to 2004 [51–53]. When these injuries are recognized early and repaired, they often do not have a major impact on the patient's functional recovery. However, delayed surgical correction or unrecognized injury may result in fistulae and local/systemic infections [52]. Ureteral injuries during RARP are reported to occur in 0.05 and 1.6 % of cases [9, 50]. In one reported single institution experience of 6442 consecutive patients undergoing RARP, three ureteral injuries (all transections) occurred, each requiring additional, robot-assisted corrective procedures, with one patient requiring readmission [50].

Blood Loss

Blood loss and transfusion requirements have not routinely been assessed as a "complication" of surgical procedures prior to the recommendations of Clavien–Dindo, Martin, and Donat [12, 18, 19, 24, 25]. In some series, surgeons performing open prostatectomy plan autologous blood transfusion and have patient's donate 2 units of blood preoperatively [8]. This lack of emphasis on bleeding and transfusion requirements as a complication of prostatectomy is illustrated in the large, comprehensive evaluation of retropubic and laparoscopic prostatectomy reported by Rabbani et al. in which blood transfusion was excluded as a complication [54]. The data in their study supports that laparoscopic prostatectomy is associated with less blood loss than open radical prostatectomy, perhaps reflecting the tamponade effect of pneumoperitoneum on small venous sinuses [12, 54, 55]. Similar to standard laparoscopic prostatectomy, RARP is associated with reduced bleeding and transfusion rates [10]. The Clavien–Dindo classification of surgical complications cites bleeding and transfusion requirements, as a class 2 complication in the grading system of severity (Fig. 24.1) [18]. The Martin–Donat criteria (Fig. 24.2), specifically addressing complications associated with urologic surgery, require quantitation of bleeding and transfusion rates [12, 18, 56]. A large, consecutive series of 3317 RARP patients reported by Agarwal et al. using Martin–Donat reporting standards and an exhaustive review of multiple datasets, confirmed that RARP was associated with a 1.7 % incidence of postoperative anemia and bleeding, which incidentally was the most common early complication of RARP [12]. This rate is slightly less than the contemporary rate of 2 % for transfusion with RARP reported by others. This includes asymptomatic, reactive transfusions delivered to patients for hematocrit below 30 [10, 12]. The imperative or symptomatic transfusion rate, in the above series of RARP is considerably less at 0.4 % [12]. The prophylactic use of heparin anticoagulant to prevent venous thrombosis and thromboembolism may increase the risk of bleeding which may be further increased, especially, if there is concomitant use of antithrombotic treatments (aspirin and other antiplatelet agents, steroids and NSAIDS, or additional anticoagulants) [28]. The availability and prompt administration of replacement colloid and/or packed red cells may minimize poor outcomes associated with uncompensated blood loss. As mentioned above, patients undergoing prostatectomy for PCa are at increased risk for thromboembolic events, and are often candidates for heparin prophylaxis [36, 37]. Many additional factors have been shown to influence intraoperative blood loss including surgical volume, operative time, and prostate size. Prostate size especially correlates with blood loss during RARP [10]. Contemporary studies reporting blood loss show a mean estimated blood loss with RARP of 166 ml (69–534) and a transfusion rate approximating 2 % (0.5–5 %) [10].

Conversion

Conversion of RARP to a standard laparoscopic or open procedure may occur for technical or patient-related reasons. Reasons for conversion include: irrevocable/critical robot malfunction, control of intraoperative bleeding, and unexpected adhesions, which may not allow surgery to progress or may compromise the safe creation of adequate pneumoperitoneum. Rarely, an anatomic anomaly or simply excessive adiposity may mandate conversion to gain adequate exposure. As surgical experience increases, the frequency of conversion of RARP to standard laparoscopic or open procedures

APPENDIX A. Classification of Surgical Complications

Grades	Definition
Grade I:	Any deviation from the normal postoperative course without the need for pharmacological treatment or surgical, endoscopic and radiological interventions.
	Acceptable therapeutic regimens are: drugs as antiemetics, antipyretics, analgetics, diuretics and electrolytes and physiotherapy. This grade also includes wound infections opened at the bedside.
Grade II:	Requiring pharmacological treatment with drugs other than such allowed for grade I complications.
	Blood transfusions and total parenteral nutrition are also included.
Grade III:	Requiring surgical, endoscopic or radiologica; intervention
Grade III-a:	intervention not under general anesthesia
Grade III-b:	intervention under general anesthesia
Grade IV:	Life-threatening complication (including CNS complication): requiring IC/ICU-management
Grade IV-a:	single organ dysfunction (including dialysis)
Grade IV-b:	multi organ dysfunction
Grade V:	Death of a patient
Suffix 'd':	If the patient suffers from a complication at the time of dischrge (see examples in Appendix B, http://Links.Lww-com/SLA/A#),\ the suffix "d" (for 'disability') is added to the respective grade of complication. This label indicates the need for a follow-up to fully evaluate the complication.

: brain hemorrhage, ischemic stroke, subarrachnoidal bleeding, but excluding transient ischemic attacks (TIA); IC: Intermediate care; ICU: INtensive care unit
www.surgicalcomplication.info

Fig. 24.1 Modified Clavien–Dindo classification system

Table 1
Martin criteria for the evaluation of article reporting complications after surgery

Criteria	Requirement
Method of accruing data defined	Prospective or retrospective accrual of data are indicated.
Duration of follow-up indicated	Report clarifies the time period of postoperative accrual of complications, such as 30 d or same hospitalization.
Outpatient information included	Study indicates that complications first identified after discharge are included in the analysis.
Definitions of complications provided	Article defines at least 1 complication with specific inclusion criteria.
Mortality rate and causes of death listed	The number of patients who died in the postoperative period of study are recorded together with cause of death.
Morbidity rate and total complications indicated	The number of patients with any complication and the total number of complications are recorded.
Procedure-specific complications included	Radical prostatectomy: anastomotic leak, lymphocele, urinary retention, obturator nerve injury, etc.
Severity grade used	Any grading system designed to clarify severity of complications, including major and minor, is reported (eg, Clavien and Dindo grading system).
Length-of-stay data	Median or mean length of stay is indicated in the study.
Risk factors included in the analysis	Evidence of risk stratification and method used is indicated by study.

Fig. 24.2 Martin classification system

usually declines, which may be secondary to better patient selection, better surgical skills, or more surgical experience [12]. Previously reported open conversion rates from RARP have ranged from 0 to 5 % with the majority of series reporting 0 % [57]. Modern reports indicate that conversion, of any type, is a rare occurrence in fully trained surgeons, and that RARP has a lower conversion rate than standard laparoscopic radical prostatectomy (LRP), reported to be 1.9 % by Bhayani et al. from multi-institutional data [39, 58]. An analysis of 82,338 patients undergoing RARP, by Weiner et al. using the National Cancer Database between 2010 and 2011, reported an open conversion rate of 0.9 % [59]. Sub-analyses demonstrated that 22.9 % of those conversions occurred at facilities contributing less than 4 % of the total cases for yearly RARP volume, emphasizing the importance of an experienced surgical team in avoiding conversions [59]. Since the potential for conversion always exists, there is continued justification for comprehensive surgical training, in *all* of the approaches to radical prostatectomy for the surgeon performing RARP [12, 57].

Postoperative

Ileus

Ileus, defined as an intolerance of solid food for at least three postoperative days (that may be accompanied by nausea, vomiting, bloating, or abdominal distention), is the most frequently reported gastrointestinal medical complication after RARP. Patients undergoing abdominal surgery have ileus rates ranging from 5 to 25 % while patients undergoing RARP have ileus rates ranging from 1.5 to 4.2 % [12, 51, 60]. Ileus may be associated with patient and/or operative factors. In a study of 228 patients having undergone transperitoneal RARP with an overall ileus rate of 2.6 %, diabetes was shown to be an independent risk factor for ileus [60]. Operative factors include visceral manipulation or trauma, anesthetic and/or perioperative analgesic medications (especially opiates), and increasingly complex procedures (e.g., concomitant lymph node dissection). Expectedly, higher rates of ileus are reported with the transperitoneal as opposed to the extraperitoneal approach to RARP [60]. Ileus has also been seen more frequently in the presence of an abdominal urine leak [10, 48, 61]. Ileus has been reported as the most common cause of readmission or unscheduled visits following an early discharge program post-radical prostatectomy [62].

Infectious complications are most common within the first 30 days following surgery [12]. It may be secondary to a medical complication, such as pneumonia, colitis, or urinary tract infection or the result of a surgical site infection. Most reports comparing complications have not separately commented on the incidence of infection between open and laparoscopic procedures. Earlier reports, reflecting initial RARP experiences reported *all* perioperative complication rates, which incorporated postoperative infections, as similar to those of retropubic prostatectomy [33, 62, 63]. This was not universally observed, however, Ficarra et al. observed significantly higher complication rates with retropubic prostatectomy, compared to RARP and standard LRP, which were similar [61]. Infection in patients undergoing RARP is reported to have an incidence of <1.0 % of patients or 5 % (20/368) of all reported complications in a recent large series [12].

In order to lower infectious complications, preoperative urinalysis with urine culture and sensitivity can easily avoid surgery on patients with infected urine. Furthermore, even if final results are not available at the time of surgery, the culture can expedite appropriate antimicrobial treatment if infection secondary to urinary contamination is causative. Postoperative fluid collections of all types (hematoma, urinoma, lymphocele) increase the risk of infection and should be promptly identified, and appropriately treated.

Lymphocele

Lymphocele development is the most common delayed complication of RARP, with an occurrence of 0.8 % [10, 12]. Rates of lymphocele and lymphorrhea in other series, have generally been reported at approximately 3.1 % (0–8 %) [10, 64]. Lymphoceles commonly develop after a lymph node dissection and the risk increases with more extensive dissections. Judicious ligation of lymphatic channels with clips may reduce its incidence.

Anastomosis Complication

Catheter dwell time has been viewed as a meaningful, albeit indirect, measure of the integrity of the urethral bladder anastomosis. In their series of RARP patients, Novara et al. identified a mean catheter duration of 6.3 days (1–6) [10]. Patients with longer catheter durations can result from prolonged urine leaks secondary to RARP performed in a salvage setting, larger prostate volumes, or a history of transurethral resection of the prostate [10, 29].

Length of Stay

Length of stay (LOS) remains a poor surrogate for overall perioperative complications and outcomes due to the multiple factors that influence it. Similar to the inaccurate and poorly defined terms "minor" and "major" complications, LOS remains a residual metric from the unstandardized reports of surgical complications that precede the Clavien–Dindo classification schema and the Martin–Donat modifications. LOS is still used as a rough estimate of complication severity, and is a parameter followed closely by economists for its correlation with inpatient costs. Keeping the issues with LOS in mind, modern rates of LOS for RARP are estimated to be 1.9 days (1–6) with many high-volume institutions discharging patients within 23 h of surgery by essentially performing RARP as a same day, out-patient procedure with 23 h of observation after surgery [10]. The current safety profile and rapid recovery associated with RARP has made the LOS metric no longer relevant for RARP, allowing current studies and reports to focus on better indices of functional and oncologic outcomes [29].

Hernia

Incisional hernia is a recognized complication of RARP with a reported incidence of 0.2–4.8 %; however, it is commonly under diagnosed given the limited follow-up in most series [65]. In a series of 577 patients who underwent RARP between 2003 and 2012, Chennamsetty et al. reported a 4 % incidence of incisional hernia repair (almost exclusively umbilical in location) diagnosed within a mean follow-up of 5 years. Similarly, a SEER (surveillance, epidemiology, and end results) database analysis revealed a 5.4 % incisional hernia repair rate following minimally invasive RP within 3.1 years postoperatively [65]. The occurrence of incisional hernia was increased in patients with larger median prostate weights (45 vs. 38 g, $P=0.001$) and was 2–3 times more common in patients having had a prior laparoscopic cholecystectomy (12.5 % vs. 4.6 %, $P=0.033$) [65].

Port site hernia is a complication that also must be addressed and represents a complication of ~1 % of laparoscopic surgeries [66]. Fascial closure is the best method of avoiding port site hernia. It was historically recommended that port sites >10 mm require fascial closure particularly when a cutting trocar was used for port placement [66]. This was difficult due to the small size of the laparoscopic port incision and was more difficult prior to the advent of fascial closure devices. They were also more common prior to the advent of blunt trocars. With blunt trocars, it may only be necessary to close port sites >12 mm [66]. Using this guideline, more modern studies report port site hernias at a rate of ~0.4 % [66].

Functional Outcomes (Incontinence/Erectile Dysfunction)

Historically, the earliest, most comprehensive, study addressing incontinence and sexual function following RP for PCa was the Prostate Cancer Outcomes Study (PCOS), conducted by the National Cancer Institute (NCI) between 1994 and 1999 [67]. This study investigated health-related quality of life (HRQOL) outcomes observed nationally in a large heterogenous cohort of patients following the initial community-based treatment of PCa. The findings confirmed important adverse sequelae of RP [67]. At ≥18 months post-RP, 8.4 % of men were incontinent and 59.9 % were impotent. Nerve-sparing procedures were helpful, reducing impotence from 66 to 56 %. However, even bilateral nerve-sparing efforts resulted in an erectile dysfunction (ED) rate of 56 %, a finding more common in older men and black patients [67]. Recognizing that surgical techniques (standard and robot-assisted laparoscopic RP) and other modalities of care are constantly evolving, there is a continual need for ongoing study and standardized reporting of HRQOL outcomes, such as recovery of continence, and erectile function.

Although there is no universally accepted definition or standard objective measurement of urinary continence (UI) and ED after RARP, it is clear that the functional outcomes of UI and ED are of paramount concern to patients. Furthermore, it should be stressed that these are not true complications of surgery and rather, are likely unintended consequences. However, they are also not justified outcomes and every effort needs to be made to prevent their occurrence when oncologically feasible. The incidence of UI and ED are confounded by multiple patient, operative, and reporting variables. Initial reports of UI provided evaluations at diverse postoperative time points and used varying definitions of continence. In other reports, continence is neither defined nor reported, but rather considered an expected result, justified in view of the surgery being performed. Likewise, the reporting of ED has been equally flawed in previous reports. Definitions are unstandardized and/or simply omitted. Several barriers exist to obtaining accurate patient data including: not documenting patient's subjective complaints, variable responses depending upon the type of query made, patient unwillingness to candidly discuss these sensitive and intimate problems, lack of standardized method of obtaining data (e.g., written or interviewer-elicited, prospective or retrospective), and the wide variation about patients and physicians as to what is considered acceptable or *normal*. These obstacles in gathering accurate information, provides some justification for the wide ranges reported for continence, (52–95 %) and potency (62–97 %) in the early literature following RARP [48, 57, 61, 68–70].

Incontinence

Stress urinary incontinence is an unfortunately common adverse event associated with RARP and is viewed by most patients as a meaningful reduction in their quality of life. At 1 month post-op from RARP, continence, defined as being free of using any absorbent pads, is estimated to be 56 % [71]. Although previous definitions of continence allowed some pad usage, current definitions of continence do not and the requirement for *any* pads to protect against inadvertent leakage of urine should be considered to be incontinence [70, 71]. Advanced age and significant lower urinary tract symptoms are associated with incontinence, though the strength of the prediction is generally low, while, lower risk disease, young age, and low comorbidities are associated with early continence after RARP [70–73]. Patient and prostate specific factors such as increased BMI and prostate gland size lower the likelihood of early continence [70–73]. Surgical experience also correlates positively with early continence post-RARP. The 1-year incontinence rate post-RARP ranges from 4 to 31 % using a *no pad* definition [73]. New, reliable predictors of early continence are recognizably sparse; a recent report suggests promise for discriminating pad-free continence at 1, 3, and 6 months post-op, with the use of uroflowmetry and a urine flow stop test at the time of urethral catheter removal [74]. This simple, noninvasive maneuver appears to improve the ability to predict early continence post recovery from RARP [74]. RARP series have reported lower rates of incontinence compared to retropubic prostatectomy and laparoscopic prostatectomy; however, large series of experienced open and laparoscopic surgeries show similar rates [73].

Nevertheless, multiple modifications have been proposed to reduce the frequency and extent of UI. Posterior musculofascial reconstruction, with or without anterior reconstruction, has been suggested as offering a slight advantage for urinary continence at 1 month postoperatively [70, 73]. In addition, recent data suggests that pelvic floor muscle training (PFMT) should also be modified. Traditionally, PFMT has focused mostly on repeated Kegel exercises pre- and post-operatively in order to obtain the muscle strength and control to prevent urine leakage during times of increased abdominal pressure. A recent study, however, objectively examined the exact times and activities associated with incontinence in 24 patients post-RARP by a single surgeon [75]. This study found that the majority of men experienced incontinence while sitting or walking at 3 and 6 weeks after RARP. They concluded that sustained functional PFMT should be promoted in order to increase endurance and prevent leakage in the most common situations [75].

Erectile Dysfunction

Preservation of erectile function is an essential component to HRQOL. However, evaluation and quantification of ED has been variable. In a large meta-analysis of RP studies with ≥1 year follow-up, only 10 % of 212 relevant studies met the minimal requirements for adequate reporting of the effects of surgery on erectile function [76]. Inconsistent definitions, incomplete data acquisition, and heterogeneous patient populations have rendered comparisons implausible between different procedures and even different series on the same procedure [76]. Despite the limitations of such data, Tal et al. found that overall recovery of erectile function was seen in the majority of men (58 %), with single-centers reporting approximately twice the recovery than reported by multicenter series (60 % vs. 33 %, RR = 1.82, P=0.001). The authors found that patients <60 years achieved greater recovery than older patients (77 % vs. 61 %, RR = 1.26, P=0.001) and revealed only minimal improvement with follow-up >18 months compared to early post-op evaluations (60 % vs. 56 %, RR = 1.07, P=0.02). Notably, laparoscopic RP showed similar recovery of erectile function to open RP (58 % vs. 58 %, respectively, pNS); both were inferior to RARP with regard to recovery of erectile function (73%, $P=0.001$ vs. open and laparoscopic RP) [76]. Despite this finding, they concluded that the superiority of any single surgical procedure was yet to be determined [76].

Nerve-sparing (NS) RARP is the most commonly used technique when attempting to maximize erectile outcomes. NS has also been shown to improve continence rates in men undergoing RARP with rates of continence positively correlated to the degree of neurovascular bundles saved [77]. There are several different levels of NS; pathologic features of the tumor and patient desire to retain potency determine the level. During RARP, the quality of NS is usually classified by laterality (none, unilateral, and bilateral) or degree (none, partial, and full). In one report, the surgeon's subjective assessment of nerve-sparing predicted time to recovery of function post-op [29, 78]. The ideal study to evaluate erectile function post-RP should be prospective, stratified for variability in surgical technique, and controlled for age, baseline erectile function, use of erectogenic therapies, and comorbidities. This type of study is yet to be completed [76].

Readmission

Readmission rates have been used as a surrogate for surgical complications. Based on this premise, the Centers for Medicare and Medicaid Services (CMS) has recently extended penalties for readmissions to hospitals for all medical conditions from a previous directive which was limited to only three medical conditions [79]. Although readmission rates have been criticized as imprecise and at times arbitrary, an extensive review of 346 hospitals in the American College of Surgeons National Surgical Quality Improvement Program (ACS NSQIP), for the year 2012 [80], revealed readmissions to be primarily attributable to surgical complications, rather than being reflective of patient and hospital characteristics or socioeconomic factors. Whether readmission rates truly reflect a quality measure in surgery remains debatable [81, 82]. In a large study of 59,273 surgical procedures performed in 112 Veterans Affairs hospitals between 2005 and 2009, Morris et al. found that readmission rates were predicted by patient comorbidities, procedural factors, and the occurrence of postoperative complications. Readmission rates were more reflective of the occurrence of *post-discharge complications*, rather than *pre-discharge* complications. The most common post-discharge complications were surgical site infections [81, 82]. Similar conclusions were drawn by Merkow et al. who assessed unplanned readmission rates for 498,875 operations [80]. Merkow concluded readmission after surgery was associated with new post-discharge complications [80]. Morris et al. suggest that readmission rates are of value for assessing trends in the frequency of surgical complications and for assessing progress in the surgical management of disease; although rates of readmission may depend more on better prevention techniques for surgical site infection than surgical techniques. [80, 82] The refinement of readmission rates, structured within the Clavien–Dindo classification of surgical complications better classifies adverse postoperative events.

Progress

As described above, improvement in outcomes, as well as more structured reporting has been seen in most new reports detailing the complications of RARP. The reasons for improved general surgery outcomes are complex and reflect more than participation in a program measuring complications, maintaining a database of practitioners and their outcomes, and efforts to mimic best practices [1, 83]. This was shown by the equally successful reduction in risk-adjusted adverse surgical outcomes observed for hospitals that did not participate in the ACS NSQIP. In addition, Osborne et al. determined no significant improvements in outcomes at 1,2, or 3 years after enrollment in the ACS NSQIP compared to the time period before enrollment. These outcomes included risk-adjusted 30-day mortality, serious complications, reoperations, and readmissions [84]. This study used national Medicare data of over 1.2 million patients undergoing general and vascular surgery in 263 participating hospitals [84]. However, there will be significant benefit in capturing complications by standardized reporting practices. The use of objective, comprehensive techniques of electronic health record data review, so-called *big data*, and dedicated software may allow the ability to capture most major and minor complications from the medical record automatically. This may exclude multiple potential areas of bias that exist with the much more tedious manual abstraction of medical records for adverse postoperative events [85].

Electronic health records (EHR) and large electronic databases have gained broad diffusion over the last several years in both the public and private sector [85]. Anderson & Chang propose automatic retrieval of prospectively identified objective variables from these electronic health records [85]. They performed separate multivariate logistic regression analyses on 745,053 general surgery patients, over a 5 year period beginning in 2005, using the NISQIP database [85]. Using 25 objective measurement variables already routinely collected, they concluded that large data analysis can be utilized in order to provide rigorous, risk-adjusted quality assessment (complication and mortality rates) that avoided time intensive and possibly incomplete or biased data retrieval [85]. These authors suggest that a wider application of their automatic data collection techniques may provide improvements to surgical outcomes and assessments of surgical quality, and may help eliminate subjectivity and bias in data collection. They provide compelling evidence that future outcomes reporting obtained from the use of "big data" show certain promise [85].

As a result many researchers are increasingly using registries to cull cases for review [86, 87]. The American Urological Association (AUA) has recently announced the creation of a specialty-wide national registry for healthcare outcomes and quality, related to the diagnosis and treatment of prostate cancer [88]. Although several university registries exist for prostate cancer care, the AUA Quality registry, (referred to as AQUA), is the first national registry. Launched in 2014, it is expected to be in full operation by July 2015. It will begin with prostate cancer and expand thereafter and will enable practitioners to benchmark their results against national database results and quantitate resource utilization. It will address oncological outcomes, functional outcomes, and complications. It may allow assessment of the course of the disease; variations in treatment, prognosis, and HRQOL resulting from PCa care patterns far in excess of that available through prospective comparative trials [86–88].

Technique Modifications

Modifications of the RARP technique have been reviewed and found to not significantly influence perioperative outcomes including: surgical approach (transperitoneal vs. extraperitoneal), preservation of the bladder neck, reconstruction of the vesicourethral junction (anterior, posterior, or complete anterior and posterior), anastomotic suture (barbed or standard monofilament suture), interfascial neurovascular dissection, and incision/ligation of the dorsal venous complex. [10, 89–94] Newer robotic platforms have improved the dexterity and adaptability of RARP procedure. At our institution, we have begun to perform the majority of RARP procedures without placing the patient in the lithotomy position, thereby reducing complications that may stem from lithotomy positioning such as nerve injuries. Technical changes will continue to alter the complication profile as time goes on.

Recommendations

Complications

Unfortunately, neither the Clavien–Dindo, Martin–Donat criteria, nor the Expanded Accordion Severity Grading System has been universally adopted [18, 20, 22, 95]. Further detracting from progress in this area is the observation that up to 35.3 % of papers published, claiming to have used the Clavien–Dindo classification system, did not use it properly [22]. Standardized reporting of surgical outcomes through the Clavien–Dindo classification allows better understanding of surgical data. The extension of this classification to urological surgery by Donat's modifications and the incorporation of the Expanded Accordion Severity Grading System which categorizes outcomes into failures, complications and sequelae, provide the ability to critically evaluate the complications of urologic surgery [95] (Fig. 24.3). Unfortunately, the challenge remains to have all surgeons adopt standardized reporting. We encourage clinical investigators, institutional review committees, and peer-reviewed journals, to request implementation of these standards.

Progress in the comprehensive reporting of postoperative complications has achieved significant milestones in the past two decades (Table 24.1). A summary of information related to the reporting and grading of complications after urological procedures was reported as an ad hoc EAU guidelines panel on the reporting method of complications after urologic procedures [22]. These researchers found that peer-reviewed manuscripts identified by a systematic review of the literature reported complications using standardized criteria in only 35 % of reports. An improvement in quality of the reporting of postoperative adverse events was demonstrated by an increase to 48.3 % of reported complications using standardized criteria, between 2009 and 2010 [22].

In the past, comparisons between ORP, LRP, and RARP have not uniformly documented and reported complications thereby limiting the ability to make comparisons. Rabbani et al. comprehensively reviewed the outcomes of 3458 patients undergoing ORP and 1134 patients who underwent LRP; however, they did not review the postoperative adverse effects of RARP [54].

RARP, the most common surgical approach for organ-confined PCa, was reviewed separately by Novara et al. Coelho et al. and Agarwal et al. [10, 12, 32] Each strived to implement the Martin–Donat criteria in their reports, thereby providing more uniform representation of complications for comparison. Limitations stemming from small patient population, failure to examine comorbidities, and follow-up limited to 6 weeks, compromised two of the studies [10, 12, 32]. The largest study providing a standardized report of complications of RARP was in 3317 consecutive patients by Agarwal et al. [12] The well-substantiated conclusions of these studies, gleaned from exhaustive clinical review and standardized reporting, is that RARP is a safe procedure with a 9.8 % rate of complications, most of which occur within the first 30 days post-op [12].

Functional Outcomes

In light of the difficulty with qualitative and quantitative characterization of problems, such as incontinence and ED, an equally important task is to standardize reporting of functional outcomes. To accomplish this, we would encourage the routine, prospective use of one comprehensive patient questionnaire in evaluating complications of urologic surgery. The tool for this assessment should be validated and universally accepted; to date, such a tool has yet to be

Table 1 Accordition classification system with seveity weights

Grade	Description	
1	Treatment of complication requires only minor invasive procedures that can be done at the bedside, such as insertion of intraveous lines, urinary catheters, and nasogastric tubes, and drainage of wound infections. Physiotherapy and antiemetics, antipyretics, analgesics, diuretics, electrolytes, and physiotherapy are permitted.	0.110
2	Complication requires pharmacologic treatment with drugs other than such allowed for minor complications, e.g. antiviotics. Blood transfusions and total parenteral nutrition are also included.	0.260
3	No general anesthesia ie required to treat the complication: requires management b an endoscopic, interventioanal procedure, or reoperation without general anesthesia.	0.370
4	General anesthesia is required to treat complication. Alternately, single-organ failure has developed.	0.600
5	General anesthesia is required to treat complication and single organ failure has developed.Alternately, multisystem organ failure (2 or more organ systems) has developed.	0.790
6	Postoperative death occured.	1.000

Fig. 24.3 Accordion complication classification system

Table 24.1 Selected studies of RARP outcomes and complications reporting method employed

Year	Author (s)	Patients (*n*)	Reporting standard	Complications (%)	Follow up (months)
2014	Jeong et al. [102]	100	MCD	56.8	6
2014	Pilecki et al. [103]	4374	NSQIP	5.62	1
2013	Maddox et al. [104]	575	MCD	16.2	1
2013	Rogers et al. [105]	69	CD	5.8	37.7
2013	Sagalovich et al. [106]	82	None	2.4	6
2013	Ou et al. [107]	148	MCD	7.4	30.6
2013	Yuh et al. [108]	406	MCD	18	NR
2012	Ahmed et al. [109]	1000	CD	9.70	1
2012	Yuh et al. [110]	30	CD	30	7
2012	Jung et al. [111]	200	CD	3	24
2012	Van der Poel et al. [112]	904	CD	14.1	>36
2012	Silberstein et al. [113]	562	None	3	NR
2011	Patel et al. [100]	1111	MCD	6.6	22
2011	Agarwal et al. [12]	3317	CD	9.80	24.2 (12.4–36.9)
2011	Jayram et al. [114]	248	CD	4	24
2011	Davis et al. [115]	261	None	5	NR
2011	Lallas et al. [116]	473	None	1.1	NR
2010	Novara et al. [117]	415	Martin + MCD	21.70	NA
2010	Jeong et al. [118]	200	CD	12	NR
2010	Coelho et al. [32]	2500	CD	5.10	25
2010	Yee et al. [119]	32	MCD	34	8.7
2010	Katz et al. [120]	94	CD	35.1	7.6
2010	Cooperberg et al. [121]	126	None	1.1	NR
2009	Ham et al. [122]	121	None	8.3	NR
2009	Zorn et al. [123]	1155	None	13	NR
2009	Feicke et al. [124]	99	None	7	NR
2009	Polcari et al. [125]	60	None	4.6	NR
2008	Patel et al. [126]	1500	None	4.3	53

CD Clavien–Dindo classification system [23], *MCD* modified Clavien–Dindo classification system [18], *NSQIP* The National Quality Improvement Program Classification System [103], *Martin* Martin classification system [19], *NR* not reported, *NA* not applicable

identified. Incontinence may be evaluated using the International Consultation of Incontinence Questionnaire-Urinary Incontinence (ICIQ-UI) [48, 96] or through the AUA Symptom score. Sexual dysfunction, including ED, may be estimated utilizing the Sexual Health Inventory for Men (SHIM) [48] or the International Index of Erectile Function (IIEF) questionnaires [97]. Once consensus can be achieved, universal questionnaires can be employed at predetermined time points.

Composite Indices (Combining Oncological, Functional Outcomes, and Complications)

A method to address oncological outcomes, complications, functional outcomes, and other areas of concern, the so-called *trifecta*, was suggested by Patel et al. [98] It was designed to represent a readily communicated index of the surgical outcomes of continence, potency, and cancer-free status. The concept of a trifecta is justified by

Patel et al. in light of the high number of younger patients who seek additional information regarding HRQOL after surgery, especially urinary, and sexual function [98, 99]. A subsequent modification of the trifecta concept has broadened the notion of an easily understood, comprehensive index to that of a *"pentafecta,"* with inclusion of no postoperative complications and negative surgical margins [100, 101]. It must be recognized, however, that a composite index is no more accurate than the accuracy of its individual components. Therefore, the individual components need to be accurately assessed and failure to do so compromises the entire comprehensive index. Consequently, reporting of each of the individual components of any composite index is still required.

Future

In the future, the parameters stored in the electronic health record may be available for extraction, thereby minimizing the cost and time-intensive process of individual chart review. This process, if routine and merged with a standardized reporting of complications, may be a prompt and objective method of determining accurate frequencies of complications. This would enable comparative effectiveness analyses between institutions, surgical procedures, and other treatment modalities for PCa.

Conclusion

- Multiple studies have shown that under most circumstances, the repetitive performance of a surgical technique results in decreased operative times and reduced complication rates [9, 27, 56]. In regards to RARP, the following conclusions can be made:
- Urologic surgery is moving toward more standardized reporting of postoperative adverse events by incorporating the classification of surgical complications of Clavien–Dindo and the modifications of Martin–Donat. This trend must be accelerated until it is universally recognized as a requisite for the reporting of complications.
- RARP is a safe procedure with most large series reporting no deaths. Overall, 10 % of patients develop complications. Most (~80 %) of these complications are evident within the first 30 days postoperatively.
- The most common early complications of RARP are postoperative anemia and bleeding requiring transfusion (<2 %).
- The most common delayed complications of RARP are bladder neck contracture (<1 %), and lymphocele formation (<1 %); both are usually treated endoscopically or with percutaneous drainage (Grade 3 by Clavien–Dindo).
- Oncological outcomes, functional outcomes, and complications represent critically important independent aspects of RARP. Each requires its own comprehensive, rational, and readily understandable standardized reporting system in order to allow accurate comparisons across surgeons, institutions, and surgical techniques.
- Functional outcomes including urinary incontinence and ED, considered as "complications" by patients, represent important aspects of RARP and should be qualitatively, and quantitatively assessed in order to accurately describe the true benefits and limitations of RARP.
- To date, a universal comprehensive method of obtaining and reporting functional outcomes is lacking. The level of concern regarding UI and ED postoperatively makes this a priority, for which a standardized reporting system is needed.

In this discussion, complications of RARP have been addressed. The implementation of a standardized urologic surgical reporting system for complications of RARP, and other urologic procedures, is a critical requirement for continued excellence in urologic patient care. Simply having systems and definitions is not enough. Researchers must advance the idea of routinely reporting complications, comprehensively, understandably, accurately, and in a standardized reporting framework. Urologists must demand this information in their investigation of new techniques, and in comparison with standard and older techniques. In answer to the question posed at the beginning of this chapter, we believe, substantial (measurable) progress, beyond that acknowledged secondary to simply advancing along the learning curve, has indeed been made in robot-assisted radical prostatectomy.

References

1. Berwick DM. Measuring surgical outcomes for improvement: was Codman wrong? JAMA. 2015; 313(5):469–70.
2. Fink AS, Campbell Jr DA, Mentzer Jr RM, et al. The National Surgical Quality Improvement Program in non-veterans administration hospitals: initial demonstration of feasibility. Ann Surg. 2002;236(3):344–53. discussion 353–344.
3. Donabedian A. The end results of health care: Ernest Codman's contribution to quality assessment and beyond. Milbank Q. 1989;67(2):233–56. discussion 257–267.
4. George AK, Srinivasan AK, Cho J, Sadek MA, Kavoussi LR. Surgical site infection rates following laparoscopic urological procedures. J Urol. 2011; 185(4):1289–93.
5. Cadiere GB, Himpens J, Germay O, et al. Feasibility of robotic laparoscopic surgery: 146 cases. World J Surg. 2001;25(11):1467–77.
6. Kaye DR, Mullins JK, Carter HB, Bivalacqua TJ. Robotic surgery in urological oncology: patient care or market share? Nat Rev Urol. 2015;12(1):55–60.
7. Barbash GI, Glied SA. New technology and health care costs—the case of robot-assisted surgery. N Engl J Med. 2010;363(8):701–4.
8. Barton MK. No cost or safety advantage to robot-assisted radical prostatectomy compared with open-procedure surgery for patients with prostate cancer. CA Cancer J Clin. 2014;64(5):293–4.
9. Schmitges J, Trinh QD, Abdollah F, et al. A population-based analysis of temporal perioperative complication rates after minimally invasive radical prostatectomy. Eur Urol. 2011;60(3):564–71.
10. Novara G, Ficarra V, Rosen RC, et al. Systematic review and meta-analysis of perioperative outcomes and complications after robot-assisted radical prostatectomy. Eur Urol. 2012;62(3):431–52.
11. Abbou CC, Hoznek A, Salomon L, et al. Remote laparoscopic radical prostatectomy carried out with a robot. Report of a case. Prog Urol. 2000;10(4):520–3.
12. Agarwal PK, Sammon J, Bhandari A, et al. Safety profile of robot-assisted radical prostatectomy: a standardized report of complications in 3317 patients. Eur Urol. 2011;59(5):684–98.
13. Guillonneau B, Rozet F, Cathelineau X, et al. Perioperative complications of laparoscopic radical prostatectomy: the Montsouris 3-year experience. J Urol. 2002;167(1):51–6.
14. Gawande AA, Thomas EJ, Zinner MJ, Brennan TA. The incidence and nature of surgical adverse events in Colorado and Utah in 1992. Surgery. 1999;126(1):66–75.
15. Pomposelli JJ, Gupta SK, Zacharoulis DC, Landa R, Miller A, Nanda R. Surgical complication outcome (SCOUT) score: a new method to evaluate quality of care in vascular surgery. J Vasc Surg. 1997;25(6):1007–14. discussion 1014–1005.
16. Veen MR, Lardenoye JW, Kastelein GW, Breslau PJ. Recording and classification of complications in a surgical practice. Eur J Surg. 1999;165(5):421–4. discussion 425.
17. Pillai SB, van Rij AM, Williams S, Thomson IA, Putterill MJ, Greig S. Complexity- and risk-adjusted model for measuring surgical outcome. Br J Surg. 1999;86(12):1567–72.
18. Clavien PA, Barkun J, de Oliveira ML, et al. The Clavien-Dindo classification of surgical complications: five-year experience. Ann Surg. 2009;250(2): 187–96.
19. Martin 2nd RC, Brennan MF, Jaques DP. Quality of complication reporting in the surgical literature. Ann Surg. 2002;235(6):803–13.
20. Gandaglia G, Trinh QD. Models of assessment of comparative outcomes of robot-assisted surgery: best evidence regarding the superiority or inferiority of robot-assisted radical prostatectomy. Urol Clin North Am. 2014;41(4):597–606.
21. Trotti A, Colevas AD, Setser A, et al. CTCAE v3.0: development of a comprehensive grading system for the adverse effects of cancer treatment. Semin Radiat Oncol. 2003;13(3):176–81.
22. Mitropoulos D, Artibani W, Graefen M, et al. Reporting and grading of complications after urologic surgical procedures: an ad hoc EAU guidelines panel assessment and recommendations. Eur Urol. 2012;61(2):341–9.
23. Clavien PA, Sanabria JR, Strasberg SM. Proposed classification of complications of surgery with examples of utility in cholecystectomy. Surgery. 1992; 111(5):518–26.
24. Donat SM. Standards for surgical complication reporting in urologic oncology: time for a change. Urology. 2007;69(2):221–5.
25. Dindo D, Demartines N, Clavien PA. Classification of surgical complications: a new proposal with evaluation in a cohort of 6336 patients and results of a survey. Ann Surg. 2004;240(2):205–13.
26. Zorn KC, Wille MA, Thong AE, et al. Continued improvement of perioperative, pathological and continence outcomes during 700 robot-assisted radical prostatectomies. Can J Urol. 2009;16(4):4742–9. discussion 4749.

27. Birkmeyer JD, Finks JF, O'Reilly A, et al. Surgical skill and complication rates after bariatric surgery. N Engl J Med. 2013;369(15):1434–42.
28. Gainsburg DM. Anesthetic concerns for robotic-assisted laparoscopic radical prostatectomy. Minerva Anestesiol. 2012;78(5):596–604.
29. Montorsi F, Wilson TG, Rosen RC, et al. Best practices in robot-assisted radical prostatectomy: recommendations of the Pasadena Consensus Panel. Eur Urol. 2012;62(3):368–81.
30. Weerakoon M, Papa N, Lawrentschuk N, et al. The current use of Active Surveillance in an Australian cohort of men: a pattern of care analysis from the Victorian Prostate Cancer Registry. BJU Int. 2015;115 Suppl 5:50–6.
31. Adams JB, Moore RG, Micali S, Marco AP, Kavoussi LR. Laparoscopic genitourinary surgery utilizing 20 mmHg intra-abdominal pressure. J Laparoendosc Adv Surg Tech A. 1999;9(2):131–4.
32. Coelho RF, Palmer KJ, Rocco B, et al. Early complication rates in a single-surgeon series of 2500 robotic-assisted radical prostatectomies: report applying a standardized grading system. Eur Urol. 2010;57(6):945–52.
33. Coelho RF, Rocco B, Patel MB, et al. Retropubic, laparoscopic, and robot-assisted radical prostatectomy: a critical review of outcomes reported by high-volume centers. J Endourol. 2010;24(12):2003–15.
34. George AK, Wimhofer R, Viola KV, et al. Utilization of a novel valveless trocar system during robotic-assisted laparoscopic prostatectomy. World J Urol. 2015;33(11):1695–9.
35. Kim SH, Yang HK, Lee JH, Lee ES. A retrospective analysis of incidence and its associated risk factors of upper urinary tract recurrence following radical cystectomy for bladder cancer with transitional cell carcinoma: the significance of local pelvic recurrence and positive lymph node. PLoS One. 2014; 9(5):e96467.
36. Geerts WH, Pineo GF, Heit JA, et al. Prevention of venous thromboembolism: the seventh ACCP conference on antithrombotic and thrombolytic therapy. Chest. 2004;126 Suppl 3:338S–400.
37. Secin FP, Jiborn T, Bjartell AS, et al. Multi-institutional study of symptomatic deep venous thrombosis and pulmonary embolism in prostate cancer patients undergoing laparoscopic or robot-assisted laparoscopic radical prostatectomy. Eur Urol. 2008;53(1):134–45.
38. Van Hemelrijck M, Adolfsson J, Garmo H, et al. Risk of thromboembolic diseases in men with prostate cancer: results from the population-based PCBaSe Sweden. Lancet Oncol. 2010;11(5):450–8.
39. Kim JY, Khavanin N, Rambachan A, McCarthy RJ, Mlodinow AS, De Oliveria Jr GS, et al. Surgical duration and risk of venous thromboembolism. JAMA Surg. 2015;150(2):110–7. doi:10.1001/jamasurg.2014.1841.
40. Tyritzis SI, Wallerstedt A, Steineck G, et al. Thromboembolic complications in 3,544 patients undergoing radical prostatectomy with or without lymph node dissection. J Urol. 2015;193(1):117–25.
41. Kilic OF, Borgers A, Kohne W, Musch M, Kropfl D, Groeben H. Effects of steep Trendelenburg position for robotic-assisted prostatectomies on intra- and extrathoracic airways in patients with or without chronic obstructive pulmonary disease. Br J Anaesth. 2015;114(1):70–6.
42. Olympio MA. Postoperative visual loss after robotic pelvic surgery. BJU Int. 2013;112(8):1060–1.
43. American Society of Anesthesiologists Task Force on Perioperative Visual Loss. Practice advisory for perioperative visual loss associated with spine surgery: an updated report by the American Society of Anesthesiologists Task Force on Perioperative Visual Loss. Anesthesiology. 2012;116(2):274–85.
44. Wen T, Deibert CM, Siringo FS, Spencer BA. Positioning-related complications of minimally invasive radical prostatectomies. J Endourol. 2014;28(6):660–7.
45. Kaushik D, High R, Clark CJ, LaGrange CA. Malfunction of the Da Vinci robotic system during robot-assisted laparoscopic prostatectomy: an international survey. J Endourol. 2010;24(4):571–5.
46. Andonian S, Okeke Z, Okeke DA, et al. Device failures associated with patient injuries during robot-assisted laparoscopic surgeries: a comprehensive review of FDA MAUDE database. Can J Urol. 2008;15(1):3912–6.
47. Chen CC, Ou YC, Yang CK, et al. Malfunction of the da Vinci robotic system in urology. Int J Urol. 2012;19(8):736–40.
48. Murphy DG, Bjartell A, Ficarra V, et al. Downsides of robot-assisted laparoscopic radical prostatectomy: limitations and complications. Eur Urol. 2010;57(5):735–46.
49. Lavery HJ, Thaly R, Albala D, et al. Robotic equipment malfunction during robotic prostatectomy: a multi-institutional study. J Endourol. 2008;22(9):2165–8.
50. Jhaveri JK, Penna FJ, Diaz-Insua M, Jeong W, Menon M, Peabody JO. Ureteral injuries sustained during robot-assisted radical prostatectomy. J Endourol. 2014;28(3):318–24.
51. Gonzalgo ML, Pavlovich CP, Trock BJ, Link RE, Sullivan W, Su LM. Classification and trends of perioperative morbidities following laparoscopic radical prostatectomy. J Urol. 2005;174(1):135–9. discussion 139.
52. Guillonneau B, Gupta R, El Fettouh H, Cathelineau X, Baumert H, Vallancien G. Laparoscopic [correction of laproscopic] management of rectal injury during laparoscopic [correction of laproscopic] radical prostatectomy. J Urol. 2003;169(5):1694–6.
53. Hung CF, Yang CK, Cheng CL, Ou YC. Bowel complication during robotic-assisted laparoscopic

radical prostatectomy. Anticancer Res. 2011;31(10): 3497–501.
54. Rabbani F, Yunis LH, Pinochet R, et al. Comprehensive standardized report of complications of retropubic and laparoscopic radical prostatectomy. Eur Urol. 2010;57(3):371–86.
55. Kowalczyk KJ, Levy JM, Caplan CF, et al. Temporal national trends of minimally invasive and retropubic radical prostatectomy outcomes from 2003 to 2007: results from the 100% Medicare sample. Eur Urol. 2012;61(4):803–9.
56. Trinh QD, Bjartell A, Freedland SJ, et al. A systematic review of the volume-outcome relationship for radical prostatectomy. Eur Urol. 2013;64(5):786–98.
57. Ficarra V, Cavalleri S, Novara G, Aragona M, Artibani W. Evidence from robot-assisted laparoscopic radical prostatectomy: a systematic review. Eur Urol. 2007;51(1):45–55. discussion 56.
58. Bhayani SB, Pavlovich CP, Strup SE, et al. Laparoscopic radical prostatectomy: a multi-institutional study of conversion to open surgery. Urology. 2004;63(1):99–102.
59. Weiner AB, Murthy P, Richards KA, Patel SG, Eggener SE. Population based analysis of incidence and predictors of open conversion during minimally invasive radical prostatectomy. J Urol. 2015;193(3):826–31.
60. Ozdemir AT, Altinova S, Koyuncu H, Serefoglu EC, Cimen IH, Balbay DM. The incidence of postoperative ileus in patients who underwent robotic assisted radical prostatectomy. Central Eur J Urol. 2014;67(1):19–24.
61. Ficarra V, Novara G, Artibani W, et al. Retropubic, laparoscopic, and robot-assisted radical prostatectomy: a systematic review and cumulative analysis of comparative studies. Eur Urol. 2009;55(5):1037–63.
62. Nelson B, Kaufman M, Broughton G, et al. Comparison of length of hospital stay between radical retropubic prostatectomy and robotic assisted laparoscopic prostatectomy. J Urol. 2007;177(3):929–31.
63. Krambeck AE, DiMarco DS, Rangel LJ, et al. Radical prostatectomy for prostatic adenocarcinoma: a matched comparison of open retropubic and robot-assisted techniques. BJU Int. 2009;103(4): 448–53.
64. Ploussard G, Briganti A, de la Taille A, et al. Pelvic lymph node dissection during robot-assisted radical prostatectomy: efficacy, limitations, and complications-a systematic review of the literature. Eur Urol. 2014;65(1):7–16.
65. Chennamsetty A, Hafron J, Edwards L, et al. Predictors of incisional hernia after robotic assisted radical prostatectomy. Adv Urol. 2015;2015:7.
66. Kang DI, Woo SH, Lee DH, Kim IY. Incidence of port-site hernias after robot-assisted radical prostatectomy with the fascial closure of only the midline 12-mm port site. J Endourol. 2012;26(7):848–51.
67. Stanford JL, Feng Z, Hamilton AS, et al. Urinary and sexual function after radical prostatectomy for clinically localized prostate cancer: the Prostate Cancer Outcomes Study. JAMA. 2000;283(3):354–60.
68. Berryhill Jr R, Jhaveri J, Yadav R, et al. Robotic prostatectomy: a review of outcomes compared with laparoscopic and open approaches. Urology. 2008; 72(1):15–23.
69. Touijer K, Eastham JA, Secin FP, et al. Comprehensive prospective comparative analysis of outcomes between open and laparoscopic radical prostatectomy conducted in 2003 to 2005. J Urol. 2008;179(5):1811–7. discussion 1817.
70. Ahlering TE, Gordon A, Morales B, Skarecky DW. Preserving continence during robotic prostatectomy. Curr Urol Rep. 2013;14(1):52–8.
71. Lavigueur-Blouin H, Noriega AC, Valdivieso R, et al. Predictors of early continence following robot-assisted radical prostatectomy. Can Urol Assoc J. 2015;9(1–2):e93–7.
72. Choi SK, Park S, Ahn H. Randomized clinical trial of a bladder neck plication stitch during robot-assisted radical prostatectomy. Asian J Androl. 2014.
73. Ficarra V, Novara G, Rosen RC, et al. Systematic review and meta-analysis of studies reporting urinary continence recovery after robot-assisted radical prostatectomy. Eur Urol. 2012;62(3):405–17.
74. El-Hakim A, Al-Hathal N, Al-Qaoud T, et al. Novel uroflow stop test at time of catheter removal is a strong predictor of early urinary continence recovery following robotic-assisted radical prostatectomy: a pilot study. NeurourolUrodyn. 2015;34(1):60–4.
75. Mungovan SF, Huijbers BP, Hirschhorn AD, Patel MI. What makes men leak? An investigation of objective and self-report measures of urinary incontinence early after radical prostatectomy. Neurourol Urodyn. 2016;35(2):225–9.
76. Tal R, Alphs HH, Krebs P, Nelson CJ, Mulhall JP. Erectile function recovery rate after radical prostatectomy: a meta-analysis. J Sex Med. 2009;6(9): 2538–46.
77. Srivastava A, Chopra S, Pham A, et al. Effect of a risk-stratified grade of nerve-sparing technique on early return of continence after robot-assisted laparoscopic radical prostatectomy. Eur Urol. 2013; 63(3):438–44.
78. Kang SG, Schatloff O, Haidar AM, et al. Does surgeon subjective nerve sparing score predict recovery time of erectile function following robot-assisted radical prostatectomy? J Sex Med. 2015;12(6): 1490–6.
79. Leape LL. Hospital readmissions following surgery: turning complications into "treasures". JAMA. 2015; 313(5):467–8.
80. Merkow RP, Ju MH, Chung JW, et al. Underlying reasons associated with hospital readmission following surgery in the United States. JAMA. 2015; 313(5):483–95.
81. Dimick JB, Ghaferi AA. Hospital readmission as a quality measure in surgery. JAMA. 2015;313(5): 512–3.
82. Morris MS, Deierhoi RJ, Richman JS, Altom LK, Hawn MT. The relationship between timing of

surgical complications and hospital readmission. JAMA Surg. 2014;149(4):348–54.
83. Etzioni DA, Wasif N, Dueck AC, et al. Association of hospital participation in a surgical outcomes monitoring program with inpatient complications and mortality. JAMA. 2015;313(5):505–11.
84. Osborne NH, Nicholas LH, Ryan AM, Thumma JR, Dimick JB. Association of hospital participation in a quality reporting program with surgical outcomes and expenditures for Medicare beneficiaries. JAMA. 2015;313(5):496–504.
85. Anderson JE, Chang DC. Using electronic health records for surgical quality improvement in the era of big data. JAMA Surg. 2015;150(1):24–9.
86. Ghani KR, Zheng K, Wei JT, Friedman CP. Harnessing big data for health care and research: are urologists ready? Eur Urol. 2014;66(6):975–7.
87. Hussein AA, Welty CJ, Broering J, Cooperberg MR, Carroll PR. National prostate cancer registries: contemporary trends of prostate cancer in the United States. Urol Pract. 2014;1(4):198–204.
88. American Urological Association to Launch the First National Level Urology Clinical Data Registry [press release]. http://www.auanet.org/advnews/press_releases/article.cfm?articleNo=332. AUA, Accessed 23 Oct 2013.
89. Chung JS, Kim WT, Ham WS, et al. Comparison of oncological results, functional outcomes, and complications for transperitoneal versus extraperitoneal robot-assisted radical prostatectomy: a single surgeon's experience. J Endourol. 2011;25(5):787–92.
90. Freire MP, Weinberg AC, Lei Y, et al. Anatomic bladder neck preservation during robotic-assisted laparoscopic radical prostatectomy: description of technique and outcomes. Eur Urol. 2009;56(6): 972–80.
91. Shikanov S, Woo J, Al-Ahmadie H, et al. Extrafascial versus interfascial nerve-sparing technique for robotic-assisted laparoscopic prostatectomy: comparison of functional outcomes and positive surgical margins characteristics. Urology. 2009;74(3):611–6.
92. Kowalczyk KJ, Huang AC, Hevelone ND, et al. Stepwise approach for nerve sparing without countertraction during robot-assisted radical prostatectomy: technique and outcomes. Eur Urol. 2011; 60(3):536–47.
93. Wu SD, Meeks JJ, Cashy J, Perry KT, Nadler RB. Suture versus staple ligation of the dorsal venous complex during robot-assisted laparoscopic radical prostatectomy. BJU Int. 2010;106(3):385–90.
94. Lei Y, Alemozaffar M, Williams SB, et al. Athermal division and selective suture ligation of the dorsal vein complex during robot-assisted laparoscopic radical prostatectomy: description of technique and outcomes. Eur Urol. 2011;59(2):235–43.
95. Strasberg SM, Linehan DC, Hawkins WG. The accordion severity grading system of surgical complications. Ann Surg. 2009;250(2):177–86.
96. Hajebrahimi S, Nourizadeh D, Hamedani R, Pezeshki MZ. Validity and reliability of the International Consultation on Incontinence Questionnaire-Urinary Incontinence Short Form and its correlation with urodynamic findings. Urol J. 2012;9(4):685–90.
97. Briganti A, Gallina A, Suardi N, et al. What is the definition of a satisfactory erectile function after bilateral nerve sparing radical prostatectomy? J Sex Med. 2011;8(4):1210–7.
98. Patel VR, Coelho RF, Chauhan S, et al. Continence, potency and oncological outcomes after robotic-assisted radical prostatectomy: early trifecta results of a high-volume surgeon. BJU Int. 2010;106(5):696–702.
99. Eastham JA, Scardino PT, Kattan MW. Predicting an optimal outcome after radical prostatectomy: the trifecta nomogram. J Urol. 2008;179(6):2207–10. discussion 2210–2201.
100. Patel VR, Sivaraman A, Coelho RF, et al. Pentafecta: a new concept for reporting outcomes of robot-assisted laparoscopic radical prostatectomy. Eur Urol. 2011;59(5):702–7.
101. Patel VR, Abdul-Muhsin HM, Schatloff O, et al. Critical review of "pentafecta" outcomes after robot-assisted laparoscopic prostatectomy in high-volume centres. BJU Int. 2011;108(6 Pt 2):1007–17.
102. Jeong CW, Lee JK, Oh JJ, et al. Effects of new 1-step posterior reconstruction method on recovery of continence after robot-assisted laparoscopic prostatectomy: results of a prospective, single-blind, parallel group, randomized, controlled trial. J Urol. 2015;193(3):935–42.
103. Pilecki MA, McGuire BB, Jain U, Kim JY, Nadler RB. National multi-institutional comparison of 30-day postoperative complication and readmission rates between open retropubic radical prostatectomy and robot-assisted laparoscopic prostatectomy using NSQIP. J Endourol. 2014;28(4):430–6.
104. Maddox M, Lasser M, Renzulli 2nd J, Haleblian G, Pareek G. An updated report on complications following robotic prostatectomy: results of an unbiased prospective database. J Endourol. 2013;27(5):554–9.
105. Rogers CG, Sammon JD, Sukumar S, Diaz M, Peabody J, Menon M. Robot assisted radical prostatectomy for elderly patients with high risk prostate cancer. Urol Oncol. 2013;31(2):193–7.
106. Sagalovich D, Calaway A, Srivastava A, Sooriakumaran P, Tewari AK. Assessment of required nodal yield in a high risk cohort undergoing extended pelvic lymphadenectomy in robotic-assisted radical prostatectomy and its impact on functional outcomes. BJU Int. 2013;111(1):85–94.
107. Ou YC, Yang CK, Wang J, et al. The trifecta outcome in 300 consecutive cases of robotic-assisted laparoscopic radical prostatectomy according to D'Amico risk criteria. Eur J Surg Oncol. 2013;39(1): 107–13.
108. Yuh BE, Ruel NH, Mejia R, Novara G, Wilson TG. Standardized comparison of robot-assisted limited and extended pelvic lymphadenectomy for prostate cancer. BJU Int. 2013;112(1):81–8.
109. Ahmed F, Rhee J, Sutherland D, Benjamin C, Engel J, Frazier 2nd H. Surgical complications after robot-

assisted laparoscopic radical prostatectomy: the initial 1000 cases stratified by the clavien classification system. J Endourol. 2012;26(2):135–9.
110. Yuh BE, Ruel NH, Mejia R, Wilson CM, Wilson TG. Robotic extended pelvic lymphadenectomy for intermediate- and high-risk prostate cancer. Eur Urol. 2012;61(5):1004–10.
111. Jung JH, Seo JW, Lim MS, et al. Extended pelvic lymph node dissection including internal iliac packet should be performed during robot-assisted laparoscopic radical prostatectomy for high-risk prostate cancer. J Laparoendosc Adv Surg Tech A. 2012;22(8):785–90.
112. van der Poel HG, de Blok W, Tillier C, van Muilekom E. Robot-assisted laparoscopic prostatectomy: nodal dissection results during the first 440 cases by two surgeons. J Endourol. 2012;26(12):1618–24.
113. Silberstein JL, Vickers AJ, Power NE, et al. Pelvic lymph node dissection for patients with elevated risk of lymph node invasion during radical prostatectomy: comparison of open, laparoscopic and robot-assisted procedures. J Endourol. 2012;26(6):748–53.
114. Jayram G, Decastro GJ, Large MC, et al. Robotic radical prostatectomy in patients with high-risk disease: a review of short-term outcomes from a high-volume center. J Endourol. 2011;25(3):455–7.
115. Davis JW, Shah JB, Achim M. Robot-assisted extended pelvic lymph node dissection (PLND) at the time of radical prostatectomy (RP): a video-based illustration of technique, results, and unmet patient selection needs. BJU Int. 2011;108(6 Pt 2):993–8.
116. Lallas CD, Pe ML, Thumar AB, et al. Comparison of lymph node yield in robot-assisted laparoscopic prostatectomy with that in open radical retropubic prostatectomy. BJU Int. 2011;107(7):1136–40.
117. Novara G, Ficarra V, D'Elia C, Secco S, Cavalleri S, Artibani W. Prospective evaluation with standardised criteria for postoperative complications after robotic-assisted laparoscopic radical prostatectomy. Eur Urol. 2010;57(3):363–70.
118. Jeong J, Choi EY, Kim IY. Clavien classification of complications after the initial series of robot-assisted radical prostatectomy: the Cancer Institute of New Jersey/Robert Wood Johnson Medical School experience. J Endourol. 2010;24(9):1457–61.
119. Yee DS, Katz DJ, Godoy G, et al. Extended pelvic lymph node dissection in robotic-assisted radical prostatectomy: surgical technique and initial experience. Urology. 2010;75(5):1199–204.
120. Katz DJ, Yee DS, Godoy G, Nogueira L, Chong KT, Coleman JA. Lymph node dissection during robotic-assisted laparoscopic prostatectomy: comparison of lymph node yield and clinical outcomes when including common iliac nodes with standard template dissection. BJU Int. 2010;106(3):391–6.
121. Cooperberg MR, Kane CJ, Cowan JE, Carroll PR. Adequacy of lymphadenectomy among men undergoing robot-assisted laparoscopic radical prostatectomy. BJU Int. 2010;105(1):88–92.
122. Ham WS, Park SY, Rha KH, Kim WT, Choi YD. Robotic radical prostatectomy for patients with locally advanced prostate cancer is feasible: results of a single-institution study. J Laparoendosc Adv Surg Tech A. 2009;19(3):329–32.
123. Zorn KC, Katz MH, Bernstein A, et al. Pelvic lymphadenectomy during robot-assisted radical prostatectomy: assessing nodal yield, perioperative outcomes, and complications. Urology. 2009;74(2):296–302.
124. Feicke A, Baumgartner M, Talimi S, et al. Robotic-assisted laparoscopic extended pelvic lymph node dissection for prostate cancer: surgical technique and experience with the first 99 cases. Eur Urol. 2009;55(4):876–83.
125. Polcari AJ, Hugen CM, Sivarajan G, et al. Comparison of open and robot-assisted pelvic lymphadenectomy for prostate cancer. J Endourol. 2009;23(8):1313–7.
126. Patel VR, Palmer KJ, Coughlin G, Samavedi S. Robot-assisted laparoscopic radical prostatectomy: perioperative outcomes of 1500 cases. J Endourol. 2008;22(10):2299–305.

Quality of Life Evaluation: What Is Published and Practical for Routine Use

25

Ashley J.F. Brandon, Matthew D. Ingham, Michael B. Williams, and Michael D. Fabrizio

Introduction

Three million men are currently living with prostate cancer in the United States alone. The 5-, 10-, and 15-year relative survival rates have risen sharply over the past 25 years to 99.7, 98.8, and 94.3 %, respectively; however one must take into account the lead-time bias stemming from the introduction of PSA testing in the late 1990s [1]. With pharmacologic and technologic advancements in treatment for both localized and metastatic prostate cancer, oncologic outcomes continue to improve. Unfortunately, most options for the treatment of prostate cancer, including active surveillance, have well-known side effects including urinary, sexual, gastrointestinal, hormonal, cardiovascular, and psychological effects. Each of these impact quality of life in the short, intermediate, and long term. As such, decision-making regarding the management for prostate cancer is complex and should take into consideration both oncologic as well as health-related quality of life (HRQOL) outcomes.

A.J.F. Brandon • M.D. Ingham, M.D.
M.B. Williams, M.D.
Department of Urology, Eastern Virginia Medical School, Norfolk, Virginia, USA

M.D. Fabrizio, M.D., F.A.C.S. (✉)
Eastern Virginia Medical School, Urology of Virginia, PLLC, Virginia Beach, VA, USA
e-mail: mfabrizio@urologyofva.net

It is well established that in men treated for localized prostate cancer, physician ratings of symptoms do not correlate well with patient self-assessments of HRQOL [2]. Therefore, numerous evaluation tools have been developed to help both patients and providers qualify and quantify these perceived effects and compare various treatment modalities. HRQOL assessments are helpful in a clinical setting but also allow for standardized comparison of various treatment modalities for research purposes and have been increasingly used as outcome measures in clinical trials.

HRQOL Assessment Tools

Health-related quality of life questionnaires have been developed to facilitate evaluation of patient's subjective perception of how treatment impacts their overall wellbeing. Unfortunately, overall patient satisfaction is difficult to measure and does not correlate well with measured HRQOL outcomes [3]. That being said, HRQOL questionnaires are routinely used in studies both pre- and posttreatment as self-assessment surveys to track HRQOL changes in order to compare treatment modalities. These tools have been increasingly shown to be both valid and reliable, making them an important supplement to traditional biologic and physiologic measures. Figure 25.1 demonstrates a model proposed by Wilson and colleagues that provides a classification scheme for

J.W. Davis (ed.), *Robot-Assisted Radical Prostatectomy*, DOI 10.1007/978-3-319-32641-2_25

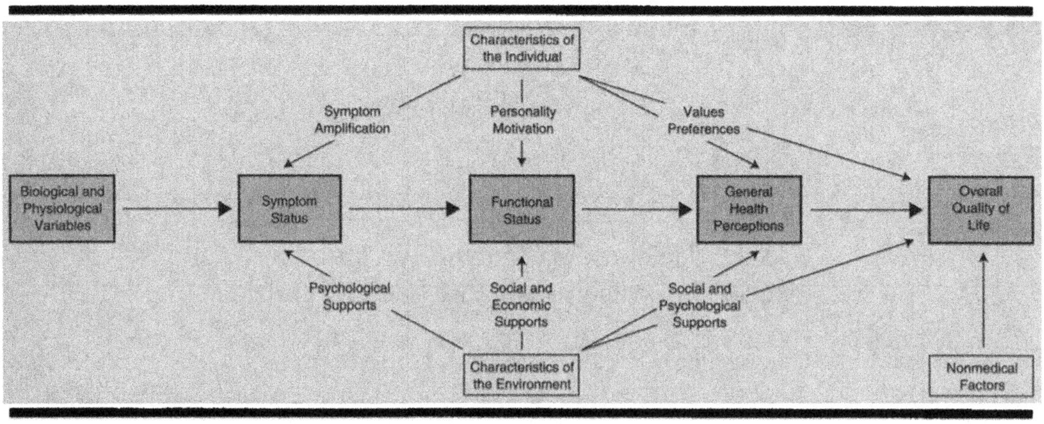

Fig. 25.1 Classification scheme for measures of health outcomes [4]

different measures of health outcomes divided into five levels: biological and physiological factors, symptoms, functional status, general health perceptions, and overall quality of life. These factors are not independent and are influenced by characteristics of the individual and environment that cannot be controlled by clinicians or the health care system [4]. As such, well-designed HRQOL assessment tools are designed to capture this interplay with the ultimate goal of improving patient-related clinical outcomes.

Original HRQOL questionnaires used in prostate cancer research were generic, being used for assessment in many diseases. Over time, these forms have been adapted for the disease-specific purpose of evaluating outcomes specific to the treatment of prostate cancer. Over the past decade, there has been a significant increase in the number of HRQOL assessment tools available, each with a specific emphasis. As such, algorithms have been proposed to assist researchers with their selection of questionnaire to fit the research goal of their specific study [5]. When comparing each HRQOL questionnaire, the quality of the tool must also be taken into consideration. A number of criteria exist, including content validity, internal consistency, criterion validity, construct validity, reproducibility, responsiveness, floor and ceiling effects, and interpretability. Utilizing these variables, Hamoen et al. evaluated the most frequently utilized HRQOL questionnaires in the literature to quantify their quality and validity (Table 25.1) [6].

Within prostate cancer research literature, the most commonly used generic HRQOL questionnaires include the European Organization for Research and Treatment of Cancer (EORTC) quality of life questionnaire core 30, Short Form-36 (SF-36), and Functional Assessment of Cancer Therapy-General (FACT-G) [6]. The three most commonly used prostate cancer-specific questionnaires include the Expanded Prostate Cancer Index Composite (EPIC), UCLA-Prostate Cancer Index (UCLA-PCI), and Functional Assessment of Cancer Therapy-Prostate (FACT-P) [6]. Hamoen et al. recommend the use of the UCLA-PCI, prostate cancer-specific questionnaire 94, or FACT-P as prostate cancer-specific instruments considering the psychometric properties [6]. However, some questionnaires are felt to be long and arduous for some patients and practicality does come into play. Based on this, recommendations for EPIC-26, PC-QOL, and UCLA-PCI stood out as the best choices with strong psychometrics and short duration [7].

The UCLA-PCI was the first prostate cancer-specific questionnaire developed and validated by Litwin et al. in the mid-1990s. It is a comprehensive measure of HRQOL for men with localized prostate cancer that can be self-administered in approximately 20 min. With primary focus on urinary, sexual, and bowel function and bother,

Table 25.1 Psychometrics of the HRQoL questionnaires used in patients with prostate cancer (method or result was rated as += good; ?=doubtful;–=poor; 0=no data available)

Instrument	Content validity	Internal consistency	Criterion validity	Construct validity	Reproducibility	Responsiveness	Floor and ceiling effects	Interpretability	Total score
General									
MOS-20	?	+	?	?	0	0	?	0	1
QLI Ferrans and Powers	+	+	?	0	+	0	0	0	3
QLI Padilla	?	+	0	0	+	0	0	0	2
SF-12	?	0	+	+	+	0	0	+	4
SF-36	?	+	0	+	0	0	–	+	2
SWLS	?	+	?	0	+	0	0	0	2
WHOQOL	?	+	?	+	+	?	0	0	3
Cancer									
CARES-SF	+	+	+	+	+	?	0	0	5
FACT-G	+	+	?	+	+	0	0	+	5
FLIC	+	+	?	0	0	0	0	0	2
QLQ-C30	?	+	0	+	0	+	0	+	4
Selby	+	+	?	0	+	?	0	0	3
Prostate cancer									
Cleary	?	+	0	?	0	0	0	0	1
EPIC	+	+	?	0	+	0	?	0	3
FACT-P	+	+	0	?	0	+	0	+	4
Pc-QoL	+	+	?	0	+	0	0	0	3
PORPUS-P	+	0	?	?	+	0	0	+	3
QLQ-PR25	+	+	?	?	0	?	–	?	1
QUFW94	+	+	0	0	+	+	0	0	4
UCLA-PCI	+	+	?	+	+	+	–	0	4

Total score was calculated as follows: each positive-rated property yielded 1 point, each doubtful property 0 points, each negative property –1 point, and when no information was available, no points were assigned

FLIC functional living index–cancer, *MOS-20* 20-item short form health survey, *Pc-Qol* prostate cancer quality of life scale, *PORPUS-P* patient-oriented prostate utility scale–psychometric, *QLQ-PR25* quality of life questionnaire for prostate cancer patients, *SWLS* satisfaction with life scale, *WHOQOL* World Health Organization Quality of Life the instrument contains six disease-targeted domains. This 20-item survey is easy to understand, has good responsiveness, demonstrates construct, and content validity, and is reproducible. Scoring for this system is based on established algorithms with scores ranging from 0 (worst) to 100 (best). Per the authors, it is best used in conjunction with the eight general domains of the SF-36 [8]. It has been validated in multiple languages and has been used in many multicenter prospective trials including the community-based Cancer of the Prostate Strategic Urologic Research Endeavor (CaPSURE) cohort [9]. This tool is free for use and downloadable with instruction on usage and scoring at http://www.proqolid.org/instruments/ucla_prostate_cancer_index_ucla_pci. See Index 25.1 for questionnaire.

The EPIC was developed and validated in 2000 and expands upon the UCLA-PCI. The original form includes 50 items and is more robust in that it also includes hormonal and urinary bother domains to facilitate a more comprehensive assessment of prostate cancer-related HRQOL [10]. This allows for assessment of HRQOL outcomes for treatment modalities such as ADT and brachytherapy. Unfortunately, the form is more time consuming for patients and thus less practical for use in a routine assessment outside of research. EPIC-26 is an abbreviated version of this questionnaire that collapses the function and bother of each domain and has been used in a few prostate cancer studies [3, 7].

QOL Outcomes Based on Treatment Modality for Localized Prostate Cancer

Brachytherapy

Brachytherapy is a good option for men with localized prostate cancer either as a monotherapy or combined with other treatment modalities such as external beam radiation or hormonal therapy. This option particularly appeals to men who are not ideal surgical candidates or those interested in a less invasive option. Most commonly reported side effects from brachytherapy include bowel irritation, voiding symptoms, and sexual side effects. More unique to this treatment modality, brachytherapy patients have a higher risk for postprocedure urinary retention with rates as high as 34 % at 1 week after the procedure, and 29, 18, and 10 % at 1, 3, and 6 months, respectively [11]. Additionally, although most acute voiding symptoms tend to peak in the first month and return to baseline after 1 year following seed placement (I-125), a transient late exacerbation of urinary symptoms has been shown to occur in up to half of all patients by 5 years [12].

Several studies using HRQOL questionnaires to compare patient-related outcomes show that brachytherapy has a statistically significant higher rate of obstructive and irritative urinary symptoms compared to other modalities [3, 13]. Specifically, large prostate size and adjuvant hormonal therapy exacerbated urinary irritation after brachytherapy or radiotherapy [3]. In contrast, another study utilizing the UCLA-PCI questionnaire showed that patients undergoing brachytherapy as a monotherapy had overall significantly better urinary bother and function scores and a threefold higher rate of return to baseline urinary function over a mean follow-up period of 24 months as compared to prostatectomy and cryoablation [14]. Both brachytherapy and external beam radiotherapy (EBRT) have higher rates of bowel-related distress and dysfunction including rectal urgency, frequency, pain, fecal incontinence, or hematochezia compared to radical prostatectomy; however, the duration of these symptoms tend to dissipate over time [3, 13, 14]. Brachytherapy has consistently shown an advantage in the sexual function domain over several longitudinal patient reported HRQOL studies and a fivefold higher rate of return to baseline function when compared to radical prostatectomy [3, 13, 14]. However, all of the reported studies have a relatively short follow-up of approximately 24 months. In the longer term, HRQOL data collected prospectively in the CaPSURE study, a nationwide prostate cancer registry, identified no significant differences in sexual function and bother between surgical and nonsurgical treatments at 5 years and beyond [15].

External Beam Radiotherapy

Like brachytherapy, EBRT is a good option for patients desiring less invasive treatment and can be used with or without hormonal therapy. As with brachytherapy, HRQOL studies indicate an increased rate of bowel-related bother and dysfunction [3, 13, 14]. Further, this is not just limited to the patient as spousal bother was significantly impacted as it related to the patient's bowel symptoms after radiotherapy [3]. Of importance for bother, short-term follow-up is the only time frame when bowel-related symptoms are identified. Following 10-years, the effects are no longer identified among any of the various treatment modalities [15]. In general, urinary symptoms were lessened and sexual function was improved after EBRT as compared to radical prostatectomy and brachytherapy [13]. Long-term recovery of sexual function was worse in patients who received androgen-suppression therapy than in those who received radiotherapy alone [3]. However, as with brachytherapy, overall sexual function was equal amongst all treatment modalities at 5- and 10-year follow-up [13].

Cryotherapy

As of 1996, the role of cryotherapy in primary treatment of localized prostate cancer was deemed an option by the AUA. An AUA Best Practice Statement published in 2008 summarizes the data on cryosurgery for the treatment of localized prostate cancer including quality of life data. Compared to other modalities for primary treatment of localized prostate cancer, there are relatively fewer patients undergoing this treatment modality and likewise fewer studies published evaluating cryotherapy in longitudinal patient reported HRQOL. One study demonstrates that cryosurgery has a higher negative impact compared to brachytherapy for both sexual and urinary function at 3 months, however after 6 months, the impact on urinary function was equivalent [16]. Similarly, cryotherapy demonstrates a threefold rate of return to baseline voiding function compared to radical prostatectomy with overall decreased urinary bother scores after 1 year [14]. In several studies, postprocedure sexual function remained comparatively poor in the cryotherapy group compared to other modalities which may be related to both poor baseline sexual function as well as physiologic properties related to the treatment itself [14, 16, 17]. In order to achieve maximal benefit from this treatment, the cryotherapy iceball must extend outside the prostatic capsule causing collateral damage to the neurovascular bundles. As such, this treatment is recommended for those patients with poor baseline erectile function or those patients not concerned about sexual function.

Radical Prostatectomy

Due to the nature of surgery, much of the negative impact on HRQOL measures such as voiding function and bother, sexual function and bother, and overall wellbeing is seen up front immediately following the procedure but tends to improve over time. As such, it is important to examine and compare the early, intermediate, and long-term effects following radical prostatectomy as they relate to quality of life when drawing comparisons between each treatment modality for localized prostate cancer.

In general, worse urinary control outcomes are noted following radical prostatectomy compared to those of brachytherapy and external beam radiation. Several longitudinal HRQOL studies comparing various treatment modalities show that patients undergoing open radical retropubic prostatectomy had lower urinary function QOL scores at a relatively short follow-up interval of approximately 24 months [13, 14]. Specifically, rates of urinary incontinence in the early postoperative period are much higher after radical prostatectomy with the most significant decline in function noted within the first year after surgery, followed by a period of recovery up to the 2-year mark, followed by a plateau. Long-term follow-up data show that this overall decrease in urinary function remains persistent at 10-years following surgery [15]. Interestingly, in the Prostate Cancer Outcomes Study (PCOS), there was no longer a difference noted between radical prostatectomy and external beam radiation at 15 years following treatment but a demonstrable overall decline in function in both treatment arms [18]. Of importance to note, both the PCOS and CaPSURE long-term HRQOL studies measured urinary function using the UCLA-PCI, which focuses primarily on urinary incontinence as a measure of function rather than irritative or obstructive symptoms. As such, the impact of surgery on urinary function is emphasized to a greater extent using this scale compared to the impact of radiation or local tumor progression [15, 18]. In men with severe preoperative lower urinary tract symptoms based on AUA symptom score, robotic prostatectomy demonstrates a statistically significant improvement in urinary symptoms and increased quality of life scores postoperatively in both short and long term [19]. This effect is not unique to robotic prostatectomy and has been demonstrated numerous times with all forms of radical prostatectomy compared to other treatment modalities including watchful waiting [3, 20]. There is no clear difference between nerve-sparing prostatectomy compared to non-nerve-sparing prostatectomy related to HRQOL voiding domains [15].

Sexual function and bother outcomes also tend to be worse for radical prostatectomy patients compared to other treatment modalities including brachytherapy, external beam radiation, watchful waiting, and active surveillance in short- and intermediate-term follow-up [3, 13–15]. These outcomes tend to be mitigated by implementation of nerve-sparing techniques [3, 15]. As expected, non-nerve-sparing surgery was associated with lower sexual function scores at all periods in time up to 5 years following prostatectomy compared to nerve-sparing procedures [15]. Analysis of long-term CaPSURE data shows, as with urinary function, there was significant decline in sexual function noted over the first year after prostatectomy, followed by a period of recovery in the second year and then a plateau in function. Interestingly, at 5-year follow-up, sexual bother was not different in nonsurgical groups compared to patients who underwent nerve-sparing radical prostatectomy [15]. Though PCOS showed an initial difference in the incidence of erectile dysfunction at 2 and 5 years following radical prostatectomy versus external beam radiation, this difference was lost at the 15 year follow-up likely due to both groups having such poor overall sexual function with erectile dysfunction rates as high as 87 and 95 %, respectively [18].

Within the domain of bowel bother and function, no significant decline was seen after radical prostatectomy with essentially immediate return to baseline function with no significant change in bother postoperatively [3, 13, 14]. However, the overall scale of impact within this domain was relatively low for all treatment modalities including brachytherapy, radiotherapy, and cryotherapy therefore there may be little clinically significant advantage to surgery in this realm [14]. Other studies with longer interval follow-up demonstrate a decreased rate of bowel urgency at 2- and 5-years following prostatectomy but no difference at 15-years between radical prostatectomy and external beam radiation [18].

Open radical retropubic prostatectomy is classically considered the gold standard of surgical management for treatment of localized prostate cancer but its overall frequency of use is decreasing as surgeons begin to embrace minimally invasive techniques. Each of these techniques require a patient to be an adequate surgical candidate, a postoperative recovery period requiring hospital admission, and Foley catheter to remain in place over a period of time postoperatively. Despite these similarities, there are notable differences between open and robotic prostatectomy that have been routinely demonstrated in nearly all studies comparing the two approaches. Robotic prostatectomy shows consistent advantages over the open procedure with shorter hospitalization, decreased blood loss, and lower transfusion rates [21]. In contrast, innumerable studies demonstrate no clear advantage to robot assisted prostatectomy vs. open radical prostatectomy from the standpoint of HRQOL and oncologic outcomes [14, 21].

Laparoscopic prostatectomy was introduced in the late 1990s but was not widely embraced by many centers due to the technical nature of the procedure and difficult learning curve. The first robotic prostatectomy was performed shortly thereafter in 2001. It quickly became popular in the United States, but was less commonly performed in Europe and Scandinavia where laparoscopic prostatectomy was embraced primarily for cost reasons. In a prospective trial performed in Oslo, Norway where laparoscopic prostatectomy was routinely performed, HRQOL data was collected comparing patients undergoing robotic vs. laparoscopic prostatectomy as the surgeons transitioned from one modality to the other. There was no significant difference in quality of life outcomes noted between the two modalities at any follow-up time interval up to 36 months [22].

As experience with robotic prostatectomy grows, modifications in techniques have been reported, some of which demonstrate improvement in quality of life-related outcomes. For example, posterior reconstruction of Denonvilliers' fascia prior to vesicourethral anastomosis, which was initially described by Rocco et al. for laparoscopic surgery, has been modified and utilized in robotic prostatectomy [23]. This technique has been shown to improve baseline score for urinary bother and function as well as AUA symptom score at 3-months with early return to baseline continence [24]. Similarly, a prospective randomized trial showed that combing posterior reconstruction with anterior suspension of the urethra during robotic prostatectomy led to improved early continence at 1- and 3-months after surgery compared to the control group, although there was no significant improvement in very early (15 days) and late (6 months) continence using UCLA-PCI HRQOL metrics [25]. Bladder neck preservation has also been described to improve mean urinary function using the EPIC urinary function scale at 4-month and 24-month follow-up (but no significant difference at 12-months) compared to traditional dissection, with no effect on positive margin rate [26].

New and modified intraoperative techniques, devices, and biologic agents continue to be developed, tested, and utilized during robotic prostatectomy in order to optimize quality of life outcomes such as sexual and urinary function. Likewise, postoperative interventions such as pelvic floor exercises and penile rehabilitation are also being employed to optimize postoperative outcomes. HRQOL metrics using validated questionnaires will help to standardize research outcome data and allow for easier comparison amongst these techniques and interventions.

Practical Clinical Assessment of Quality of Life

Urologists routinely underestimate the impact of treatment for prostate cancer by consistently under recognizing its impairment of the patient's quality of life. Significant differences are noted in physicians' reports of patient outcomes compared to patient self-reported outcomes using validated HRQOL questionnaires [2, 27]. This was seen in all clinical domains from sexual, urinary, and bowel function, to fatigue to bone pain; however, greater discordance was seen in the realm of pain and fatigue symptoms as this is often under assessed in the clinical setting [2]. Long-term follow-up of CaPSURE patients shows that this trend in symptom minimization persists over time [2]. Validated patient self-reporting tools will be critical in making accurate assessments regarding impact on quality of life as the number and life expectancy of prostate cancer survivors increases.

For the purposes of prostate cancer research, standardized HRQOL questionnaires such as UCLA-PCI and EPIC are comprehensive and validated tools that provide reasonably accurate assessments of each domain related to bowel, bladder, and sexual function and bother. For practical and routine use, these questionnaires are time consuming for the patients and practitioners to score and analyze in order to be useful tools to assess HRQOL and individualize treatment-related decisions. As such, efforts have been made to modify existing tools by decreasing the complexity and length of the questionnaires while still maintaining the overall integrity, validity, and predictive qualities of the patient-related outcomes questionnaire. EPIC-CP is a validated 16-question single page questionnaire that takes patients only 2–5 min to complete and is designed specifically for clinical point of care use. Compared to EPIC-26, which takes 15 min to complete, the scoring system is far less complex with scores ranging from 0 to 12 (compared to 0–100) and can be easily scored in the office setting. Minimal important differences have been defined within each domain including urinary incontinence, urinary obstruction, bowel, sexual, and vitality/hormonal which are indicative of a clinically meaningful change [28].

Other validated questionnaires such as ISI (Incontinence Symptom Index), AUA symptom index, IIEF (International Index of Erectile Function) and SHIM (Sexual Health Inventory for Men) are also routinely used in clinical practice to monitor and trend patient-related outcomes each relating to a single specific domain. For further simplification, some investigators have proposed a shift from the complex questionnaire to a single surrogate interview-based question. In one particular study, patients were asked to score their erectile function on a scale of 1–5 scale as follows: (1) normal, full erection, always capable of penetration; (2) full erection, but diminished from normal, always capable of penetration; (3) partial erection, occasionally satisfactory for intercourse; (4) partial erection, unsatisfactory for intercourse; and (5) absence of any erection. These responses were then compared to use of IIEF in patients who underwent radical prostatectomy and were found to be highly correlative with the IIEF erectile function domain score [29]. In contrast, another study comparing patient interview scores with questionnaire-based domains for continence and erectile function found poor correlation between the two with evidence of underreporting in the interview-based format [30]. Although the above instruments may be more practical for routine clinical use, the focus of each tool is relatively narrow and is not specifically designed to fully capture the broader assessment of HRQOL measures associated with the treatment of localized prostate.

Summary/Conclusions

Within the changing landscape of health care, HRQOL assessments may not only be important for helping patients and providers with medical decision making, but may also eventually be tied to monetary reimbursement in a "pay-for-performance" model. In this model, clinicians are financially incentivized to optimize outcomes by improving measurable improvements in patient health. In the realm of treatment of localized prostate cancer, given that the oncologic outcomes for each given treatment modality are similar, HRQOL may become the measurable differentiating factor used by third parties to gauge outcomes and distribute financial reimbursement. In addition, patient-related outcomes for an individual provider might eventually be disclosed to the public much like the push to disclose surgical complication rates and overall patient satisfaction data in an effort to allow patients to make an informed decision when selecting a provider. As such, the evaluation of, and focus on, health-related quality of life must not be underemphasized.

References

1. DeSantis CE, Lin CC, Mariotto AB, Siegel RL, Stein KD, Kramer JL, et al. Cancer treatment and survivorship statistics, 2014. CA Cancer J Clin. 2014;64(4):252–71.
2. Sonn GA, Sadetsky N, Presti JC, Litwin MS. Differing perceptions of quality of life in patients with prostate cancer and their doctors. J Urol. 2009;182(5): 2296–302.
3. Sanda MG, Dunn RL, Michalski J, Sandler HM, Northouse L, Hembroff L, et al. Quality of life and satisfaction with outcome among prostate-cancer survivors. N Engl J Med. 2008;358(12):1250–61.
4. Wilson IB, Cleary PD. Linking clinical variables with health-related quality of life. A conceptual model of patient outcomes. JAMA. 1995;273(1):59–65.
5. Luckett T, King MT. Choosing patient-reported outcome measures for cancer clinical research—practical principles and an algorithm to assist non-specialist researchers. Eur J Cancer. 2010;46(18):3149–57.
6. Hamoen EH, De Rooij M, Witjes JA, Barentsz JO, Rovers MM. Measuring health-related quality of life in men with prostate cancer: a systematic review of the most used questionnaires and their validity. Urol Oncol. 2015;33(2):69.
7. Rnic K, Linden W, Tudor I, Pullmer R, Vodermaier A. Measuring symptoms in localized prostate cancer: a systematic review of assessment instruments. Prostate Cancer Prostatic Dis. 2013;16(2):111–22.
8. Litwin MS, Hays RD, Fink A, Ganz PA, Leake B, Brook RH. The UCLA Prostate Cancer Index:

development, reliability, and validity of a health-related quality of life measure. Med Care. 1998;36(7):1002–12.
9. Hu JC, Elkin EP, Pasta DJ, Lubeck DP, Kattan MW, Carroll PR, et al. Predicting quality of life after radical prostatectomy: results from CaPSURE. J Urol. 2004;171(2 Pt 1):703–7. discussion 7–8.
10. Wei JT, Dunn RL, Litwin MS, Sandler HM, Sanda MG. Development and validation of the expanded prostate cancer index composite (EPIC) for comprehensive assessment of health-related quality of life in men with prostate cancer. Urology. 2000;56(6):899–905.
11. Locke J, Ellis W, Wallner K, Cavanagh W, Blasko J. Risk factors for acute urinary retention requiring temporary intermittent catheterization after prostate brachytherapy: a prospective study. Int J Radiat Oncol Biol Phys. 2002;52(3):712–9.
12. Cesaretti JA, Stone NN, Stock RG. Urinary symptom flare following I-125 prostate brachytherapy. Int J Radiat Oncol Biol Phys. 2003;56(4):1085–92.
13. Litwin MS, Gore JL, Kwan L, Brandeis JM, Lee SP, Withers HR, et al. Quality of life after surgery, external beam irradiation, or brachytherapy for early-stage prostate cancer. Cancer. 2007;109(11):2239–47.
14. Malcolm JB, Fabrizio MD, Barone BB, Given RW, Lance RS, Lynch DF, et al. Quality of life after open or robotic prostatectomy, cryoablation or brachytherapy for localized prostate cancer. J Urol. 2010;183(5):1822–9.
15. Punnen S, Cowan JE, Chan JM, Carroll PR, Cooperberg MR. Long-term health-related quality of life after primary treatment for localized prostate cancer: results from the CaPSURE registry. Eur Urol. 2015;68(4):600–8.
16. Ball AJ, Gambill B, Fabrizio MD, Davis JW, Given RW, Lynch DF, et al. Prospective longitudinal comparative study of early health-related quality-of-life outcomes in patients undergoing surgical treatment for localized prostate cancer: a short-term evaluation of five approaches from a single institution. J Endourol. 2006;20(10):723–31.
17. Hubosky SG, Fabrizio MD, Schellhammer PF, Barone BB, Tepera CM, Given RW. Single center experience with third-generation cryosurgery for management of organ-confined prostate cancer: critical evaluation of short-term outcomes, complications, and patient quality of life. J Endourol. 2007;21(12):1521–31.
18. Resnick MJ, Koyama T, Fan K-H, Albertsen PC, Goodman M, Hamilton AS, et al. Long-term functional outcomes after treatment for localized prostate cancer. N Engl J Med. 2013;368(5):436–45.
19. Gordon A, Skarecky DW, Ahlering T. Long-term outcomes in severe lower urinary tract symptoms in men undergoing robotic-assisted radical prostatectomy. Urology. 2014;84(4):826–31.
20. Steineck G, Helgesen F, Adolfsson J, Dickman PW, Johansson JE, Norlen BJ, et al. Quality of life after radical prostatectomy or watchful waiting. N Engl J Med. 2002;347(11):790–6.
21. Alemozaffar M, Sanda M, Yecies D, Mucci LA, Stampfer MJ, Kenfield SA. Benchmarks for operative outcomes of robotic and open radical prostatectomy: results from the health professionals follow-up study. Eur Urol. 2015;67(3):432–8.
22. Berge V, Berg RE, Hoff JR, Wessel N, Diep LM, Karlsen SJ, et al. A prospective study of transition from laparoscopic to robot-assisted radical prostatectomy: quality of life outcomes after 36-month follow-up. Urology. 2013;81(4):781–6.
23. Rocco B, Gregori A, Stener S, Santoro L, Bozzola A, Galli S, et al. Posterior reconstruction of the rhabdosphincter allows a rapid recovery of continence after transperitoneal videolaparoscopic radical prostatectomy. Eur Urol. 2007;51(4):996–1003.
24. Brien JC, Barone B, Fabrizio M, Given R. Posterior reconstruction before vesicourethral anastomosis in patients undergoing robot-assisted laparoscopic prostatectomy leads to earlier return to baseline continence. J Endourol. 2011;25(3):441–5.
25. Hurtes X, Roupret M, Vaessen C, Pereira H, Faivre d'Arcier B, Cormier L, et al. Anterior suspension combined with posterior reconstruction during robot-assisted laparoscopic prostatectomy improves early return of urinary continence: a prospective randomized multicentre trial. BJU Int. 2012;110(6):875–83.
26. Freire MP, Weinberg AC, Lei Y, Soukup JR, Lipsitz SR, Prasad SM, et al. Anatomic bladder neck preservation during robotic-assisted laparoscopic radical prostatectomy: description of technique and outcomes. Eur Urol. 2009;56(6):972–80.
27. Litwin MS, Lubeck DP, Henning JM, Carroll PR. Differences in urologist and patient assessments of health related quality of life in men with prostate cancer: results of the CaPSURE database. J Urol. 1998;159(6):1988–92.
28. Chipman JJ, Sanda MG, Dunn RL, Wei JT, Litwin MS, Crociani CM, et al. Measuring and predicting prostate cancer related quality of life changes using EPIC for clinical practice. J Urol. 2014;191(3):638–45.
29. Tal R, Rabbani F, Scardino PT, Mulhall JP. Measuring erectile function after radical prostatectomy: comparing a single question with the International Index of Erectile Function. BJU Int. 2012;109(3):414–7.
30. van der Poel HG, Tillier C, de Blok WM, Acar C, van Muilekom EH, van den Bergh RC. Interview-based versus questionnaire-based quality of life outcomes before and after prostatectomy. J Endourol. 2013;27(11):1411–6.

Positive Surgical Margins: How to Self-Evaluate and Improve

26

Stephen B. Williams, Christopher E. Bayne, and Brian F. Chapin

Introduction

Robot-assisted laparoscopic radical prostatectomy (RALRP) has become the most common approach to radical prostatectomy (RP) in the United States. With nearly 90 % of radical prostatectomies being performed robotically, some argue RALRP has become the new standard of care [1, 2]. Robot assistance has been shown to reduce operative time compared with laparoscopic radical prostatectomy (LRP) and, in general, it has liberated LRP to non-fellowship-trained urologists at non-high-volume centers [3, 4]. Several reports have attempted to characterize the "learning curve" associated with RALRP. Metrics used to characterize the RALRP learning curve have ranged from operative time and blood loss to positive surgical margin (PSM) rate. Learning curves have been reported to range from 30 to over 200 cases [5, 6]. Although a comprehensive learning curve for open radical retropubic prostatectomy (RRP) was recently delineated by a high-quality, multicenter study, a comprehensive RALRP-specific learning curve has not been clearly defined [7–9].

PSM status is a significant predictor of biochemical recurrence (BCR) after RP and has implications in quality and cost of care [10]. Unlike other predictors of BCR, such as prostate-specific antigen (PSA) velocity and tumor grade and stage, surgical technique influences PSM status. PSM is defined as cancerous cells present at the inked margin and can be considered iatrogenic if the PSM occurs at a location without extraprostatic extention (EPE) of the tumor. As such, PSMs after RP in cases of organ-confined prostate cancer (PCa) may serve as a surgical quality indicator and introduce the need for otherwise unnecessary adjuvant therapy. Level 1 evidence demonstrates a survival advantage when adjuvant radiotherapy is administered following RP with PSM [11]. Consequently, PSMs increase the cost of treating PCa not only at the time of BCR but also in the adjuvant setting.

Aside from single center studies, literature comparing surgical margin outcomes in minimally invasive RP to open RRP is limited [12]. Some have contended tactile sensation permitted during RRP allows better assessment of the tumor extent than with minimally invasive approaches, potentially resulting in fewer PSMs and better cancer control [13].

With RALRP so rapidly adopted, surgeons and trainees must develop ways to assess and improve their technique. PSM is an ideal model for assessment as it is often a consequence of

S.B. Williams, M.D.
Department of Urology, The University of Texas MD Anderson Cancer Center, Houston, TX, USA

C.E. Bayne, M.D.
Department of Urology, The George Washington University, Washington, DC, USA

B.F. Chapin, M.D. (✉)
Department of Urology, The University of Texas MD Anderson Cancer Center, Houston, TX, USA

1515 Holcombe Blvd, Unit 1373,
Houston, TX 77030, USA
e-mail: bfchapin@mdanderson.org

J.W. Davis (ed.), *Robot-Assisted Radical Prostatectomy*, DOI 10.1007/978-3-319-32641-2_26

surgical technique and has direct oncologic implications. The central objective of this chapter is to explore mechanisms by which surgeons can learn to improve their surgical margin positivity via individual benchmarks for improvement.

RP Surgical Margin Variability

RP is a complex procedure with a series of calculated steps. The goals of the procedure, whether performed open or with robot assistance, are cancer control, preservation of urinary continence and erectile function, and avoidance of perioperative complications. While the literature contains several publications addressing the subject of PSM rates following RALRP and RRP, controversy exists as to whether either approach lead to a higher PSM rate. At high-volume centers, PSM rates have been reported to be between 9 to 16.7 % and 14.7 to 23 % for RALRP and RRP, respectively [12, 14, 15]. While these studies reported incidence of margins stratified by surgical technique, only one study to date has controlled for all the known preoperative clinical predictors for PSM in addition to BMI, surgical experience, era and whether or not nerve-sparing approach was utilized [16].

Surgeon and patient factors both impact surgical margin status. Prior multicenter studies have shown higher surgeon volume is associated with lower PSM rates [17]; however, individual surgeon characteristics and heterogeneity also affect PSM. While surgeon volume has been noted to be significant predictor for PSM, surgeon volume was no longer a predictor of surgical margin status after excluding the highest volume surgeon from one study [18]. Moreover, PSM rates for RRP surgeons at high volume, academic referral centers vary widely from 11 to 48 % in other studies [19]. Interestingly, a multicenter study discovered significant heterogeneity in cancer recurrence following RP after adjusting for both surgeon experience and tumor characteristics [17]. In a large population-based assessment of determining PSM predictors, Williams et al. identified PSM outcomes were associated with final pathology [20]. Men with pT2 tumors experienced a PSM rate of 14.9 % compared to PSMs in 42 % of men with pT3a tumors ($p<0.001$). Moreover, surgeons incurring more than three PSMs in ten cases of pT2 disease performed below the 25th percentile. Notably, neither surgical approach nor surgeon volume was significantly associated with PSM rate. While the above study provides a population-based benchmark for surgeon self-assessment there is much needed reinforcement and improvement in surgical technique in order to optimize oncologic outcomes [12, 14, 15].

Preoperative Clinical and Radiographic Assessment

The decision to pursue nerve-sparing surgical techniques during RP can increase the risk of PSM. Traditionally, preoperative factors contributing to the decision to perform a nerve-sparing RP opposed to non-nerve-sparing RP with wide excision include the digital rectal exam (DRE), Gleason score, tumor length/volume on biopsy, PSA, and baseline erectile function. These factors contribute to a surgeon's assessment of individual risk of EPE and resultant PSMs at the time of a nerve-sparing operation. While the clinical picture likely will always have a role in operative planning, prostate imaging has become a tool used in preoperative evaluation and surgical planning for PCa. Multiparametric MRI (MP-MRI) allows visual confirmation of an abnormal exam, identification of tumor volume and location, and identification of potential areas of EPE. While prospective studies of MP-MRI in all patients undergoing RP for prostate cancer have not shown significant improvement in surgical margin status [21], it is unclear if MP-MRI could potentially be more beneficial to limiting PSMs in cases of high risk PCa (Figs. 26.1 and 26.2).

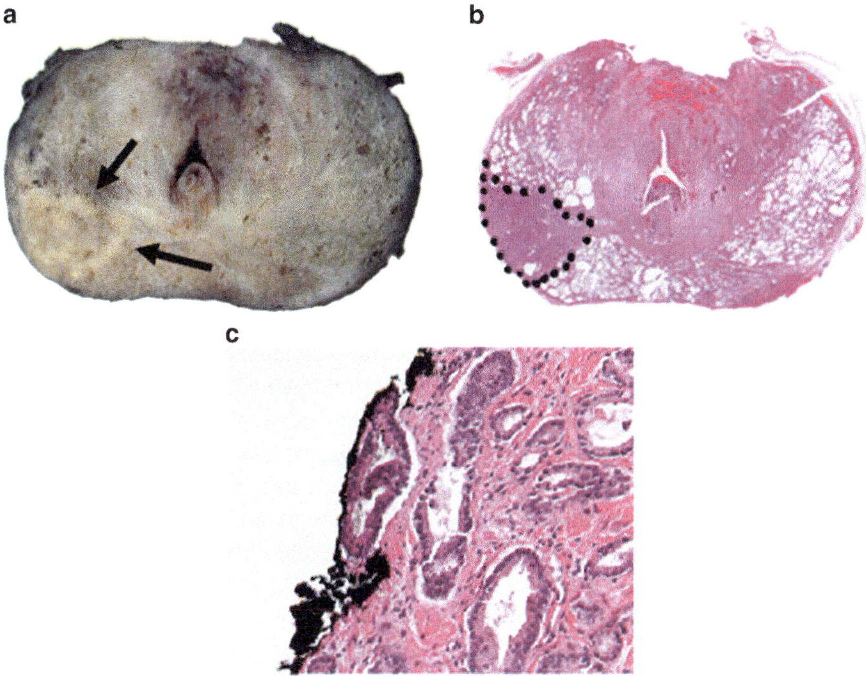

Fig. 26.1 Whole mount (**a**) with cancer at the *black arrows*. Many prostate tumors are very close to the capsule—(**b**)—and may touch the inked margin with no extraprostatic tissue to evaluate—(**c**). This is pT2+. Yossepowitch O, Bjartell A, Eastham JA, et al. Positive surgical margins in radical prostatectomy: outlining the problem and its long-term consequences. Eur Urol 2009; 55: 87–99

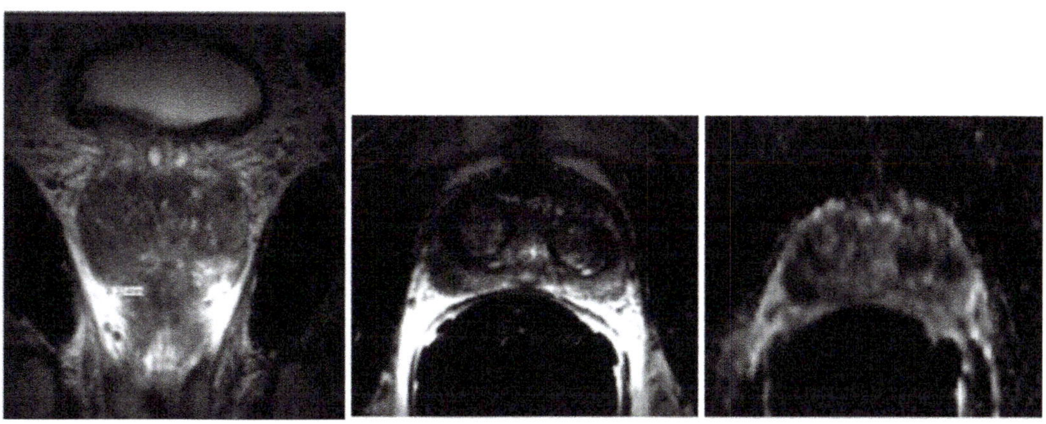

Fig. 26.2 Multiparametric MRI (MP-MRI) with 1.5T magnet and endorectal coil shows large volume disease from the right apex to base with possible EPE at the right apex (*left side* coronal). The cross sectional T2 (*center*) and diffusion weighted image map (*right*) show the dominant lesion measuring 1.4 × 0.9 cm. Standard 12-core prostate biopsy prior to the MP-MRI showed six cores of Gleason 3+4 prostate cancer on the right side. Surgical pathology showed pT3a disease with negative margin—a 20 % partial margin was taken on the side

Retrospective review of MP-MRI findings and surgical pathologic specimens with colleagues in pathology and radiology can provide the surgeon with opportunity to better understand and utilize radiographic and pathologic assessments in various clinical scenarios. This can also be a practical means of cross-disciplinary education for all parties, with consensus terminology and descriptions leading to better cross-disciplinary communication and overall improved oncologic outcomes.

Positive Margin Assessment

Oncologic efficacy following prostatectomy is measured most appropriately by metastasis-free and cancer-specific survival. However, because most cases of prostate cancer progress slowly, surrogate markers are commonly used to indirectly measure efficacy more immediately. Surgical margin status and BCR are the two most common surrogate markers used for measuring post-prostatectomy oncologic efficacy. A bulk of evidence suggests PSM confers a negative prognosis and is therefore used as a measure of surgical quality [20]. Both overall and pathologic stage-specific PSM rates have been shown to decrease with surgeon experience [17]. Therefore, critical assessment of determinants at decreasing PSM status are needed in order to improve oncologic outcomes. This is particularly true in case of organ-confined prostate cancer (pT2) where PSMs are often due to technical error and not as affected by tumor characteristics.

Pathology Self-Assessment

It is our belief that surgeons must review their pathology specimens and have a working relationship with the genitourinary pathologists at their institutions. Depending on the pathologic processing, the specimen will be processed either by whole mount or cross section. We recommended surgeons review a standard preparation of the prostate specimen with their pathologists to better understand how the specimen is sectioned. Following standard overnight processing (fixation), the prostate is embedded in paraffin with sections of tissue stained with hematoxylin and eosin. Slides can be examined histologically to determine presence of tumor, Gleason grade, EPE status, surgical margin status, and seminal vesicle involvement. When reviewing the pathology slides it is imperative to observe evidence of capsular incision as well as capsular denudation in addition to PSM. Both capsular incision as well as capsular denudation suggest surgeon error and potential for refinement in technique. Indeed, refinement of surgical technique through pathologic self-assessment has been shown to improve the incidence of PSM [22] (Figs. 26.3, 26.4, 26.5, and 26.6).

Operative Review and Refinement

Prior studies have suggested surgeons can improve their surgical skills and decrease their learning curve through reviewing videos of their own or other surgeons' techniques. Birkmeyere et al. recently demonstrated that surgical tech-

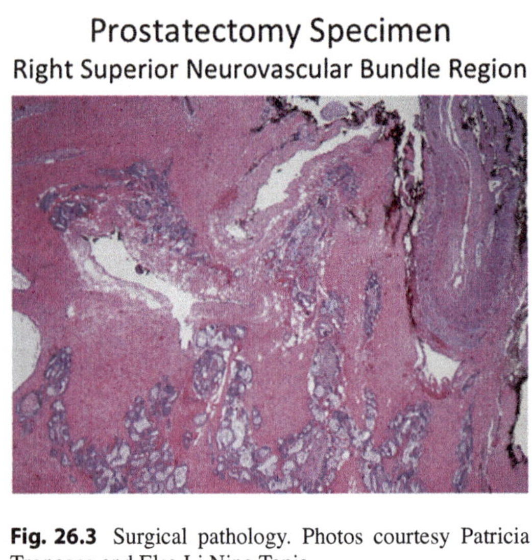

Fig. 26.3 Surgical pathology. Photos courtesy Patricia Troncoso and Elsa Li Ning Tapia

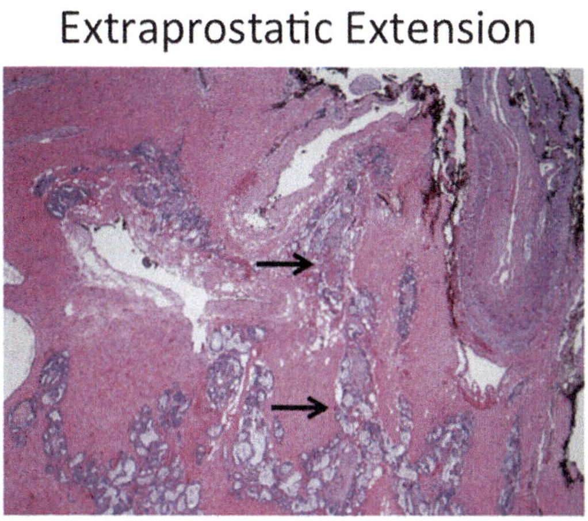

Fig. 26.4 Extraprostatic extension—tumor touching adipose tissue. Photos courtesy Patricia Troncoso and Elsa Li Ning Tapia

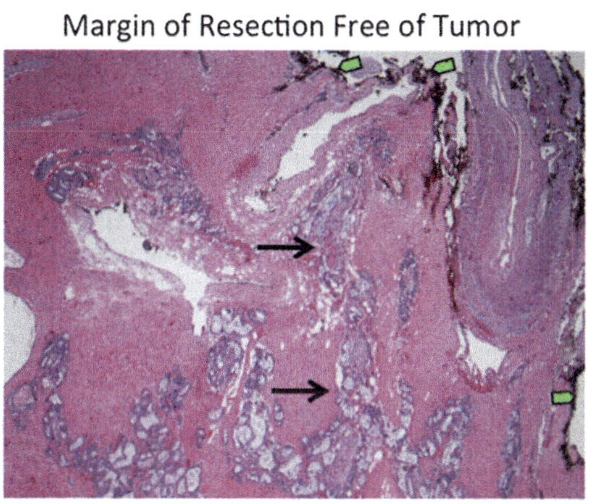

Fig. 26.5 Inked margins are free of tumor but very close. Photos courtesy Patricia Troncoso and Elsa Li Ning Tapia

nique improved through video review was associated with improved surgical outcomes [23]. As compared with patients treated by surgeons with high surgical skills ratings, patients operated by low skill ratings had increased mortality, increased risk of complications, and need for additional procedures [23]. One may argue, as with athletics, review of surgeries much like review of football game films in preparation for the upcoming game will only improve preparation and lead to optimal outcomes [23].

Modern surgical training has harnessed prior knowledge of enhanced laparoscopic techniques among video game users and applied that knowledge to surgical simulators [24]. Prior studies have been unable to demonstrate that this knowledge has enhanced acquisition of robotic techniques. Thus, the technical refinement in robotic skills in order to improved outcomes remains to be discerned.

Recent research has examined the feasibility of video-based peer feedback through social networking to facilitate robotic surgical skill acquisition [25]. Resident physicians of similar baseline surgical skills were randomized after performing the Tubes (Da Vinci Intuitive Surgical, Sunnyvale, CA) robotic simulator exercise to peer feedback versus no feedback of video-recorded performance through a social networking Web page. There were noted significant improvements in simulator exercise scores, time to completion, comfort, and satisfaction with robotic surgery simulation among the peer-reviewed cohort. Thus it appears that not only video review but critical third party assessment may improve robotic surgical skills and decrease the robotic learning curve. Further research in live surgeries followed by surgeon and third party review are needed in order to elucidate these findings.

Final Words

RALRP is a challenging procedure with multiple nuanced steps critical to optimal oncologic and functional outcomes. Surgeon self-assessment includes preoperative radiologic and pathologic evaluation in order to determine nerve-sparing feasibility and ensure adequate cancer extirpation. Moreover, postoperative pathologic review, including prostate specimen analysis, and video review of the procedure are additional methods at improving outcomes.

Conflict of Interest None

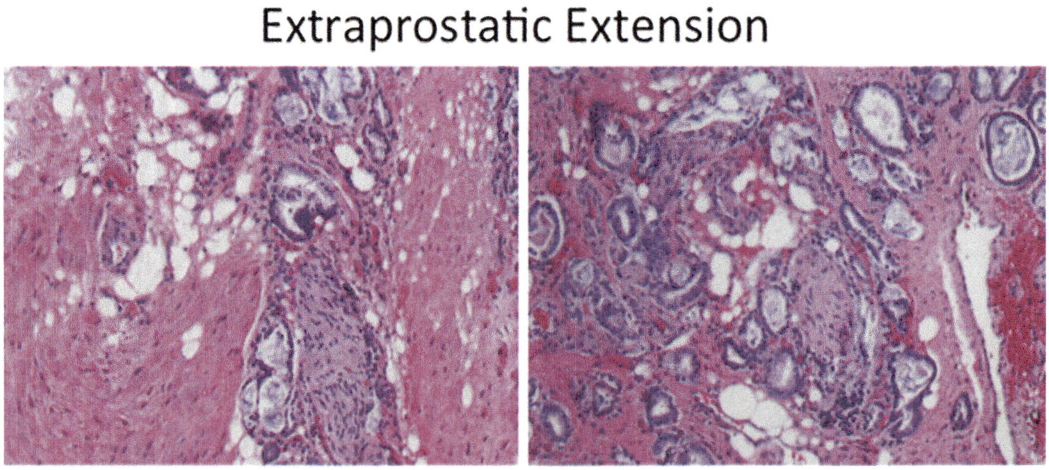

Fig. 26.6 Extraprostatic extension at higher magnification. Photos courtesy Patricia Troncoso and Elsa Li Ning Tapia

References

1. Williams SB, Prasad SM, Weinberg AC, et al. Trends in the care of radical prostatectomy in the United States from 2003 to 2006. BJU Int. 2011;108(1):49–55.
2. Tsui C, Klein R, Garabrant M. Minimally invasive surgery: national trends in adoption and future directions for hospital strategy. Surg Endosc. 2013;27(7):2253–7.
3. Jaffe J, Castellucci S, Cathelineau X, et al. Robot-assisted laparoscopic prostatectomy: a single-institutions learning curve. Urology. 2009;73(1):127–33.
4. Hakimi AA, Blitstein J, Feder M, Shapiro E, Ghavamian R. Direct comparison of surgical and functional outcomes of robotic-assisted versus pure laparoscopic radical prostatectomy: single-surgeon experience. Urology. 2009;73(1):119–23.
5. White MA, De Haan AP, Stephens DD, Maatman TK, Maatman TJ. Comparative analysis of surgical margins between radical retropubic prostatectomy and RALP: are patients sacrificed during initiation of robotics program? Urology. 2009;73(3):567–71.
6. Atug F, Castle EP, Srivastav SK, Burgess SV, Thomas R, Davis R. Positive surgical margins in robotic-assisted radical prostatectomy: impact of learning curve on oncologic outcomes. Eur Urol. 2006;49(5):866–71. discussion 871–862.
7. Vickers AJ, Savage CJ, Hruza M, et al. The surgical learning curve for laparoscopic radical prostatectomy: a retrospective cohort study. Lancet Oncol. 2009;10(5):475–80.
8. Ou YC, Yang CR, Wang J, et al. The learning curve for reducing complications of robotic-assisted laparoscopic radical prostatectomy by a single surgeon. BJU Int. 2011;108(3):420–5.
9. Novara G, Ficarra V, Mocellin S, et al. Systematic review and meta-analysis of studies reporting oncologic outcome after robot-assisted radical prostatectomy. Eur Urol. 2012;62(3):382–404.
10. Swindle P, Eastham JA, Ohori M, et al. Do margins matter? The prognostic significance of positive surgical margins in radical prostatectomy specimens. J Urol. 2005;174(3):903–7.
11. Thompson IM, Tangen CM, Paradelo J, et al. Adjuvant radiotherapy for pathological T3N0M0 prostate cancer significantly reduces risk of metastases and improves survival: long-term followup of a randomized clinical trial. J Urol. 2009;181(3):956–62.
12. Smith Jr JA, Chan RC, Chang SS, et al. A comparison of the incidence and location of positive surgical margins in robotic assisted laparoscopic radical prostatectomy and open retropubic radical prostatectomy. J Urol. 2007;178(6):2385–9. discussion 2389–2390.
13. Ellis WJ, Lange PH. Point: open radical prostatectomy should not be abandoned. J Natl Compr Canc Netw. 2007;5(7):685–8.
14. Han M, Partin AW, Chan DY, Walsh PC. An evaluation of the decreasing incidence of positive surgical margins in a large retropubic prostatectomy series. J Urol. 2004;171(1):23–6.
15. Menon M, Shrivastava A, Kaul S, et al. Vattikuti Institute prostatectomy: contemporary technique and analysis of results. Eur Urol. 2007;51(3):648–57. discussion 657–648.
16. Williams SB, Chen MH, D'Amico AV, et al. Radical retropubic prostatectomy and robotic-assisted laparoscopic prostatectomy: likelihood of positive surgical margin(s). Urology. 2010;76(5):1097–101.
17. Bianco Jr FJ, Vickers AJ, Cronin AM, et al. Variations among experienced surgeons in cancer control after open radical prostatectomy. J Urol. 2010;183(3):977–82.

18. Chun FK, Briganti A, Antebi E, et al. Surgical volume is related to the rate of positive surgical margins at radical prostatectomy in European patients. BJU Int. 2006;98(6):1204–9.
19. Eastham JA, Kattan MW, Riedel E, et al. Variations among individual surgeons in the rate of positive surgical margins in radical prostatectomy specimens. J Urol. 2003;170(6 Pt 1):2292–5.
20. Williams SB, D'Amico AV, Weinberg AC, Gu X, Lipsitz SR, Hu JC. Population-based determinants of radical prostatectomy surgical margin positivity. BJU Int. 2011;107(11):1734–40.
21. Rud E, Baco E, Klotz D, et al. Does preoperative magnetic resonance imaging reduce the rate of positive surgical margins at radical prostatectomy in a randomised clinical trial? Eur Urol. 2015;68(3):487–96.
22. Vickers AJ, Bianco FJ, Gonen M, et al. Effects of pathologic stage on the learning curve for radical prostatectomy: evidence that recurrence in organ-confined cancer is largely related to inadequate surgical technique. Eur Urol. 2008;53(5):960–6.
23. Birkmeyer JD, Finks JF, O'Reilly A, et al. Surgical skill and complication rates after bariatric surgery. N Engl J Med. 2013;369(15):1434–42.
24. Lynch J, Aughwane P, Hammond TM. Video games and surgical ability: a literature review. J Surg Educ. 2010;67(3):184–9.
25. Carter SC, Chiang A, Shah G, et al. Video-based peer feedback through social networking for robotic surgery simulation: a multicenter randomized controlled trial. Ann Surg. 2015;261(5):870–5.

27 High Risk Pathology: State-of-the-Art Post-operative Radiation Recommendations and Integration of Novel Genomic Risk Biomarkers

Vladimir Mourviev, D. Telonis, Vipul R. Patel, and David M. Albala

In 2014, it is estimated that there would be 233,000 new cases of prostate cancer and an estimated 29,480 men will die of the disease in the United States [1]. The US Food and Drug Administration (FDA) approved the use of prostate-specific antigen (PSA) in 1986 to monitor prostate cancer (PCa) in men who had already been diagnosed. In 1994, approval was expanded for use as a screening tool along with digital rectal exam (DRE) in asymptomatic patients [2] Evidence of overtreatment and over diagnosis of PCa has led the US Preventive Services Task Force (USPSTF) to recommend against PSA-based screening as of 2012 [3]. The limitations of PSA testing are found in its overall sensitivity and specificity. Most men with an elevated PSA are not diagnosed with PCa, while many men with no elevation in PSA are found to be harboring cancer. While PSA can be elevated from a number of benign conditions, including but not limited to benign prostatic hyperplasia (BPH) and prostatitis, it remains a gold standard for early detection, treatment monitoring, and prognosis. Therefore, due to the dramatic decrease in usage of this test, one should expect a reverse of stage migration of PCa toward an increase of amount of patients with high-risk disease. This will have an effect on radical prostatectomy (RP) rates, positive margins, and, ultimately, the issue of adjuvant radiation therapy (ART) vs. salvage radiation therapy (SRT).

According to the literature, 15–25% of men undergoing RP for the treatment of organ-confined disease will develop a biochemical recurrence (BCR) with subsequent local or systemic relapse [4, 5]. However, not all patients with BCR necessarily experience tumor progression that requires the need for ART [6–10]. The major objective for clinicians in this patient population is to identify which patients will require and benefit from ART. Novel genomic markers have been used in this patient population to help identify those patients that are at highest risk for progression and possibly death. This chapter highlights the latest developments in how we can improve treatment outcomes of high-risk patients undergoing RP and determine the role of ART in this patient population.

Dilemma of Post-radical Prostatectomy RT: Radiate or Wait Until Evidence of Progression

In spite of a recent publication by the American Urologic Association (AUA) and the American Society for Radiation Oncology (ASTRO), there

V. Mouraviev
Global Robotics Institute, Celebration Health, Orlando, FL, USA

D. Telonis
Associated Medical Professionals, Syracuse, NY, USA

V.R. Patel
Global Robotics Institute, Florida Hospital-Celebration Health, University of Central Florida College of Medicine, Orlando, FL, USA

D.M. Albala (✉)
Department of Urology, Crouse Hospital, Syracuse, NY, USA
e-mail: dalbala@ampofny.com

J.W. Davis (ed.), *Robot-Assisted Radical Prostatectomy*, DOI 10.1007/978-3-319-32641-2_27

is a great deal of controversy on the role of radiation therapy in patients after RP in high-risk patients. Consensus practice guidelines, with its subsequent endorsement by American Society of Clinical Oncology, have been developed to help clinicians with these patients. These official guidelines were based on three-phase 3 prospective clinical trials demonstrating the benefit vs. harm of ART compared to observation in patients with adverse final pathological features such as extraprostatic disease or positive margins (Table 27.1). Wiegel et al. (ARO 9602) presented data that suggested ART almost halved the risk of biochemical recurrence in patients with undetectable PSA following surgery [9]. Bolla et al. (EORTC 22911) demonstrated a similar decrease in biochemical recurrence [8]. In both studies, the cohorts of patients seeming to benefit the most were those with positive margins. Neither study showed any improvement in overall survival (OS), PCa-specific survival, or metastasis-free survival (MFS). However, both trials had a limited median follow-up as of only 5 years and there is a high possibility that with longer follow-up and more events, differences in survival would be more obvious. The third study (SWOG 8794) clearly demonstrated that ART improved not only biochemical recurrence but also more strict end points such as MFS and OS [6, 7].

While these trials demonstrated a significant benefit of ART, two of them (SWOG 8794 and EORTC 22911) enrolled patients prior to the widespread use of PSA or required an undetectable PSA at the time of randomization [6–8].

Table 27.1 Randomized clinical phase 3 randomized prospective trials on adjuvant RT vs. initial observation after RP followed by SRT

Authors, study, reference	No. pts	Entry criteria	Type and dose of RT	Median follow-up (years)	bDFS	OS	Results
Thompson et al. SWOG 8794 [6, 7]	425	pT3 N0 Mo R0/1 (29 % post-RP PSA ≥ 0.2 ng/ml)	2D planned 60–64 Gy	12.6	HR = 0.43 p < 0.001	HR = 0.72 p = 0.023	Improved PSA control, DM-free survival RT, and OS. 1/3 pts a received salvage RT with a same magnitude of benefit
Bolla et al. EORTC22911 [8]	1005	pT2 R1, pT3NoMo R0/1 (30 % post-RP PSA ≥ 0.2 ng/ml)	2D planned 60 Gy	10.6	HR = 0.49 p < 0.0001	HR = 1.18 p = 0.2024	Improved PSA control and local failure, did not affect OS, DM free survival, or clinical progression-free survival, did benefit pts with positive surgical margins
Wiegel et al. ARO 9602 [9]	388	pT3-T4N0 MO R0/1 (post-RP PSA undetectable)	3D planned 60 Gy	4.5	HR = 0.53 P-0.0015	N/A	Improved PSA control, limited events to assess DM and survival end points, did benefit pts with positive surgical margins

Contrary to this, both studies had almost a third of patients with detectable PSA at the time of randomization. Thus, this patient cohort was at extremely high risk for recurrence, metastasis, and death. Under contemporary requirements, any arm of the study would not be considered acceptable treatment for a patients unless their PSA decreased to <0.2 ng/ml after surgery. The Weigel study (ARO 902 l) most closely reflects current practice and treatment requirements because all patients had undetectable PSA at the time of randomization [9].

The main reason why the urological oncology community remains reluctant to widely accept and implement post-RP ART into practice is that treatment outcomes can vary, and many men will be subjected to unnecessary ART [6–10]. In all the above-mentioned prospective, randomized clinical trials examining ART (defined as treatment at the time of undetectable PSA), approximately 50 % of patients randomized to observation never developed BCR, even though some patients had detectable PSA after RP [6–10]. Even in the Weigel study (ARO 9602), which most closely resembles contemporary treatment recommendations, the vast majority of untreated patients did not progress [9]. At a median follow-up of 5 years, the clinical progression rate was only 2 % in study group vs. 3 % in control group [9]. Although hypothetically this situation can be changed with longer follow-up, one can see the limitations of the currently existing definition of high risk, as it is unable to predict a patient population at high risk for relapse at 5 years.

Clinical Utilization of Salvage Radiation Therapy as a Single Modality: Can It Prolong Survival?

To date, no randomized trials have been conducted to demonstrate the efficacy of salvage Radiation Therapy (SRT). The largest retrospective studies are presented in Table 27.2. Boorjian et al. examined 2657 men with high-risk disease, according to the D'Amico classification, who underwent RP at the Mayo Clinic between 1987 and 2003 and 856 of them received SRT [11]. Although the risk of death from PCa was almost 12 times higher in the high-risk group, 10-year biochemical-disease free survival (bDFS), metastasis-free survival (MFS), and PCa-specific survival (PCa-SS) were 55, 89, and 95 %, respectively. On multivariate analysis, SRT significantly reduced the incidence of subsequent local recurrence. However, SRT did not significantly decrease mortality compared to those not receiving SRT following BCR (5- and 10-year survival rates: 92 % vs. 91 % and 70 % vs. 69 %, respectively).

In contrast, Trock et al. followed outcomes in 635 patients who had either a biochemical or local recurrence following RP [12]. At the time of their recurrence, patients were managed with observation (63 %), SRT alone (25 %), or SRT in combination with hormonal therapy (12 %). Cancer-specific survival was significantly prolonged in patients who underwent SRT, with or without androgen-deprivation therapy (ADT), compared to observation (96 and 96 % vs. 88 % at 5 years, and 82 and 86 % vs. 62 % at 10 years). In summary, investigators demonstrated a threefold reduction in the risk of death from PCa with SRT. This risk reduction was most pronounced in patients with rapid PSA doubling time and early recurrence, two factors that are known to predict risk of death from PCa in patients who fail surgery.

Cotter et al. reported that RT appeared to prolong survival in a series of 519 men who had a BCR after RP. SRT was given, either alone or as part of a combined approach that included ADT, in 219 (37 %) of these patients [13]. At a median follow-up of 11.3 years, multivariate analysis demonstrated a significant decrease in all-cause mortality both in those with a PSA doubling time <6 months and in those with a PSA doubling time >6 months. The results of these retrospective studies provide reasonable evidence that SRT shortly after biochemical relapse may alter the natural history of prostate cancer. However, longer-term follow-up data are needed to draw further conclusions. For instance, Stephenson et al. analyzed 1962 patients who were considered to have high-risk disease using the D'Amico definition [10]. Although PCa mortality was a relatively low 8 % at 10 years, it had increased to 19 % at 15 years.

Table 27.2 Large single and multi-institutional retrospective trials on whether SRT as a single modality following PSA increase after RP can prolong survival

Authors, study, reference	No. pts	Entry criteria	Type and dose of RT	Median follow-up (years)	BCR or Local recurrence	PCa-SS or OS	Results
Boorjan et al. Mayo clinic [11]	2657	pT3 N0 Mo R0/1 (All post-RP PSA ≥ 0.2 ng/ml)	2D planned 60–64 Gy	12.6	HR = 0.13 95 % CI: 0.06–0.28	5- and 10-years: 92 % vs. 91 and 70 % vs. 69 %	Significantly decreased local recurrence, did not affect survival
Trock et al. John Hopkins [12]	635	pT2 R1, pT3NoMo R0/ (all post-RP PSA ≥ 0.2 ng/ml) with or w/o with ADT	2D planned 60 Gy	10.6	HR = 0.49 p < 0.0001	5-Years: 96 % vs. 96 % (with HT) and 88 % (w/o HT); 10-years 82 and 86 % vs. 62 %, respectively	PCa survival was significantly prolonged
Cotter et al. Duke [13]	519	pT3-T4 N0 MO R0/1 (all post-RP PSA ≥ 0.2 ng/ml) with (37 %) or w/o (63 %) ADT	3D planned 60 Gy	11.3	HR = 0.53 P-0.0015	HR = 0.53 (PSADT < 6 months) and =0.53 (PSADT > 6 months)	Significantly decrease OS
Stephenson et al. MSKCC, Cleveland clinic, U of Michigan [10]	1540- SRT	pT3 N0 M0 (14 % with ADT for 4 months)	2D planned 60 Gy	6	6-Years bDFS: 48 % when PSA ≤ 0.5 vs. 18 % when PSA > 1.5	PCa mortality- 8 % (10-years), 19 % (15-years)	Ability to control recurrent disease in 50 %
Briganti et al. Italy, Belgium, Germany, Canada [15]	390-ART, 500-initial observation	pT3 pN0 R0/1 — match-controlled adjuvant RT vs. observation followed by early salvage RT	2D and 3D planned 65-66 Gy	4.5	5-Years bDFS-78.4 % for ART vs. 81.8 %; p = 0.9	NA	No differences in 5-years bDFS were found even when pts were stratified according to pT3 sub-stage and surgical margin status
Trabulsi et al. multicenter trial [16]	211-ART, 238-SRT	pT3-4 pN0	2D planned Standard dose	6.1	5-Years bDFS rate: 73 % vs. 50 %; p = 0.007	NA	ART significantly reduced the risk of long-term BCR after RP compared with SRT
Ost et al. Ghent, Belgium, [17]	144-ART, 134-SRT	pT3-4 pN0	3D planned standard dose	3	5-Years bDFS: 85 % for ART vs. 65 % for SRT IMRT; p = 0.002	NA	ART significantly reduced the risk of long-term BCR after RP compared with SRT

A recent meta-analysis of two matched control studies and 16 retrospective studies including a total of 2629 cases was identified (1404 cases for ART and 1185 cases for SRT) comparing the efficacy of ART and SRT. This study demonstrated 3-year and 5-year bDFS, local and systemic DFS advantages in favor of ART [14]. The most valuable finding of this meta-analysis revealed an overall survival benefit of ART. The authors also found that MFS was considerable with no significant differences in both groups. The analysis suggested an impact of ART and SRT on survival after RP. It is well established that ART provides improved OS, bDFS, DFS for patients with adverse pathological factors (APFs) (e.g. positive surgical margins, seminal vesicle invasion, extra capsular extension, and higher Gleason scores) following a RP compared with SRT. These researchers concluded that ART can offer a safe and efficient alternative to SRT, with better OS and DFS at 3-and 5-year follow-up especially for patients with adverse pathological features. In fact, ART may reduce the overall need for SRT in this patient population.

Briganti et al. stratified 890 men with pT3pN0, PCa who underwent RP from a European multi-institutional cohort into two groups: ART vs. initial observation followed by early SRT (eSRT) in cases of relapse [15]. Propensity-matched analysis was employed, and patients were stratified into two groups: ART vs. observation and eventual eSRT, defined as RT given at a postoperative serum prostate-specific antigen (PSA) $\geq$0.5 ng/ml at least 6 months after RP. BCR, defined as PSA >0.20 ng/ml and rising after administration of RT, was compared between ART and initial observation followed by eSRT in cases of relapse. Overall, 390 (43.8 %) and 500 (56.2 %) patients were treated with ART and initial observation, respectively. Within the latter group, 225 (45.0 %) patients experienced BCR and underwent eSRT. In the propensity-matched cohort, the 2- and 5-years BCR-free survival rates were 91.4 and 78.4 % in ART group vs. 92.8 and 81.8 % in patients who underwent initial observation and eSRT in cases of relapse, respectively (p=0.9). No differences in the 2- and 5-years bDFS rates were found, even when patients were stratified according to pT3 sub-stage and surgical margin status (all $p \geq 0.4$). These findings were also confirmed in a multivariable analyses (p=0.6). Similar results were achieved when the cut-off to define eSRT was set at 0.3 ng/ml (all $p \geq 0.5$) [15].

Other studies have addressed a similar topic. Trabulsi et al., using a multi-institutional database of 211 ART vs. 238 SRT pT3-4N0 patients, demonstrated that ART significantly reduced the risk of long-term BCR after RP compared with SRT (5-years bDFS rate: 73 % vs. 50 %; p=0.007) [16]. Similar results were reported by Ost et al., who showed a 5-years BCR-free survival rate of 85 % for ART patients vs. 65 % for salvage intensity-modulated RT (p=0.002) [17]. However, when subgroup matching was performed in a cohort of 76 patients receiving either ART or eSRT (given at a PSA level <0.5 ng/ml), no significant difference in the 3-years BCR-free survival rates was found.

Three ongoing randomized trials are underway to define what modality is better: adjuvant or early salvage RT [18]. The TROG RAVES 0803 trial will examine 470 men with undetectable PSA and either pT3N0M0 or pT2N0M0 with positive margins. The patients are being randomized to immediate RT vs. RT for a rising PSA. The end point of this study is biochemical recurrence. The GETUG-17 trial is enrolling 718 men with pT3-4N0M0 disease with positive margins and undetectable PSA to immediate RT with androgen-deprivation therapy (ADT), vs. salvage RT with ADT. The composite end point includes clinical progression, biochemical progression, and death at 5 years. The last and most ambitious trial is RADICALS. In this 2600-patient trial, men with PSA <0.2 ng/ml plus pT3/4, Gleason 7–10, preoperative PSA $\geq$10 ng/ml, or positive margins will be randomized to immediate vs. delayed RT. The end point of this trial is PCa-specific survival.

The different prognostic tools developed in order to improve a selection of appropriate candidates for ART vs. SRT include ultrasensitive PSA-assay, the Stephenson nomogram, the risk score, and others [4, 15, 19, 20]. For instance, recent validation of the risk score in 7616 patients with pT3/4N0/1 treated with RP in the US,

Canada, and Europe demonstrated value of this tool that was associated with increasing 5- and 10-year PCs-specific mortality rate [20]. This validation confirmed that presence of two or more of the following adverse pathologic factors (Gleason score 8–10, pT3b/4, and lymph node invasion) should be considered to identify patients who benefit from early ART. However, this and other predictive systems have not been widely implemented due to their limitation to elucidate progression of PCa after RP in patients with high-risk features.

Complications of ART and SRT After RP

The concern with side effects after ART is another obstacle for increased utilization of this modality. In the SWOG 8796 trial, the risk of complications was acceptable and treatable but was clearly higher in the treated arm [6, 7]. Overall, RT was associated with a 23.8 % complication rate compared to 11.9 % in the control arm ($p=0.002$; rectal complications: 3.3 % vs. 0 % [$p=0.02$]; urethral strictures: 17.8 % vs. 9.5 % [$p=0.02$]; total urinary incontinence: 6.5 % vs. 2.8 % [$p=0.11$]). Although the reported complications in EORTC 22922 and ARO 9602 are much lower, this was not an endpoint in the study design and therefore may be underreported. As ART does not appear to be necessary in all patients and has unintended side effects, an alternative strategy is to treat only patients most likely to benefit, maximizing cure and minimizing side effects.

Subset analysis of EORTC 22911 revealed that the patients most likely to benefit were those with positive margins [8]. These patients are not only at higher risk of recurrence but, importantly, at higher risk for local recurrence and therefore will benefit from a targeted local therapy. It may even be possible to further define groups that are at risk for residual local disease and, therefore, who will benefit. Cao et al. examined a role of positive surgical margins in 294 patients by measuring the linear millimeters of tumor at the margin [21]. They revealed that the longer the margin, the more likely the recurrence. At approximately 7.5 years of follow-up, 70 % of patients with 3–6 mm of margin and 100 % of the patients with ≥6 mm of margin had recurred. These findings provide a strong rationale for utilizing adjuvant radiation in this patient cohort.

The AUA/ASTRO guideline emphasized what should be told to patients about complications undergoing and after RT [22]. During radiotherapy and in the immediate post-RT period of 2–3 months, mild to moderate genitourinary and gastrointestinal side effects may occur that can require the use of medication for treatment. Table 27.3 summarizes the acute complications by grade of ART and SRT after RP while Table 27.4 examines the late complication. In some studies, over 90 % of patients experienced either genitourinary or gastrointestinal side effects [23]. The more serious toxicity effects of radiotherapy, including those requiring aggressive medication management, outpatient procedures, or hospitalization, however, are uncommon or rare, with most studies reporting rates of ≤5 %. The lowest acute toxicity rates have been reported with use of IMRT radiotherapy techniques. As to late toxicity, mild to moderate late side effects may happen more than 90 days post-RT and are commonly reported, with some studies documenting rates as high as 79 % [22]. Serious late toxicities, however, are relatively uncommon, with most studies reporting rates of 10 % or less.

Table 27.3 Acute complications (Grade 3–4 Grade 3–4 according to RTOG or CTCAE grading systems) of ART vs. SRT after RP

Study arm type	% Genitourinary	% Gastrointestinal
Adjuvant	2.0–8.0	0.0–2.0
Salvage	0.0–6.0	0.0–2.2
Mixed	0.0–3.0	0.0–1.3

Modified from Thompson et al. [22]

Table 27.4 Late complications (Grade 3–4 according to RTOG or CTCAE grading systems) of ART vs. SRT after RP

Study arm type	% Genitourinary	% Gastrointestinal
Adjuvant	0.0–10.6	0.0–6.7
Salvage	0.0–6.0	0.0–18.0
Mixed	0.0–17.0	0.0–4.3

Modified from Thompson et al. [22]

Some cases of toxicities that are moderate to major may emerge at 4–5 years post-RT and continue beyond that point. These toxicities are more likely to include GU symptoms (up to 28 % of patients) than to include GI symptoms (up to 10.2 % of patients). The use of newer RT techniques such as IMRT decreases cumulative rates of late GU (up to 16.8 % of patients) and GI (4.0 % of patients) toxicities [22].

The rates and severity of urinary incontinence in patients who have had RP and then adjuvant RT are generally similar to rates for patients who have had RP only. Regarding sexual function, studies indicate that the majority of men who present for RT post-RP already have compromised erectile function, and thus, the impact of RT remains unclear. There is also a potential for developing secondary malignancies after RT, but these data are still inconclusive [22].

ART and SRT After RP: AUA/ASTRO Guideline

The AUA/ASTRO guideline endorsed by ASCO [22, 23] included four major principals:

1. Patient counseling.
2. Use of RT in the adjuvant and salvage setting.
3. Definitions of biochemical recurrence.
4. Conduct of restaging evaluation.

The key elements of the guidelines statements are the following:

1. Patients who are being considered for management of localized prostate cancer with radical prostatectomy should be informed of the potential for adverse pathologic findings that portend a higher risk of cancer recurrence and that these findings may suggest a potential benefit of additional therapy after surgery *(Clinical Principle).*
2. Patients with adverse pathologic findings including seminal vesicle invasion, positive surgical margins, and extraprostatic extension should be informed that adjuvant radiotherapy, compared to radical prostatectomy alone, reduces the risk of biochemical (PSA) recurrence, local recurrence, and clinical progression of cancer. They should also be informed that the impact of adjuvant radiotherapy on subsequent metastases and overall survival is less clear; one of two randomized controlled trials that addressed these outcomes indicated a benefit but the other trial did not demonstrate a benefit *(Clinical Principle).*
3. Physicians should offer adjuvant radiotherapy to patients with adverse pathologic findings at prostatectomy including seminal vesicle invasion, positive surgical margins, or extraprostatic extension because of demonstrated reductions in biochemical recurrence, local recurrence, and clinical progression *(Standard; Evidence Strength: Grade A).*
4. Patients should be informed that the development of a PSA recurrence after surgery is associated with a higher risk of development of metastatic prostate cancer or death from the disease. Congruent with this clinical principle, physicians should regularly monitor PSA after radical prostatectomy to enable early administration of salvage therapies if appropriate *(Clinical Principle).*
5. Clinicians should define biochemical recurrence as a detectable or rising PSA value after surgery that is >0.2 ng/ml with a second confirmatory level >0.2 ng/ml *(Recommendation; Evidence Strength: Grade C).*
6. A restaging evaluation in the patient with a PSA recurrence may be considered *(Option; Evidence Strength: Grade C).*
7. Physicians should offer salvage radiotherapy to patients with PSA or local recurrence after radical prostatectomy in whom there is no evidence of distant metastatic disease *(Recommendation; Evidence Strength: Grade C).*
8. Patients should be informed that the effectiveness of radiotherapy for PSA recurrence is greatest when given at lower levels of PSA *(Clinical Principle).*
9. Patients should be informed of the possible short-term and long-term urinary, bowel, and sexual side effects of radiotherapy as well as of the potential benefits of controlling disease recurrence *(Clinical Principle).*

The Value of Novel Biomarkers

The AUA/ASTRO guideline has suggested a great need for prognostic biomarkers [22]. As a background for this, in SWOG 8794, the only randomized controlled trial finding a survival benefit to ART (median follow-up of 12.6 years and up to 20 years of follow-up overall) metastases were reported in only 37 of 211 RP only patients and in 20 of 214 ART patients [7]. Although a high-risk population, most men did not develop metastases or die of cancer. Ideally, ART or SRT should be given only to the carefully selected patients predisposed to the development of PCa recurrence. New genomic markers have been developed for serum and tissue specimens which may be implemented to help with treatment, monitoring, and providing prognostic information. These tests can be used along with clinical pathological information to better understand the natural history of the disease (Table 27.5).

Biomarkers of First Generation

Prolaris® (Myriad Genetics)

Prolaris is a prognostic genomic assay that measures the RNA expression level of 46 genes, including cell cycle progression (CCP) genes, which are known to correlate with PCa cell proliferation. A key distinguishing factor between cancerous and noncancerous cells is the increase in CCP gene mutations [24, 25]. This test can be used in both the biopsy setting to provide information that may help with active surveillance decisions and in the post prostatectomy setting. In the post-prostatectomy setting, Prolaris can help to identify those patients that have a high risk for biochemical recurrence. The test uses a minimal tissue sample from formalin-fixed paraffin-embedded prostatectomy specimens and provides information on 10-year biochemical recurrence rates.

Table 27.5 The genomics markers applicable to prostatectomy tissue analysis

Marker	Clinical value	Cost ($)
CCP-Prolaris® (Myriad)	• Risk stratification • PCa-specific survival • Recurrence	3400
GPS (OncotypeDX® Genomic Health)	• Prediction of metastases or death in high-grade tumors	3800
GC (Decipher®, Genome Dx)	• Recurrence probability • Prediction of metastasis	4200

CCP cell-cycle progression, *GPS* genomic prostate score, *GC* genomic classifier

Cuzick et al. tested CCP in a retrospective cohort of 366 patients who had undergone radical prostatectomy [25]. Results showed that the CCP signature was a highly significant predictor of outcome after prostatectomy. The authors were able to predict biochemical recurrence in univariate analysis (Hazard ratio (HR) for a one unit change in CCP (doubling) = 1.89; 95 % CI (1.54, 2.31) $\chi^2=34\times0$, 1*df*, $p=5\times6\times10-9$) and multivariate analysis (HR = 1.74; 95 % CI (1.39, 2.17) $\chi^2=21\times65$, 1*df*, $p=3\times3\times10-6$) (Fig. 27.1a, b).

Cooperberg and colleagues obtained samples from 464 PCa patients who had undergone RP without or with ADT [26]. The hazard ratio for each unit increase in CCP score (range, −1.62 to 2.16) was calculated to be 2.1 (95 % CI, 1.6–2.9). These researchers concluded that with an adjustment for the calculated CAPRA-S score, the HR was 1.7 (95 % CI, 1.3–2.4). The score was able to sub-stratify patients with low clinical risk as defined by CAPRA-S ≤ 2 (HR, 2.3; 95 % CI, 1.4–3.7), demonstrating that the CCP score has significant prognostic accuracy and may improve the accuracy of risk stratification in patients with clinically localized PCa. Furthermore, the addition of the CCP score to a previously calculated CAPRA-S score was shown to allow for patients to be stratified in terms of risk of recurrence at 10 years across a broad range of risk subgroups defined by Gleason score, PSA level, and CAPRA-S score.

Genomic Prostate Score (GPS) (OncotypeDX®, Genomic Health)

Many men who are diagnosed with prostate cancer will have indolent disease that will not spread aggressively. These men are good candidates for

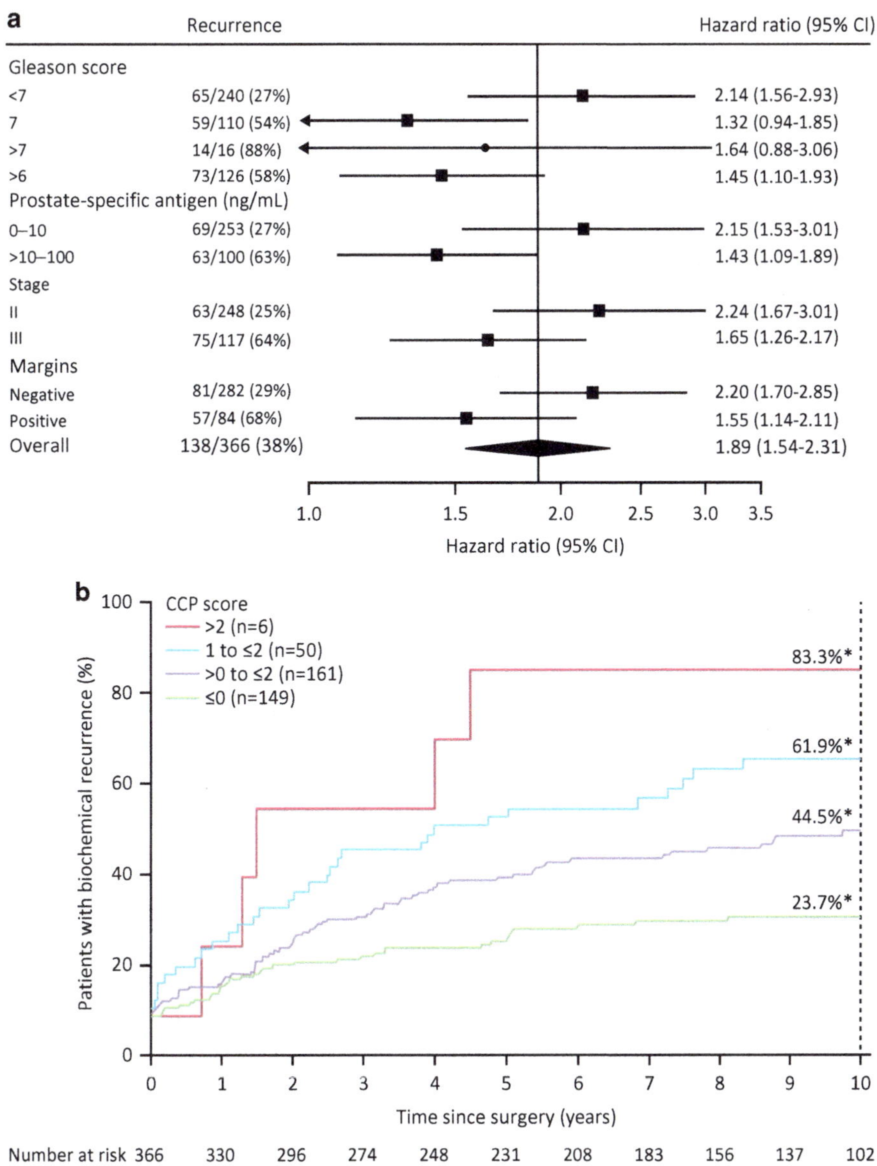

Fig. 27.1 Analysis of the CCP score in the radical prostatectomy cohort. (**a**) Forest plot graphing the CCP score hazard ratio (HR) in different clinical subgroups. The recurrence rate for each subgroup is also given (recurrences/size), and the size of the each box is proportional to the number of recurrences within that patient subgroup. The thin lines indicate the 95 % CI for each HR. The diamond at the bottom is the 95 % CI of the HR for the entire cohort. (**b**) Kaplan-Meier plot of recurrence vs. time for patients grouped by integer values of CCP score. Each bin corresponds to a twofold increase in CCP expression. The *green line* (149 patients). Adopted from Cuzick et al. [25]

active surveillance (AS) instead of definitive treatment (prostatectomy or radiation therapy) which can lead to incontinence, impotence, and other side effects that can greatly compromise overall quality of life [27]. OncotypeDX uses five reference genes (ARF1, ATP5E, CLTC, GPS1, PGK1) and 12 genes representing four biological pathways, including androgen signaling (FAM13C, KLK2, AZGP1, SRDSA2), cellular organization (FLNC, GSN, TPM2, GSTM2), stromal response (BGN, COL1A1, SFRP4), and proliferation (TPX2) [28]. Patients with very low-, low-, and low-intermediate risk disease receive an individualized GPS score, which is used to predict adverse pathology [28]. This test, which is used primarily in the biopsy setting for selecting AS patients, may provide useful information in patients that undergo definitive therapy and have unfavorable pathological features at RP.

Klein et al. identified and validated a biopsy-based gene expression GPS-signature that predicts clinical recurrence, prostate cancer (PCa) death, and adverse pathology [29]. Gene expression was quantified by reverse transcription–polymerase chain reactions for the prostatectomy study ($n = 441$). Decision-curve analysis and risk profiles were then used together with clinical and pathologic characteristics to evaluate clinical utility. In decision-curve analysis (Fig. 27.2), a greater net benefit was realized for each end point through the combination of clinical (CAPRA) and genomic (GPS) information compared with clinical information alone. Over a range of threshold probabilities, incorporation of GPS would be expected to lead to initiation of early ART in patients who have unfavorable pathology at RP.

Prostate Cancer Genomic Classifier (Decipher®, Genome DX)

The Decipher-genomic classifier (GC) (GenomeDx Biosciences, San Diego, CA) uses a whole transcriptome microarray assay from formalin-fixed, paraffin-embedded PCa specimens. This assay is used to predict the risk of disease progression after a patient undergoes a radical prostatectomy. The test measures the expression of 22 RNA biomarkers in prostate cancer specimens [30]. Decipher may help physicians determine which patients are best suited for multimodality therapy, such as adjuvant radiation therapy. The biomarker panel was derived from a genome-wide search of PCa in more than 500 patients from the Mayo Clinic Tumor Registry [31]. The markers represent multiple oncogenic pathways, including cell cycle progression, cell adhesion, motility, migration, and immune-system modulation. This signature was developed and validated as a predictor for clinical metastases after RP in a cohort of men with adverse clinical and pathologic features. Further, it was shown to more accurately predict metastases than individual clinical variables or nomograms.

Ross et al. evaluated the GC score for predicting metastatic disease progression in clinically high-risk patients ($N = 85$) with BCR after RP. In the GC low-score and high-score groups, 8 and 40 % of patients developed metastases after BCR, respectively ($p < 0.001$) [32]. The area under the curve (AUC) for predicting metastasis after BCR was 0.82. In a multivariate model, the risk for metastasis increased by 49 % for each 0.1-point increase in GC score (HR, 1.49: $p < 0.001$) (Fig. 27.3a, b). Compared with standard clinical and pathologic variables, the GC score was a better predictor of metastasis, suggesting its potential use as a valuable tool to identify patients who require earlier initiation of ART at the time of predicted BCR.

Den at al. tested how incorporation of the GC in clinical models would more accurately predict biochemical failure (BF) and distant metastases (DM) in 139 patients after receiving post-RP RT who had either pT3 disease or positive margin and who did not receive ADT [33]. The authors assessed the GC performance for predicting BF and DM after post-RP RT in comparison with clinical nomograms. The area under the receiver operating characteristic curve of the Stephenson model was 0.70 for both BF and DM, with the addition of GC, it significantly improved the area under the receiver operating characteristic curve to 0.78 and 0.80, respectively. The authors validated the value of quantitative GC for three previously reported GC score risk groups. In multivariate analysis, the hazard ratio (HR) for intermediate and high GC was 2.9 and 8.1 in comparison to the low GC risk group being most significant risk factors for postoperative RT. These data suggest a clinical utility and additional value of the GC score in shared decision-making. As it has been shown before, implementation of this marker altered the decision making process in almost 50 % of cases. Furthermore, a combined use of GC and clinical and final pathological parameters can enhance the predictive value for BF and DM development.

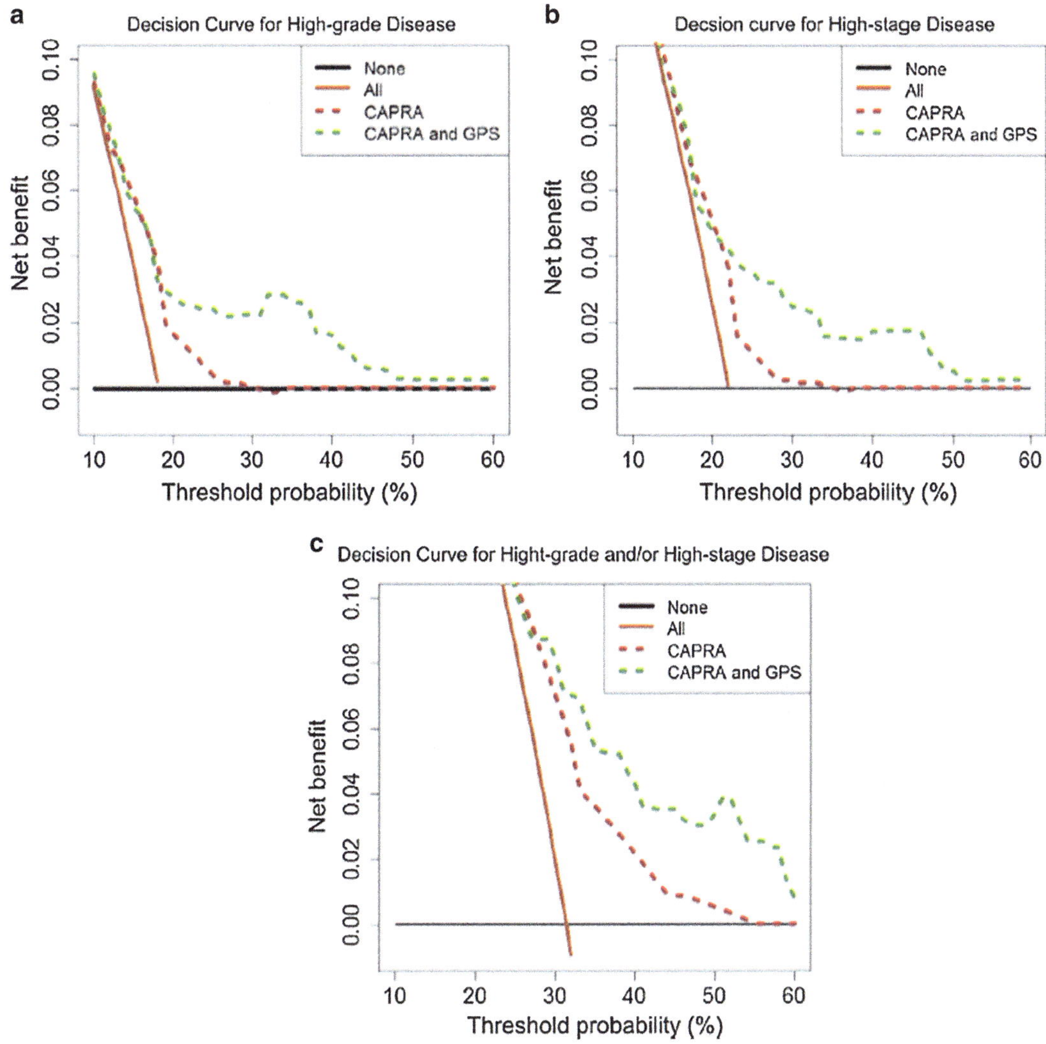

Fig. 27.2 For the outcomes of (**a**) high-grade disease (Gleason pattern I4+3), (**b**) high-stage (pT3a) disease, and (**c**) high-grade and/or high-stage disease, decision curves are presented comparing a model based on clinical and pathologic characteristics summarized by the Cancer of the Prostate Risk Assessment (CAPRA) score to a model combining the CAPRA score with genomic information represented by the Genomic Prostate Score (GPS). For each analysis, the combined CAPRA plus GPS model yielded greater net benefit than the CAPRA score alone, indicating improved discrimination and calibration. *CAPRA* cancer of the prostate risk assessment, *GPS* genomic prostate score. Adopted from Klein et al. [29]

Biomarkers of Second Generations

Noncoding RNAs

The revolutionary development of first generation molecular markers in prostate cancer has brought about next generation sequencing platforms [35]. The advanced genome-wide association studies (GWAS) have emerged as a new approach to identify alleles associated with prostate cancer risk in an unbiased fashion, i.e., without prior knowledge of their position or function [34]. The use of noncoding RNAs as novel biomarkers in prostate cancer was reported by Ronnau and colleagues [37] The use of this approach, in the ENCODE project, has revealed that a much larger proportion of the genome

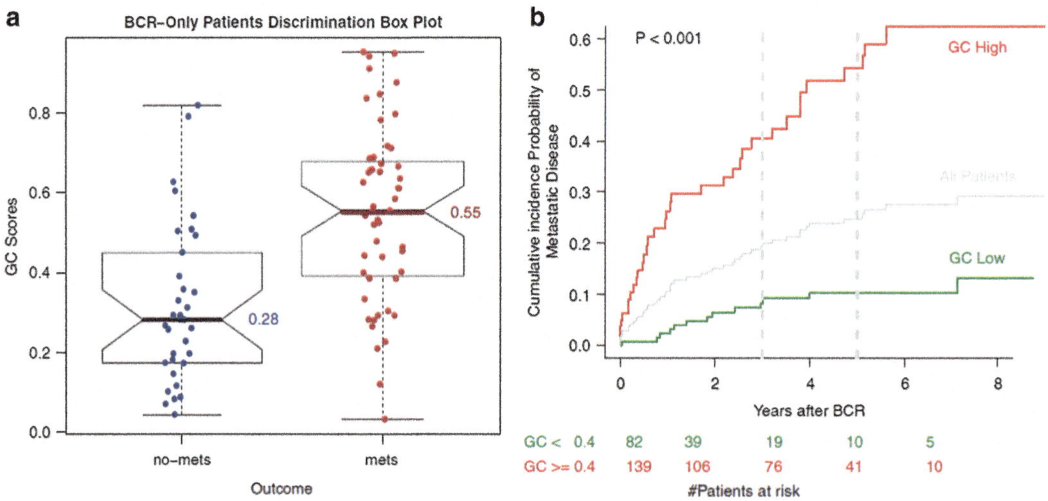

Fig. 27.3 Influence of genomic classifier (GC) score on metastatic progression in patients with biochemical recurrence (BCR) following radical prostatectomy. (**a**) Box plots demonstrating the distribution of GC among patients who progressed to metastasis following BCR (mets) vs. those who did not. (**b**) Cumulative incidence of clinical metastasis based on GC risk groups. Adopted from Ross et al. [32]

(70 %) is transcribed as non-protein coding (nc) RNA, including long (lnc) RNAs (over 200 bps long) [36]. The latest GENCODE project has annotated 14,880 lncRNAs from 9277 loci, but only a few of them are characterized [37]. Although the biological roles of lncRNA (the "dark matter of the genome") are not nearly as well-understood as the protein coding mRNAs, it became clear that they play important roles in almost every aspects of cancer biology. Apoptosis, proliferation, cell cycle progression, and cell growth all suggest a possible role for long lncRNA as a novel PCa marker [38, 39] (Table 27.6).

A new entity of lncRNA molecules is of particular interest because of its high tissue-and tumor-specificity, and therefore can be considered as a new generation of biomarkers. Further identification of abundant lncRNA in humans demonstrated their role as critical components of cancer biology promoting these molecules to play a "cutting edge" role cancer research. LncRNAs are expressed at much lower levels and with much higher cell-type specificity than mRNAs. Currently, several lncRNAs are identified to play critical roles in the development and progression of PCa (Table 27.7). Lee at al. reported a group of prostate cancer-specific lncRNAs that are up-regulated in PC3 cell lines and in PCa patient samples compared with nonmalignant prostate epithelial and matched normal (healthy) patient prostate tissues [38]. Six prostate cancer up-regulated lncRNAs (AK024556, XLOC_007697, LOC100287482, XLOC_005327, XLOC_008559, and XLOC_009911) were characterized in PCa

Table 27.6 Multivariate Cox proportional hazards analysis of most significant risk factors for postoperative RT biochemical failure and distant metastasis

Risk factor	Biochemical failure HR (95 % CI) *P*	Distant metastasis HR (95 % CI) *P*
GC intermediate	2.88 (1.21–6.85) 0.02	2.15 (0.18–39.48) 0.55
Gleason score high	8.13 (3.40–19.46) <0.0001	14.28 (2.13–210.38) 0.005
Pre- RP PSA (log_2)	1.49 (1.06–2.10) 0.02	2.69 (1.33–5.65) 0.007
Pathological GS (Ref ≤ 7)	2.21 (1.07–4.56) 0.03	2.13 (0.30–14.99) 0.4
Detectable PSA (Ref.: undetectable)	3.23 (1.49–6.98) 0.003	0.92 (0.08–10.42) 0.91

Modified from Den et al. [33]
AAM African American Men, *CI* confidence interval, *HR* hazard ratio, *GC* genomic classifier, *GS* Gleason score, *RP* radical prostatectomy, *Ref* referent

Table 27.7 Long noncoding RNA as novel biomarkers

lncRNA	Function	PCa phenotype
PCA3	Biomarker	Not known
PTENP1	Biomarker, tumor suppressor	Binds PTEN-suppressing miRNAs
SChLAP1	Biomarker	Predict PCa-progression after RP promoting invasion and metastasis
SPKY4-IT1	Biomarker	Promotes cell proliferation and invasion, inhibits cell apoptosis, predicts PCa-progression after RP

tissue samples (Gleason score >6.0) and compared with matched normal tissues. Investigators found that these markers can be detected in patient's urine samples and that they are up-regulated when compared with normal urine. Molecular function of one of the up-regulated lncRNAs, AK024556 (SPRY4-IT1) was highly up-regulated in human prostate cancer cell line PC3 but not in LNCaP, and siRNA knockdown of SPRY4-IT1 in PC3 cells inhibited cell proliferation and invasion and increased cell apoptosis. A RNA chromogenic in situ hybridization (CISH) assay was developed to detect long noncoding RNAs in primary PCa. The results of this tissue array demonstrated the specificity of expression in PCa. SPRY4-IT1 expression was easily detected in all prostatectomy specimens [Gleason scores 6 (3+3), 7 (3+4 and 4+3), 8 (4+4), 9 (5+4 and 4+5), and 10 (5+5)] vs. no staining of normal prostatic tissue (Fig. 27.4). A quantitative analysis of the tissue array further confirmed the higher staining intensity in tumor tissues compared with normal tissues. These results indicate that SPRY4-IT1 expression is specific to PCa and can be detected using standard clinical staining procedures [38].

Conclusion

Ultimately, the decision to proceed with ART for locally advanced PCa with adverse pathological features or to postpone it for only those who develop biochemical failure is a difficult one. While both debating sides found consensus to find a tailored approach that identifies and treats the patients at risk for death from disease, other patients can choose watchful waiting with less risk for morbidity of treatment. Ongoing randomized trials may eventually shed some light at the end of the tunnel, but for now and at least for the next few years, the joint AUA/ASTRO guidelines with ASCO panel endorsement look very reasonable. First of all, careful and thorough discussions between the patient and multiple health care professionals can facilitate a shared decision making process with a tailored approach. The treatment chosen is based on the patient's individual risk of local recurrence and his concern with reasonable balance between cancer control and side effects of treatment that can affect quality of life issues. As such, many clinicians advocate for SRT as a more selective approach rather than ART. At present, there is no level 1 evidence to support the hypothesis that ART and early SRT can provide patients with the same treatment outcome. It is also clear that even among a high-risk patient population based on standard clinical features, there remain a significant proportion of patients who may benefit from additional local therapy, whereas others may require systemic therapy. Conversely, some large-scale studies have shown that there also exist a significant proportion of patients for whom disease progression is indolent and who derive little benefit from post-RP RT.

Finally, novel biomarkers allow predictive capability and clinical utility beyond clinicopathologic characteristics and better decision-making. The use of genomic signatures has been demonstrated to change clinical decision making process in approximately 50 % of cases. Furthermore, the combined use of genomic scores and clinical/pathological parameters will synergistically enhance each other to guide the treatment decision for ART vs. SRT. Taking into considerations cost/efficacy ratio for any kind of RT, avoidance of unnecessary or untimely or inadequate treatment would have major implications for healthcare systems all over the world. This could significantly reduce potential overtreatment of patients who will not progress and also impact survival.

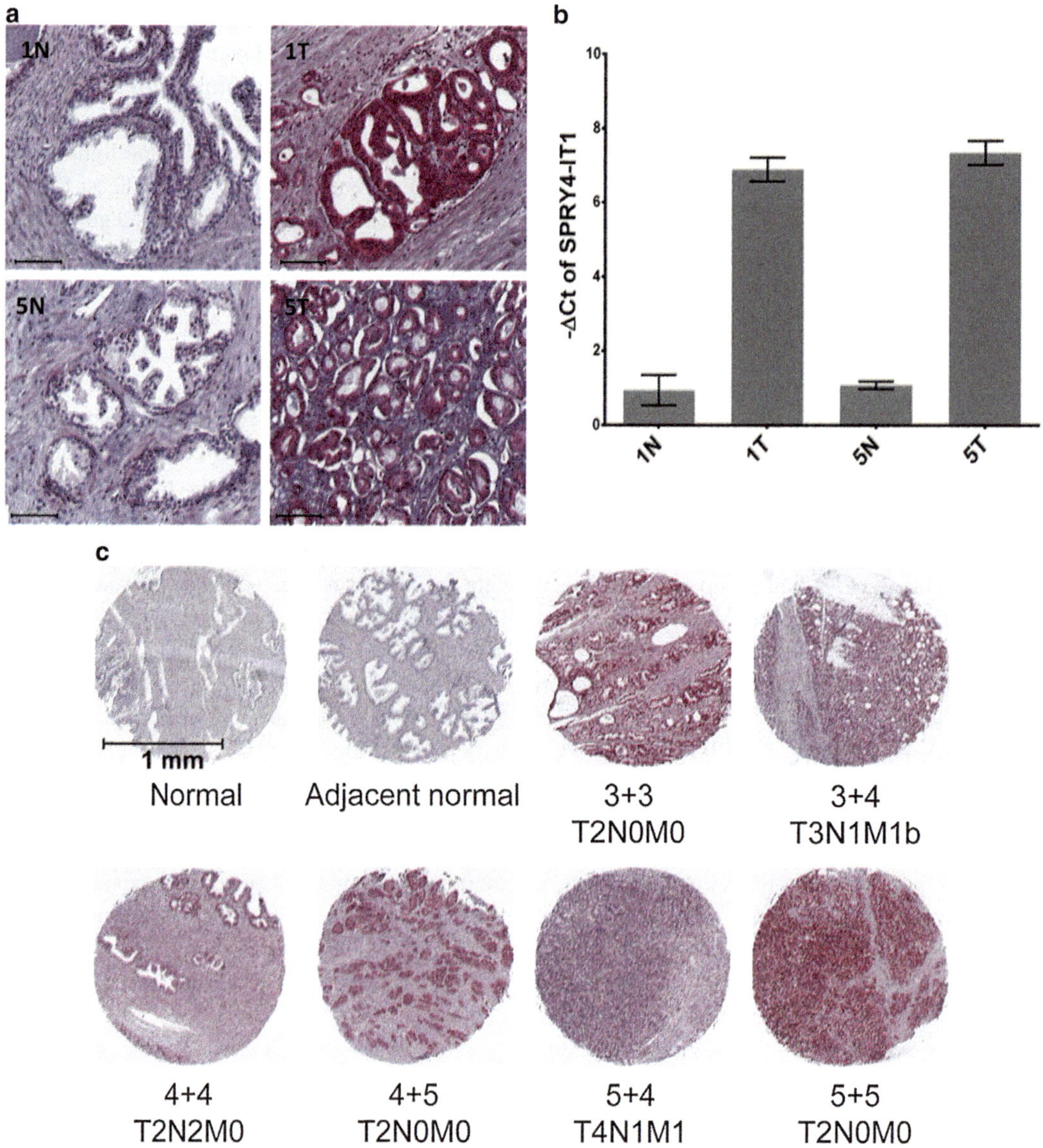

Fig. 27.4 RNA chromogenic in situ hybridization (CISH) analysis of SPRY4-IT1. (**a**) RNA-CISH staining of SPRY4-IT1 in tumor samples and matched normal tissues (formalin-fixed, paraffin-embedded (FFPE) samples). Expression was visualized using alkaline phosphatase-labeled probes. (**b**) qPCR of SPRY-IT1 expression in tumor and matched tissue samples (FFPE samples in **a**). (**c**) RNA-CISH staining of SPRY4-IT1 expression in human prostate cancer tissue array. Tissue samples include normal prostate, adjacent normal, and prostate cancer samples indicated by Gleason scores: 6 (3+3), 7 (3+4 and 4+3), 8 (4+4), 9 (5+4 and 4+5), and 10 (5+5). Expression is visualized using alkaline phosphatase-labeled probes. Scale bar Z 100 mm (**a**). *N* normal patient, *T* prostate cancer patient. Adopted from Lee et al. [38]

References

1. Howlader N, Noone AM, Krapcho M, Garshell J, Miller D, Altekruse SF, et al. SEER cancer statistics review, 1975–2011 Bethesda, MD: National Cancer Institute; 2014 (updated April 2014; cited 2014). http://seer.cancer.gov/csr/1975_2011.
2. Institute TNC. Prostate specific antigen (PSA) test Bethesda, MD2012 (cited 2014). http://www.cancer.gov/cancertopics/factsheet/Detection/PSA.
3. Moyer VA. Screening for prostate cancer: U.S. Preventive Services Task Force recommendation statement. Ann Intern Med. 2012;157(2):120–34.
4. Stephenson AJ, Scardino PT, Eastham JA, Bianco Jr FJ, Dotan ZA, DiBlasio CJ, et al. Postoperative nomogram predicting the 10-year probability of prostate cancer recurrence after radical prostatectomy. J Clin Oncol. 2005;23(28):7005–12.
5. Kupelian PA, Elshaikh M, Reddy CA, Zippe C, Klein EA. Comparison of the efficacy of local therapies for localized prostate cancer in the prostate-specific antigen era: a large single-institution experience with radical prostatectomy and external-beam radiotherapy. J Clin Oncol. 2002;20(16):3376–85.
6. Thompson Jr IM, Tangen CM, Paradelo J, Lucia MS, Miller G, Troyer D, et al. Adjuvant radiotherapy for pathologically advanced prostate cancer: a randomized clinical trial. JAMA. 2006;296(19):2329–35.
7. Thompson IM, Tangen CM, Paradelo J, Lucia MS, Miller G, Troyer D, et al. Adjuvant radiotherapy for pathological T3N0M0 prostate cancer significantly reduces risk of metastases and improves survival: long-term follow-up of a randomized clinical trial. J Urol. 2009;181(3):956–62.
8. Bolla M, van Poppel H, Collette L, van Cangh P, Vekemans K, Da Pozzo L, et al. Postoperative radiotherapy after radical prostatectomy: a randomised controlled trial (EORTC trial 22911). Lancet. 2005;366(9485):572–8.
9. Wiegel T, Bottke D, Steiner U, Siegmann A, Golz R, Storkel S, et al. Phase III postoperative adjuvant radiotherapy after radical prostatectomy compared with radical prostatectomy alone in pT3 prostate cancer with postoperative undetectable prostate-specific antigen: ARO 96-02/AUO AP 09/95. J Clin Oncol. 2009;27(18):2924–30.
10. Stephenson AJ, Scardino PT, Kattan MW, Pisansky TM, Slawin KM, Klein EA, et al. Predicting the outcome of salvage radiation therapy for recurrent prostate cancer after radical prostatectomy. J Clin Oncol. 2007;25(15):2035–41.
11. Boorjian SA, Karnes RJ, Crispen PL, Rangel LJ, Bergstralh EJ, Blute ML. Radiation therapy after radical prostatectomy: impact on metastasis and survival. J Urol. 2009;182(6):2708–14.
12. Trock BJ, Han M, Freedland SJ, Humphreys EB, DeWeese TL, Partin AW, et al. Prostate cancer-specific survival following salvage radiotherapy vs observation in men with biochemical recurrence after radical prostatectomy. JAMA. 2008;299(23):2760–9.
13. Cotter SE, Chen MH, Moul JW, Lee WR, Koontz BF, Anscher MS, et al. Salvage radiation in men after prostate-specific antigen failure and the risk of death. Cancer. 2011;117(17):3925–32.
14. Chen C, Lin T, Zhou Y, Li D, Xu K, Li Z, et al. Adjuvant and salvage radiotherapy after prostatectomy: a systematic review and meta-analysis. PLoS One. 2014;9(8):e104918.
15. Briganti A, Wiegel T, Joniau S, Cozzarini C, Bianchi M, Sun M, et al. Early salvage radiation therapy does not compromise cancer control in patients with pT3N0 prostate cancer after radical prostatectomy: results of a match-controlled multi-institutional analysis. Eur Urol. 2012;62(3):472–87.
16. Trabulsi EJ, Valicenti RK, Hanlon AL, Pisansky TM, Sandler HM, Kuban DA, et al. A multi-institutional matched-control analysis of adjuvant and salvage postoperative radiation therapy for pT3-4N0 prostate cancer. Urology. 2008;72(6):1298–302. discussion 302–4.
17. Ost P, De Troyer B, Fonteyne V, Oosterlinck W, De Meerleer G. A matched control analysis of adjuvant and salvage high-dose postoperative intensity-modulated radiotherapy for prostate cancer. Int J Radiat Oncol Biol Phys. 2011;80(5):1316–22.
18. Kibel AS. Treat now or later: the dilemma of postoperative radiotherapy. Eur Urol. 2012;61(3):452–4.
19. Moul JW. When should we pull the trigger for post-radical prostatectomy radiotherapy? Eur Urol. 2012;62(3):488–90.
20. Gandaglia G, Karakiewicz PI, Briganti A, Trudeau V, Trinh QD, Kim SP, et al. Early radiotherapy after radical prostatectomy improves cancer-specific survival only in patients with highly aggressive prostate cancer: validation of recently released criteria. Int J Urol. 2015;22(2):88–95.
21. Cao D, Humphrey PA, Gao F, Tao Y, Kibel AS. Ability of linear length of positive margin in radical prostatectomy specimens to predict biochemical recurrence. Urology. 2011;77(6):1409–14.
22. Thompson IM, Valicenti RK, Albertsen P, Davis BJ, Goldenberg SL, Hahn C, et al. Adjuvant and salvage radiotherapy after prostatectomy: AUA/ASTRO guideline. J Urol. 2013;190(2):441–9.
23. Freedland SJ, Rumble RB, Finelli A, Chen RC, Slovin S, Stein MN, et al. Adjuvant and salvage radiotherapy after prostatectomy: American Society of Clinical Oncology clinical practice guideline endorsement. J Clin Oncol. 2014;32(34):3892–8.
24. Crawford ED, Ventii K, Shore ND. New biomarkers in prostate cancer. Oncology (Williston Park). 2014;28(2):135–42.
25. Cuzick J. Prognostic value of a cell cycle progression score for men with prostate cancer. Recent Results Cancer Res. 2014;202:133–40.
26. Cooperberg MR, Simko JP, Cowan JE, Reid JE, Djalilvand A, Bhatnagar S, et al. Validation of a cell-cycle progression gene panel to improve risk

stratification in a contemporary prostatectomy cohort. J Clin Oncol. 2013;31(11):1428–34.
27. Knezevic D, Goddard AD, Natraj N, Cherbavaz DB, Clark-Langone KM, Snable J, et al. Analytical validation of the Oncotype DX prostate cancer assay—a clinical RT-PCR assay optimized for prostate needle biopsies. BMC Genomics. 2013;14:690.
28. Klein EA, Cooperberg MR, Magi-Galluzzi C, Simko JP, Falzarano SM, Maddala T, et al. A 17-gene assay to predict prostate cancer aggressiveness in the context of gleason grade heterogeneity, tumor multifocality, and biopsy undersampling. Eur Urol. 2014;66(3): 550–60.
29. Klein EA. Precision medicine approaches to the diagnosis and management of prostate cancer. Oncology (Williston Park). 2014;28(2):143–4. C3.
30. Badani K, Thompson DJ, Buerki C, Davicioni E, Garrison J, Ghadessi M, et al. Impact of a genomic classifier of metastatic risk on postoperative treatment recommendations for prostate cancer patients: a report from the DECIDE study group. Oncotarget. 2013;4(4):600–9.
31. Karnes RJ, Bergstralh EJ, Davicioni E, Ghadessi M, Buerki C, Mitra AP, et al. Validation of a genomic classifier that predicts metastasis following radical prostatectomy in an at risk patient population. J Urol. 2013;190(6):2047–53.
32. Ross AE, Feng FY, Ghadessi M, Erho N, Crisan A, Buerki C, et al. A genomic classifier predicting metastatic disease progression in men with biochemical recurrence after prostatectomy. Prostate Cancer Prostatic Dis. 2014;17(1):64–9.
33. Den RB, Feng FY, Showalter TN, Mishra MV, Trabulsi EJ, Lallas CD, et al. Genomic prostate cancer classifier predicts biochemical failure and metastases in patients after postoperative radiation therapy. Int J Radiat Oncol Biol Phys. 2014;89(5):1038–46.
34. Chung CC, Hsing AW, Edward Y, Biritwum R, Tettey Y, Adjei A, et al. A comprehensive resequence-analysis of 250 kb region of 8q24.21 in men of African ancestry. Prostate. 2014;74(6):579–89.
35. Ronnau CGH, Verhaegh GW, Luna-Velez MV, Shalken JA. Noncoding RNAs as novel biomarkers in prostate cancer. BioMed Res Int. 2014; Epub 2014 Aug 28.
36. Djebali S, Davis CA, Merkel A, Dobin A, Lassmann T, Mortazavi A, et al. Landscape of transcription in human cells. Nature. 2012;489(7414):101–8.
37. Derrien T, Johnson R, Bussotti G, Tanzer A, Djebali S, Tilgner H, et al. The GENCODE v7 catalog of human long noncoding RNAs: analysis of their gene structure, evolution, and expression. Genome Res. 2012;22(9):1775–89.
38. Lee B, Mazar J, Aftab MN, Qi F, Shelley J, Li JL, et al. Long noncoding RNAs as putative biomarkers for prostate cancer detection. J Mol Diagn. 2014;16(6):615–26.
39. Pickl JMA, Heckman D, Ratz L, Klauck SM, Sultman H. Novel RNA markers in prostate cancer: functional considerations and clinical translation. BioMed Res Int. 2014; Epub 2014 Aug 28.

Long-Term Oncologic Outcomes of Robot-Assisted Radical Prostatectomy

28

Newaj Abdullah, Tae-Kyung Kim, and James O. Peabody

Introduction

Prostate cancer (PCa) is the most common noncutaneous malignancy and is the second leading cause of cancer-related death in men in the United States [1]. Radical prostatectomy is the preferred treatment choice over active surveillance for organ-confined disease [2, 3]. Robot-assisted radical prostatectomy (RARP) is a novel approach to radical prostatectomy. The first structured program for RARP was developed at the Vattikuti Urology Institute of the Henry Ford Health System in 2000 [4]. Since then, RARP has been adopted by many centers in the United States, Europe, and the rest of the world. Singh et al. [5] estimated that up to 80 % of radical prostatectomies in the United States are performed using the robotic approach. Since RARP is a novel innovation of this millennium, the long-term oncological outcomes of RARP are still being gathered. While the well-documented long-term oncological control of open radical prostatectomy and laparoscopic radical prostatectomy exist, only a handful of early adopters of RARP are now reporting their mid- and long-term experiences with this technique. This chapter not only summarizes the recent findings on the long-term oncological outcomes of RARP, but also presents the long-term oncological outcomes of open and laparoscopic prostatectomy, and compares these findings to that of RARP.

N. Abdullah, M.D. • J.O. Peabody, M.D., F.A.C.S. (✉)
Vattikuti Urology Institute, Henry Ford Health System, 2799 West Grand Boulevard, Detroit, MI 48202, USA
e-mail: jpeabod1@hfhs.org

T.-K. Kim, B.S.
Department of Urology, University of Michigan Health System, Ann Arbor, MI, USA

Measurement of Long-Term Oncological Outcome

Commonly reported measures of the long-term oncological outcomes of radical prostatectomy are biochemical recurrence-free survival (BCRFS), metastasis-free survival (MFS), and cancer-specific survival (CSS). The time from prostatectomy to the detection of metastasis describes metastasis-free survival, and the number of individuals who have not died of cancer in a specific time period refers to cancer-specific survival. Unlike MFS and CSS, the definition of BCRFS is not uniform in literature [6]. The descriptive variation is an important consideration because the definition utilized can alter the outcome of the research. For example, a number of investigations demonstrated varying disease progression rates—up to 35 %—depending on the utilized BCR definition [7–9]. Table 28.1 shows the various definitions of BCRFS reported in literature.

J.W. Davis (ed.), *Robot-Assisted Radical Prostatectomy*, DOI 10.1007/978-3-319-32641-2_28

Table 28.1 Definitions of biochemical recurrence reported in literature

BCR definition	Description
Single PSA ≥0.6	Single PSA value of 0.6 ng/ml or higher
Single PSA ≥0.4	Single PSA value of 0.4 ng/ml or higher
Single PSA ≥0.2	Single PSA value of 0.2 ng/ml or higher
PSA ≥0.4 and rising	PSA ≥0.4 ng/ml followed by a value higher than the first by any amount
PSA ≥0.2 and rising	PSA ≥0.2 ng/ml followed by a value higher than the first by any amount
PSA ≥0.1 and rising	PSA ≥0.1 ng/ml followed by a value higher than the first by any amount
Two successive rises, final ≥0.2	Two successive (not necessarily consecutive) rises by any incremental amount, final PSA value ≥0.2
Three successive rises	Three successive (not necessarily consecutive) rises by any incremental amount
Three successive rises ≥0.1	Three successive (not necessarily consecutive) incremental PSA rises of 0.1 ng/ml or greater
Three consecutive rises	Three consecutive PSA rises by any incremental amount

All BCR definitions were based on PSA measurements more than 1 month after radical prostatectomy

PSA prostate-specific antigen

Adapted from Stephenson et al. *J Clin Oncol.* 2006 Aug 20;24(24):3973–8

Long-Term Oncological Outcome After RARP

There are a limited number of studies that investigate the long-term oncological outcome following RARP—Table 28.2. A short follow-up period limited early studies. Badani et al. [10] reported on 2766 patients undergoing RARP with a median follow-up period of 22 months and found the overall BCR rate to be 7.3 %. Barocas et al. [11] followed 2132 patients with a median follow-up period of 8 months, and estimated the 3-year BCRFS rates to be 93.1 and 55.4 % for pT2 and pT3 disease, respectively. Menon et al. [12] reported the first longer-term oncologic outcomes in 2010 while following 1384 patients with median follow-up period of 5 years. Of the 1384 followed patients, 189 patients experienced BCR—defined as a confirmed value of PSA ≥0.2 ng/ml, 13 patients developed metastasis, and seven patients died of PCa. The actuarial BCRFS rates were 90.7, 86.8, and 81.0 % at 3-year, 5-year, and 7-year time point, respectively. When stratified by D'Amico risk group, the BCRFS rate was 96.8, 95.1, and 92.6 % in low-risk group; 86.7, 80.2, and 69.8 % in intermediate-risk group; and 78.2, 72.0 and 67.5 % in high-risk group at 3-year, 5-year, 7-year following RARP, respectively. This study also identified preoperative and postoperative factors that independently predict the risk of BCR. They found that pathologic Gleason grade 8–10 and pathologic stage T3b/T4 are the strongest predictors of BCR.

Following the US study by Menon et al., Suardi et al. [13] reported the long-term oncological outcomes on 184 patients from a single European center. Unlike the patient population in the US study who were secondary-treatment naïve for the entire duration of the study, 10.3 % of patients in this European study received adjuvant radiation therapy 3 months following their RARP. Suardi et al. followed the patients for a median follow-up period of 5.6 years, and defined BCR as a confirmed value of PSA ≥0.2 ng/ml. The overall BCRS rate was 94, 86, and 81 % at 3-year, 5-year, and 7-year time point, respectively. When stratified by pathological state, the BCRS rates were 97, 93, and 85 % for patients with pT2 disease; 94, 84, and 84 % for patients with pT3a disease; and 69, 43, and 43 % in patients with pT3b disease at 3-year, 5-year, 7-year following RARP, respectively. With regard to pathologic Gleason score, the BCRFS rate was 97, 98, and 88 % for patients with pathologic Gleason score ≤6; 90, 86, and 75 % for patients with pathologic Gleason score 7; and 85, 65, and 65 % for patients with pathologic Gleason score 8–10 at 3-year, 5-year, and 7-year following RARP. Suardi et al. identified the presence of seminal vesicle invasion and pathologic Gleason score 8–10 as strong independent predictors of BCR.

Table 28.2 Biochemical recurrence-free survival rates in robot-assisted radical prostatectomy series

First author	Year	Cases, *n*	Follow-up, month	Overall BCRFS rate
Menon et al.	2010	1384	60	3 Year: 90.7 % 5 Year: 86.8 % 7 Year: 81.0 %
Suardi et al.	2012	184	67	3 Year: 94 % 5 Year: 86 % 7 Year: 81 %
Soorakumaran et al.	2012	944	76	5 Year: 87.1 % 7 Year: 84.5 % 9 Year: 82.6 %
Diaz et al.	2014	483	120	10 Year: 73.1 %
Abdollah et al.[a]	2015	1100	120	10 Year: 50 %

BCRFS biochemical recurrence-free survival
[a]Abdollah et al. evaluated BCRFS exclusively in D'Amico high-risk prostate cancer

In 2012, Soorakumaran et al. [14] published the second European study on the long-term oncological outcomes of 944 patients undergoing RARP for PCa—defining BCR as a confirmed value of PSA ≥0.2 ng/ml. The overall BCRFS rate was 84.8 % at median follow-up period of 6.3 years. The BCRFS rate for all patients was 87.1, 84.5, and 82.6 % at 5-year, 7-year, and 9-year following RARP. In this study, 9 patients died of PCa—resulting in cancer-specific survival rate of 98.0 %. Soorakumaran et al. study demonstrates that surgeon volume is an independent risk factor for BCR. Increased risk of BCR is seen for surgeons who have operated on fewer than 150 patients. Other predictors of BCR include preoperative PSA >10 ng/ml, pathological stage of pT3a and pT3b, and pathological Gleason score >6.

Diaz et al. [15] recently published on oncological outcomes 10 years following RARP—representing the longest surveillance data following RARP to date. Diaz et al. followed 483 patients to assess BCRFS, MFS, and CSS at the 10-year time point. These patients were part of the discovery and early learning curves of their institution. The study utilized the American Urological Association Localized Prostate Cancer Update Panel report's definition of BCR and includes a confirmed value of PSA ≥0.2 ng/ml, a PSA ≥0.4 ng/ml, or by receipt of salvage therapy. There were 108 BCR, 11 metastases, and 6 deaths from PCa during the median 10-year follow-up period. The overall actuarial BCRFS, MFS, and CSS rates were 73.1, 97.5, and 98.8 % at 10 years following RARP. When stratified by D'Amico risk groups, the 10-year BCRFS rate was 85.7 % for low-risk group, 62.4 % for intermediate-risk group and 43.2 % for high-risk group. Additionally, Diaz et al. demonstrated that D'Amico risk groups or pathologic Gleason grade, pathologic stage, and margin status are strong predictor of BCR.

Abdollah et al. [16] recently investigated the long-term outcomes in clinically high-risk prostrate canter treated with RARP using data from three multinational institutions. This study only evaluated patients with D'Amico high-risk disease. Biochemical chemical recurrence was defined as a confirmed value of PSA ≥0.2 ng/ml. Based on this study, the over BCRFS rate was 50 % at 10-year time point. In order to address heterogeneity within the D'Amico high-risk disease, this study further stratified patients into five risk groups using regression analysis: RG1, very low risk (GS ≤ 6); RG2, low risk (PSA ≤ 10 ng/ml and GS = 7); RG3, intermediate risk (PSA ≤10 ng/ml and GS ≥10 ng/ml); RG4, high risk (PSA > 10 ng/ml and GS = 7) and RG5, very high risk (PSA >10 ng/ml and GS ≥8). In these RGs, 10-year BRCFS was 86, 70, 36, 31, and 26 %, respectively. Cancer-specific survival at 10-year was 99, 96, 85, 67, and 55 % from the very low-risk groups to high-risk groups, respectively.

Long-Term Oncological Outcome After Open and Laparoscopic Radical Prostatectomy

Two alternatives to RARP are open radical prostatectomy and laparoscopic radical prostatectomy. The long-term oncological outcomes following these procedures have been documented in literature and compares to that of RARP. Dorin et al. [17] evaluated 10-year BCR after open radical retropubic prostatectomy by following 2487 patients. The median follow-up time was 7.2 years. Biochemical recurrence was defined as a rise in PSA above the undetectable level and was verified by two consecutive increases in patients with a postoperatively undetectable PSA, with an interval of 3–4 months between PSA draws. During the 10-year follow-up period, a total of 279 patients developed BCR and 49 patients died of prostate cancer, resulting in an 11 % BCR rate and a 2 % CSS rate. In this study, all patients were stratified into low-, intermediate-, and high-risk group based on D'Amico risk stratification scheme. The 10-year BCRFS was 92, 83, and 76 % for low-, intermediate- and high-risk group, respectively. In another series, Touijer et al. [18] followed 1422 patients with clinically localized prostate cancer who underwent laparoscopic radical prostatectomy over 10-year period. Of the 1422 patients, 153 experienced BCR. In this study, the overall BCRFS rate was 78 and 71 % at 5-year and 8-year time point. When stratified into low-, intermediate-, and high-risk groups based on pretreatment prostate cancer nomogram BCRFS probability of >90 %, 89–71 %, and <70 %, BCRFS rate at 5-year was 91, 77, and 53 %, respectively.

Conclusions

Robot-assisted radical prostatectomy has become the predominant surgical treatment for clinically localized prostate cancer since its introduction in 2000. The first structured high-volume programs were developed in the early part of this century. These programs are only recently able to publish 5-year and now 10-year outcomes data. The results in these publications demonstrate relative equivalence of the measured outcomes of BCRFS and CSS for RALP and open and laparoscopic prostatectomy. Factors predictive of recurrence include higher Gleason score, pathologic stage, and PSA.

Disclosure None of the authors report conflicts of interest.

Editorial Comment: John W. Davis

Any novel procedure in oncology needs long-term follow-up. An exciting alternative to standard therapy for favorable risk disease is focal therapy using cryotherapy, laser, or other source of ablation. These represent very new techniques and deserve careful scrutiny as to their safety and efficacy. Anecdotal failures are more difficult to analyze—errors in patient selection, technique, follow-up care? Just this past month, I have diagnosed two impressive failures from focal laser ablation—one lymph node metastatic and one locally advanced. Such events happen after robotic prostatectomy as well; however, we have a full pathology report to help us understand what happened. Ultimately, robotic surgery is just a tool to accomplish what we know and have studied for decades in open surgery.

Nevertheless, long-term oncologic outcomes are important, and the Henry Ford group presents an excellent review of the long-term outcomes from this procedure that they started. I would also highlight their work as reported by Sukumar and Rogers [19]. The final cohort consisted of 4803 patients with a median 26 months follow-up—IQR 1.2–54.6. The overall biochemical recurrence rate was 9.8 %. The actuarial 8-year results were 81 % biochemical recurrence free, 98.5 % metastasis free, and 99.1 % cancer-specific survival. This is a non-comparative study that occurred at the first high volume center and included their learning curve. Nevertheless, the overall and detailed statistics provided certainly support a consistent oncologic outcome compared to open technique.

Another key recent study by Hu et al. [20] is often referred to as robotic outcomes—"2nd generation." In a more established cohort using

SEER/Medicare and propensity-based analyses, RARP had fewer positive margins than open—13.5 % versus 18.3 % and less additional cancer therapy within the first six postoperative months. If cases continue to be condensed toward fewer, high-volume referral surgeons, then perhaps oncologic control may be a benefit at this endpoint. Overall, surgeons will utilize their robotic pT2 and pT3a positive margin rates for early quality assessment. The question as to whether a pT2 Gleason 3+4 negative margin or any other combination of stage, grade, and margin status behaves in the exact same manner using similar definitions of failure and length of follow-up. The data presented would support this notion, although prospective controlled trials are lacking. The early pathologic staging seems satisfactory to most robotic surgeons to make a full-scale switch to the technique, compared to the dilemma of the ablative treatments that need much longer outcomes before recommending broad usage.

References

1. Center MM, Jemal A, Lortet-Tieulent J, Ward E, Ferlay J, Brawley O, Bray F. International variation in prostate cancer incidence and mortality rates. Eur Urol. 2012;61(6):1079–92. doi:10.1016/j.eururo.2012.02.054.
2. Bill-Axelson A, Holmberg L, Ruutu M, Garmo H, Stark JR, Busch C, Nordling S, Haggman M, Andersson SO, Bratell S, Spangberg A, Palmgren J, Steineck G, Adami HO, Johansson JE. Radical prostatectomy versus watchful waiting in early prostate cancer. N Engl J Med. 2011;364(18):1708–17. doi:10.1056/NEJMoa1011967.
3. Thompson I, Thrasher JB, Aus G, Burnett AL, Canby-Hagino ED, Cookson MS, D'Amico AV, Dmochowski RR, Eton DT, Forman JD, Goldenberg SL, Hernandez J, Higano CS, Kraus SR, Moul JW, Tangen CM. Guideline for the management of clinically localized prostate cancer: 2007 update. J Urol. 2007;177(6):2106–31. doi:10.1016/j.juro.2007.03.003.
4. Menon M, Tewari A, Peabody J. Vattikuti Institute prostatectomy: technique. J Urol. 2003;169(6):2289–92. doi:10.1097/01.ju.0000067464.53313.dd.
5. Singh I, Hemal AK. Robotic-assisted radical prostatectomy in 2010. Expert Rev Anticancer Ther. 2010;10(5):671–82. doi:10.1586/era.10.35.
6. Stephenson AJ, Kattan MW, Eastham JA, Dotan ZA, Bianco Jr FJ, Lilja H, Scardino PT. Defining biochemical recurrence of prostate cancer after radical prostatectomy: a proposal for a standardized definition. J Clin Oncol. 2006;24(24):3973–8. doi:10.1200/jco.2005.04.0756.
7. Amling CL, Bergstralh EJ, Blute ML, Slezak JM, Zincke H. Defining prostate specific antigen progression after radical prostatectomy: what is the most appropriate cut point? J Urol. 2001;165(4):1146–51.
8. Gretzer MB, Trock BJ, Han M, Walsh PC. A critical analysis of the interpretation of biochemical failure in surgically treated patients using the American Society for Therapeutic Radiation and Oncology criteria. J Urol. 2002;168(4 Pt 1):1419–22. doi:10.1097/01.ju.0000029729.26315.fd.
9. Kuban DA, Thames HD, Shipley WU. Defining recurrence after radiation for prostate cancer. J Urol. 2005;173(6):1871–8. doi:10.1097/01.ju.0000157682.40869.65.
10. Badani KK, Kaul S, Menon M. Evolution of robotic radical prostatectomy: assessment after 2766 procedures. Cancer. 2007;110(9):1951–8. doi:10.1002/cncr.23027.
11. Barocas DA, Salem S, Kordan Y, Herrell SD, Chang SS, Clark PE, Davis R, Baumgartner R, Phillips S, Cookson MS, Smith Jr JA. Robotic assisted laparoscopic prostatectomy versus radical retropubic prostatectomy for clinically localized prostate cancer: comparison of short-term biochemical recurrence-free survival. J Urol. 2010;183(3):990–6. doi:10.1016/j.juro.2009.11.017.
12. Menon M, Bhandari M, Gupta N, Lane Z, Peabody JO, Rogers CG, Sammon J, Siddiqui SA, Diaz M. Biochemical recurrence following robot-assisted radical prostatectomy: analysis of 1384 patients with a median 5-year follow-up. Eur Urol. 2010;58(6):838–46. doi:10.1016/j.eururo.2010.09.010.
13. Suardi N, Ficarra V, Willemsen P, De Wil P, Gallina A, De Naeyer G, Schatteman P, Montorsi F, Carpentier P, Mottrie A. Long-term biochemical recurrence rates after robot-assisted radical prostatectomy: analysis of a single-center series of patients with a minimum follow-up of 5 years. Urology. 2012;79(1):133–8. doi:10.1016/j.urology.2011.08.045.
14. Sooriakumaran P, Haendler L, Nyberg T, Gronberg H, Nilsson A, Carlsson S, Hosseini A, Adding C, Jonsson M, Ploumidis A, Egevad L, Steineck G, Wiklund P. Biochemical recurrence after robot-assisted radical prostatectomy in a European single-centre cohort with a minimum follow-up time of 5 years. Eur Urol. 2012;62(5):768–74. doi:10.1016/j.eururo.2012.05.024.
15. Diaz M, Peabody JO, Kapoor V, Sammon J, Rogers CG, Stricker H, Lane Z, Gupta N, Bhandari M, Menon M. Oncologic outcomes at 10 years following robotic radical prostatectomy. Eur Urol. 2015;67(6):1168–76. doi:10.1016/j.eururo.2014.06.025.
16. Abdollah F, Sood A, Sammon JD, Hsu L, Beyer B, Moschini M, Gandaglia G, Rogers CG, Haese A, Montorsi F, Graefen M, Briganti A, Menon M. Long-term cancer control outcomes in patients with clinically high-risk prostate cancer treated with

robot-assisted radical prostatectomy: results from a multi-institutional study of 1100 patients. Eur Urol. 2015. doi:10.1016/j.eururo.2015.06.020.
17. Dorin RP, Daneshmand S, Lassoff MA, Cai J, Skinner DG, Lieskovsky G. Long-term outcomes of open radical retropubic prostatectomy for clinically localized prostate cancer in the prostate-specific antigen era. Urology. 2012;79(3):626–31. doi:10.1016/j.urology.2011.09.051.
18. Touijer K, Secin FP, Cronin AM, Katz D, Bianco F, Vora K, Reuter V, Vickers AJ, Guillonneau B. Oncologic outcome after laparoscopic radical prostatectomy: 10 years of experience. Eur Urol. 2009;55(5):1014–9. doi:10.1016/j.eururo.2008.10.036.
19. Sukumar S, Rogers CG, Trinh QD, et al. Oncologic outcomes after robot-assisted radical prostatectomy: long-term follow-up in 4,803 patients. BJU Int. 2014;114:824–31.
20. Hu JC, Gandaglia G, Karakiewicz PI, et al. Comparative effectiveness of robot-assisted versus open radical prostatectomy cancer control. Eur Urol. 2014;66:666–72.

Part IV

Patient Education

Personalized Versus Generic Patient Handouts: Tools to Improve Patient Knowledge on Treatment Options and Perioperative Care

29

John W. Davis

Introduction

Early in my practice, I noted that patient's spouses had fairly consistent lines of questioning, both in the decision making process, and in the logistics of getting through surgery process. I started with a generic handout of "frequently asked questions" and over a decade expanded it into a full-scale patient handout that is updated periodically. In this chapter I include much of its content straight on (**Italics portion**) but modify parts personal to me in a way that you can use to modify it for your practice. I talk a lot in clinic, so my clinic runs late and patients compliment me on its content, and it does give them a task during the waiting.

Step 1: Establish an Introduction to Your Practice

Who are you? Who is on your team? What should they expect as they negotiate your clinic or institution?

J.W. Davis, M.D. (✉)
Department of Urology, Uro-surgical Prostate Cancer Program, The University of Texas M.D. Anderson Cancer Center, Houston, TX, USA
e-mail: jdhdavis@aol.com

I start out with a table of contents for the whole handout and then go into a welcoming statement:

> ***Thank you for choosing to visit us at the Genitourinary Center at the University of Texas M. D. Anderson Cancer Center. This guide was originally written in 2003 as a guide to post-operative care for prostate cancer surgery, and has since been expanded to a broader scope with updates as needed. If you are being seen for prostate cancer screening, this guide may be a bit beyond the scope of your interests, but look for the sections on global health screening, diet, and prevention. A secondary guide to screening and diagnosis is in development, as there are so many new developments in this area. A significant portion of the content of this handout derives from the many hours I've spent with patients and their families discussing the topic of prostate cancer. When similar questions are frequently asked, I try and insert more content to address them. Thus, this guide is more of a joint written "blog" between physician, patient, and family, rather than a static document such as a published book. If you have a suggestion for new content, a correction, or clarification, please let me know and you'll be in the next version.***
> ***The vision of the institution as a whole is to "be the premier cancer center in the world, based on the excellence of our people, our research-driven patient care and our science. We are Making Cancer History." To accomplish this vision in prostate cancer, we have multiple tasks to perfect: identification of ideal candidates for active surveillance, highly efficacious treatments with minimal side effects for patients with more threatening tumors, and combination treatments for the higher risk cases. Meanwhile, we must consider the whole patient and not just the***

J.W. Davis (ed.), *Robot-Assisted Radical Prostatectomy*, DOI 10.1007/978-3-319-32641-2_29

cancer. In fact, most men with prostate cancer die of something else (heart disease is #1).

You could insert your brief CV at this point, but I would suggest putting it at the end so as not to lead off the document with yourself emphasized. They will certainly find it later.

Step 2: Walk Them Through a New Patient Encounter

Consultation Outline

1. *At the beginning of your visit, we will review the records from your other involved providers—inside or outside of MDACC. In addition, all new patients to MDACC are asked to complete the "New Patient Database." Recently, this has become an online form that you can do in advance. What we are looking for are general facts about your medical condition, medications, allergies, and fitness for various treatment options. Please think through your medication list carefully and including all prescribed and "over-the-counter" medications, vitamins, supplements, i.e., anything you ingest that is not food. Also include anything you ingest on an "as needed" basis, which we denote as "PRN." In some cases, there are features of your medical condition or prostate anatomy that may be a contraindication to certain treatments. If so, we will evaluate and focus on alternatives. Any outside ultrasound and biopsy reports are helpful. Outside biopsy materials are reread at MDACC, but in some cases your visit occurs before this is completed. A well-organized PSA history (year, value, etc.) is very valuable.*
2. *A physical examination is an essential element to any new patient visit. Naturally, this exam will be focused upon potentially relevant findings to prostate cancer screening or treatment. Therefore, our exam should not be viewed as a substitute for a more thorough physical examination by your primary physician, and we are not necessarily trying to perform comprehensive cancer screening. In most cases, the physical exam is first performed by physician's assistant who is specifically trained for the initial screening exam, and I may double check pertinent findings or anything you would like me to address. If you have no complaints specific to the exam, I often spend the visit on the counselling component.*
3. *An important goal of the visit is to communicate back to you our assessment of your disease risk. A prostate cancer risk classification is an estimate of the likelihood of the disease progressing despite attempted curative therapy. The best information to determine risk classification starts with the PSA, clinical stage, and biopsy Gleason score. In intermediate to higher risk cases, imaging studies such as an MRI, CT, and/or bone scan may be needed. Additional details from the biopsy report are helpful such as the number of cores positive, and the size of the tumor foci present (some are reported by actual length of a tumor foci and others as a percentage).*
4. *Next, we will discuss treatment options. The standard options may include active surveillance, surgery (open or robotic), or radiation therapy (IMRT, proton, or brachytherapy (seeds)). Alternate treatment options may include cryotherapy or HIFU (high intensity focused ultrasound). In general, a treatment option is considered alternative if the available published literature on outcomes is limited to less than 10 years of follow-up.*
5. *At the end of our discussion, there are several possible conclusions.*
   (a) *Pending status. This means you have opted to review options presented to you and no definitive decisions have been made. It is up to you to contact us for any further consultation or treatment. If you elect for treatment elsewhere, I would appreciate knowing your decision, but that is up to you. You can easily leave us an email through your mymdanderson.org account (more on that later).*
   (b) *Further diagnostic testing. For laboratories or simple tests, we can send you right over. For imaging studies such as CT scan, bone scan, or MRI, you will need an appointment that will take us between 1*

and 3 days to complete. Usually, you can leave the clinic and my scheduler will contact you with these appointments. Be sure we have a cell phone or local contact number.

(c) *Further consultation—medical oncology, radiation oncology. If we feel you need to visit with one of these specialists, we will request a consult, and usually we can determine availability by the next day. However, the appointment itself could be the next day or a few days later.*

(d) *Treatment scheduled. If you are ready to schedule surgery, we can usually give you a surgery date, and at that point, may request an IMPAC clinic appointment. This is a medical clinic that does a complete assessment of your health and any surgical risk factors. They will order appropriate labs, EKG, and possibly heart stress testing. If you have minimal medical problems, you probably will not need this step.*

6. *Please note that we are happy to serve in any of several roles.*
   (e) *We can be your primary treatment and follow-up center.*
   (f) *We can be your primary treatment center, and arrange follow-up in your local area.*
   (g) *We can be a second opinion resource, and you arrange treatment and follow-up elsewhere.*
7. *Post-Visit Communication.*
   (h) *You should receive a cover sheet with contact telephone information. However, moving into the modern era, MD Anderson now has a multipurpose Web-tool for patient use called MyMDAnderson.org. You can establish an account by using your MDACC medical record number and then setting up a password by answering security questions. The server can do a number of things:*
   - *Medical Chart—all of your pathology, transcribed doctor notes, labs, and X-ray reports are all available. Lab and pathology are not seen until 7 days after finalized so the teams can discuss results. Dictations are not seen until signed by the provider.*
   - *Appointments—you can see all upcoming appointments. Hardcopies are still mailed.*
   - *Secure messaging—you can send messages to your team and back. My clinic has two different addresses—"Davis Clinical," and "Davis Scheduling." Use the clinical address for questions for myself, physicians assistant, and/or nurse. Use scheduling for requests to the scheduler—change appointments, etc. Note that all correspondence goes on your medical chart, so we can refer back later—thus a better service than emails that can be deleted.*
   - *As a general rule, I prefer you correspond with the mymdanderson server as it is quicker for us to respond, and multiple team members can see them. Voice mails take too long to listen to, and only go to one address, and are not part of the medical record. If you have an emergency, then call the triage line in the clinic during normal hours, or hospital operator after hours.*

Step 3: Prostate Cancer Key Facts

Give the patient some of your own favorite facts useful in the decision making process. Since the document is dynamic, you can review it and add new information as it becomes available. As with many things, patient questions will generate new ideas for inclusion/revision.

1. *Prostate cancer is very common with a 1 in 6 lifetime risk. The risk begins as early as the 4th decade and continues lifetime.*
2. *Prostate cancer mortality is less common—1:40. This means many patients die of other causes either with nonlethal cancer, or with treated cancer.*
3. *The top three causes of death in men are cardiovascular disease, cancer, and accidents. Cardiovascular disease is the top cause of*

death in men with and without prostate cancer. Another way to think of this is that if prostate cancer is your greatest risk of death, and we cure you, then whatever was number two now moves up to the top position, and it is likely to be cardiovascular disease. It is somewhat convenient that all preventative measures for cardiovascular disease are also helpful for prostate health—with or without cancer. These measures are probably familiar to you: lose weight, control your blood pressure, control your cholesterol, eat a low-fat diet, exercise, lift weights, etc. More on this later in the guide.

4. *The exact causes of prostate cancer are not known, but are probably multiple. Risks we know about include heredity, high fat diet, and having the male hormone testosterone in your blood for so many years (i.e., if you remove the testicles before puberty, the prostate will not grow and you will not develop prostate cancer. I wouldn't recommend this prevention strategy!)*
5. *A simplified approach to thinking about prostate cancer is to describe four distinct groups of cancers by their biologic potential, i.e., how they may behave currently and in the future.*
   (a) *Low volume/Low grade tumors.*
   - *The challenge of this group is that we see a small amount of low-grade tumor on the biopsy, but these tumors don't always behave like cancers in the traditional sense. These tumors may remain nonactive for many years of decades. Local treatments are very successful, because the cancers are not very threatening. Active surveillance may be an appropriate strategy, and we have a protocol for this. Recent protocols are evaluating alternative treatment concepts such as HIFU (high intensity frequency ultrasound) and focal cryotherapy. In some cases, immediate standard treatment (surgery or radiation) is appropriate and selected.*
   - *For those who have read about the "controversies" of PSA screening, this area of low volume/low grade tumor is an important component. These tumors were likely never detected before PSA, and seem to be a unique entity. It remains unknown/unclear whether or not the more lethal prostate cancers develop that way "de novo" or rather develop from low grade tumors that progress. Either way, the problem from the public health care debate is that approximately 90 % of men in the USA choose to treat these tumors despite the risk of side effects and despite minimal to no mortality from these tumors.*
   - *The only real threat we see in low volume/low grade tumors is that fact that a small percentage (approximately 10–15 %) may have higher grade/volume tumors present, and a few—3 %—may have several steps higher. So we prefer to just re-biopsy to look for these and possible imaging.*

   (b) *Early stage/lethal potential tumors/complete response to treatment.*
   - *These are tumors that show signs of lethal potential, such as intermediate grade, higher volume, higher PSA (>10). In this category, active treatment aims to eliminate the tumor permanently. Many treatment modalities such as surgery, radiation, brachytherapy, and cryotherapy can accomplish this goal.*

   (c) *Locally advanced stage/lethal potential tumors/failed local therapy.*
   - *These are tumors that may look just like category two; however, months to years after treatment, the disease becomes active again as evidenced by a rising PSA. For surgical patients, sometimes the pathologic staging predicts for this possibility, such as with non organ-confined tumors. As many as 15–30 % of patients treated for local disease may suffer a relapse in the future. Surgical patients may be salvaged with follow-up radiation. Radiation patients may be salvaged with surgery (higher side effects, however), or cryotherapy.*

Hormone treatment may play a role as well. It is possible that a second local therapy may succeed months to years after a failed initial therapy. In my way of thinking, this means that some cancers have the ability to locally invade in the pelvis, but lack the ability to spread beyond into the bones.

(d) *Advanced disease.*
   - *With PSA screening, we do not see as many patients at diagnosis with advanced disease, meaning disease in the lymph nodes or bones. Some patients with localized disease may progress to this stage years later. Hormonal therapy plays a key role. In some cases, local therapy may be added. Chemotherapy is available if hormonal therapy stops working—both taxotere and carbazitazel improve survival. Recently, the FDA has approved the vaccine therapy Sipeulecel (trade name Provenge, by Dendreon), Abiraterone, and Enzalutamide for treatment of castrate-resistant prostate cancer.*

(e) *Putting it together.*
   - *The challenge of prostate cancer evaluation is that there can be tremendous overlap between the four categories listed above. Someone can look like #1 but actually be #3. Someone can look like #3 but be #2, etc. A primary goal of our visit will be to put all available information into perspective for you and help make the best decision, knowing that we don't have perfect information going in. Research at the institution focuses on trying to improve our ability to predict prostate cancer biologic potential.*

(f) *How do I choose between multiple treatment options?*
   - *It is important to emphasize that there are no randomized clinical trials to answer the question as to which local therapy is the best. Each has their advantages and disadvantages and must be weighed individually. The goal of this handout is to cover the straightforward facts of prostate cancer treatment so our consult time can focus on this question. At the conclusion of our meeting, it is very common to find that more than one treatment can be recommended. We will do our best to make a best recommendation for you.*
   - *Of interest, the American Urological Association has updated guidelines on prostate cancer treatment. The only two randomized clinical trials they quote are:*
     - *Compared to watchful waiting, radical prostatectomy may improve survival.*
     - *Radiation therapy, if selected, should be given at higher dose to decrease risk of recurrence.*
     - *Currently, comparisons of treatment options (using randomized trials as evidence) are not possible for the purposes of determining superiority.*
     - *Here is the Web link for the AUA patient guide:*
       http://www.auanet.org/guidelines/patient_guides/pc08.pdf.
     - *Here is the Web link for the full AUA prostate cancer guidelines:*
       http://www.auanet.org/guidelines/main_reports/proscan07/content.pdf.

Step 4: Introduce Your Robotic Surgery Program

In the early years, many programs cut and pasted promotional materials from Intuitive Surgical on the benefits of robotic surgery. There is no longer a vacuum of information to continue such practices. Patients want to see your own data, volumes, and experiences. The more details, the better, and the less time you will have to spend in clinic answering the same data points. Here is my version:

Robotic Assisted Radical Prostatectomy

We are proud to offer the robotic prostatectomy procedure. MDACC currently owns three daVinci Si systems, and one daVinci Xi. As of June, 2015 I have performed >2000 robotic and >100 laparoscopic (manual) prostatectomy procedures. I perform 6 cases in a full workweek. Here are some robotic case/volume milestones:

Date	*# procedures/other milestones*
8/4/2004	*1 (Norfolk, Virginia)*
3/2006	*150 (from Virginia)*
4/13/2006	*Began practice at MDACC*
4/29/2006	*1st Houston case, at Memorial Hermann*
7/5/2006	*1st robotic case at MDACC*
9/14/2006	*200*
4/12/2007	*300*
10/18/2007	*400*
12/15/2007	*2nd daVinci system installed at MDACC*
3/24/2008	*500*
11/7/2008	*652*
7/17/2009	*787 3rd daVinci at MDACC*
12/4/2009	*900*
6/1/2011	*1200*
11/9/2011	*1300*
10/1/2012	*1500*
6/30/2015	*2000 4 systems running at MDACC*

During the time course of this case experience, the procedure times have decreased. For example two similar cases were performed: 5/4/2007 in 4 h 17 min (complete surgery time), and 5/5/2008 in 2 h 38 min. As of 2011, further refinements have the prostatectomy times down to 60–75 min, anastomosis 15 min (2 layers), and extended pelvic lymph node dissection (if indicated) in 30–40 min. There have been numerous technical revisions—>13 total—to decrease the use of cautery (thermal heat) around the nerve bundles and urinary control muscles. We use clips and sutures to control vessels and try and guide the dissection as close to the prostate as safe and minimize trauma to the surrounding critical structures.

For organ-confined cancers, the negative margin rate (complete cancer removal) has been 93–95 % which is very competitive with the best of open and robotic series. In the last 100 procedures, the negative margin rate has increased to >97 %, perhaps from more experience and/or lower volume of disease from PSA screening. By contrast, the steady rate of negative surgical margins from open surgery by multiple surgeons at MDACC between 2003 and 2008 was 90 %. Therefore, this technology has been introduced in a safe manner allowing us to improve upon the standard results of open surgery. Recovery of urinary function occurs in >95 % of men using a loose definition (dry to mild/occasional stress incontinence) and 85 % if using a stricter definition. The timing of urinary function recovery is mostly within the first 6–12 weeks with potential improvement seen out to 1 year. Sexual function is a much more complex topic and not adequately expressed as a single statistic. The determinates of sexual function after surgery are patient age, health history, medications, smoking history, sexual function before surgery, number of nerve bundles spared, surgeon technique/experience. In the ideal circumstance of the patient 50 years old, perfect function, no health history or medications, and expert surgery with bilateral nerve sparing, the potency rate may be as high as 90 % after 1–2 years of follow-up. For the typical patient, the rate may be 50 %, and if there are several adverse predictors, it may be 0–20 %. The time to recovery of sexual function is much longer than urinary function. Most early function is at 6 months, with improvement to 2 years and longer.

Regarding sexual function and nerve preservation, I have found it safe to spare all or most of neurovascular bundle tissue in most patients. At this point in my experience I know exactly how to spare nerve bundles when appropriate and I use a technique in which no cautery (thermal heat) is used near the nerve bundle tissue. In the ideal patient, we often observe early erections even in the 1st 6 weeks. MDACC provides me with a travel budget, which I use to go to national and international meetings in search of any technical refinements to this operation, so I am confident in providing you with the best possible operation.

Now that MDACC has the latest technologies in surgery (robots) and radiation therapy (protons) we are conducting a clinical evaluation of quality of life after all treatments and will be the first comparison of its kind to include these recent technologies.

Here are some frequently asked questions regarding this minimally invasive procedure.

1. *What are the advantages?*
   (a) *The most consistent outcome advantage is reduced blood loss during the procedure, and reduced hospital stay. Reduced pain and scaring is possible, but not as clear a difference as many patients do very well with low midline incisions. Recent reports are demonstrating that major and minor complications are reduced with robotic surgery—especially the chance of scarring of the urinary tract. It was recently highlighted by the US Preventative Services Task Force that "up to 1 in 200 men may die after prostate cancer surgery." This is an alarming statistic, but based on 1990s data, mostly collected in Medicare age (65 and up) patients. We have recently reviewed a large hospital network of over 70,000 cases from 2004-2010 and found 1:1100 operative mortality ratio for open surgery and 1:3900 for robotic—likely even smaller for expert robotic surgeons.*
   (b) *Cancer control, urinary function recovery, sexual function recovery in experienced hands are equal to high quality open surgery results. The weight of available evidence does not support superiority at this time. Ultimately, the skill and experience of the surgeon translates into better outcomes more than the technique itself. From strictly an engineering perspective, the robotic instrumentation (reduced size, range of motion) and magnified 3D vision is superior to open surgery, and therefore with time it may be possible to train a larger number of expert surgeons with the robot compared to open. Recent studies has shown that open surgeons, even after expert training, required approximately 250 cases to complete their learning curve. It remains to be proven whether robotic surgeons can achieve high benchmarks earlier. A post learning curve consecutive series of 100 cases showed only two patients had a positive surgical margin, and 1 was organ confined and 1 was not. This is significantly better than my rates from 2003–2006 to 2006–2007. In addition, theses rates would be better than many open series from experienced surgeons. As mentioned, we have made a comparison of open surgery, laparoscopic surgery, and robotic surgery and are preparing the results for publication. The conclusions are that the laparoscopic technique resulted in higher positive margins compared to open, while the robotic technique resulted in lower positive margins.*
   (c) *Compared to laparoscopic prostatectomy, the vision is improved through the 3D camera, and the instruments have 7° of freedom allowing mini-wrist movements at the tips of the instruments.*
   (d) *Robotic prostatectomy is minimally invasive, but unlike radiation and cryotherapy treatments, it provides complete pathologic staging, and the opportunities for secondary radiation should the disease recur.*
2. *Why do you prefer this technique?*
   (a) *There are mild advantages in blood loss, pain, and scaring (Fig. 29.1). As we move forward it is my hope and goal that this procedure will allow top results to be obtained by more surgeons, and in fewer cases then the literature suggests occurs with open surgery.*
   (b) *The comfort and ergonomic advantages provided to the surgeon are very noticeable. The images below is a close-up of a robotic needle driver, demonstrating how the instrument can articulate in 7° like a human hand on a small scale. The shaft of the instrument is only 8 mm in diameter.*

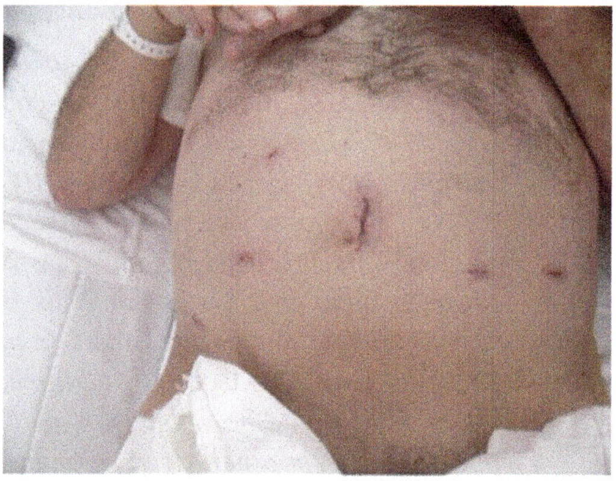

Fig. 29.1 Incisions for robotic surgery

3. *What if I am overweight?*
   (a) *The robotic camera and instruments can access the pelvis very well in most men, even up to 350 pounds, so this procedure may be an advantage in this circumstance. That said, if the body mass index is >40, we have observed greater difficulty with ventilation during surgery and reduced quality of the results. In these circumstances, it may be best to loose significant weight or look for a different option. If you do not know your BMI, we will have it in our computer system, or you can Google out "BMI calculator" and input your height and weight. Anything <40 generally does fine.*
4. *What about prior surgery?*
   (a) *In most cases, laparoscopic instruments can mobilize prior scar tissue and proceed with the case. We are also developing the skill set to perform "extraperitoneal" access in such situations as do open surgeons.*
5. *How often do you perform this surgery?*
   (a) *A typical work week includes.*
      - *Mondays—block time for 2–3 cases at MDACC.*
      - *Tuesday—Clinic all day.*
      - *Wednesday—Research and meetings related to the prostate program.*
      - *Thursday—two cases if help available.*
      - *Friday—block time 2–3 cases at MDACC.*
6. *Where are the incisions?*
   (a) *One is near the belly button and the largest as this is where the prostate is removed. The remaining 5 are 8 mm or less and in the lower abdomen. I used to try and curve the incision around the inner left side of the belly button so it will be less noticeable once healed. However, we observed a small but noticeable incidence of delayed hernias—often 6 or more months after the operation. Therefore, this access may introduce a weakness to the abdominal wall. I now use two alternatives: (1) incise and extract the prostate through an incision right above the umbilicus, or (2) place the camera below the umbilicus, but extend and extract through the right lateral port. Umbilical hernias, if already present, can be fixed during the closure.*
7. *How long in the hospital?*
   (a) *One night is the goal. The pattern is usually.*
      - *Post operative night: ambulate, clear liquid diet.*
      - *Day 1, regular breakfast, ambulate.*
      - *Home mid-day.*
8. *How long does the catheter stay in?*
   (a) *Seven days if you are <2 h from us. Otherwise 9–10 days.*
   (b) *The nursing ward provides a video and training class on care and removal of the catheter.*
   (c) *The catheter can be removed in the clinic, a local physician, or the most convenient is to learn to remove it yourself.*
   (d) *Airline travel with a catheter works very well—even international.*
9. *Can the catheter come out sooner?*
   (a) *This questions has been asked and research at other centers. In summary:*
      - *Catheter removal at 3 days is possible if a cystogram xray shows no leak at the anastomosis (approximately 80 % of cases). However 15 % of patients will then experience urinary retention and require urgent replacement—a stressful experience.*

- *One center is reporting early results from a strategy of placing a suprapubic catheter (through the lower abdominal wall), and then removing the standard urethral catheter the day after surgery. The suprapubic catheter then comes out between 4 and 7 days when the patient demonstrates adequate bladder emptying. The surgeons at this center are reporting less overall patient discomfort and equal urinary control results. At this time I am not doing this as I have concerns over placing additional holes in the abdomen and bladder just to save a few days of catheter time. Therefore, I would like to see more studies and follow-up results.*

10. *How much pain is involved?*
    (a) *One to two days of incision soreness, needing a few pain pills.*
    (b) *Mild perineal, scrotal swelling and soreness can linger for a week or so. If a lymph node dissection is performed, the scrotal swelling can be quite large—softball size. This will go away and is not harmful, but certainly generates some phone calls with concern. It's ok to show your friends. Related to the surgery is the possibility that the testicles become more sensitive to touch for a few weeks—sensory nerves travel near the operative site and can be irritated. This also goes away.*
    (c) *Our current bladder reconstructive technique helps restore continence at an earlier time. However in about 10 % of cases, patients report a few days of bladder spasms that generally resolve. Medications are provided for this problem.*
11. *Return to activities?*
    (a) *Walking: day 1.*
    (b) *Stairs: day 1.*
    (c) *Light exercise: 2nd week.*
    (d) *Work: 2nd week.*
    (e) *Bicycle riding in 6 weeks (unless a recumbent seat—can be sooner).*
    (f) *No restrictions at all after 6 weeks.*
12. *Can you perform a lymph node dissection?*
    (a) *Yes. Most will have a lymph node dissection—the extent depends upon the disease risk. For lower risk disease, we can discuss skipping it, which could make recovery faster. If the primary tumor is found to be much larger and/or higher grade than the biopsies showed, it is possible to return for a lymph node dissection later, but this would likely be a <10 % risk.*
13. *What happens to the prostate gland?*
    (a) *We place it in a bag and remove through the belly button area intact. It is analyzed by a pathologist the same as for open surgery.*
14. *Can you spare nerves?*
    (a) *Yes—the technique works very well for this. We will discuss if it is appropriate for you.*
    (b) *The Gleason score helps us determine this as well as PSA and DRE. Here is the breakdown from my last 200 cases of organ confined disease by Gleason score, assuming a PSA <10.*
        - *Gleason 3 + 3, organ confined 100 %.*
        - *Gleason 3 + 4, organ confined 90 %.*
        - *Gleason 4 + 3, organ confined 60 %.*
        - *Gleason 4 + 4 or higher, organ confined 30 %.*
    (c) *Thus, most all patients with 3 + 3 and 3 + 4 should be candidates for bilateral nerve sparing. For Gleason 4 + 3 or higher, select patients can have nerve sparing, and most can at least have 1 nerve bundle spared. In addition, we now recognize the possibility to perform a "partial" or "incremental" nerve sparing procedure, i.e., take a custom designed wider margin around a specific area, but try and leave the majority of the nerve tissue intact.*
    (d) *In approximately 4–5 % of cases, our assessment of your cancer risk is way off, i.e., significant increase in Gleason grade or staging seen on final pathology of the prostate. This problem is universal, and*

speaks to the need for more research for new biomarkers.

15. *Can you assess the prostate during the procedure?*
    (a) *We can do frozen section biopsies at selected areas of concern, but not the whole gland.*
16. *What about tactile feedback?*
    (a) *Opinions on this subject have changed in recent years. In the late 1990s the majority of expert open surgeons made it clear at our meetings that "feeling" the prostate during the surgery was not useful and often misleading. A few surgeons claimed they could "feel" the neurovascular bundles and then decide whether to take them or leave them. Most disagreed, as most extensions of cancer outside the prostate are a matter of a millimeter—not something anyone can feel through a gloved finger. Now that the robotic technique is very popular, the opinion that an open surgeon can "feel" and assess the tumor with his/her finger is being voiced more often. From my open surgical background, I always thought it was mostly misleading and the biopsy data the most important.*
    (b) *Believe it or not, the robot has tactile feedback. It is actually more of a resistance feedback in that the hand controls transmit resistance when you pull or push on something. When combined with the magnified 3D vision, your brain actually starts to simulate tactile feedback, so when you lift or touch something, you feel it on the controls and see it with your eyes. As a result, fine, delicate maneuvers are quite possible with the robot.*
17. *How long is the procedure?*
    (a) *Anesthesia induction, IV lines, arterial line—20–30 min.*
    (b) *Laparoscopic access, robot docking—5 min.*
    (c) *Work time at console.*
        - *Prostatectomy: 60–70 min.*
        - *Anastomosis: 15 min.*
        - *Pelvic lymph node dissection (if needed): 30–45 min.*
    (d) *Extract prostate, close incisions: 15 min.*
    (e) *Anesthesia: wake up, transport to recovery: 15 min.*
    (f) *Total room time—3–3.5 h for most cases, add 30–45 min if lymph node dissection, add more time for obesity, or very large prostates.*
18. *What about "add-on" procedures?*
    (a) *I routinely reconstruct the posterior layer of the bladder/urethra before doing the standard anastomosis and reconstruct the top of the bladder to the pubovesicle ligaments. These add-ons give the reconstruction more strength, and we collect quality of life surveys to determine if urinary continence is restored sooner. I consider these steps standard.*
    (b) *Inguinal hernias—if we encounter one I generally will use a mesh plug/match to repair the defect, as otherwise the hernia becomes worse from our accessing the pelvis through the abdomen. So it's really just part of the closure and may save having to undergo a separate hernia surgery in the future.*
19. *How many do you do in a day?*
    (a) *As many as 3.*
    (b) *I'm not tired for the afternoon case.*
    (c) *I always get a good night sleep before surgery.*
        - *On that note, I generally go to the gym every morning between 5 a.m. and 6:15 a.m. for a cardio and/or strength workouts and time my arrival to the MDACC parking lot right at 7 a.m. when anesthesia will start the first case. Therefore, if you are a first start case, you won't see me until afterwards, so try and get questions settled ahead of time.*
20. *What about safety procedures?*
    (a) *MDACC is fairly quick to adopt any known improvements in patient safety—often ahead of final national recommendations. We perform a Universal Protocol or "time-out" to identify correct patient, correct procedure, correct antibiotics and allergies. The nurses will put you through*

a number of identify checks before surgery. In addition, I have a laptop computer by the console with instant access to your medical records so I can look at your biopsy reports, and any imaging we've done to be sure we do the correct nerve sparing, and lymph node dissection (if needed). In the future, this setup may be viewed as primitive as I think robotics in the future will continue to evolve into comprehensive information tools. In addition to viewing and controlling the operative field, the robot itself can display tests results, and images. Current research at some institutions is trying to figure out how to match up a radiology image with the surgeon's view.

21. *Does the robot ever break down? About every 6 months the robot may unexpectedly need servicing that may result in needing to reschedule a procedure. This may cause travel and logistical inconvenience for the patient. The robot can be repaired in 1–2 days but the rescheduling may take longer to arrange. It is very rare for the robot to have a problem during the case as it goes through very sensitive diagnostic procedures during boot-up phase (like a computer). If it did breakdown, the case may be completed with one less working arm, or possibly the procedure converted to an open approach. The former situation has happened to me once and the latter has not.*
22. *Which robot models do you have?*
    (a) *As of 2015, the program has 4 systems: a dual console SI, two single console SI, and an Xi. All are upgraded systems with high definition three-dimensional video.*
    (b) *Our robotics suite is also equipped with overhead audio and wireless microphones to improve communication between surgeon and assistant.*
23. *When you remove the prostate, can you tell if you "got it all?"*
    (a) *For the most part, the prostate cancer is invisible, and blends in with the normal gland. Thus, our goal is to remove the prostate and to avoid the surrounding structures. The final pathology is what matters the most.*
24. *When will the final pathology be ready?*
    (a) *If a group of pathologist reads the prostatectomy cases, and they prepare and average sampling of the gland, reports can be completed in 1–2 weeks. At MDACC, we have a single pathologist reading all cases, and she prepares a very detailed sampling of the gland to read. Her reports detail not only Gleason grade, stage, and margin status, but individually characterize the size and location of each focus of tumor.*
    (b) ***As a result of the detailed, consistent analyses from a single pathologist, the reports are not finalized until the 6 week clinic follow-up visit.***
    (c) *Occasionally, reports are available earlier and I will have my PA call the results, but in most cases, we just discuss this at the 6-week visit.*
    (d) *With mymdanderson.org you can check ahead to see if it's ready.*
        - *A pathology report will detail a lot of information, but the highlights are:*
            - *Stage—is it confined to the prostate, or extraprostatic extension, or seminal vesical invasion?*
            - *Gleason grade—a new Gleason is given, unless taking hormones.*
            - *Margin status—does the cancer touch the edge of resection? If so, the margin is measured in millimeters.*
            - *Lymph node status.*
            - *Note that the combination of the above can predict the chance of the PSA going up again, but it's just a prediction—our long-term plan is a combination of the pathology report and the PSA measurements.*
25. *How long do I have to be in Houston for surgery?*
    (a) *The entire trip including preoperative clinic visit, surgery, and recovery can be done in 6 days.*
    (b) *You may leave the hospital on the day after surgery, but remain in Houston*

until the 3rd day. You may depart by car or plane.

(c) *To avoid blood clots in the legs, avoid sitting in the same position for more than 1 h, i.e., take frequent rest stops to stretch.*

26. *What have you improved about the operation at MDACC?*

    (a) *I recognize 11 different steps of the operation and have adjusted as follows:*

    - *Dropping the bladder. We spare the midline attachments to keep the peritoneum intact and hopefully keep the bowel from migrating into the pelvis. This way we can still use radiation later if needed.*
    - *Dividing the endopelvic fascia. For disease clinically localized to the prostate, we can preserve most of the endopelvic fascia with the lateral prostatic fascia. This keeps the lateral nerve bundles more protected. In about 10 % of cases, accessory arteries travel right over the prostate on the way to the penis. We have learned to preserve these arteries in most cases. You never know just how much blood supply the penis needs for a quality erection. We preserve the pubovesical ligaments (see #3) to decrease manipulation of the rhapdosphincter muscles needed for urinary control.*
    - *Dorsal vein ligation. We suture this large vein complex under the pubovesical ligaments and then anchor up to the pubic bone. This keeps it ligation tight and minimizes trauma to the urinary control muscles.*
    - *Anterior bladder neck division. We keep a "middle third cautery rule" meaning only thermal heat in the midline. At the lateral thirds, we use clips and bipolar ligation to minimize heat to the nerve bundles. We do not try and make the bladder neck ultra small as this does not affect continence. We make a generous bladder opening so the margins are ok, and reconstruct it later.*
    - *Posterior bladder neck division. Again, middle third cautery only. This is mainly an experience factor as to how to divide bladder from prostate and stay in the proper plane without getting into prostate or bladder.*
    - *Seminal vesicle/Vas. The key is to keep cautery away from the tips of the seminal vesicles as these are right on the nerve bundles. The arteries to the seminal vesicles need careful clipping as they will bleed.*
    - *Nerve bundle. The technique is called "symmetry." Basically you divide the dorsal vein bundle, lateral prostatic fascia, and then work your way into the plane between the nerve bundle and prostate wherever it looks easiest. Work right, left, front, back, etc. No cautery. If veins bleed that's ok, you sew them over at the end if needed. For nerve sparing we go right to the capsule, and modify for any partial nerve sparing or non nerve-sparing.*
    - *Apex. The key is the squeeze the dorsal vein complex—whatever squeezes is not prostate. We sharply cut without burning. The next key is the line up the dissections of the dorsal vein with the nerve bundles, and the lateral sphincter muscles. The goal is complete preservation of the urethra without getting into prostate tissue, and without damaging the nerve bundles passing very close to this dissection.*
    - *Pelvic lymph node dissection. We used to do the standard Obturator Fossa dissection which takes 15 min and yields around 8 lymph nodes. Now we do an more extensive node template that includes hypogastric lymph nodes and sub-Obturator lymph nodes. The median yield is*

18–20 nodes and it takes around 45 min. The percent yield has increased from 2–3 % to 10–15 % (25 % if high risk). Therefore, we are taking more lymph nodes and finding more positive, i.e., the right lymph nodes. Removing lymph nodes that are positive may help stage a patient better for subsequent therapy, and may have a higher cure rate.

- *Posterior anastomosis. We start with a posterior reconstructive stitch of Denonvilliers' fascia to rhabdosphincter, i.e., a "Rocco" stitch named by the Italian surgeons. This gives more backbone to the reconstruction and takes tension off. The bladder neck is sutured smaller to match the urethra. Then a running suture line is performed.*
- *Anterior anastomosis. The top line is completed and checked for water tightness. A final anterior reconstructive stitch is placed for more strength, and support.*

27. *With these various changes and experience, the major complication rate has decreased from 5 to 1.3 %, and the minor complication rate 14 to 4.5 %. Of all of the early complications, 45 % are now avoided by specific changes to technique. The remaining are continued risk of having a surgery and/or patient selection features, i.e., cardiac disease.*
28. *We have also been using endorectal coil MRI to help stage intermediate to high risk cases. In the high risk cohort, the MRI has found to be 83 % accurate and provide the surgeon with 87 % helpful information. We are working on adding up the results with intermediate risk disease.*
29. *As discussed previously, the overall positive margin rate has declined to 2 % with 1.2 % for organ confined disease.*
30. *A comprehensive functional outcome metric will be completed this summer. I can estimate for you in clinic.*
31. *Anything I left out—I can add to the guide.*

Step 5: Personal Profile

Here are sample bullet items you can fill in for yourself:

1. Personal.
   (a) Birthplace, parents, spouse, children and their interests.
   (b) Your favorite mug shot.
2. High School.
3. College.
4. Medical School.
5. Graduate training.
6. Licensing/boards.
7. Fellowships.
8. Job history.
9. Titles.
10. Clinical interests.
11. Research interests.
12. Web links to content of interest featuring you or your team.

People absolutely will read these details. At a certain point, I mention that I try and "train" for long OR days and do morning exercise as preferred to trying to go after work. At least once a week a patient asks me how my morning workout went.

Step 6: Institution or Group Profile

What can you tell your patient about your intuition, group practice, *etc.*? Given them your own take. In my situation, patients often ask "why MD Anderson?" "Why travel too far?" Here is my take:

The Genitourinary Cancer Center at M.D. Anderson: Resources for Your Health

The Genitourinary Cancer Center (GU center) is designed to be a comprehensive, team approach to eliminating cancer of the genitourinary tract. We have 10 faculty urologists, 13 medical oncologists, and 5 radiation oncologists who focus on GU tumors. We have excellent support from pathology and radiology to properly stage and evaluate patients. We are active in designing clinical trials to improve patient care. We have a large staff of nurses and scheduling staff to make your visit here as beneficial as possible.

For patients who have a particularly challenging situation, we have a weekly conference attending by all specialties during which we review the key facts and discuss the optimal treatment plan.

The center employs a patient advocacy team to help address any complaints or compliments you may have.

Adjacent to the GU center are other excellent facilities in our Ambulatory Care Building such as diagnostic radiology, laboratory, anesthesia, and outpatient surgery. Most of your outpatient care can all occur on this South side of the campus.

How did M.D. Anderson become the number 1 ranked Cancer Center in America? A center like ours certainly needs the best faculty and staff. In addition, we need resources and our best sources have been clinical revenue, competitive grants, and philanthropy. Unfortunately, clinical revenue and grants are shrinking over time and philanthropy has become a major source for developing cutting edge clinical and research programs. If you are interesting in finding out how to support our center I would be happy to put you in contact with our development office. We also have a special program dedicated towards minimally invasive surgery called MINTOS (Minimally Invasive New Technology in Oncologic Surgery) that needs support. See our website at http://www.mdanderson.org/topics/mis/.

Research and Training at M.D. Anderson.

We have a number of clinical trials available and I will discuss if any would be useful to your care. The department trains residents from the University of Texas Houston, and fellows in urologic oncology who are fully trained urologists seeking advanced experience in our field.

Step 7: Logistics of Surgery

If they have read that far and like your team, they may schedule surgery and be trying to figure out how to coordinate with the rest of their schedule and lives. Go over your expectations on how to get through surgery with attention to safety and efficiency.

Surgery at M.D. Anderson—the logistics.

During the evaluation trip, you will undergo a primary medical evaluation followed by appropriate laboratory tests, radiology tests, and evaluation by anesthesia. Some patients may need advanced imaging such as MRI, and some may need medical or cardiology clearance.

When you return for surgery, there is a preoperative visit on Tuesday, followed by surgery Wed or Friday. You can usually return home by Sunday or Monday. Thus, the trip for surgery is usually less than 1 week.

The business center can assist with travel needs.

Stopping Medicines Before Surgery.

It is critical to remember to stop taking Aspirin, Plavix, Coumadin, and any other blood thinners 1 week prior to scheduled surgery. If you are unclear as to whether any of your medicines need to be discontinued prior to surgery please ask during your appointment or call my physician assistant in advance. Most patients undergo their preoperative appointment the Tues of the week of their surgery, so if they are still taking Aspirin, Plavix, etc. the procedure will have to be rescheduled. Some oral diabetic medicines need to be stopped.

It is also a good idea to stop all over the counter supplements and vitamins the week before, because some have potential blood thinning abilities.

Other medications for blood pressure, diabetes, cholesterol, thyroid disorders, prostate enlargement, and others can generally be taken up until the night before surgery. Your anesthesia team will go over last minute medication instructions during their consultation with you.

Step 8: Your Provider Team

In a busy practice, you cannot survive if patients perceive you to be a solo operation. Most large practices will have mixtures of nurses, schedulers, physician assistants, and perhaps trainees.

Introduce them to your team and list contact procedures. Give them a guide to which team member is best able to handle questions and the unexpected.

Here is my team with the names deleted:

Dr. John W. Davis' team at M.D. Anderson

Nurse

___ is my nurse and can help with many aspects of your evaluation, post-operative care, and follow—up. Please contact her for any issues relating to catheter care, temperature elevation, wound care, etc. She can advise you on minor health concerns. For any serious health concerns, contact my physician assistant and/or arrange emergency center evaluation. If you are near the GU center, call as soon as possible, and it is possible to be seen in clinic as an add-on.

Scheduler

___ is my scheduler and is responsible for entering all orders, testing, and consults into our system so that all evaluations are arranged. Please contact her with any scheduling issues.

Mid-Level Providers

We have a pool of physician assistants and nurse practitioners that assist in the clinic and can assist with medication orders and hospital workups. The dedicated physicians assistant for my clinic is ___, who started with us in ___. His/her specialty will be working with the patients undergoing robotic prostatectomy. ___ is a nurse practitioner who will be specializing in working with patients undergoing active surveillance for prostate cancer, and patients being screened for prostate cancer.

Please note that all members of my team work with other physicians as well. Everyone has voice mail and will return messages as soon as possible. For urgent matters, ask for the triage nurse in the clinic, and they can help locate members of my team or someone covering for them in their absence.

Fellows and Residents

We train four urologic oncology fellows per year and are fortunate to have up to 12 different urology residents from the University of Texas-Houston. In the clinic, they may assist with your visit. They assist in surgery and inpatient care.

Step 9: Establish a "Blog" Feel to Your Handout: Up To Date, Dynamic

As you return from various meetings and read new studies, consider writing up a paragraph on your interpretation. For steps 1–8 you have a basic handout, so now expand it with new topics. New questions from patients can go on as new entries. You could also give them a recommending Web page reading list. Here is a sample of blog updates from 2009 to 2012:

Additional FAQ's—2009–2012 updates

At this point, many patients and families have read this handout and naturally have further questions pertinent to their situation. Obviously we should discuss these face to face, but I'll add a few written comments to the most common questions for you to consider as well.

1. *What are the best arguments in favor of surgery?*
   (a) *No peer-reviewed, guideline based organization that has looked at the comprehensive body of literature of prostate cancer treatment outcomes has been able to recommend one therapy as superior to another. The 10-year disease control rates measured by PSA are similar between surgery and radiation, and mostly predicted by your pretreatment risk factors such as PSA, biopsy Gleason, and clinical stage. The functional quality of life outcomes differ in severity in certain functions, but in global assessments are not different. Surgery has more stress incontinence. Radiation has more bowel/bladder irritation. Surgery has an early pattern of erectile dysfunction with a pattern of healing. Radiation has a more delayed onset of erectile dysfunction risk. Surgery requires the catheter, anesthesia, short term pain medications, and leave from work. Radiation requires multiple trips to the center and induces bothersome fatigue during therapy.*
   (b) *That said, the main difference in my view is* ***knowledge.*** *A surgically removed prostate is a uniquely valuable source of tissue*

for research to improve care of this disease. The pathologic examination becomes a new set of staging information that will help us understand your future risk of recurrence, and possible need for follow-up treatment. After the surgery, the PSA should be undetectable at <0.1 ng/mL. Therefore, the monitoring of your treatment success is clear and easy to perform, i.e., does not require extensive imaging or examinations unless the PSA becomes detectable at >0.2 ng/mL. If that were to occur, or the prostate tumor appears to have advanced outside of the gland, it is feasible to apply radiation after surgery with acceptable side effects. By contrast, a radiation pathway produces no further tissue, no further pathologic staging, detectable PSA levels that are harder to interpret, and repeat prostate examinations. Surgery performed for a radiation failure has a higher complication rate than the other way around, but can be performed if absolutely necessary.

2. *Why is there no clinical study to answer these questions?*
   (a) *In the culture of the US health care system and male population, there has been limited interest to participate in a randomized clinical trial. Both sides of the equation are culpable: treatment providers generally provide only one of the treatments and are less likely to recommend the one they don't perform, and to further complicate the picture, US men generally do not like to give up the choice of treatment, given that they are so different. Attempts to randomize the treatments have been funded and approved, but not accrued enough patients to answer the question. In England, a large government sponsored study has successfully enrolled enough patients to compare active surveillance, radiation, and surgery, but early results may not be available until 2015.*
3. *Why should I have my surgery at MDACC?*
   (a) *It is common for a patient and his family to visit multiple surgeons' and to try and collect as much information as possible to compare them. Published studies have confirmed what you would probably guess on your own: higher volume surgeons and hospitals produce greater numbers of favorable outcomes than lower volume surgeons and hospitals. This does not mean that lower volume centers don't have high quality outcomes, but as a group perform lower than high volume. It is also possible for a few high volume centers to have inadequate outcomes. However, there is no good data to tell us how to compare high volume centers to each other. Everyone you meet with, including myself, will naturally want to present their experience in the best possible light. I will cede the possibility that other high volume robotic surgeons can do the procedure as well as I can. However, I've seen enough live surgery from the best to know that no one is doing anything superior to me. It is fair to point out that I am on a straight salary at MDACC that is not directly tied to the number of cases performed. I have no investment interests in any of the technology we use (I would alert you to the fact that an increasing number of urology and primary care physicians in community practice are investors in radiation and cryotherapy technology, which may influence their advise). I try and keep a busy schedule, but am not required to fill the schedule with so many cases that I am rushing or overly fatigued. I slow down the case when necessary to give you every opportunity for an ideal outcome. Beyond that, I think the best argument in favor of treatment at MDACC is the highly experienced nature of the whole team of doctors in pathology, diagnostic radiology, radiation oncology, and medical oncology. Take a look through the institution's website and read its mission statement—this is truly a unique place.*
4. *What would you do if this were you? Your father?*

(a) *I will go on record to state that I would strongly consider surgery all the way up into my 70s. After age 70 or so, I would consider brachytherapy if thought to be a candidate. However I would do so only with the plan that I would take my chances on success and not consider salvage therapy if it fails—too many side effects. For my theoretical father, I would plan the same. For my actual father, he has relative contraindications to elective surgery and no contraindications to radiation, so would probably have the latter. If the cancer were limited to 1 small core of Gleason 3 + 3 cancer, I would consider surveillance for the situation of myself or father. And yes, I've had my PSA checked.*

5. *The US Preventative Services Task Force recently recommended against routine screening—did I do the right thing checking my PSA and having a biopsy?*
   (a) *The findings of the Task Force were certainly controversial and not without its critics. The document is actually written very well, with sound methodology in many respects, and the potential harms of screening do need to be addressed—such biopsy risks, and morbidity/mortality from treatment. The Task Force considered mostly large randomized trials and other large population based studies to determine what the average result might be from screening. Although screening can save lives, it can also lead to unnecessary treatment, and potential harms from treatment. However to not screen subjects many men from having lethal potential disease grow beyond the point of cure. So in my mind, the way to be smart about screening is to start it when you are young and the potential benefit is greatest. If screening leads to a low volume/low grade tumor then consider surveillance. If you need treatment, then go to a high volume center. These are the things you can control—knowledge, sound decisions, and high quality treatment team.*
6. *What about the PIVOT trial?*
   (a) *The PIVOT trial reported that radical prostatectomy produced no survival benefit compared with observation. This trial was also controversial in that it was severely under-recruited—less than 300 patients in each group completed their assigned therapy. It was also carried out at mostly Veterans hospitals, and was a much older age group than I operate on, and their 10 year overall survival was not very good. That said, the study supports the notion that prostatectomy is not required for everyone, and is of questionable benefit for older patients with lower grade disease. On the other hand the study showed benefits for higher-grade disease.*

Step 10: Broaden Your Horizons: There Is More Than Just the Robot

Once patients are in your clinic, there are many other possible topics where they may want your expertice. Years ago, it impressed me listening to Mark Moyad that all of this work we do in prostate cancer is still a lesser source of mortality than cardiac disease. Patients need help in this area, and so do I. So I added a diet/nutrition section giving full credit to Dr. Moyad's books. This is an expansion of the blog session and almost like a detailed book review. In the future, I may consider a similar approach to related topics such as imaging, biomarkers, and novel systemic therapy.

Supplement: Prostate Cancer and Nutrition

Key reference:

Promoting Wellness: for Prostate Cancer Patients.

Author Mark A. Moyad, MD, MPH

Copyright 2009: Ann Arbor Michigan media group, LLC

Inquiries: www.annarbormediagroup.com re: ISBN: 978-1-58726-565-5

Dr. Moyad is a urologist with an interest in nutrition and supplements that started even before he trained as a urologist. His book can be found online. Chapters 1 and 2 deal with diet and supplements and are worth summarizing in this guide. I recommend obtaining your own copy if you have a serious interest in this area. I will abstract key facts from this book in the form of common questions asked in the clinic—some that you are asking and some that you are not asking but should be. The sample format:

1. *Question*
   (a) ***Dr. Moyad fact***
   - *JWD comments*
2. *What are the top six causes of death in US men?*
   (a) ***Cardiovascular disease, cancer, accidents, lung disease, diabetes, pneumonia/flu.***
      - *In fact, cardiovascular disease is the most common cause of death in men with and without prostate cancer. Since prostate cancer is such a slow growing problem, it is a better strategy to plan preventions and interventions that address prostate cancer and your overall health.*
      - *Another way to think of this list is as follows. At any given time, we have a list of several possible causes of our own deaths. It may be the case that prostate cancer is at the top of the list, and that with our expert care we can remove that from the list. Unfortunately this means that whatever was number 2 on the list moves up to number 1, and so on. As a colleague of mine once pointed out—even the famous figures in the New Testament of the Bible who were cured by one of Jesus' miracles.....have since died.*
      - *Most preventative medicine are tips you have heard before: control your blood pressure, control your cholesterol, wear a seatbelt in a car, wear a helmet when riding a bike, don't smoke, avoid obesity—a top cause of diabetes and other problems, get a flu shot, etc.*
3. *How do we measure Cholesterol?*
   (a) ***Measure your total, LDL ("bad"), HDL ("good"), and triglycerides. In addition, the test "high sensitivity C-Reactive Protein" can predict additional risk of cardiovascular disease (CVD) despite normal cholesterol. In addition, measure your blood pressure.***
   - *Dr. Moyad provides tables to interpret these tests, which I won't reproduce, but they can be found with a simple google search, and discuss with your primary care physician (PCP).*
   - *A major theme of the book, is that most all dietary measures that help your cholesterols and blood pressure also help lower your risk of prostate cancer, and may be helpful even if you have it.*
4. *What is a reasonable weight?*
   (a) ***Weight can be measured by the body mass index (BMI) which accounts for your height and weight. Most of us cannot control our height anymore, so the only input you can control is the weight. An ideal BMI <25, 25–29 is overweight, and ≥30 is obese. Additional measures include the waist circumference, and waist-to-hip ratio.***
      - *I recommend the BMI scale, and with google you can find it at a National Institutes of Health web page. I think it is very hard for most to diet all the way from obese to normal weight, but the overweight BMI of 25–29 is probably reasonable.*
5. *Is there a pill I can take to reduce my risk of serious health problems?*
   (a) ***Yes. There is such a pill. It will reduce by 25% or more your risk of Alzheimer's disease, colon cancer, depression, erectile dysfunction, heart disease, osteoporosis, premature death, prostate cancer, prostatitis, and prostate enlargement.***
   (b) ***The cost of the pill varies from free to very expensive depending on which one you buy.***
   (c) ***The side effects may include addiction to the pill, and a variety of orthopedic injuries depending upon your choices.***

(d) ***Yes, you guessed it—it's exercise: 30 min a day, including weight lifting.***
- *I've heard Dr. Moyad present this at meetings and always gets a good laugh. But seriously, it is probably impossible for any diet or supplement to help you achieve your health goals without including exercise. I lot of my patients say they "walk" a lot when asked about exercise. I suppose this is better than sitting on a sofa scanning channels. However, walking only minimally affects your metabolic weight for the amount of time involved. Ideally, choose an aerobic that elevates your heart rate to 70 % or so of maximum. There are detailed methods of determining this, that account for your age—any health club will have resources to help you with this. You have to establish a resting heart rate when you wake up in the morning. So for example in my case, my resting is 61. Sitting here on an airplane typing this guide supplement for you it is 81, or 40 % of maximum. If I go on an elliptical machine, I usually sustain a heart rate of 130–140, or 70–80 % of max. Sometimes I do a spin class and we "sprint" for a segment that pushes it to 150–155. I've also noticed that if you work out for only 15 min, you spend half of that time just building your heart rate, so only 7–8 min of exercise at your 70 % max rate. Whereas if you do 30 min, you still spend 7–8 min building but nearly twice the time at 70 % max, and nearly twice the calories burned. As for the weight lifting, Dr. Moyad points out that reducing osteoporosis, heart, and other risks require this. Thus, exercise daily and alternate aerobic with weight lifting, you are more complete. Finally, my personal observation from the clinic and from my health club, is that the most consistent exercisers generally are tied to training for a sport (Tennis) or an event (cycling race, marathon). Sorry, but golf even without a cart probably doesn't count—but better than none). Exercise just to exercise has a higher drop out rate. Some experts state that morning exercise is more habitual and reliable than after-work.*

6. *Why is obesity such a problem in the USA? What do I change?*
   (a) **Higher portion sizes, higher fat content, higher calories.**
   (b) **Learn to read nutrition labels and recognize the "bad" fats, which are the saturate fats (non-lean meat, dairy, fast food), and the trans fats (aka. partially hydrogenated fats, from margarine, fast foods, snack foods, deep-fried foods). Lower saturated fats may correlated with less risk of prostate cancer, and less risk of recurrence for treated patients. The better fats are the monounsaturated fats (plant based cooking oils), polyunsaturated fats (plant based cooking oils, flaxseed, fish, nuts, soybeans.**
   (c) **While learning to read labels and limit your "bad" fat food choices, note that most any diet can have more vegetables and fruit. However, be cautious that fruit/vegetable juices do not have the same nutritional benefits as the actual substance, and can have enormous calorie content. For example an 8 oz. mixed fruit smoothie can have 200–250 calories, while light beer only has 70–80! It is easy to read labels and note that diet drinks, coffee, tea, water are all <50 calories.**
   (d) **Consume more omega-3 fatty acids. Best bets are from herring, mackerel, oysters, salmon, snapper, and trout. Caution with halibut and some forms of tuna as they have high mercury content.**
   (e) **Consume more plant estrogen from soy and flaxseed.**
   (f) **Go nuts! Most have good fats, omega-3 fatty acids. Caution with calorie content, however.**

(g) ***More fiber—best sources are beans, fruit, vegetables, bran cereals, flaxseed, whole grains, and oats. Take home message here: 1st choice is to do this with cereal, fruit, and flaxseed. Fiber pills not recommended.***

(h) ***Diet programs—most are probably fine and engineered to trick you into cutting out 200 calories per day. They just do it differently: weight watchers make you do the math and give group support; South Beach cuts carbs, etc.***

(i) ***Read labels and cut back on sodium.***

(j) ***Alcohol in moderation may be healthy—for men 1–2 servings/day. In excess—damaging. Note the calorie contents of your choices. Biggest weight gainer is hard alcohol in mixers.***

- *If you have serious interest in this topic, I would get the book. If you want me to suggest some priorities, I would do the exercise first, and the basic dietary changes: cut unnecessary calories with simple substitutions (diet soda for regular, etc.) and add more fruit/vegetable content. If you're ready for the next level, then learn the fat content, fish content information. If you can accomplish these two, then move on to the fiber, flaxseed, sodium type details. I recommend being quite strict about the exercise programs. However, for diet, I think it's reasonable to eat the foods you really like from time to time, i.e., celebrate with a nice steak on a weekend night but don't eat red meat three times a day.*

Final Steps: Images

We are all visual by nature. I left one image in this chapter on the port placement as an example, but there are several more I use that you could consider to add more flair:

1. Pictures of the robotic system—use your own rather than Google images.
   (a) Console, articulating instruments, dual consoles.
2. Pictures of your team/institution/department members.
3. Pictures of technique.

The problem to solve next is resolution. I note that my handout gets copied and recopied and the images are often worthless. Moving forward, I would recommend looking at a cloud storage of high quality images with Web links—if so inclined, links to YouTube clips of the surgery. Many patients are looking for this content anyway so they might as well see yours rather than another's.

Active Surveillance and Patient Support Intervention

30

Patricia A. Parker, Jeri Kim, and David M. Latini

Prostate cancer is the most common cancer, apart from skin cancer, among American men. The American Cancer Society forecasts that in 2015 220,800 men will be diagnosed with prostate cancer and that 27,540 will die of the disease [1]. Widespread prostate-specific antigen (PSA) screening has identified more men with localized prostate cancer earlier in the disease process than was previously possible, resulting in the detection of prostate cancer in many men who are unlikely to die of it [2]. The findings from an evaluation of PSA screening by the U.S. Preventive Services Task Force led to revised national screening recommendations [3].

Active surveillance (AS) is a viable option for many men with early stage disease or very slow-growing prostate cancer [4–6]. AS allows men diagnosed with prostate cancer to avoid unnecessary treatment and its side effects, including impotence and incontinence, which can dramatically reduce quality of life (QOL). AS involves regular monitoring with PSA evaluation, digital rectal examination, and biopsy, although the optimal timing and schedule for monitoring remains under investigation. Careful selection of criteria for AS may allow men who qualify for it to delay or potentially avoid debilitating long-term side effects of such aggressive treatments as surgery or radiation [7–10]. Men on AS who show early signs of disease progression can receive early intervention and do not have poorer pathological outcomes than men receiving immediate treatment [6, 11, 12]. Additionally, a recent cost-effectiveness analysis found that observation (watchful waiting [WW] and AS) slightly improved quality-adjusted life expectancy and is less expensive than treatment for men 65–75 years of age with localized prostate cancer [13]. The terms AS and WW are sometimes used interchangeably; however, WW was originally used for older patients who were not considered candidates for treatments such as surgery or radiation and who may or may not have opted for an aggressive monitoring schedule, whereas AS typically refers to the active monitoring schedule as described above. In this chapter, we will focus on AS.

P.A. Parker, Ph.D. (✉)
Department of Psychiatry & Behavioral Sciences, Memorial Sloan-Kettering Cancer Center, New York, NY
e-mail: pparker@mdanderson.org

J. Kim, M.D.
The University of Texas MD Anderson Cancer Center Houston, TX, USA

D.M. Latini, Ph.D., M.S.W.
Baylor College of Medicine, Houstony, TX, USA

Impact of AS on Psychosocial Adjustment and QOL

Compared with the number of studies of men on active treatment, the number of studies that have examined the psychosocial impact of the surveillance process is relatively low. Some have suggested that being on AS may create uncertainty, anxiety,

J.W. Davis (ed.), *Robot-Assisted Radical Prostatectomy*, DOI 10.1007/978-3-319-32641-2_30

and distress for men with prostate cancer, inasmuch as many cancer patients have difficulty with the emotional burden of living with an untreated cancer [14, 15] and anxiety may be one reason men choose immediate treatment instead of AS [16–18]. Undergoing PSA monitoring has been found to be associated with increased anxiety [19]; thus, men on AS may have varying levels of anxiety, rising during monitoring and falling at other times; however, longitudinal analyses that specifically assess the timing of anxiety around monitoring and at other times have not been done. A cross-sectional study of men on AS found that 16 % of men met criteria for anxiety and 6 % for depression on the Hospital Anxiety and Depression Scale [20]. Higher anxiety was significantly associated with younger age and longer time since diagnosis. Higher depression was associated with longer time since diagnosis. There were no significant differences between men on AS, controlling for age and time since diagnosis, and men who were undergoing immediate treatment or who already had treatment. Men on AS or who had radiation therapy completed measures of general and disease-specific QOL 5–10 years after diagnosis [21]. Men on AS had better bowel function, less bother with bowel function, and fewer problems getting an erection than did men who underwent radiotherapy but had similar general and cancer-specific QOL. A recent review indicated that anxiety and uncertainty were two prevalent responses from men when they are on AS [22]. However, other studies have found that anxiety was not higher in men on AS than it was in nonclinical norms [23].

Kasperzyk et al. reported on the QOL of prostate cancer survivors in the Physicians' Health Study [24]. Of the 1230 men diagnosed with localized prostate cancer, 125 were initially treated with WW. At follow-up (mean, 7.3 years), 41 % of men on WW remained free of treatment, 34 % had received radiation therapy, 16 % underwent hormonal therapy, and 10 % had surgery. Younger age, higher clinical stage, higher Gleason score, and higher PSA level at diagnosis predicted progression to treatment. In univariate analyses, a comparison of men on WW and those on treatment reported significantly less urinary incontinence (3.5 % vs. 10 %) and erectile dysfunction (68 % vs. 78 %) but more obstructive urinary symptoms (22 % vs. 13 %). After adjusting for age at diagnosis, comorbidity score, and time from diagnosis to QOL assessment, investigators found men on WW remained less likely to report urinary leakage/incontinence and erectile dysfunction than those initially treated.

In a study comparing distress 8 years after surgery or entry into WW, men who had surgery reported more urinary leakage, more impaired erectile functioning, a greater decrease in libido, but fewer obstructive urinary symptoms than did men who were on WW [25]. What is important, however, is that 30–40 % of men in both groups reported that prostate cancer negatively affected their daily activities in areas such as health-related distress, worry, feeling low, and insomnia. In a comparison of AS with brachytherapy and robot-assisted laparoscopic prostatectomy, men on brachytherapy and those undergoing prostatectomy reported decreased QOL compared with men on AS, whereas the three groups reported a similar overall QOL [26]. Other studies have found no difference in anxiety, depression, or distress between men on AS and men undergoing surgery [20, 27].

Predictors of QOL

Although the overall QOL of men on AS appears to be high, there are factors associated with better and poorer QOL among this population. Bellardita et al. [28], for example, examined predictors of QOL and adjustment to prostate cancer during AS. They found that not having a partner and having poorer mental health scores were associated with poorer QOL. Additionally, being on AS longer was associated with better QOL. Anderson et al. [23] found that anxiety and fear of recurrence predicted overall and prostate-specific QOL.

Barriers to Acceptance of AS

Pickles et al. [29] conducted a review to identify barriers to AS. They identified psychosocial issues faced by men on AS as similar to those reported by others and reported the issues included anxiety about not having an intervention, uncertainty related to loss of control, and dissatisfaction with the lack of patient education and support. They recommended increasing AS education and improving communication and interventions to reduce anxiety and uncertainty as well as to boost peer support.

One factor that has been identified as affecting the decision to go from AS to treatment is anxiety. Controlling for baseline demographic and clinical characteristics and disease progression, Latini et al. [18] found that anxiety change rate predicted having active treatment. A qualitative study of 21 men diagnosed with localized prostate cancer found that 19 of them did not want AS. Reasons provided for preferring treatment over AS were anxiety, fear of cancer spreading, family persuasion to seek treatment, and lack of knowledge about AS [16].

Unique Issues of Men on AS

What is unique about being on AS in contrast with choosing active treatment is the ongoing nature of the decision-making process. Relatively little is known about the choice of AS for men with prostate cancer. A small qualitative study of men on AS in Canada found that they perceived their cancer was not an immediate threat to their health or life and they wanted to avoid the side effects of treatment [30]. Another important factor that affected the decision making was the physician's recommendation. A recent qualitative study explored views of AS among men diagnosed with localized prostate cancer [31]. Men who chose AS viewed their cancer as low risk and as a way to have time to decide about treatment and avoid the side effects of treatment. Men on AS did substantial research on their own about options but also valued physician input. Penson [32] characterized factors that influence patients' acceptance and adherence to AS. Factors that influence choice of treatment or AS include desire for cancer control or cure, concerns about side effects of treatment, and age at diagnosis. Physician recommendation, opinion of family and friends, and overall decisional uncertainty also affect the decision.

O'Callaghan et al. conducted a qualitative study of men with localized prostate cancer who either had treatment or were on AS [33]. Partners were also included. Decisions about whether to go on AS or get treatment were influenced by the satisfaction from information gathered from the physician and other sources and by their emotional reactions, their cancer-related memories, and lifestyle factors. Stressors for men on AS included fears about disease progression and about "not doing anything."

A recent study examined the perceptions of radiation oncologists and urologists about AS [34]. Researchers found that 72 % of respondents indicated that AS is effective, and 80 % reported it was underutilized; however, 71 % reported that their patients were not interested in this option. These results differed by specialty, with urologists more likely to agree than radiation oncologists that AS is effective and to report comfort recommending it in low-risk cases. Radiation oncologists were also more likely to report that patients were not interested. In response to a case scenario of a 60-year-old healthy man diagnosed with low-risk prostate cancer, most physicians recommended radical prostatectomy (45 %) or brachytherapy (35 %). Only 22 % endorsed AS. This highlights the fact that despite physicians' belief that AS is effective and underutilized, they continue to recommend treatment to patients with low-risk cancer who would be well suited for AS.

A recent study examined posts from a variety of Internet sites and online support groups to examine perceptions of AS [35]. Analysis of these Internet conversations indicated 30 % were classified as positive, 30 % as negative, and 41 % as neutral. Before 2008, patient perception of WW or AS was overwhelmingly negative, but positive perception has increased since that time. This increase appeared to be related to increased patient emphasis on QOL factors and endorsement of AS by national medical organizations. Unmet needs regarding AS included the desire for more information on long-term outcomes of AS and for more information from unbiased specialists.

Effect of Repeated Biopsies on Erectile Function

One potential concern that has been identified in the AS literature is the effect of repeated biopsies on erectile functioning. Braun et al. [36], for example, examined erectile functioning in men on AS. Among the 342 men, the mean age was 64 years, the mean follow-up on AS was 3.5 years, and the median number of biopsies was five. During the first 4 years on AS, erectile function decreased 1 point per year on the International Index of Erectile Function (scale, 1–30). Results were similar when data were stratified by comorbidities and number of biopsies.

Interventions and Potential Targets for Intervention for Men with Prostate Cancer on AS

Physical and disease-specific QOL is generally higher for men on AS than for men on treatment, while the data on distress is somewhat mixed. For these reasons, QOL interventions for men on AS have focused on the psychological impact of AS. One intervention that has been developed specifically for men with prostate cancer on AS focuses on uncertainty management [37]. This intervention is based on Mishel's Uncertainty in Illness Theory, which posits that uncertainty disrupts individuals' usual routines and their sense of order and structure and that chronic illness causes uncertainty to spread from uncertainty about the disease to uncertainty about broader life issues. Men who had been on AS for 1–124 months (mean, 10.3 years) were randomized to usual care or a five-session telephone-delivered intervention designed to help men integrate uncertainty into their lives by cognitively reframing how they viewed their illness and the uncertainty it produced. Results indicated that men in the intervention group were significantly more likely to view their lives in a new light and experience a decrease in confusion as well as improvements in QOL.

Oliffe et al. [38] conducted a qualitative study to examine self-management strategies of men on AS, which identified uncertainty as the predominant stressor. Main themes of uncertainty focused on mortality, the potential for cancer to spread beyond the prostate, the potential imminent need for treatment, and how men might cope with treatment-related morbidities. In addition, men's uncertainty was time sensitive and peaked leading up to scheduled monitoring visits and receipt of PSA and biopsy results. The way in which men managed the uncertainty varied. Focusing on living a normal life helped some men manage their uncertainty. Men also reported "doing something extra" through researching treatment options, including making lifestyle changes to improve their well-being and/or using complementary and alternative medicine approaches.

Stress management skills and one's confidence in employing these coping skills may be important predictors of adjustment among men on AS. A recent study found that men who were more confident in their ability to cope with prostate cancer had fewer intrusive thoughts about their cancer than men who were less confident in their ability to cope [39]. While these results are descriptive, they point to the need for interventions that provide both coping skills and greater confidence in using these skills to manage the potential uncertainty of AS.

An exception to this focus on the psychological impact of AS is a comprehensive lifestyle intervention that includes a stress management component, a low-fat vegan nutritional intervention, and physical exercise. In one lifestyle study, participants were randomized to receive either the lifestyle intervention or standard care [40]. A year after enrollment, participants who achieved a better lifestyle reported enhanced physical QOL, lower stress, and better sexual functioning. Over a 2-year period, significantly fewer participants in the lifestyle intervention group underwent conventional prostate cancer treatment [41] than chose that option in other AS studies. A third paper reported 5-year follow-up data for a subset of participants enrolled in the original study. Men who completed the lifestyle intervention were shown to have longer relative telomere length [42] than the control peers, which was a positive development inasmuch as shortened telomere length is associated with aging and morbidity. An ongoing study (Men's Eating and Living [MEAL] study) is examining a telephone-based counseling intervention to assess the effectiveness of a high-vegetable diet in men with prostate cancer on AS. Participants will be followed over 24 months. The primary outcome in this study is clinical progression and secondary outcomes include anxiety and QOL.

Impact on Partners

A diagnosis of prostate cancer not only affects the man who is diagnosed, but also affects his spouse/partner and others close to him. There is some evidence that partners of men who are diagnosed with cancer are more distressed than the men diagnosed [43]. In addition, the AS process may also create additional anxiety. Seiler et al. [44] examined retrospectively anxiety levels in men with prostate cancer on AS and their partners and found that, although partners had significantly higher anxiety scores than the men with prostate cancer, the scores were not clinically elevated. Factors associated with significant anxiety were the lower general health status of the men and lower emotional functioning.

Conclusions and Future Directions

Overall, men on AS have been found to have good overall QOL, comparable to that of men receiving immediate treatment. Most studies, however, have examined QOL for only 1–2 years after being on AS. Studies with outcomes based on longer terms are needed to determine if there are changes in QOL in subsequent years. Future work is also needed to evaluate how PSA, biopsy, and other monitoring might affect anxiety levels or other types of distress. Additional work is also needed to evaluate how having treatment following AS affects QOL and psychosocial adjustment.

Physician/surgeon characteristics may also be important factors contributing to who goes on AS and satisfaction with the decision. This is an area that warrants further study.

Editorial Comment

This chapter may seem off-topic for a textbook on robotic prostatectomy. However, a successful robotics program has to be acknowledged as experts in the whole disease rather than just technicians. Active surveillance continues to increase as our understanding of low-grade cancer improves. Our surgical rate for low-grade cancer is currently in the 15 % range compared to 30 % a decade ago. However, anywhere from 10 to 30 % of active surveillance patients may at some point be reclassified to higher risk and move on to treatment. The chapter by Parker, Kim, and Latini provides a unique service a comprehensive prostate cancer program can add—patient counseling and support for active surveillance. The remaining checklist for a modern prostate clinic (beyond our agenda) would be active surveillance inclusion criteria, monitoring strategies, and threshold for delayed treatment. Related will be the rapidly expanding fields of tissue based biomarkers reclassification and advanced imaging with fusion biopsies—both designed to risk reclassify and identify treatment candidates who initially looked like surveillance candidates.

References

1. American Cancer Society. Cancer facts and figures 2015. Atlanta: American Cancer Society; 2015.
2. Dall'Era MA, Cooperberg MR, Chan JM, Davies BJ, Albertsen PC, Klotz LH, et al. Active surveillance for early-stage prostate cancer: review of the current literature. Cancer. 2008;112:1650–9. doi:10.1002/cncr.23373.
3. Moyer VA, U.S. Preventive Services Task Force. Screening for prostate cancer: U.S. Preventive Services Task Force recommendation statement. Ann InternMed.2012;157:120–34.doi:10.7326/0003-4819-157-2-201207170-00459.
4. Zerbib M, Zelefsky MJ, Higano C, Carroll PR. Conventional treatments and localized prostate cancer. Urology. 2008;72:25–35. doi:10.1016/j.urology.2008.10.005.
5. Singer EA, Kaushal A, Turkbey B, Couvillon A, Pinto PA, Parnes HL. Active surveillance for prostate cancer: past, present and future. Curr Opin Oncol. 2012;24:243–50. doi:10.1097/CCO.0b013e3283527f99.
6. Venderbos LD, Bokhorst LP, Bangma CH, Roobol MJ. Active surveillance: oncologic outcome. Curr

Opin Urol. 2013;23:268–72. doi:10.1097/MOU.0b013e32835efe8f.
7. Sanda MG, Dunn RL, Michalski J, Sandler HM, Northouse L, Hembroff L, et al. Quality of life and satisfaction with outcome among prostate-cancer survivors. N Engl J Med. 2008;358:1250–61. doi:10.1056/NEJMoa074311.
8. Soloway MS, Soloway CT, Eldefrawy A, Acosta K, Kava B, Manoharan M. Careful selection and close monitoring of low-risk prostate cancer patients on active surveillance minimizes the need for treatment. Eur Urol. 2010;58:831–5. doi:10.1016/j.eururo.2010.08.027.
9. Resnick MJ, Koyama T, Fan K-H, Albertsen PC, Goodman M, Hamilton AS, et al. Long-term functional outcomes after treatment for localized prostate cancer. N Engl J Med. 2013;368:436–45. doi:10.1056/NEJMoa1209978.
10. Bergman J, Litwin MS. Quality of life in men undergoing active surveillance for localized prostate cancer. J Natl Cancer Inst Monogr. 2012;2012:242–9. doi:10.1093/jncimonographs/lgs026.
11. van den Bergh RC, Roemeling S, Roobol MJ, Aus G, Hugosson J, Rannikko AS, et al. Outcomes of men with screen-detected prostate cancer eligible for active surveillance who were managed expectantly. Eur Urol. 2009;55:1–8. doi:10.1016/j.eururo.2008.09.007.
12. Warlick C, Trock BJ, Landis P, Epstein JI, Carter HB. Delayed versus immediate surgical intervention and prostate cancer outcome. J Natl Cancer Inst. 2006;98:355–7.
13. Hayes JH, Ollendorf DA, Pearson SD, Barry MJ, Kantoff PW, Lee PA, et al. Observation versus initial treatment for men with localized, low-risk prostate cancer: a cost-effectiveness analysis. Ann Intern Med. 2013;158:853–60.doi:10.7326/0003-4819-158-12-201306180-00002.
14. Bailey Jr DE, Wallace M, Mishel MH. Watching, waiting and uncertainty in prostate cancer. J Clin Nurs. 2007;16:734–41.
15. Wallace M. Uncertainty and quality of life of older men who undergo watchful waiting for prostate cancer. Oncol Nurs Forum. 2003;30:303–9.
16. Xu J, Dailey RK, Eggly S, Neale AV, Schwartz KL. Men's perspectives on selecting their prostate cancer treatment. J Natl Med Assoc. 2011;103:468–78.
17. van den Bergh RC, Essink-Bot ML, Roobol MJ, Wolters T, Schroder FH, Bangma CH, et al. Anxiety and distress during active surveillance for early prostate cancer. Cancer. 2009;115:3868–78. doi:10.1002/cncr.24446.
18. Latini DM, Hart SL, Knight SJ, Cowan JE, Ross PL, Duchane J, et al. The relationship between anxiety and time to treatment for patients with prostate cancer on surveillance. J Urol. 2007;178(3 Pt 1):826–31. discussion 31–2.
19. Roth AJ, Weinberger MI, Nelson CJ. Prostate cancer: psychosocial implications and management. Future Oncol. 2008;4:561–8. doi:10.2217/14796694.4.4.561.
20. Burnet KL, Parker C, Dearnaley D, Brewin CR, Watson M. Does active surveillance for men with localized prostate cancer carry psychological morbidity? BJU Int. 2007;100:540–3.
21. Thong MS, Mols F, Kil PJ, Korfage IJ, van de Poll-Franse LV. Prostate cancer survivors who would be eligible for active surveillance but were either treated with radiotherapy or managed expectantly: comparisons on long-term quality of life and symptom burden. BJU Int. 2010;105:652–8. doi:10.1111/j.1464-410X.2009.08815.x.
22. Kazer MW, Psutka SP, Latini DM, Bailey DEJ. Psychosocial aspects of active surveillance. Curr Opin Urol. 2013;23:273–7. doi:10.1097/MOU.0b013e32835eff24.
23. Anderson J, Burney S, Brooker JE, Ricciardelli LA, Fletcher JM, Satasivam P, et al. Anxiety in the management of localized prostate cancer by active surveillance. BJU Int. 2014;114 Suppl 1:55–61. doi:10.1111/bju.12765.
24. Kasperzyk JL, Shappley III WV, Kenfield SA, Mucci LA, Kurth T, Ma J, et al. Watchful waiting and quality of life among prostate cancer survivors in the Physicians' Health Study. J Urol. 2011;186:1862–7. doi:10.1016/j.juro.2011.06.058.
25. Bill-Axelson A, Garmo H, Holmberg L, Johansson JE, Adami HO, Steineck G, et al. Long-term distress after radical prostatectomy versus watchful waiting in prostate cancer: a longitudinal study from the Scandinavian Prostate Cancer Group-4 randomized clinical trial. Eur Urol. 2013;64:920–8. doi:10.1016/j.eururo.2013.02.025.
26. Acar C, Schoffelmeer CC, Tillier C, de Blok W, van Muilekom E, van der Poel HG. Quality of life in patients with low-risk prostate cancer. A comparative retrospective study: brachytherapy versus robot-assisted laparoscopic prostatectomy versus active surveillance. J Endourol. 2014;28:117–24. doi:10.1089/end.2013.0349.
27. Punnen S, Cowan JE, Dunn LB, Shumay DM, Carroll PR, Cooperberg MR. A longitudinal study of anxiety, depression and distress as predictors of sexual and urinary quality of life in men with prostate cancer. BJU Int. 2013;112(2):E67–75. doi:10.1111/bju.12209.
28. Bellardita L, Rancati T, Alvisi MF, Villani D, Magnani T, Marenghi C, et al. Predictors of health-related quality of life and adjustment to prostate cancer during active surveillance. Eur Urol. 2013;64:30–6. doi:10.1016/j.eururo.2013.01.009.
29. Pickles T, Ruether JD, Weir L, Carlson L, Jakulj F. Psychosocial barriers to active surveillance for the management of early prostate cancer and a strategy for increased acceptance. BJU Int. 2007;100(3):544–51.
30. Davison BJ, Oliffe JL, Pickles T, Mroz L. Factors influencing men undertaking active surveillance for the management of low-risk prostate cancer. Oncol Nurs Forum. 2009;36:89–96. doi:10.1188/09.ONF.89-96.
31. Volk RJ, McFall SL, Cantor SB, Byrd TL, Le YL, Kuban DA, et al. "It's not like you just had a heart

attack": decision-making about active surveillance by men with localized prostate cancer. Psychooncology. 2014;23:467–72. doi:10.1002/pon.3444.
32. Penson DF. Factors influencing patients' acceptance and adherence to active surveillance. J Natl Cancer Inst Monogr. 2012;2012(45):207–12. doi:10.1093/jncimonographs/lgs024.
33. O'Callaghan C, Dryden T, Hyatt A, Brooker J, Burney S, Wootten AC, et al. What is this active surveillance thing? Men's and partners' reactions to treatment decision making for prostate cancer when active surveillance is the recommended treatment option. Psychooncology. 2014;23:1391–8. doi:10.1002/pon.3576.
34. Kim SP, Gross CP, Nguyen PL, Smaldone MC, Shah ND, Karnes RJ, et al. Perceptions of active surveillance and treatment recommendations for low-risk prostate cancer: results from a national survey of radiation oncologists and urologists. Med Care. 2014;52:579–85. doi:10.1097/MLR.0000000000000155.
35. Mishra MV, Bennett M, Vincent A, Lee OT, Lallas CD, Trabulsi EJ, et al. Identifying barriers to patient acceptance of active surveillance: content analysis of online patient communications. PLoS One. 2013;8:e68563. doi:10.1371/journal.pone.0068563.
36. Braun K, Ahallal Y, Sjoberg DD, Ghoneim T, Dominguez Esteban M, Mulhall J, et al. Effect of repeated prostate biopsies on erectile function in men on active surveillance for prostate cancer. J Urol. 2014;191:744–9. doi:10.1016/j.juro.2013.08.054.
37. Bailey DE, Mishel MH, Belyea M, Stewart JL, Mohler J. Uncertainty intervention for watchful waiting in prostate cancer. Cancer Nurs. 2004;27:339–46.
38. Oliffe JL, Davison BJ, Pickles T, Mroz L. The self-management of uncertainty among men undertaking active surveillance for low-risk prostate cancer. Qual Health Res. 2009;19:432–43. doi:10.1177/1049732309332692.
39. Yanez B, Bustillo NE, Antoni MH, Lechner SC, Dahn J, Kava B, et al. The importance of perceived stress management skills for patients with prostate cancer in active surveillance. J Behav Med. 2015;38:214–23. doi:10.1007/s10865-014-9594-1.
40. Daubenmier JJ, Weidner G, Marlin R, Crutchfield L, Dunn-Emke S, Chi C, et al. Lifestyle and health-related quality of life of men with prostate cancer managed with active surveillance. Urology. 2006;67:125–30.
41. Frattaroli J, Weidner G, Dnistrian AM, Kemp C, Daubenmier JJ, Marlin RO, et al. Clinical events in prostate cancer lifestyle trial: results from two years of follow-up. Urology. 2008;72(6):1319–23. doi:10.1016/j.urology.2008.04.050.
42. Ornish D, Lin J, Chan JM, Epel E, Kemp C, Weidner G, et al. Effect of comprehensive lifestyle changes on telomerase activity and telomere length in men with biopsy-proven low-risk prostate cancer: 5-year follow-up of a descriptive pilot study. Lancet Oncol. 2013;14:1112–20. doi:10.1016/S1470-2045(13)70366-8.
43. Kornblith AB, Herr HW, Ofman US, Scher HI, Holland JC. Quality of life of patients with prostate cancer and their spouses. The value of a data base in clinical care. Cancer. 1994;73(11):2791–802.
44. Seiler D, Randazzo M, Leupold U, Zeh N, Isbarn H, Chun FK, et al. Protocol-based active surveillance for low-risk prostate cancer: anxiety levels in both men and their partners. Urology. 2012;80:564–9. doi:10.1016/j.urology.2012.04.053.

A Return to Key Surgical Technique: Neurovascular Bundle Sparing with Antegrade Technique

31

Mathew Goland-Van Ryn, Avinash Reddy, Eric Moskowitz, Ash Tewari, and Thomas Bessede

Introduction

Prostate cancer is one of the most common malignancies to affect men across the globe and remains a leading cause of cancer-related death [1]. However, treatment for this disease has developed to the point where it can be successfully managed without life altering side effects. In the PSA screening era, the focus has transitioned to minimizing the morbidity associated with prostate cancer treatment. While multiple options remain for the treatment of prostate cancer, the most central to the practicing Urologist is the radical prostatectomy. Three parameters are fundamental to the modern surgical management of prostate cancer: oncological outcome, urinary continence, and erectile function. While the first is of primary importance, the latter two can now be achieved without compromising safety through new technologies and modern nerve-sparing techniques.

M.G.-V. Ryn • A. Reddy • E. Moskowitz
A. Tewari (✉) • T. Bessede MD, PhD
Mount Sinai Health System, New York, NY, USA
e-mail: ash.tewari@moutsinai.org

Scientific Foundations of Nerve Sparing in Radical Prostatectomy

The guiding principles for our approach at nerve sparing (NS) are based in the neuroanatomy of the human prostate. Until recently, the vast and complex network of innervating fibers was not fully understood. While initial work by Walsh and Donker was critical to understanding the importance of NS in radical prostatectomy, research has now demonstrated a more complex pattern of nerve supply providing potency and contributing to continence in men [2].

Periprostatic nerves, rather than coursing in one orientation around the prostatic capsule, form a hammock providing neurovascular support for the prostate from the base, across the posterolateral aspect and down to the apical tissue [2]. This neural hammock is clearly illustrated in Fig. 31.1. Three distinct regions comprise the hammock: the proximal neurovascular plate (PNP), predominant neurovascular bundle (PNB), and accessory distal neural pathways (ANP).

The PNP provides integration for all neural signals abutting the prostate. The anatomical location is lateral to the bladder neck, seminal vesicles (SVs), and inferior vesicle vessel branches extending posterolaterally to the prostatic base

J.W. Davis (ed.), *Robot-Assisted Radical Prostatectomy*, DOI 10.1007/978-3-319-32641-2_31

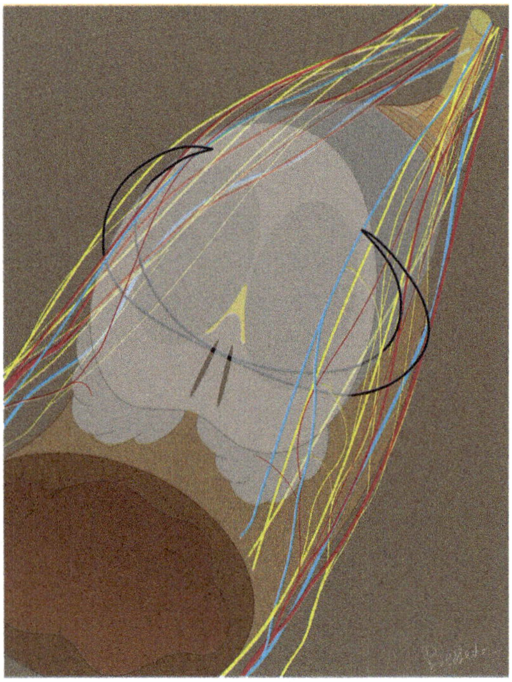

Fig. 31.1 Neural hammock of the prostate

where it is joined by branches to the cavernous nerve. It then becomes the traditional neurovascular bundle with some branches extending through the fascia and capsule as accessory pathways [2].

The PNB provides the primary route for innervation to the cavernous tissue as well as the urethral sphincter and levator ani muscle. It is found in the lateral pelvic fascia (LPF) posterolateral to the prostate. The bundle's greatest width is at the prostatic base with variation in direction and diameter as it approaches the apex [2].

The ANP comprises accessory nerves distributed throughout the LPF anterolateral and posterior to the prostate. Some studies have found as much as 20 % of these fibers are along the ventral border of the prostate [3]. An apical plexus can occasionally be observed and comprises fibers from the ANP and PNB. It penetrates the rectourethralis muscle and may provide innervation for cavernous tissue as well as the urinary sphincter [2].

A more detailed anatomic diagram of prostatic neurovascular supply has led to the development of an incremental grading system for NS in RALP. Based on preoperative parameters including PSA, Clinical Stage (CS), Gleason Score (GS), and tumor presence on Multiparametric (MP) eMRI a specific level of NS is attempted. Grades on NS are based on anatomic principles and are further described below in our section on NS.

Surgical Techniques for NS in RALP

Critical to any surgery are the general techniques utilized when handling delicate tissue. RALP in particular requires careful handling of tissue. Any injury to the nerve fibers can delay or eliminate the ability of men to regain sexual function after surgery. While performing the NS dissection care should be taken to avoid cautery throughout. This includes all aspects of dissection from the delivery of the SVs to the reconstruction of the bladder neck. Sharp dissection with robotic scissors should replace mono- and bipolar current.

An additional principle is the avoidance of excessive traction during this stage of RALP. Bruising and avulsion of nerve fibers can contribute to erectile dysfunction following surgery. While adequate exposure of surgical planes is critical to successful removal of the prostate, this can and should be accomplished without unnecessary torque being applied to the NVB as it courses along the outside of the prostatic capsule.

Preoperative Planning

Traditional preoperative planning relies upon well-established nomograms which take into account the clinical features of prostate cancer (i.e., GS, serum PSA, and CS) in order to determine the extent of the cancer. Supplementing this information with preoperative imaging in the form of MRI enhances our decision making in fine-tuning the NS approach most appropriate for each patient.

The ideal MRI for prostate cancer detection and staging comprises T1 and T2 weighted imaging along with functional imaging, specifically diffusion weighted and dynamic contrast enhanced imaging. A pelvic phased-array coil is used along with an endorectal coil on a high field-strength magnet, ultimately optimizing the ability to detect extraprostatic extension or SV invasion. This assessment of the risk of extraprostatic extension enables an approach where the grade of NS is individualized for each patient. As the risk of extraprostatic extension increases, the grade of NS is adjusted accordingly without compromising oncological efficacy.

Despite thorough preoperative planning, intraoperative adjustments are often made to accommodate texture changes, which can occur secondary to a variety of insults or diseases. A patient's prior exposure to multiple biopsies, inflammation, thrombophlebitis, or prostatitis impacts intraoperative decision making regarding the opportunity for preservation or need for excision of nerves. The ability to nerve spare during robotic prostatectomy in the setting of thrombophlebitis, a history of multiple biopsies, or prior radiation therapy relies upon visual cues such as changes in color, texture, bulging and irregularity of surface, stickiness of planes, and obvious views of the tumor. The absence of tactile feedback is counteracted by the visual information afforded in a highly magnified, well-lighted, and three-dimensional color field.

Steps for NS

NS surgery involves preservation of the three previously discussed neuronal zones that are surgically identifiable: the PNP, PNB, and ANP. Injury to these nerves can occur during opening of the endopelvic fascia (EPF), dissection of the SVs, and prostatic dissection. Our main principles of NS surgery include athermal technique and traction free, gentle manipulation of tissue when in proximity to neurovascular tissue. Careful dissection using clips to control individual vessels minimizes the risk of crush injury or thermal damage to nerve fibers and ganglions.

Preservation of EPF and Puboprostatic Ligaments

After developing the space of Retzius, the EPF and puboprostatic ligaments (PPL) are exposed by mobilizing the overlying adipose and connective tissue. The EPF is not incised routinely, due to the risk of damaging accessory nerve branches and distal neuronal pathways of the broad neuronal zones. However, there are circumstances where incision of the EPF is indicated. They include moderate to high risk of T3 cancer, large volume of disease at the apex, very large or very small prostatic volume, or technical difficulty encountered intraoperatively. Incisions of the EPF should be made near the prostatic capsule as proximal and lateral incisions increase the risk of nerve injury.

Division of Bladder Neck

Mobilization of the adipose tissue anterior to the prostate and bladder facilitates identification of the bladder neck. The consistency of the adipose tissue changes at the bladder neck and becomes more adherent to the bladder than the prostate. The anterior bladder neck is incised using a 0° lens, Maryland forceps, and monopolar scissors

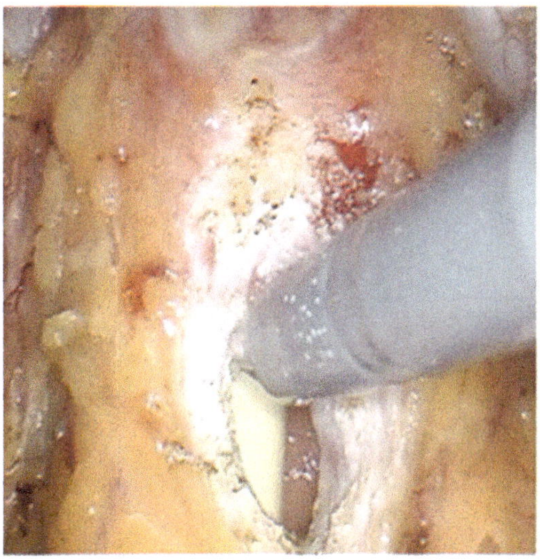

Fig. 31.2 Division of the bladder neck

until the Foley catheter is identified (Fig. 31.2). The Foley catheter is then delivered out of the bladder and firmly retracted anteriorly to provide traction. The posterior bladder neck is then incised to reveal the retrotrigonal tissue layer. This is a consistent fibrovascular tissue layer that overlies the vas deferens and SVs. Division of this layer exposes the vas and SVs.

SV Dissection

Preservation of the PNP is the focus during dissection of the vas deferens and SVs. Proximal plate fibers travel lateral to the tips of the SVs and are at risk for thermal damage during dissection of both the vas deferens and SVs. The vas deferens is divided after the associated artery is clipped. The cut end of the vas is then lifted to provide traction to facilitate dissection of the SVs. The use of electrocautery is permissible while dissecting near the midline but must be avoided when progressing laterally and toward the tips of the SVs. We first dissect directly onto the SVs medially and continue this plane laterally until the SVs are completely dissected and the SV pedicle controlled (Fig. 31.3). This approach facilitates identification and clipping of individual perforating vessels.

Nerve Sparing

Prostatic dissection is performed in a 360° fashion beginning at the posterior medial avascular plane. Thermal energy is avoided and dissection is performed exclusively with clips and sharp division. We dissect a plane between the prostatic fascia and Denonvilliers' fascia and follow this distally toward the apex. This plane is relatively avascular and may be dissected with minimal bleeding. Dissection is initially performed along the midline to develop a working space. We continue the dissection laterally and proximally until the prostatic pedicles are encountered. The depth of the dissection plane within the layers of periprostatic fascia is determined during the initial preoperative planning. The pedicles are clipped and sharply divided. Once the pedicles are released, we proceed with lateral and apical dissection. Continuing in the previously determined plane, we dissect laterally along the prostate to the level where the EPF joins the LPF. We then dissect medial to the PPL to complete the apical nerve release.

In addition to sparing the PNBs, we have developed a grading scheme that correlates to the level of dissection within the four compart-

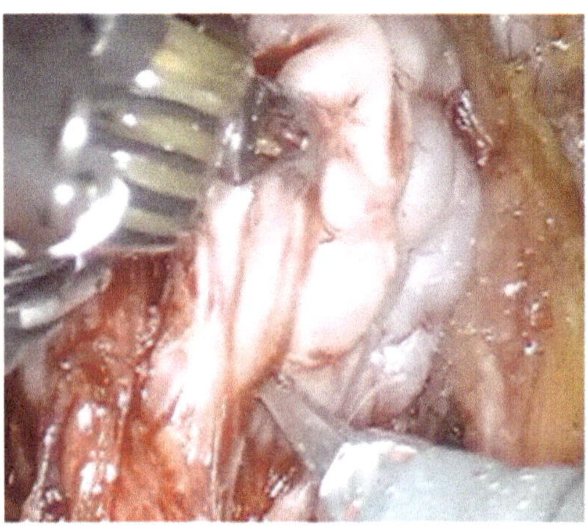

Fig. 31.3 Delivery of seminal vesicles

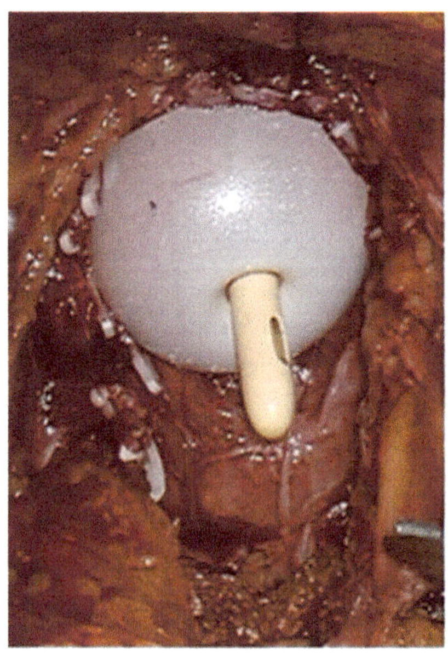

Fig. 31.4 Neurovascular bundle after removal of prostate

ments of the periprostatic tissue. The grade of NS is determined preoperatively based on the risk of extraprostatic extension based on the aforementioned preoperative risk stratification algorithm. Modifications may be made according to intraoperative visual cues. Intraoperative frozen sections are performed on the margins to verify oncologic efficacy of the procedure. Figure 31.4 shows the neurovascular bundle after removal of the prostate.

Grade 1: Maximal NS is performed for patients with essentially no risk of EPE. Grade 1 is achieved by dissecting just adjacent to the prostatic capsule. Laterally, dissection is performed between the prostatic capsule and the paraprostatic veins, which can be referred to as the medial venous plane, to maximally preserve the neural hammock. Posterior dissection is performed between the prostatic capsule and Denonvilliers' fascia (Fig. 31.5).

Grade 2: For patients with low risk of EPE, Grade 2 dissection is performed outside of the paraprostatic veins laterally to preserve the main neural trunks and within the superficial

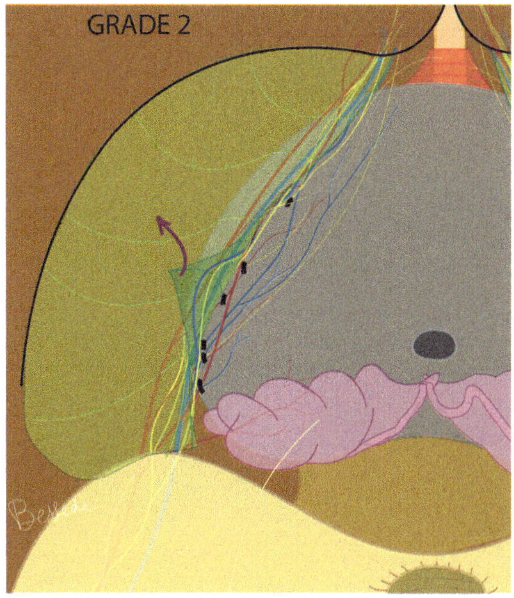

Fig. 31.6 Grade 2 nerve sparing

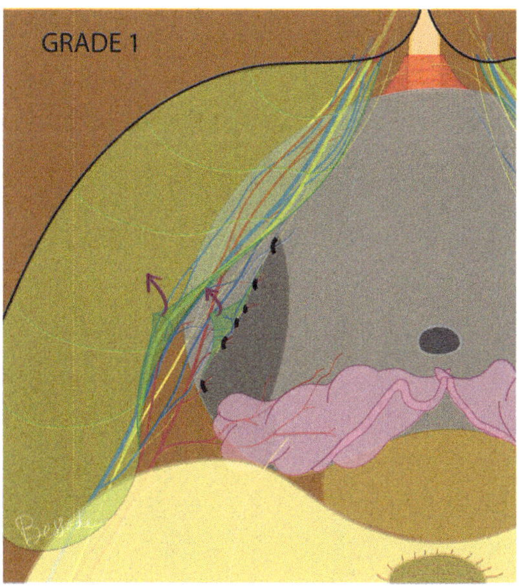

Fig. 31.5 Grade 1 nerve sparing

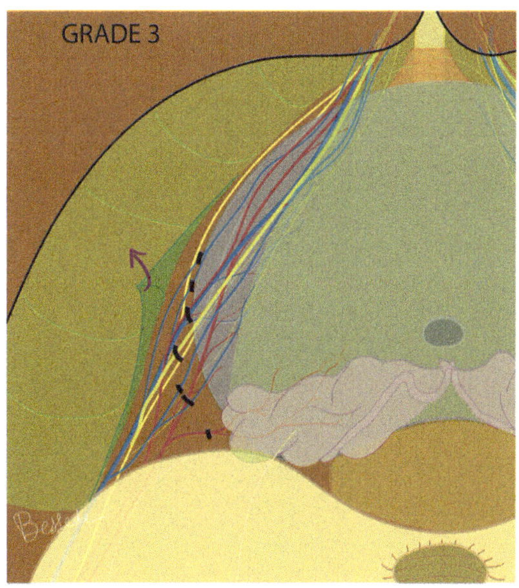

Fig. 31.7 Grade 3 nerve sparing

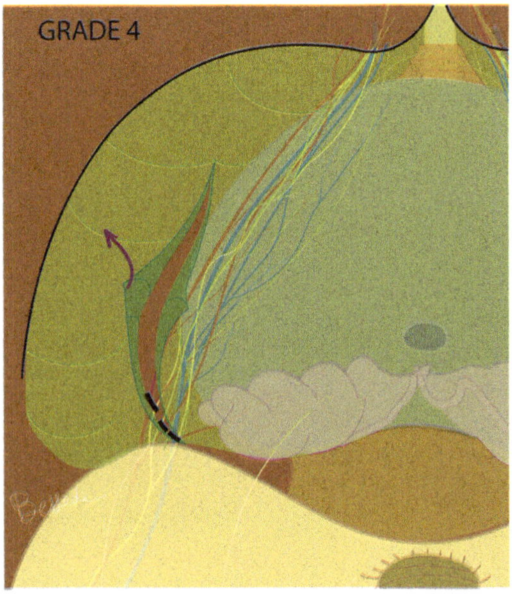

Fig. 31.8 Grade 4 nerve sparing

Denonvilliers' fascia posteriorly. Dissecting transluminally across the veins can aid with identification of this plane (Fig. 31.6).

Grade 3: For patients with moderate risk of EPE, this dissection is performed in an incremental fashion to preserve the lateral nerve fibers but not the medial fibers. Dissection is performed laterally within the layers of the LPF. The levator fascia is left intact. Denonvilliers' fascia is excised posteriorly along with the specimen (Fig. 31.7).

Grade 4 (non-NS): Grade 4 does not spare nerves. It is utilized in patients with high risk for EPE. Wide excision of the LPF including the levator fascia and Denonvilliers' fascia is performed, containing most of the neurovascular tissue [4]. This ca n be observed in Fig. 31.8.

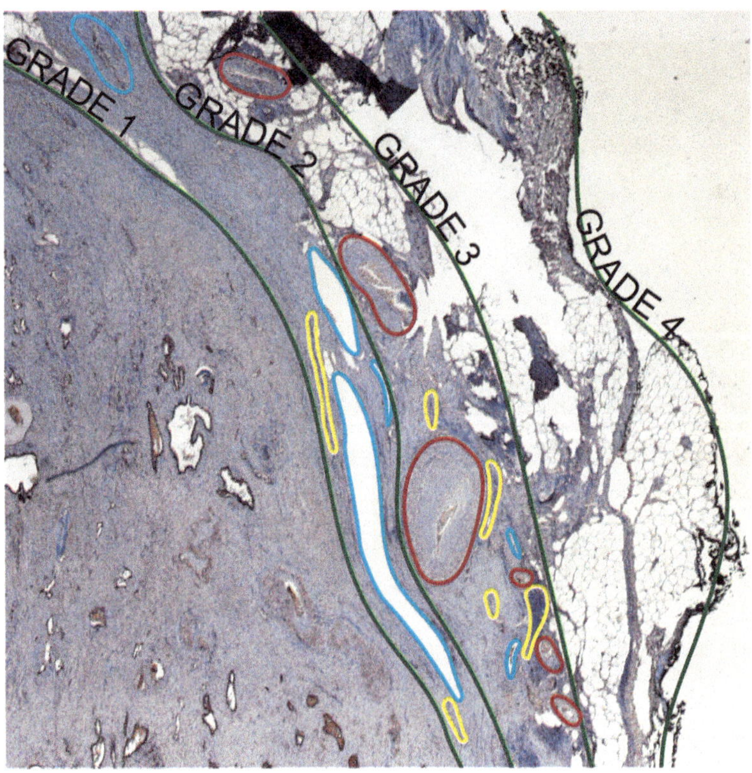

Fig. 31.9 Histological planes of Nerve-Sparing prostatectomy

Future of NS in Robotic-Assisted Laparoscopic Radical Prostatectomy

Radical prostatectomy has changed dramatically since the surgery was initially described. NS in particular has developed into an anatomically driven surgery based on the most modern imaging modalities available. However, there is still the potential for further developments within this field of surgery. Hypothermic cooling has recently been applied through both irrigation and endorectal cooling balloons to decrease inflammation associated with NS during RALP. Initial studies show promise with regards to improvements in early continence following surgery [5]. Newly published research has also investigated the use of amniotic/chorionic tissue wrapped around the neurovascular bundle during RALP to accelerate continence and potency after surgery [6]. While modern NS RALP provides progress, it is clear that continued research is warranted to ensure further improvements in erectile quality and continence are achieved.

References

1. Jemal A, Bray F, Center MM, Ferlay J, Ward E, Forman D. Global cancer statistics. CA Cancer J Clin. 2011;61(2):69–90.
2. Takenaka A, Tewari A. Anatomic basis for carrying out state-of-the-art radical prostatectomy. Int J Urol. 2012;19:7–19.
3. Eichelberg C, Erbersdobler A, Michl U, et al. Nerve distribution along the prostatic capsule. Eur Urol. 2007;51:105–10.
4. Tewari A, Ali A, Metgud S, Theckumparampil N, Srivastava A, Khani F, Robinson B, Gumpeni N, Shevchuk M, Durand M, Sooriakumaran P, Li J, Leung R, Peyser A, Gruschow S, Asija V, Harneja N. Functional outcomes following robotic prostatectomy using athermal, traction free risk-stratisfied grades of nerve sparing. World J Urol. 2013;31:471–80.
5. Finley D, Osann K, Skarecky D, Ahlering T. Hypothermic nerve-sparing radical prostatectomy: rationale, feasibility, and effect on early continence. Urology. 2009;73:691–6.
6. Patel V, Samavedi S, Bates A, Kumar A, Coehlo R, Rocco B, Palmer K. Dehydrated human amnion/chorion membrane allograft nerve wrap around the prostatic neurovascular bundle accelerates early return to continence and potency following robot-assisted radical prostatectomy: propensity score-matched analysis. Eur Urol. 2015;67(6):977–80.

Afterword: The Unwritten Chapters

John W. Davis

Thank you for reading this textbook and I hope you find it a useful resource. I thank the many authorship groups who contributed their time (uncompensated) and expertise to help all of us continue our learning process. I particularly enjoyed the creativity many authorship groups demonstrated. Text chapters do not carry the same degree of significance for academic promotion compared to peer reviewed articles, but as you have seen, these chapters provide more space and more room for inclusion of ideas and experiences than is possible in a peer-reviewed original article. Ultimately, text chapters are all about education and quality outcomes rather than academic promotion.

What is it like to edit a textbook? It starts with an idea and a set of meetings and correspondence with the publisher to set an agenda and unique focus for the project. Then at some point, you just have to start listing as many chapter ideas as possible, as many quality authors as possible, and then start matching them up. Many of these authors saw the whole book outline and chose their topics, and a few contributed their own ideas. I wrote some chapters intended that way all along and a few that remained "unclaimed." Overall the acceptance rate among invited authors was very high, and as stated in the introduction, many of us work together at various CME meetings and association congresses.

Behind the scenes, however, some chapters had to be dropped for various reasons—unclaimed, claimed but work never completed, and in some cases, perhaps the data is just too preliminary. For this afterword, I outline a few of these ideas that remain unwritten chapters, but perhaps stronger topics for the future. These are mostly projects I've led or participated in, so I apologize in advance for the shameless self-referencing.

The Cost-Effectiveness of Robotic Surgery

Of course there is no way you can spend millions of capital budget dollars on robotic surgery platforms, and additional many thousands on disposable drapes and instruments and say this is a "cost savings" venture. Any operating room administrator can tell you a lot more than I can about the hidden costs of robotic surgery—scopes, instruments, drapes, special sterilizer units, maintenance contracts, scope repairs, schedule disruptions for robot service calls, instrument breakage, and premature termination. There are different personnel costs associated with figuring out robot calendars and utilization rules, training staff, maintaining disposable inventory. Robots have to go into larger rooms (600 sq ft is ideal), and standard laparoscopic gear and external monitors are required. At the end of the day, robotic systems need a lot of storage space that is secure and minimizes movement of the system. Equipment techs have to be trained on system setup, troubleshooting, and storage. Sometimes rooms have to be set up for a robotic case, and then converted to another setup later in the day for an open procedure.

So where is the value? At the beginning of the robotic expansion phase, the promise was that oncologic, potency, and continence data would be better, and I would argue that the data is supe-

J.W. Davis (ed.), *Robot-Assisted Radical Prostatectomy*, DOI 10.1007/978-3-319-32641-2 rior compared to standard laparoscopic with all of its ergonomic and instrumentation challenges. However, there is not much data to prove superiority compared to open technique—assuming expert surgeons either way. Over time, however, the data is stronger in the areas of efficiency and complications. In a study with Raju Thomas from Tulane University and Usha Kraeden from Intuitive's Medical Affairs department [1], we looked at a large insurance database called Premier Perspective. This database spanning 2004–2010 included over 70,000 cases from thousands of surgeons and over 300 hospitals. Although operating room time was higher for robotic, it improved with experience, and hospital stay, transfusion rates, and complications were better with robotic cases. Unfortunately, this database had inconsistent reporting of costs, especially whether or not the amortized capital expense per case was included, pro-rated, or not included. Therefore we had to leave it out. In another study using insurance data, my colleague Tina Shih [2] also found fewer complications for robotic cases. The hospitalization costs were higher at discharge by $1574. However by 90 days when factoring the costs of complications, that delta decreased by more than half. In an internal study performed at MD Anderson that looked at full 1 year cost of care, robotic surgery was less expensive than open by $1235, IMRT by $24,010, and proton therapy by 47,949. These methodologies are still being refined, but the point was well taken by our business planning group that high volume robotic surgery can be cost-competitive when factoring beyond the day of surgery expense ratios. These arguments, of course, are more difficult to construct with lower volume procedures that are more straightforward than radical prostatectomy. This area of cost analysis will certainly be dynamic in the future and a worthy niche for rising stars in academics.

Other Nerve Sparing Techniques

The chapter by Patel's group is certainly excellent and emphasizes their retrograde nerve release method that uses a capsular artery as a key landmark. I must admit, I've been chasing this technique for years and can sometimes find the landmark artery. Often I just set up the retrograde release and if I get into bleeding or cannot complete the plane back to the median space, then I just go back to an antegrade release to finish. The orientation points are very clear even if you do part of the retrograde release. The point is that there are other ways to release nerves, and other authors can take you down their own step-by-step approach. Two alternates would be a pure antegrade release, the composite as described, and an effort to preserve more of the anterior nerve tissue for continence—the veil technique. Figure 1 shows a setup for a veil technique—the release point has to be very high and some of the vein plexi from the Santorini's has to be clipped and divided to get to the capsule. I find it useful to divide some of the anterior bladder neck for more orientation. Figure 2 shows a right nerve sparing technique by Markus Graefen at the Martini Klinik in Hamburg, Germany. The technique goes straight antegrade and tries to pick out each major arterial branch going from the pedicle to the prostate base and to clip with small 3 mm titanium clips.

Overall, the key to nerve sparing technique is to avoid cautery, to minimize stretch injury, and to maintain the integrity of the nerve bundle. The portion at the base is vulnerable to disorientation and excising too much tissue. My recommendation is to study all of these techniques and employ them as the individual anatomy allows.

Imaging

A competing concept to the Neurosafe chapter authored by the Martini group is to use MRI imaging to predict pT3 stage. I have used this technique for nearly a decade. Our early experience with T2 weighted images only was published by my colleague TJ Pugh in radiation oncology [3]. His emphasis was to use the surgical pathology and imaging prediction to assist in brachytherapy dosimetry. The sensitivity for EPE prediction was only 51 %; however, with a 2 mm window of error, the accuracy was 97 % when combined with cT1c and a negative MRI. Certainly the bulk of evidence on MRI relates to biopsy tech-

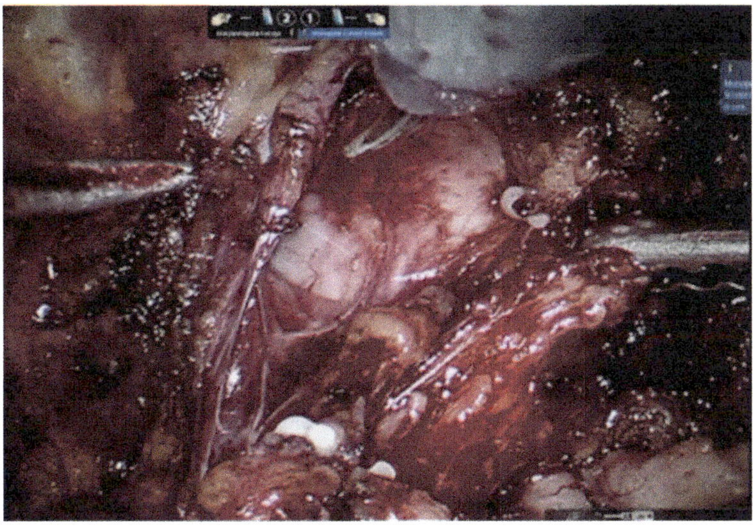

Fig. 1 A left nerve sparing technique with anterior veil technique—the endopelvic fascia to the left is preserved and the dissection goes from just off midline of the Santorini's plexus straight to the capsule. The bladder neck is partial divided to find this plane. The apex and DVC are often left until later in the procedure as more nerve release is required to get to the DVC compared to a standard plane through the endopelvic fascia. Photo—John Davis

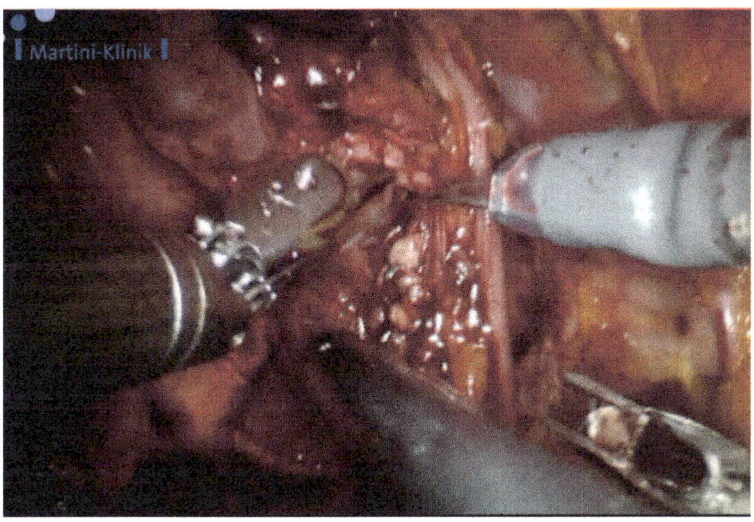

Fig. 2 Straight antegrade nerve sparing with 3 mm titanium clips. Courtesy Markus Graefen, Hamburg, Germany. Note that the neurovascular bundle is mobilized in the midline and laterally. In this step, the pedicle is being taken off of the base in an antegrade method. Note the array of small 3 mm clips on the patient side where individual perforating vascular branches have been identified, clipped, and divided cold

nique and fusion platforms. There is hope for this line of prediction, and hopefully a cost and efficiency comparison for this versus Neurosafe. We recently examined our expanded experience including multiparametric technique. In the subset of men at risk for pT3a disease, the confirmed pT3a positive margin rate was 10 % imaged and 30 % non-imaged [4].

Neoadjuvant Therapy with Novel Agents

It is well known and reported by treatment guidelines that neoadjuvant androgen deprivation therapy (ADT) does not make a significant difference in recurrence rates for higher risk disease. We may still use the strategy when there is an expected delay in therapy or very bulky disease that is not a candidate or preference for radiation. The next wave of studies is harnessing our emerging library of therapies for castrate resistant disease. In the study by Taplan et al. [5], men with high risk, non-metastatic disease were treated with 3 months of ADT with a 1:1 randomized cohort also receiving 3 months of abiraterone acetate, and then both cohorts received abiraterone/ADT for another 3 months. The primary objective was more pharmacokinetic—significantly improved reductions in intraprostatic androgens for the combination versus ADT alone. However, there was a low rate of complete responses. A forthcoming study from our institution has a fully randomized cohort of ADT only versus ADT/abiraterone for 3 months, i.e., a true control group. Approximately 20 % of the combination group will have significant reductions in residual tumor (presented at 2012 ASCO—Efsthathiou et al.). I highly recommend reading Eric Small's editorial that accompanies the Taplin article as a guide to understanding the neoadjuvant space and its challenges. Current agents clearly reduce PSA and tumor burdens, but there are resistance mechanisms at play. Abiraterone may represent the ultimate in androgen suppression, but additional agents may be required for a meaningful response, and other clinical trials are looking at the neoadjuvant chemotherapy question (CALGB 90203). Therefore, novel neoadjuvant therapy remains in the clinical trial space rather than routine clinical practice.

References

1. Davis JW, Kreaden US, Gabbert J, Thomas R. Learning curve assessment of robot-assisted radical prostatectomy compared with open-surgery controls from the Premier Perspective Database. J Endourol. 2014;28:560–6.
2. Shih YT, Ward JW, Pettaway CA, Xu Y, Matin SF, Davis JW, Thompson BP, Etling LS. Comparative effectiveness, cost, and utilization of radical prostatectomy among young men within managed care insurance plans. Value in Health. 2012;15:367–75.
3. Pugh TH, Frank SJ, Achim M, Kuban DA, Lee AK, Hoffman KE, McGuire SE, Swanson DA, Kudchadker R, Davis JW. Endorectal magnetic resonance imaging for predicting pathologic T3 disease in Gleason score 7 prostate cancer: Implications for prostate brachytherapy. Brachytherapy. 2013;12:204–9.
4. Bozkurt Y, Achim M, Davis JW. Nerve sparing radical prostatectomy planning using endorectal magnetic resonance imaging before robot-assisted radical prostatectomy. Presented at the 11th Turkish Endorurology Society, Apr 2015, Antalya, Turkey.
5. Taplin ME, Montgomery B, Logothetis CJ, Bubley GJ, Richie JP, Dalkin BL, et al. Intense androgen-deprivation therapy with abiraterone acetate plus leuprolide acetate in patients with localized high-risk prostate cancer: results of a randomized phase II neoadjuvant study. J Clin Oncol. 2014;32:3705–15.

Index

J.W. Davis (ed.), *Robot-Assisted Radical Prostatectomy*, DOI 10.1007/978-3-319-32641-2

Q

Printed by Printforce, the Netherlands